DRUG-INDUCED SUFFERINGS

DRUG-INDUCED SUFFERINGS

MEDICAL, PHARMACEUTICAL AND LEGAL ASPECTS

Proceedings of the Kyoto International Conference Against Drug-Induced Sufferings, 14–18 April, 1979, Kyoto International Conference Hall, Kyoto, Japan

Edited by T. Soda

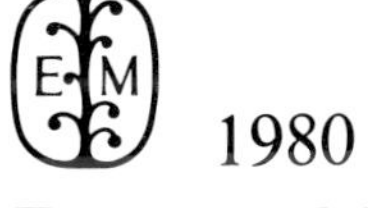

1980
Excerpta Medica, Amsterdam-Oxford-Princeton

International Congress Series No. 513

ISBN Excerpta Medica 90 219 0441 1
ISBN Elsevier North-Holland 0 444 90140 X

Library of Congress Cataloging in Publication Data

Kyoto International Conference Against Drug-Induced
Sufferings, 1979.
Drug-induced sufferings.
(International congress series ; no. 513)
Includes index.
1. Drugs--Side effects--Congresses. 2. Drugs--
Toxicology--Congresses. 3. Drugs--Law and legislation--
Congresses. I. Soda, Takemune, 1902- II. Title.
III. Series. [DNLM: 1. Iatrogenic disease--Congresses
2. Drug therapy--Adverse effects--Congresses. W3 EX89
no. 513 1979 / QZ42 K99d 1979]
RM302.5.K96 1979 363.1'94 80-10565
ISBN 0-444-90140-X (Elsevier)

Publisher:
Excerpta Medica
305 Keizersgracht
1000 BC Amsterdam
P.O. Box 1126

Sole Distributors for the USA and Canada:
Elsevier North-Holland Inc.
52 Vanderbilt Avenue
New York, N.Y. 10017

Printed in The Netherlands by Casparie bv, Amsterdam

The Kyoto International Conference Against Drug-Induced Sufferings (KICADIS)
14–18 April, 1979

Chairman	T. Soda
Organizing Committee	H. Izumi R. Kono A. Sakuma I. Shigematsu S. Sunahara
Secretariat	M. Kukuminato S. Shibata H. Suzuki H. Tamashiro S. Tomizawa E. Totsuka

Preface

Even after the severe lessons of the thalidomide tragedy, a widespread outbreak of subacute myelo-optico-neuropathy (SMON) occurred with the number of patients reaching a total of more than 10,000. We, Japanese physicians, pharmacists and lawyers, were deeply ashamed of these repeated drug-induced sufferings and decided therefore to hold the Kyoto International Conference Against Drug-Induced Sufferings (KICADIS) in the hope of preventing future drug disasters.

This Conference was held from April 14 to 18, 1979, in Kyoto. Many physicians, pharmacists, authorities concerned with drug affairs and administration, and lawyers engaged or interested in drug-induced sufferings were invited to take part and useful reports were made and fruitful discussions held.

This endeavor by KICADIS aroused a large response from the public and the publication of the proceedings of the meeting was obviously required to make available the contents of the Conference not only to the participants, but also to many other people. Hence, through the cooperation of Dr. M.N.G. Dukes, who was one of the participants in the Conference, the Organizing Committee of KICADIS decided to have the proceedings published by Excerpta Medica.

We hope that this book will be widely used for the prevention of drug-induced sufferings as well as for the relief of those who are suffering as a result of these disasters.

Takemune Soda
Chairman, Organizing Committee,
KICADIS

Speakers and Contributors

Shintaro Asakura, M.D.

Professor, Department of Public Health, Osaka University Medical School, 4–3–57 Nakanoshima, Kita-ku, Osaka, 530 Japan

John C. Ballin, Ph.D.

Director, Department of Drugs, American Medical Association, 535 North Dearborn Street, Chicago, IL 60610, U.S.A.

Mildred G. Ballin, M.D.

46 South County Line Road, Hinsdale, IL 60521, U.S.A.

Hirokuni Beppu, M.D.

Head, Department of Neurology, Tokyo Metropolitan Hospital of Fuchu, 2–9–2 Musashidai, Fuchu-City, Tokyo, 183 Japan

Lennart Berggren, M.D.

Professor, Department of Ophthalmology, University Hospital, S–750 14 Uppsala 14, Sweden

Lars E. Böttiger, M.D.

Professor and Head, Department of Internal Medicine, Karolinska Institute and Hospital, S–104 01, Stockholm 60, Sweden

Benjamin D. Cabrera, M.D.

Professor of Parasitology and Dean, Institute of Public Health, University of the Philippines, 625 Pedro Gil Street, Ermita, P.O. Box EA 460, Manila, The Philippines

Iwan Darmansjah, M.D.

Professor, Department of Pharmacology, University of Indonesia Medical School, P.O. Box 358, Salemba 6, Jakarta, Indonesia

Maurice N.G. Dukes, M.D.

Head, Department of Pharmacotherapy, Central Inspectorate for Drugs, Ministry of Health, Dokter Reijersstraat 10, Leidschendam, The Netherlands

Kazuo Fukutomi, D.Sc.

Senior Researcher, Department of Public Health Statistics, The Institute of Public Health, 4–6–1 Shirokanedai, Minato-ku, Tokyo, 108 Japan

Rokuro Hama, M.D.

Department of Internal Medicine, Hannan Central Hospital, 3–3–28 Minami-Shinmachi, Matsubara-City, Osaka, 580 Japan

Ryoichi Hanakago, M.D.

Department of Neurology, Tokyo Metropolitan Hospital of Fuchu, 2–9–2 Musashidai, Fuchu-City, Tokyo, 183 Japan

Manabu Hanano, Ph.D.

Professor, Faculty of Pharmaceutical Sciences, University of Tokyo, 7–3–1 Hongo, Bunkyo-ku, Tokyo, 113 Japan

Paul Hangartner, M.D.

Veterinarian, 5, Marc-Dufour, CH–1007 Lausanne, Switzerland

Olle Hansson, M.D.

Associate Professor, Department of Pediatrics, University of Gothenburg, East Hospital, S–416 85 Gothenburg, Sweden

Freya Hermann, M.S.

Associate Professor of Pharmaceutical Science, School of Pharmacy, Oregon State University, Corvallis, OR 97331, U.S.A.

Andrew Herxheimer, M.B.

Senior Lecturer in Clinical Pharmacology and Therapeutics, Charing Cross Hospital Medical School, London W6 8RF, U.K.

Toshio Higashida, M.D.

Professor, Department of Public Health, Kansai Medical University, 1 Fumizono-cho, Moriguchi-City, Osaka, 570 Japan

Yoshio Hiramatsu

Department of Pharmacological Research, Teikoku Zoki Co., Ltd., 1604 Shimosakunobe, Takatsu-ku, Kawasaki-shi, 213 Japan

Tsu-Pei Hung, M.D.

Professor, Department of Neurology and Psychiatry, National Taiwan University Hospital, Taipei, Taiwan 100

William H.W. Inman, M.B.

Principal Medical Officer, Committee on Safety of Medicines, Finsbury Square House, 33/37A Finsbury Square, London EC2A 1PP, U.K.

Takashi Ishizaki, M.D.

Chief, Division of Clinical Pharmacology, Clinical Research Institute, National Medical Center Hospital, Toyama-cho 1, Shinjuku-ku, Tokyo, 162 Japan

Hiroshi Izumi

Attorney-at-Law, 5th Floor, Yamaichi Building, 3–11 Yotsuya, Shinjuku-ku, Tokyo, 160 Japan

Anita Johnson

Attorney, 1791 Lanier Place, N.W., Washington, D.C. 20009, U.S.A.

Shigekoto Kaihara, M.D.

Associate Professor, Hospital Computer Center, University of Tokyo Hospital, 7–3–1 Hongo, Bunkyo-ku, Tokyo, 113 Japan

Hiroshi Kaneda

Tokyo 2nd Group of Plaintiffs for SMON Litigation, 7 Rokuban-cho, Chiyoda-ku, Tokyo, 102 Japan

Kiyohiko Katahira, Ph.D.

Assistant, Department of Clinical Pharmacology, Medical Research Institute, Tokyo Medical and Dental University, 2–3–10 Kanda Surugadai, Chiyoda-ku, Tokyo, 101 Japan

Ryuichi Kato, M.D.

Professor, Department of Pharmacology, School of Medicine, Keio University, 35 Shinanomachi, Shinjuku-ku, Tokyo, 160 Japan

Takashi Kawachi, M.D.

Vice-Director, National Cancer Center Research Institute, 5–1–1 Tsukiji, Chuo-ku, Tokyo, 104 Japan

Hitoshi Kawai

Assistant, Hospital of Kyoto University, 76–13 Chino-cho, Ogoto, Otsu-City, 520–01 Japan

Tsutomu Kigasawa

Tokyo 2nd Group of Plaintiffs for SMON Litigation, 7 Rokuban-cho, Chiyoda-ku, Tokyo, 102 Japan

Karl H. Kimbel, M.D.

Secretary General, Drug Commission of the German Medical Profession, Haedenkampstrasse 5, 5000 Cologne 41, Federal Republic of Germany

Takeshi Kojima, LL.D.

Professor, Faculty of Law, Chuo University, 2–39–2–301 Sendagaya, Shibuya-ku, Tokyo, 160 Japan

Reisaku Kono, M.D.

Director, Central Virus Diagnostic Laboratory, National Institute of Health, 326 Nakafuji, Musashimurayama-shi, Tokyo, 190–12 Japan

Michio Kukuminato

Attorney-at-Law, 2–19–7 Soto-kanda, Chiyoda-ku, Tokyo, 101 Japan

Yukio Kurahashi

Associate Professor, Faculty of Medicine, Okayama University, 135–4 Maruyama, Okayama, 703 Japan

Birgitta Lannek, M.D.

Veterinarian, Stångberga Gård, 18040 Brottby, Sweden

Widukind Lenz, M.D.

Professor, Institut für Humangenetik der Universität Münster, Vesaliusweg 12–14, 44 Münster/Westf., Federal Republic of Germany

Åke Liljestrand, M.D.

Director, Department of Drugs, National Board of Health and Welfare, Box 607, S–751 25 Uppsala, Sweden

N.D.W. Lionel, M.B.

Associate Professor, Department of Pharmacology, Faculty of Medicine, University of Sri Lanka, Colombo Campus, Kynsey Road, Colombo 8, Sri Lanka

Per Knut M. Lunde, M.D.

Associate Professor in Clinical Pharmacology, University of Oslo and Head, Division of Clinical Pharmacology and Toxicology, The Central Laboratory, Ullevål Hospital, Oslo, Norway

Mia Lydecker, M.A.

Consultant, National Commission on Arthritis and on Epilepsy (NIH), Menlo Commons, 2140 Santa Cruz Ave. E102, Menlo Park, CA 94025, U.S.A.

M.L. Mashford, M.B.

Chairman, Adverse Drug Reactions Advisory Committee, Department of Medicine, St. Vincent's Hospital, Fitzroy, Victoria 3065, Australia

Motosaburo Masuyama, D.Sc.

Professor, Science University of Tokyo, 1–3 Kagurazaka, Shinjuku-ku, Tokyo, 162 Japan

Junichi Matsunami

Attorney-at-Law, 15–25 Nakagawa-motomachi, Takaoka-City, 933 Japan

Renzo Matsushita

Executive Vice-President, The Green Cross Corporation, 1–1–47 Chuoh, Joto-ku, Osaka, 536 Japan

Kenneth L. Melmon, M.D.

Professor and Chairman, Department of Medicine, Stanford University School of Medicine, Stanford, CA 94305, U.S.A.

Nobuo Motohashi, Ph.D.

Councillor for Pharmaceutical Affairs, Ministry of Health and Welfare, 1–2–2 Kasumigaseki, Chiyoda-ku, Tokyo, 100 Japan

Tsuneji Nagai, Ph.D.

Professor of Pharmaceutics, Hoshi Institute of Pharmaceutical Sciences, Hoshi College of Pharmacy, 2–4–41 Ebara, Shinagawa-ku, Tokyo, 142 Japan

Kantaro Nagano

Attorney-at-Law, 402 15th Mori Building Bekkan, 2–7–6 Toranomon, Minato--ku, Tokyo, 105 Japan

Shuhji Nakamura

Attorney-at-Law, Niigata Godo Law Office, Jiho-Kaikan, 280 Niban-cho, Higashi-Nakadori, Niigata, 951 Japan

Koichi Nishida

Attorney-at-Law, Nishida, Fuketa and Endo Law Office, 7th Floor, Nankai Tokyo Building, 5–51–1 Ginza, Chuo-ku, Tokyo, 104 Japan

Yasuhiro Noguchi

Nagoya Pharmacology Laboratory, Pfizer Taito Co., Ltd., 5–2 Taketoyo-cho, Chita-gun, Aichi-ken, 470–23 Japan

Godfrey P. Oakley, Jr., M.D.

Chief, Birth Defects Branch, Chronic Diseases Division, Bureau of Epidemiology, Center for Disease Control, 1600 Clifton Road N.E., Atlanta, GA 30333, U.S.A.

Kengo Ohashi

Attorney-at-Law, 506 Bengoshi Building, 1–21–8 Nishi-Shimbashi, Minato-ku, Tokyo, 105 Japan

Yukio Onishi

Attorney-at-Law, Nishi-Ginza Law Office, 5th Floor, Ginza Sunny Building, 3–4–16 Ginza, Chuo-ku, Tokyo, 104 Japan

Junri Ozaki

Attorney-at-Law, Kioicho Law Office, 920 Kioicho-TBR Building, 5–7 Kojimachi, Chiyoda-ku, Tokyo, 102 Japan

Douglas B. Payne

Attorney-at-Law, Ishii Law Office, 623 Fuji Building, 3–2–3 Marunouchi, Chiyoda-ku, Tokyo, 100 Japan

Mohd. Zaini B. Abdul Rahman, M.B.

Head, Division of Biochemistry, Institute for Medical Research, Jalan Pahang, Kuala Lumpur 02–14, Malaysia

Akira Sakuma, Ph.D.

Professor, Department of Clinical Pharmacology, Medical Research Institute, Tokyo Medical and Dental University, 2–3–10 Kanda Surugadai, Chiyoda-ku, Tokyo, 101 Japan

Akiyoshi Satake

Editor, National News Division, Asahi-shinbun, Yuraku-cho, Chiyoda-ku, Tokyo, 100 Japan

Shigeo Shibata, M.D.

Chief, Section of Adult Disease, Department of Epidemiology, The Institute of Public Health, 4–6–1 Shiorkanedai, Minato-ku, Tokyo, 108 Japan

Itsuzo Shigematsu, M.D.

Director, Department of Epidemiology, The Institute of Public Health, 4–6–1 Shirokanedai, Minato-ku, Tokyo, 108 Japan

Kazuo Shiino

Pharmacist, 2–42–7 Nanmei-cho, Chigusa-ku, Nagoya, 464 Japan

Haruko Shimojima

Attorney-at-Law, 5th Floor, Hatori Building, Chuo-ku, Tokyo, 104 Japan

Hyun-Duk Shin, Ph.D.

Associate Professor, Department of Environmental Science, Kyung Hee University, Seoul 131, Korea

Milton Silverman, Ph.D.

Senior Faculty Member, Health Policy Program, School of Pharmacy and Medicine, University of California, San Francisco, CA, U.S.A.

Takemune Soda, M.D.

Consultant (Former Director), The Institute of Public Health, 4–6–1 Shirokanedai, Minato-ku, Tokyo, 108 Japan

Kyoichi Sonoda, M.Soc.

Associate Professor, Department of Health Sociology, School of Health Sciences, Faculty of Medicine, University of Tokyo, 7–3–1 Hongo, Bunkyo-ku, Tokyo, 113 Japan

Hidehiro Sugisawa

Student, Tokyo Pharmaceutical University, 3 Kiryu Flat, 6–19–8 Hirayama, Hino-shi, Tokyo, 191 Japan

Shigeichi Sunahara, M.D.

Director Emeritus, Tokyo National Chest Hospital, 2–31–25 Kichijojihonmachi, Musashino-shi, Tokyo, 180 Japan

Fumio Suzuki

Tokyo 2nd Group of Plaintiffs for SMON Litigation, 7 Rokuban-cho, Chiyoda-ku, Tokyo, 102 Japan

Hidero Suzuki, M.D.

Professor and Chairman, Department of Internal Medicine, University of Occupational and Environmental Health, School of Medicine, Yahata Nishi-ku, Kitakyushu, 807 Japan

Hiroshi Suzuki

Attorney-at-Law, Ebashi Law Office, 314, Marunouchi-yaesu Building, 2–6–2 Marunouchi, Chiyoda-ku, Tokyo, 100 Japan

Katsuya Takahara

Attorney-at-Law, Okayama Law Center, 5th Floor, Shakai-Bunka-Kaikan, 5–7 Yumino-cho, Okayma, 700 Japan

Tetsuo Takano

Lecturer, Ritsumeikan University, 2–9–50 Akeboshi-cho, Uji-shi, 611 Japan

Toshiaki Takasu, M.D.

Lecturer in Neurology and Neurotoxicology, University of Tokyo; Chief Neurologist, Outpatient Division, University of Tokyo Hospital; Department of Neurology, Institute of Brain Research, Faculty of Medicine, University of Tokyo, 7–3–1 Hongo, Bunkyo-ku, Tokyo, 113 Japan

Hidehiko Tamashiro, Ph.D.

Research Fellow, Section of Adult Disease, Department of Epidemiology, The Institute of Public Health, 4–6–1 Shirokanedai, Minato-ku, Tokyo, 108 Japan

Zenzo Tamura, Ph.D.

Professor and Director, Hospital Pharmacy, Faculty of Medicine, University of Tokyo, 7–3–1 Hongo, Bunkyo-ku, Tokyo, 113 Japan

Jun Tateishi, M.D.

Chairman and Professor of Neuropathology, Neurological Institute, Faculty of Medicine, Kyushu University 60, Maidashi, Fukuoka, 812 Japan

Peck Chuan Teoh, M.D.

Associate Professor, Department of Medicine, University of Singapore, c/o Singapore General Hospital, Outram Road, Singapore 3, Republic of Singapore

Kugahisa Teshima

Graduate Student, Department of Health Sociology, School of Health Sciences, Faculty of Medicine, University of Tokyo, 7–3–1 Hongo, Bunkyo-ku, Tokyo, 103 Japan

Gianni Tognoni, M.D.

Head, Laboratory of Clinical Pharmacology, 'Mario Negri' Institute for Pharmacological Research, Via Eritrea 62, 20157 Milan, Italy

Setsuo Tomizawa, M.D.

Professor, Department of Pharmacology, School of Pharmaceutical Sciences, Kitazato University, 5–9–1 Shirokane, Minato-ku, Tokyo, 108 Japan

Etsro Totsuka

Attorney-at-Law, 5th Floor, Yamaichi Building, 3–11 Yotsuya, Shinjuku-ku, Tokyo, 160 Japan

Tadao Tsubaki, M.D.

Professor, Department of Neurology, Brain Research Institute, Niigata University, Asahimachi 1, Niigata, 951 Japan

Michio Tsunoo, M.D.

Professor of Pharmacology, Nippon Medical School, 1–1–5 Sendagi, Bunkyo-ku, Tokyo, 113 Japan

Michael Tuveson

Attorney-at-Law, Erik Tuvesons Advokatbyrå, Österbrogatan 4, 23100 Trelleborg, Sweden

Boris Velimirovic, M.D.

Chief, Field Office U.S. – Mexico Border, Pan-American Sanitary Bureau, World Health Organization, 509 U.S. Court House, El Paso, TX 79901, U.S.A. *Present Address:* Regional Officer for Communicable Diseases, World Health Organization, Regional Office for Europe, Scherfigsvej 8, 2100 Copenhagen Ø, Denmark

Alexander M. Walker, M.D.

Epidemiologist, Boston Collaborative Drug Surveillance Program, Boston University School of Medicine, 400 Totten Pond, Road, Waltham, MA 02154, U.S.A.

Barbro Westerholm, M.D.

Director General, National Board of Health and Welfare, 106 30 Stockholm, Sweden

Hachiro Yaginuma

Attorney-at-Law, Toranomon Law Office, 3rd Floor, 2nd Bunsei Building, 1–11–7 Toranomon, Minato-ku, Tokyo, 105 Japan

Morris L. Yakowitz

Former Drug Control Officer, United States Food and Drug Administration and Drug Control Advisor at the American Regional Office of the World Health Organization, 4133 E. Pima Street, Tucson, AZ 85712, U.S.A.

Yoichiro Yamakawa

Attorney-at-Law, Koga, Yoshikawa, Yamakawa and Nakagawa Law Office, 5th Floor, Kyosho Building, 1–9–3 Hirakawa-cho, Chiyoda-ku, Tokyo, 102 Japan

Seizaburo Yamaoka, Ph.D.

President, Nihon Medi-Physics Co., Ltd., 4–2–1, Takatsukasa, Takarazuka-City, 665 Japan

Kiyoshi Yamashita

Attorney-at-Law, Osaka Kyodo Law Office, 6th Floor, No. 1 Kita Building, 4–7–1 Nishi-Tenma, Kita-ku, Osaka, 530 Japan

Tomoji Yanagita, M.D.

Director, Preclinical Research Laboratories, Central Institute for Experimental Animals, 1433 Nogawa, Takatsu-ku, Kawasaki, 213 Japan

Izumi Yasuhira

Student, Faculty of Medicine, Kyoto University, 12–2 Nishiyama, Matsugasaki, Sakyo-ku, Kyoto, 606 Japan

Masayuki Yokota

Research Staff, Central Laboratory, Meiji Seika Co., Ltd., Morooka-cho, Kohoku-ku, Yokohama-shi, 222 Japan

Kozaburo Yoshikawa

Attorney-at-Law, 7th Floor, Ukigai Building, 1–14 Kandanishiki-cho, Chiyoda-ku, Tokyo, 101 Japan

Contents

Introductory remarks

TAKEMUNE SODA

Institute of Public Health, Tokyo, Japan

In planning this Kyoto International Conference Against Drug-Induced Sufferings (KICADIS), it was the aim of the Organizing Committee to invite many specialists from Japan and abroad, administrators, social workers, jurists and others. I would like to explain the background of our efforts and plans and the objectives of this Conference.

It is a contradiction and even a tragedy in human society that some kinds of drugs, invented and produced with the purpose of alleviating the pain and worry caused by disease and injury, cause more serious sufferings or even intensify them, e.g. the prevalence in many countries of phocomelia due to thalidomide and the subacute myelo-optico-neuropathy (SMON) epidemic due to the intake in Japan of clioquinol and allied compounds for the treatment of intestinal disorders.

Several international symposia and meetings have already been held in recent years to exchange the various experiences gained in different countries and to promote more organized cooperation as a means of finding effective measures to rid us of such a contradiction and tragedy. A number of peculiar experiences were reported; ingenious ideas were exchanged; appeals for relief by the sufferers from drug-related inflictions were repeated; and many basic problems were nearly settled in principle, by almost all scientists in medicine and pharmaceutics, health administrators, lawyers, social workers, etc. They recognized the necessity for strict checks on the safety of new drugs before their release on the market, on the basis of sound scientific reasoning and a number of animal experiments and practical tests. Much progress has been made in the methods of pre-marketing safety tests. However, the present situation is still far from satisfactory, demanding the powerful development of effective monitoring systems of the adverse effects of various drugs after their release on the market. Recent progress in epidemiological methods and the information sciences should be more skillfully introduced to ensure completeness and to increase the speed of reporting and of data retrieval.

The Japanese Committee for the Organization of KICADIS is interested rather in problems of a scientific and technical nature. However, it recognizes, at the same time, the importance of the practical application of the results of scientific and technological research to governmental administrative practice, which should have the largest share of actual responsibility in the combat against the adverse effects of drugs. It is indispensably useful for mankind as a whole.

The Committee is also well aware of the fact that the campaign against drug-induced diseases is a very complicated matter which cannot achieve a victory without considerable assistance from many groups of people at the present time. In this connection, the Committee provided a session for the discussion of social movements of various kinds, such as the mass-movement of sufferers from drug-induced diseases for their relief, official and private relief institutions and organizations for the sufferers, various problems relating to lawsuits for compensation, the role of informative circles in the promotion of public understanding of the correct use of drugs, etc.

Fortunately, a sufficient number of speakers have sent their reports to be presented at the three Sessions of this Conference, and an accompanying Panel Discussion on SMON. In thanking them for their kind cooperation, The Japanese Organizing Committee wishes the Conference every success.

KEYNOTE REPORTS

Drugs and drug-induced sufferings

SHIGEICHI SUNAHARA

Tokyo National Chest Hospital, Tokyo, Japan

The development of new drugs in recent years has brought immeasurable benefit to mankind. Compared with physicians 50 years ago a recent medical graduate treats many patients more successfully, as a result of more efficient drugs. The average life span exceeds 70 years in many civilized countries, a fact probably related to the improved living standards, labor conditions and nutrition; the contribution of highly effective medicines recently developed cannot be ignored, however. The extended life span in Japan after World War II largely reflects the use of various antibiotics to overcome dysentery and pneumonia in infants and tuberculosis in adolescents. There remain illnesses difficult to cure including cancer, neuromuscular disease, and various geriatric problems. Progress in biomedicine depends on the drug industry and scientists making every effort to produce more effective drugs and governments should encourage them while the public should appreciate that the development of new drugs requires cooperation with the investigators.

Recent tragic drug-induced suffering must not be forgotten. In particular it is noteworthy that SMON, quadriceps contracture after intramuscular injection in infants, sudden death after oral administration of drugs in ampoules for the common cold etc., were mostly restricted to Japan. It is however pertinent that the latter two accidents resulted from unreasonable use rather than from the drugs themselves.

Drugs, being foreign to the human body, only by chance evolve therapeutic value and it is more or less inevitable that they harbor some undesirable effects.

To prevent drug-induced suffering, the following 4 caveats are essential: (1) develop a drug with the least possible hazards; (2) collect as detailed information as possible about adverse reactions to the drug even after careful screening; (3) find the safest way of drug administration based on the above-mentioned information; (4) always be alert for unknown risks.

PRE-MARKETING CONTROL OF DRUG SAFETY

The impact of the thalidomide affair on administration cannot be overemphasized. It led to the Kehauver-Harris Amendment in the U.S.A., followed by many countries, including Japan, in which administrative measures were taken, as a matter of convenience rather than revising the Drug Laws themselves: The intervention of administrative authorities in drug development has been strengthened and detailed pre- and post-marketing procedures to confirm drug safety have been requested.

Animal species, size of sample etc. in preclinical tests have been assessed and improved, but variations among species remain serious. Even very sophisticated animal tests cannot replace clinical research; they are indispensable preparatory stages for a clinical trial. In other words, animal tests only suggest hypotheses for clinical medicine and conclusions must be reconfirmed and modified by clinical investigation consisting of pre-marketing trials of Phase I through Phase III and post-marketing surveillance or Phase IV trial. This avoids the error inherent in direct extrapolation of animal data to man. The considerable ethical difficulties in administering a new chemical substance, the safety of which is unknown in man, in order to develop a safe drug are obvious. All those concerned with developing new drugs consider this ethical dilemma and there is no easy solution. The Declaration of Helsinki revised in Tokyo in 1975 must be adhered to, in particular the procedures of informed consent and peer review. As no scientist has the right to use a human being as an experimental subject in the name of human welfare or progress of science, no clinical trial should be carried out without informed consent; however, the informed consent of a layman cannot justify the experiment from the scientific and ethical points of view and peer review by an independent committee consisting of qualified scientists is essential. In other words, both individual investigators and medical science or the professional society should guarantee the propriety of the plan and experimental design. These ethical procedures are prerequisites for drug development.

POST-MARKETING SURVEILLANCE

Although marketing of a new drug after satisfactory confirmation of its safety is desirable, the final evaluation of safety is only possible after it has been administered to a variety of patients. The approval of the administrative authorities is thus only a parole and the process for safety testing continues throughout the whole life of a drug. This is why post-marketing surveillance has been stressed, although very few countries are satisfied with the efficiency of the existing spontaneous monitoring system. Reports from physicians and hospitals are often incidental and capricious, and cases in which a causal relationship is difficult to establish often remain unreported. In Japan, annual reports number a few hundred, varying from slight reactions such as fever, exanthema, etc. to death, the latter numbering 2 or 3 in a year. The discrepancy between the small number of reported adverse reactions and the large number of cases of drug-induced suffering reported in the newspapers is surprising. The reduced efficiency of spontaneous monitoring, it is believed, is due both to the lack of a physician's confidence in establishing causal relationships between the symptom and the drug, and to his fear of evoking the patients' grievance. Physicians must be conscious of their responsibility in the monitoring procedure, for they are the important members of the team for drug safety control. To improve the quantity and quality of spontaneous monitoring, an intensive monitoring system such as the Boston Collaborative Drug Surveillance Project is highly desirable and the registered release suggested by Dr. Dollery is another important consideration.

Most serious drug-induced suffering in the past was discovered by epidemiological study. Starting with patients with unusual symptoms, causes were sought retrospectively and conclusions finally related the suffering to the drug. The prospective activity of adverse reaction monitoring did not contribute at all. In a sense, this devalues the post-marketing surveillance system. In future, efforts should aim to discover almost all drug-induced sufferings, earlier or later, in the course of adverse reaction monitoring.

The documents required for new drug applications are increasingly voluminous; if the seventies are compared with the sixties, it takes 4 times longer to approve a new drug from the start of the clinical trial while the cost for the development of a new drug increased 10 times in the U.S.A., and the number of new chemical entities approved decreased to one third. Not only has the financial burden on the drug industries become severe but the problem of so-called 'drug lag' has become serious. It is frequently suggested that clinical trials should be simplified and the priority given to post-marketing surveillance, since even very intensive and time-consuming pre-marketing investigations rarely produce ideal information about drug safety. Since, however, a reduction in the level of pre-marketing trials cannot be justified, future efforts should focus on the intensification of post-marketing surveillance.

Another important problem is the influence of long-term administration of drugs such as antihypertensives, hypoglycemics, oral contraceptives etc. The toxic manifestations of such drugs are very difficult to distinguish from the symptoms of baseline disease, or from a new disease. The prognosis of life compared with the untreated population is often the only measure. The large-scale Phase IV clinical trials on several thousand subjects for more than 5 years such as UGDP and CDP in the U.S.A. and the clofibrate trial in Europe were carried out at enormous expense for these very reasons.

DRUG ADMINISTRATION

Drugs as products of capitalism should not be left to free competition, for they directly influence life, and their usefulness cannot readily be compared with other products. The so-called 'time test' may be applicable to drugs but it often takes too long, and may produce disasters such as thalidomide and clioquinol.

Drugs in origin closely related to public welfare are now more widely used and are mass-produced and consumed in bulk. It is thus essential to know how such drugs modify human health and influence subsequent generations. Drugs are now 'environmental chemicals' so that individual industries as well as governments must monitor safety.

In Japan, the administrative authorities have been preoccupied with the settlement and making excuses for successive drug-induced injuries. As a result, positive preventative approaches and the development of new drugs have been slow. At present, the Japanese Government proposes a revision of the Drug Affairs Act but compared, for example, with the proposed revision in the U.S.A., it is slight, the basic philosophy being ambiguous and deficient in technical scrutiny. Drug administration should not merely be control or regulation, rather ethics and scientific progress must be the central consideration. It is indispensable for the efficacy and safety of drugs that clinical-pharmacological training and research and National Centers of Clinical Pharmacology be established. The Japanese Drug

Affairs Bureau must urgently increase the number of personnel, for, at present, the examination of drugs is a part-time exercise of experts in medical schools, normally engaged in other work. Without change, meddling with the Act will be ineffective.

Administrations should not only apply legal sanctions, but also earmark sufficient research funds to develop safe and effective new drugs; easily developed drugs have already appeared, so that future progress will be more difficult. In addition, large-scale Phase IV clinical trials are too expensive for individual companies and governmental support is necessary.

The chemicals industry may now be stagnant, but the drug sections are still relatively profitable. For humanitarian reasons the industries should strictly observe and comply with established standards and always be cautious of unforeseen hazards of old and new drugs.

Drugs may be safe on the shelves of the drug houses and pharmacies, but their toxicity only becomes apparent when they come into contact with the human body!

It is difficult to predict drug safety in man since the relationships between experimental animal and human responses are discontinuous. Scientists are well aware of the weaknesses and shortcomings, but beyond their own specialties, their opinions are limited. Clinicians tend to accept the chemical and pharmacological assertions regarding the development of the drug, while the chemists and pharmacologists tend to believe that the clinicians can readily determine the efficacy and safety of a drug in man. However, adverse reactions often resemble the symptoms of 'base-line' diseases, and with so many drugs in use today, it is difficult to identify hazardous drugs; thalidomide and clioquinol are apt examples. The intensified animal tests and clinical trials following the Kehauver-Harris Amendment, have largely removed extensive drug-induced disease, but cases such as the recent proctatol incident in Great Britain are pertinent reminders.

Medical science, still far from perfect, aims for perfection by gradual modification. The drug industries are responsible for both preclinical and clinical trials and are ethically responsible for any unforeseen consequence of widely used drugs. The development of new and genuinely useful drugs demands unrestricted creative scientific energy, incisive criticism from the physicians and heavily self-critical attitudes.

The descriptive literature on drugs, concerning details of adverse reactions and contraindications, is often too extensive, sometimes giving the impression of prepared excuses for all eventualities. On the other hand, advertisements tend to emphasize only the beneficial actions. More close and frank communication between the physician and the industries is essential.

CLINICAL SAFETY

Adverse reactions to drugs are related not only to the drug per se, but also to the condition of the patients – sex, age, race, constitution, environment, etc. To obviate drug-induced suffering, reasonable ways must be developed to reduce the toxicity of the drug itself. The clinical safety of the drug should encompass the information supplied by the manufacturer as well as the suggestion that the physicians communicate to the industry; this will ensure continuous modification of the information regarding drug safety. In other words, physicians, unlike patients, are not mere consumers of the drugs; rather they are important and effective members of the development team. Other kinds of merchandise may pass directly to the consumers without special knowledge, not so drugs. Experts must ensure that the general public are protected from unfamiliar and potentially harmful drugs. The physician not only treats patients but he must protect them from drug-induced suffering.

Whether physicians are currently aware of these responsibilities remains questionable however. Medical education itself needs improvement in this respect. Indeed medical training today perhaps emphasizes diagnosis and pathological physiology, and the attitude that 'Any fool can treat' is too prevalent. Biomedical progress and the development of the chemical industry may render the effect of drugs more acute in the future; at the same time, potential drug-induced suffering will increase. Clinical-pharmacological training must be intensified; at present there are only 2 or 3 departments of clinical pharmacology in Japanese university medical schools.

DRUG-INDUCED SUFFERING IN JAPAN

Although a very difficult task, I would like to try and explain why there have been so many cases of drug-induced suffering in Japan. Firstly, ever since the development of drug industries began in Japan after the Meiji restoration about a hundred years ago, the drug industries have endeavored to catch up with Western countries by importing already finished drugs. At the same time, they were also preoccupied with the manufacture of similar drugs already marketed in other countries, taking advantage of the processing patent system used until recently. In other words, Japanese pharmaceutical companies in the past employed synthetic chemists, not biologists. Accordingly, as they marketed those drugs which had been used already and were believed to be safe in other countries, they lacked the acute sense of responsibility for safety that creators of new drugs must have.

The second point is related to 'poly-pharmacy'. The fact that almost 40% of total expenditure in medical care is on drugs is almost unique. Historically, Japanese physicians were called 'Kusushi' (drug-man), medical treatment being synonymous with drug therapy. In addition, the idea of separating medical practice from drug dispensation has been talked of but not implemented; meanwhile, the present social insurance system places more emphasis upon drugs than on physician's skill. Japanese physicians have thus become accustomed to easy use of drugs. These aspects and factors such as increased daily dosages, frequency and duration of drug administration have all contributed to producing drug-induced suffering, as regards both scale and the adverse effects of drug interaction. The medical care system in general must be improved, the industries must refrain from exaggerated advertising, and the physicians must not use drugs of obscure clinical-pharmacological indications if drug misuse is to be eliminated.

Another point concerns racial differences in pharmacokinetics. In the case of INH, for example, the clearly established racial differences in metabolism are closely related to the frequency of adverse effects such as polyneuritis, liver toxicity and SLE in different countries. Because of the large number of SMON cases in Japan, it is thus reasonable to suppose a relationship with race although at present firm evidence is lacking. But before automatically thinking of genetically determined racial differences, it is necessary to compare the quantity of the drugs used, their routes of administration and the adverse-reaction reporting systems in the different countries.

Finally I would like to examine the changes in doctor-patient relationships of recent years. In the past, physicians were obliging and, at the same time, authoritative persons in the local community, and even if a drug caused suffering, the victim tended to let the matter drop. However, as mass production of drugs in modern factories has inevitably increased the scale of drug-induced suffering, people have become more aware of their rights. These are considered to be the reasons why drug-induced suffering has become such a serious social problem today. However, it must be pointed out that, in Japan, individual litigations are fewer than mass litigations. This may partly be because of the huge number of people involved and of the necessity for specialized knowledge of the law, but it may also reflect an insufficient awareness of individual rights.

In conclusion, the progressive increase in drug-induced disease is endangering the mutual trust between the doctors and patients. To restore this relationship, doctors must always strive for the patient, and patients, in turn, must understand that drug treatment and medical care in general always entail degrees of risk.

Trends and lessons of SMON research

REISAKU KONO

Central Virus Diagnostic Laboratory, National Institute of Health, Tokyo, Japan

SMON along with thalidomide was one of the most severe man-made disasters induced by drug abuse. There are many valuable lessons to be learned and it behoves us to appreciate them to prevent a repetition. The Kyoto International Conference against Drug-Induced Sufferings is organized and convened against this background.

A battle may be seen as a sequence of errors and mistakes by allies and enemies, victory being in the hands of those with fewer mistakes. Our SMON Research Commission certainly produced good results, but there were also many faults. Toward the end of the 1960s, SMON was prevalent throughout Japan, and in Okayama Prefecture it took a particularly severe, epidemic form. The government could not ignore the incidence, and had to take practical measures; thus the SMON Research Commission was formed.

As virologist, I was nominated chairman of a commission to examine a drug-induced disease. This reflected the strongly suspected feeling that SMON was a new virus disease.

When new epidemic diseases broke out, a microbial etiology, especially viral, used to be suspected. Pellagra is a classic example: it was once believed to be a communicable disease and, as is well known, Goldberger swallowed fecal extracts of the patients to destroy this notion. Minamata disease is now known to be the result of intoxication by organic mercury compounds, but initially it was no exception when it first appeared in an epidemic fashion. We were still within grasp of the ghosts of Pasteur and Koch!

I first saw a sufferer with SMON in Mie University Hospital in 1959. The patient was a woman in mid-fifties displaying paraplegia of both legs. Professor Takasaki had seen several similar cases and there was a small outbreak. I was at that time engaged in poliovirus research, so I suspected such a virus to be the cause. No virus could be isolated, however. Many subsequent attempts to isolate viruses from various materials of patients with SMON have also failed. In 1965, Shingu et al. successfully isolated echovirus type 21 from feces of SMON patients and claimed that it was a causative agent (1). About this time, the first SMON study group was organized by the government and was chaired by the late Professor Maekawa of Kyoto University. Dr. Shingu and I participated in the study group and tried to confirm Shingu's findings but were unsuccessful. The study group was dissolved without success. One reason for the failure was the small amount of research funds provided by the government – less than 5000 U.S. dollars. In contrast, the second study group, namely the SMON Research Commission established in 1969, got 30,000,000 yen or 83,000 U.S. dollars for the first year and equivalent amounts thereafter. Apparently, the success of the SMON Research Commission was in part due to more generous funding. This is a good lesson for the Japanese Ministry of Health and Welfare. The results of the SMON study provoked other projects covering various other malignant or hard-to-cure diseases; they now include 43 study projects with total research funds of about 1.2 billion yen. As noted, until 1969 a viral etiology was thought to be the most plausible cause of SMON. In the SMON Research Commission (2), four major lines of research were pursued: (1) an epidemiological study involved a nationwide survey of SMON prevalence in 1967 and 1968, a follow-up survey, and a special investigation of environmental conditions in Akita, Aichi and Okayama Prefectures where the disease was prevalent; (2) the cause of the illness was explored using virological, bacteriological and toxicological approaches; (3) extensive neuropathological investigations were conducted on all autopsied cases throughout Japan; (4) clinical aspects (including diagnosis, laboratory studies on metabolic disorders, nutritional deficiencies, etc.) and improvement of therapeutic measures were examined. During the research, these lines were modified and new ones added so that the approach to the problem by the SMON Research Commission was multidisciplinary. In the event of outbreaks of a new disease in the future, such a multidisciplinary approach must be applied. In 1971, for example, the Commission consisted of 6 sections: epidemiology, microbiology, pathology, therapy and rehabilitation, clioquinol, and sociomedical studies. The clioquinol section was established because it was found that the drug had a close connection with the etiology of the neurological disorders. From 1972 onwards, hardly any cases of SMON occurred, and the Commission (the Committee as of 1972) therefore shifted the emphasis of its work towards the rehabilitation and treatment of SMON patients and towards the study of the mode of action of clioquinol in relation to the development of SMON. To this end, an Executive Committee was formed, consisting of 12 members from each of the 6 sections all of whom were nominated by the chairman. All study projects were assessed by this Committee, and their progress was reviewed approximately every 3 months. As soon as clioquinol had emerged as an important etiological factor in the second year, studies were promptly directed towards this agent.

The government's decision to suspend sales of clioquinol was made on 8th September, 1970, on the basis of the investigations carried out by the SMON Research Commission, in the course of which evidence implicating clioquinol in the etiology of SMON was presented. Eighteen months later at a General Assembly of the SMON Commission held on 13th March, 1972, a tentative verdict on the etiology of the disease was officially announced; the Commission concluded that the majority of the patients clinically diagnosed as having SMON were suffering from neurological disorders as a result of clioquinol (3). This conclusion has since received confirmation, and no contrary findings have emerged.

Meanwhile, I continued research along the lines that SMON was a slow virus infection on the basis of its clinical, pathological and epidemiological features. Some workers felt, however, that from a neuropathological point of view a viral etiology was unlikely. Neuropathology alone cannot however exclude a slow virus etiology of a disease; if such were the case, Dr. Gajdusek could not have established a slow virus etiology for kuru and Creutzfeldt-Jakob disease.

In the end, the slow virus etiology was finally rejected after experiments in our laboratory in collaboration with Dr. Gajdusek. Monkeys and mice were inoculated with materials from the CNS of SMON patients and observed for over a year; nothing happened. The same materials were inoculated into chimpanzees by Dr. Gajdusek and again no neuropathological changes were observed after 3 years (4).

During these studies, several viruses were suggested as causes of SMON. To date, only Inoue's agent has been supported by Tanabe Pharmaceutical Co., Ltd. (5), but it has not been extensively confirmed during the past 10 years (4). Indeed its very existence is now considered doubtful.

The discovery of a so-called SMON virus by Dr. Inoue was given sensational newspaper coverage in 1970, and aroused shock in both patients and the public, as well as social turmoil among families, because people feared infection. A number of patients committed suicide. This is an unfortunate example of how imprudent presentation of science and its sensational treatment by the mass media can elicit a social problem; it is also a valuable lesson for scientists to be aware of the social implications of scientific discovery. Although freedom of scientific research and freedom of the press must be maintained, all of us should remember our social responsibilities.

The SMON Research Commission was established on September 2, 1969, and it took 11 months for Professor Tsubaki to discover the causal relationship between intake of clioquinol and SMON. However, during this period there are several interesting anecdotes. Elucidation of clioquinol action came from the studies of the green pigment seen in SMON patients.

In the fall of 1969 Takasu et al. noticed that the fur of the tongue showed a green discoloration in some SMON patients (6). In May, 1970, Igata et al. found that two patients had excreted greenish urine (7). It was then soon discovered by Yoshioka and Tamura that the green pigment observed in the urine and feces of SMON patients was the iron chelate of clioquinol (5-chloro-7-iodo-8-hydroxyquinoline) and also that the urine contained a large amount of crystals of free clioquinol (7). Ikeda found high iron and zinc concentrations in the green fur of the tongue (9). Later, Imanari and Tamura confirmed the presence of clioquinol in the green fur by gas chromatography (10). Tsubaki was the first neurologist to suspect, on the basis of clinico-epidemiological studies, that SMON was caused by intake of clioquinol (11). A new etiological hypothesis ascribed SMON to intoxication resulting from treatment with drugs containing clioquinol.

Why had research on the etiology of SMON not hit upon clioquinol until 1970? There were at least two occasions when physicians suspected that clioquinol might have something to do with SMON. I know of a certain professor rebuking one of his staff physicians for connecting clioquinol with SMON. In 1967 the study group of the National Hospitals on SMON reported as follows: Entero-vioform, mesaphylin, Emaform (home produce of clioquinol), chloromycetin and Ilosone were often prescribed to SMON patients but no link was found between Entero-vioform and SMON (12). This report referred to Entero-vioform in particular so that clioquinol must have been suspected by someone in the study group. Dr. Tsugane, who was responsible for the survey, said that the survey was not thorough enough to unearth clioquinol as a causative agent. One of the reasons could have been that clioquinol had been used as a drug for the intestinal disorders of SMON, and it was hard to believe that clioquinol was toxic rather than a remedy. It is now known that there are two kinds of intestinal disorders in SMON; the first has variable etiology and provoked clioquinol administration; the second appears later and is now considered to be clioquinol-induced (13). In animals, clioquinol increases small intestinal contractions as a result of its central nervous actions, explaining the second abdominal symptom of SMON (14).

There were many intramural outbreaks of SMON in hospitals (15, 16). In one instance the multiple cases in one ward were considered to reflect the infectious nature of SMON (17). It is regrettable that epidemiological surveys of these hospital outbreaks were always inconsistent and thorough investigation of drug administration became difficult particularly after the clioquinol hypothesis was published because the hospitals did not cooperate. If the surveys had been comprehensive, clioquinol would have been discovered much earlier. Thorough epidemiological investigations of all the factors on such occasions should be mandatory.

Once the neurotoxicity of clioquinol was strongly suspected, the Japanese Central Pharmaceutical Affairs Council advised the Ministry of Health and Welfare on 7th September, 1970, to suspend sales and production of clioquinol and broxyquinoline (2). But for the bitter lessons of thalidomide, these measures would not have been implemented so quickly.

In addition, it initiated a kind of prospective field experiment on the clioquinol hypothesis, although – for obvious ethical reasons – no control group could be provided. The dramatically decreased incidence of new SMON cases after the suspension of sales of the two drugs is extremely strong supportive evidence for the etiological role played by clioquinol in SMON (18) (Fig. 1).

As a virologist, I applied Koch's postulate to the SMON-clioquinol relationship, in a review article (2). Koch's postulate is useful to determine a causal relationship between an agent and a disease, provided there is a 1 : 1 correspondence between the two. Such application suggests a rather simple SMON-clioquinol relationship.

Many modifications of Koch's postulate and the criteria to determine the causes

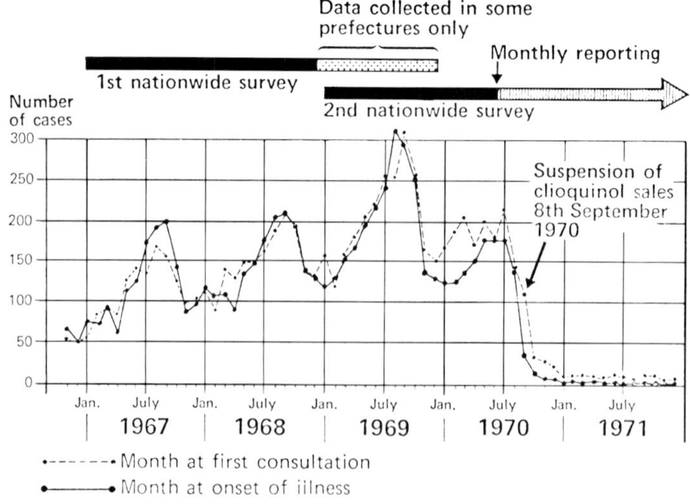

Fig. 1. Number of SMON cases recorded in Japan by year and by month.

TABLE 1. *Criteria for causation: a unified concept (A.S. Evans)*

1. The prevalence of the disease should be higher in those exposed than those not exposed
2. Exposure to the putative cause should be present more commonly in those with the disease than those without the disease
3. The incidence should be higher in persons who are so exposed than in those not exposed as shown in prospective studies
4. Exposure to the suspected factor should precede the disease
5. There should be a measurable spectrum of host responses
6. Experimental reproduction of the disease should be demonstrated
7. Elimination of the putative cause should decrease the incidence of the disease
8. Prevention or modification of the host response should decrease or eliminate the expression of the disease

TABLE 2. *Incidence rates of SMON among clioquinol takers and non-takers*

Groups of patients surveyed	Clioquinol administered	No. of SMON cases (%)	Total no. of patients studied
A. In-patients of a surgical hospital	Yes	34(44)	78
	No	0(0)	77
B. Patients in the medical department of a general hospital	Yes	29(11)	263
	No	0(0)	706
C. Out-patients of a general hospital	Yes	17(3.2)	532
	No	4(0.1)	3,789
D. In-patients of a T.B. hospital	Yes	5(4.4)	114
	No	0(0)	217

of a disease have been suggested. One set of criteria proposed by Evans (19) may be applied to the SMON-clioquinol relationship, item by item. Table 1 shows 8 criteria proposed by Evans, for No. 1 of which several case-history studies can be applied in Table 2. Figure 2 shows the rate of clioquinol intake: 80% by patients with SMON; 23% by those with ordinary gastrointestinal disorders; and 8% by outpatients as a whole in a hospital, representing item No. 2. The dramatic drop of SMON incidence after the banning of sales of clioquinol applies to items No. 3 and 7 (Fig. 1). Of Evans' proposed 8 criteria, 7 are fulfilled; No. 8 is applicable only to a microbial agent.

If a drug is a causative agent of an epidemic like SMON, it is possible to estimate the exact quantities consumed in a hospital, sold in prefectures geographically and produced in chronological time; it will thus become possible to compare the incidence of the disease in question with the distribution of the drug in time and space. This is unique to a drug-induced disease but rarely applicable to outbreaks of microbial disease. There is abundant evidence showing such geographical and chronological relationships between SMON and clioquinol (Figs. 3 and 4).

Initially, it was of great concern from both the medical and public health viewpoints, whether or not SMON was infectious. The epidemiological evidence (Table 3) seemed to support the infectious nature of SMON; on the other hand, it was hardly considered to be infectious on clinical and pathological grounds (Table 4). At the time these contradictory findings were amalgamated to reach general conclusions on the pathogenesis of SMON. The clioquinol theory has achieved such unification.

The toxic action of clioquinol on nerves is now being elucidated, and thus the problems concerning etiology and pathogenesis are almost solved. A remaining problem is why SMON was so prevalent in Japan. Abuse of clioquinol is considered to be an important cause but racial and genetic predisposition cannot be disregarded. It is regrettable that little progress has been made in the treatment of SMON in spite of strenuous efforts. It is most difficult to cure visual impairment

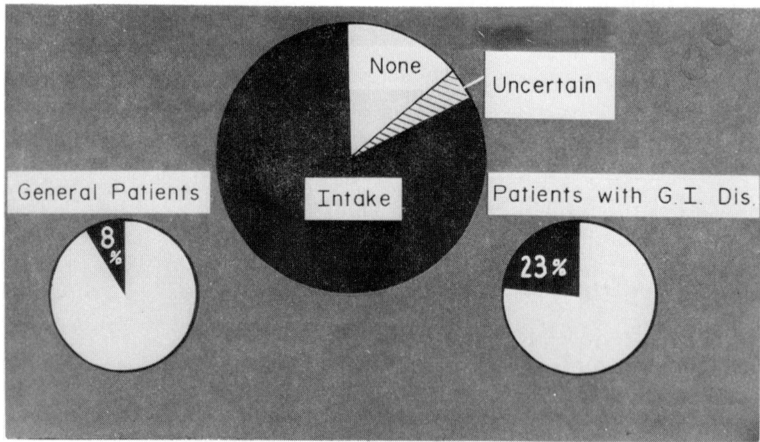

Fig. 2. Clioquinol intake (%) by SMON patients and others (1970).

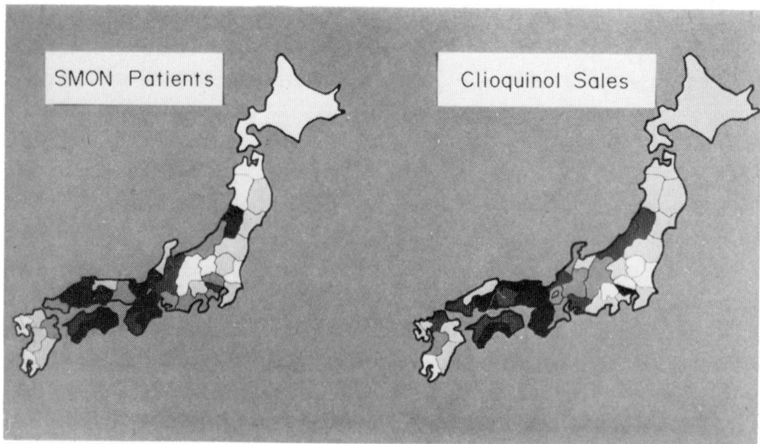

Fig. 3. Prevalence of SMON patients and amount of clioquinol sales by prefecture.

TABLE 3. *Phenomena suggesting infectious nature of SMON*

1. Epidemic occurrence in some areas
2. Sometimes familiar aggregation of cases
3. Hospital outbreaks frequent
4. Higher incidence rates in medical and paramedical profession
5. Higher prevalence in summer

TABLE 4. *Phenomena inexplicable by infection hypothesis*

1. Route of transmission not clear
2. In most areas cases were sporadic and it was hard to trace contact between them
3. Morbidity higher in women over middle age; rare in children
4. Clinically: Patients have no fever, rash and other signs suggesting infection
5. Laboratory findings: No gross changes in blood and CSF pictures
6. Pathologically: Axonal degeneration and demyelination of spinal cord, optic and peripheral nerves. Topography of lesions most closely resembled subacute combined degeneration of the spinal cord

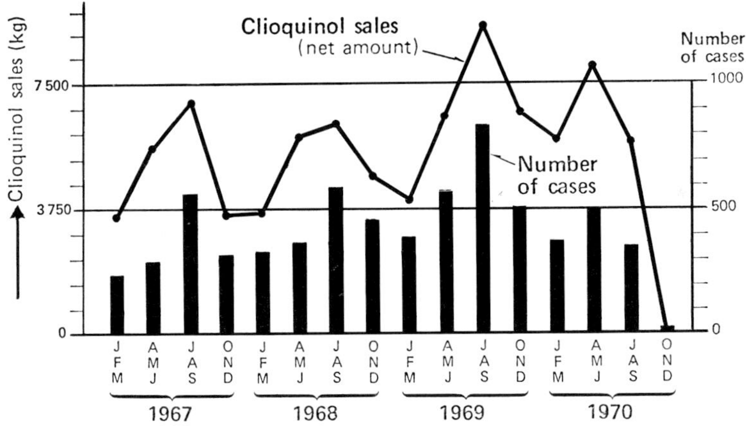

Fig. 4. Relationship between quarterly clioquinol sales and number of SMON cases.

and to alleviate severe pain and tingling sensations in the affected limbs. On the other hand, studies on rehabilitation contribute to the understanding of SMON dysfunction and disability, and to the improvement of motor function which is based on muscle physiology. The achievements in rehabilitation of SMON will be applicable to rehabilitation of other neural diseases.

Scientific achievements made by the SMON Research Commission and the SMON Research Committee, as organized by the foremost authorities from various fields in Japan, are as great as one can expect under existing circumstances, although there are some criticisms. What is insufficient was the dissemination of studies by the SMON Research Commission and SMON Research Committee to countries outside Japan. This occasion when we have many guests from abroad may allow worldwide transmission of our results and information on SMON and clioquinol.

Lastly, regarding the legal aspects, SMON patients started a suit against the government and three pharmaceutical companies. In court the results of the SMON Research Commission and the SMON Research Committee are central. Generally speaking, both the judges and the lawyers studied the results carefully and there were no major scientific errors in the judgement. The general public is apt to think that problems like either clioquinol or viruses are finally decided in court. The notion that scientific matters can be judged by jurists is unacceptable. Such trials will increase in number in the future, however, so that perhaps there are better ways in which scientific specialists can directly take part in judgement. Other countries have different and perhaps better systems than the Japanese. The medico-legal aspects require further debate.

REFERENCES

1. Shingu, M., Nakagawa, Y., Takedasu, H. and Okuda, K. (1965): Isolation of echotype 21 virus from patients with 'infectious column myelitis' following abdominal signs. *Nippon Densenbyo Gakkai Zasshi (J. Jap. Ass. infect. Dis.), 39,* 139 (in Japanese with English summary).
2. Kono, R. (1978): A review of SMON studies in Japan. In: *Epidemiological Issues in Reported Drug-Induced Illnesses – SMON and Other Examples,* p. 121. Editors: M. Gent and I. Shigematsu. McMaster University Library Press, Hamilton, Ontario.
3. Kono, R. (1972): Summarizing report. *Report of SMON Research Commission, No. 12,* p. 45 (in Japanese).
4. Kono, R. (1975): The SMON virus theory (correspondence). *Lancet, 2,* 370.
5. Inoue, Y.K., Nishibe, Y. and Nakamura, Y. (1971): Virus associated with SMON in Japan. *Lancet, 1,* 853.
6. Takasu, T., Igata, A. and Toyokura, Y. (1970): On the green tongue observed in SMON patients. *Igaku no Ayumi (Progr. Med.), 72,* 539 (in Japanese).
7. Igata, A., Hasebe, M. and Tsuji, T. (1970): On the green pigment found in SMON patients; two cases excreting greenish urine. *Nippon Iji Shimpo (Jap. med. J.), 2421,* 25 (in Japanese).
8. Yoshioka, M. and Tamura, Z. (1970): On the nature of the green pigment found in SMON patients. *Igaku no Ayumi (Progr. Med.), 74,* 320 (in Japanese).
9. Ikeda, Y. (1971): Toxicological investigation of SMON etiology. *Nippon Rinsho (Jap. J. clin. Med.), 29,* 766 (in Japanese).
10. Imanari, T. and Tamura, Z. (1970): Detection of chinoform from green fur of the tongue of SMON patients. *Igaku no Ayumi (Progr. Med.), 75,* 547 (in Japanese).
11. Tsubaki, T., Homma, Y. and Hoshi, M. (1971): Neurological syndrome associated with clioquinol. *Lancet, 1,* 696.
12. Tsuganezawa, M. (1967): Epidemiologic data and consideration. In: *Report of SMON Research by National Hospital Study Group,* p. 4 (in Japanese).
13. Sobue, I. (1978): Clinical features of SMON. In: *Epidemiological Issues in Reported Drug-Induced Illnesses – SMON and Other Examples,* p. 137. Editors: M. Gent and I. Shigematsu. McMaster University Library Press, Hamilton, Ontario.
14. Tateishi, J., Kuroda, S., Ikeda, H. and Otsuki, S. (1977): Experimental subacute myelo-optico-neuropathy. In: *Neurotoxicology, Vol. 1,* p. 658. Editors: L. Roizin, H. Shiraki and N. Grcevic. Raven Press, New York.
15. Nakae, K. and Shibata, T. (1978): A hospital survey on SMON in the Japanese town of Yubara. In: *Epidemiological Issues in Reported Drug-Induced Illnesses – SMON and*

Other Examples, p. 216. Editors: M. Gent and I. Shigematsu. McMaster University Library Press, Hamilton, Ontario.

16. Aoki, K. and Ohtani, M. (1978): Hospital survey on the relationship between SMON and clioquinol. In: *Epidemiological Issues in Reported Drug-Induced Illnesses – SMON and Other Examples*, p. 238. Editors: M. Gent and I. Shigematsu. McMaster University Library Press, Hamilton, Ontario.
17. Serizawa, H. Suzawa, H., Fukushima, M., Yokoyama, T. and Kitahara, T. (1971): Experiences of SMON outbreak in Emrei Hospital, Okaya City. In: *Report of Surveys on SMON in Nagano Prefecture*, p. 6. (in Japanese). Nagano Medical Association.
18. Yanagawa, H. (1978): Observations on the decrease in SMON cases in Japan before the suspension of clioquinol sales. In: *Epidemiological Issues in Reported Drug-Induced Illnesses – SMON and Other Examples*, p. 196. Editors: M. Gent and I. Skigematsu. McMaster University Library Press, Hamilton, Ontario.
19. Evans, A.S. (1978): Causation and disease: a chronological journey. *Amer. J. Epidemiol.*, *108*, 249.

The voice of the consumer

OLLE HANSSON

University of Gothenburg, Department of Pediatrics, East Hospital, Gothenburg, Sweden

I am a doctor. However, like most of us, I will probably also at some time be a patient and drug consumer. It is in the role of the well-informed and concerned drug consumer that I am speaking now.

I am aware of the fact that the problems concerning drugs are very complex. I am aware of the huge economic stakes in the search for new drugs. I am aware of the painstaking control by the medical authorities. But, I am also aware of the power of profit and the effectiveness of marketing departments. And I am also aware of the improbability of a drug which is not only effective but also harmless and without unwanted effects.

As a consumer I am very selfish. I want the best possible drug, and I want to be completely sure that my drug has been developed and investigated with the highest possible scientific skill and thoroughness. I also want my doctor to be fully informed about the benefits and risks of the drug and, finally, I want this information explained to me.

Can I get all this today? Frankly, I really don't know. But I do know that there are many undisputable and disturbing facts concerning drugs. And this worries me as a consumer. I will mention some of those facts, and I hope that this conference will answer some questions that they raise.

UNDISPUTABLE AND DISTURBING FACTS

When asked to comment on the manuscript of this speech a friend of mine said that in his opinion it seemed too shrill. 'You could make exactly the same points in a cooler, matter-of-fact tone.' That is certainly true. But it is also true that it is not an easy thing for a well-informed consumer to keep cool – for ever. So, what I am going to say might sound provocative to those who are not informed. This very conference, however, is sad proof of the present repugnant state of things.

Unscrupulous drug companies

The first and most disturbing fact is the existence at the present time of a number of unscrupulous drug companies around the world. This is particularly disturbing as it is quite difficult to find a drug company which does not deserve to be criticized. High esteem by doctors, a famous international reputation, prestige and worldwide marketing are no guarantees for the consumer. We do not have to look for examples. All of us know what Chemie Grünenthal and thalidomide stand for.

We know the way that chloramphenicol has been, and perhaps still is, marketed in Latin America, for example, by Parke-Davis, Winthrop, McKesson, Boehringer and others. Chloramphenicol is a life-saving drug indicated only in a few severe infectious diseases because its potential adverse effects may kill the patient. The risk-benefit evaluation therefore has to be extremely strict. This is in complete contrast to the free sale and soft indications given by the marketing departments of the drug companies. We also know the way in which anabolic steroids have been marketed to children in the poor countries on indications such as 'thinness', 'underweight', 'loss of appetite', 'lack of strength', 'general weakness' etc. by companies such as Ciba-Geigy, Winthrop, and Schering. And we know what Entero-Vioform and Ciba-Geigy stand for, like many other drug companies selling hundreds of other drugs containing oxyquinolines. More examples will be given during this conference.

It is often claimed that a drug is 'free from all side-effects' despite the fact that the producer knows that this is just not true! The drug companies often try to say that these claims are made locally by agents or medical authorities without their approval. If so, these companies who must have an adequate knowledge of their own drugs should of course refuse to sell them to agents who they know make irresponsible claims.

Laws for protection of drug producers

The second fact is that in most countries the laws seem to be written for the protection of the drug producers, not for the consumers. Even in countries thought to have very strict drug regulations – such as Sweden and Great Britain – the legal situation for the consumer is unsatisfactory. In Sweden, all documents concerning drugs in the hands of the medical authorities are by law considered confidential for 20 years if the documents contain facts thought to be harmful, in the broadest sense, to the drug producers.

In Sweden, as in many other countries, it is very difficult for the medical authorities to ban a registered drug which has been proved useless in practice and which no longer fulfils modern standards for documentation of efficacy. In such a case it is *not* up to the producer to prove the efficacy claimed. On the contrary, the medical authorities have to give scientific proof that the drug is useless – which, in fact, is a rather peculiar double-blind investigation for medical authorities to make, not to mention the ethical aspects.

In 1965, a panel of British experts assessing the therapeutic effectiveness of 2,241 out of 3,000 products judged 35% of them to be ineffective, obsolete or irrational combinations. In 1971, a similar investigation of 2,000 products by a panel of the American Food and Drug Administration found that 60% lacked evidence for their therapeutic claims. Some of these were ordered off the US market, but most have found ready markets elsewhere, in Third World countries, where regulations governing toxicity and efficacy of drugs may be rudimentary or non-existent.

In Britain about 20,000 branded medicines are estimated to be on the market; in West Germany there are 24,000 drugs, in Italy 21,000, and in France 8,500.

In India, a government committee has estimated that the country's basic pharmaceutical needs can be satisfied by 116 generic drugs, which is less than 1% of the 15,000 brand drugs sold there at present. A Brazilian government agency, which provides drugs free or at very low cost to the poorer sections of the population, deals with a list of just 108 generic pharmaceutical products, of which 52 are classified as essential. On the open market in Brazil, some 14,000 branded drugs are available.

A WHO document says that 'the range of medicinal products marketed in various countries varies from more than 30,000 to less than 2,000'. How many do consumers need? WHO has prepared a model list of essential drugs to help the developing countries draw up their own lists. It contains about 190 'essential drugs' and about 30 'complementary drugs'.

Many of the drugs lacking evidence for the therapeutic claims are potentially dangerous. Entero-Vioform is one of these. In Great Britain, Entero-Vioform has not been formally banned but is intended for prescription only. It is in fact not marketed at present, so no one can obtain it on prescription either. Therefore no official indications are established and no data-sheet is available because, according to British law, this is not needed if the drug is not promoted!

This is great – especially for the marketing department in the headquarters of Ciba-Geigy in Basle! 'Entero-Vioform is not banned in Britain, it is on prescription only!' – that is the truthful information from Ciba-Geigy to the countries in the Third World. The annual sales of Entero-Vioform and other clioquinol-containing products by Ciba-Geigy were recently said to be $40 million worldwide.

In many countries, inadequate laws and regulations are combined with incompetence on the part of the medical authorities. The recent statement by Mr Arsenio Regala, of the Philippine Food and Drug Administration, is an extreme example. Last year he said that clioquinol-based drugs marketed as Entero-Vioform or Mexaform do not produce adverse effects in Philippinos because of their 'genetic characteristics'. He cited chloramphenicol as another example of a drug which has caused reactions in Americans, but is well tolerated in the Philippines.

Association between medical profession and drug industry

Thirdly, in all countries there are unhealthy bonds between doctors and the drug industry. It is not exaggerated to speak of a 'medico-industrial complex' in analogy to the 'military-industrial complex'.

The bonds are not only at the individual level. It is not only drinks, dinners, conferences at home and abroad, and even other things at the drug companies' expense. Medical journals depend on the income from drug advertisements. The drug industry also exerts influence through direct support to institutions, medical societies and postgraduate education.

An inquiry into associations between leading physicians and the drug industry in Finland recently showed that a relationship was common (41%). Medical teachers had the highest frequency of relationship. But also those on the National Board of Health who had controlling functions over drug information, had relationships. The most common form of connection was membership of the administrative or scientific board of a drug company. The investigators concluded that the frequent connections between the medical elite and the pharmaceutical industry may have important influences on medical practice and health policy.

The Finnish situation is apparently valid also for other countries. In my country it is often stated that a small country like Sweden does not have sufficient competent physicians to serve the universities and the drug industry separately. I do not believe that this is the whole truth, however.

The medico-industrial complex also may have direct implications for the consumers. One example is the screening for and treatment of hypertension in the USA. Ciba-Geigy describes its own role in the following way: 'Ciba has made a major and continuing commitment to add its expertise to the growing number of organizations devoting much time and effort in the fight against high blood pressure. We are playing a leading role in many of the activities of the National High Blood Pressure Education Program serving on several of its advisory and resource committees.' In this connection, it might be pertinent to remind you that hypertension was the theme for the World Health Day on April 7, 1978. From the commercial point of view this very suitably puts the beta-blockers in focus for especial interest at a time when markets are growing and indications widening. To what extent we are looking at a sound development can be doubted, but it will only be possible to evaluate this in the future. What is beyond doubt, however, is the effectiveness of the drug industry in 'cooperating' with leading doctors and in marketing their best-sellers. Hopefully the information given to the prescribers is based on scientific documentation only and not on the futuristic speculations which occupy some of the brains of the industry.

A hint of what we can expect was given by the head of the Ciba-Geigy Adverse Drug Reaction Center, Dr. Oliver de S. Pinto, in a speech at an internal Ciba-Geigy meeting (Ciba-Geigy Pharma Registration Symposium, Fürigen, March 15, 1977): 'Our long term trials with beta-blockers in hypertension concern the Primary Prevention of heart attacks, strokes and other episodes that are manifestations of degenerative processes. There are more and more old people and the potential markets in these indications are enormous. As far as beta-blockers are concerned, we will have to explore the possibilities of an even greater market and provided safety can be confirmed for very long term treatment there are already good arguments to suggest all or many men over the age of 40 could obtain considerable protection from the long term prophylactic administration of beta-blockers even if they do not have hypertension. This not only raises the need to define ways in which such a hypothesis can be proved but also poses additional problems for drug health authorities as well as ourselves since it is entirely foreseeable that, as has already happened with oral contraceptives, health authorities will have to take decisions about permitting the use of such drugs in normal people. This is not dreaming and although not something for this year it is a major consideration for the near future, which is based upon reasonably well established knowledge and the needs of the community. It's logical too: if you are a woman and premenopausal, if you wish to avoid getting pregnant and if you are not frigid, and if you are heterosexual, the chances are you will take the pill, which has some risks but they are rare. If you have community responsibility and the birth rate is too high (or the abortion rate a problem) you will encourage use of the pill. If you are over forty and perfectly healthy, your cardiovascular system and especially the blood vessels to your heart and brain will be subjected to considerable stresses with their attendant risks. If you have community responsibility you will, at least in many countries, be faced with the dilemma of an ageing population that needs to be kept healthy so it can be productive and less of a burden upon the younger members of your society. There is good evidence that at least some beta-blockers could provide multifaceted protective effects for such people. Side effects are certainly rare although with equal certainty we can say we do not know enough about them yet. It is entirely logical to consider studies aimed at demonstrating a protective effect of beta-blockers if they are taken early enough by healthy people who are potentially at risk. Obviously such research is of acute interest to our marketing colleagues as well as ourselves. One can even dream a little: it is not entirely illogical to consider a combination of Trasicor (oxprenolol) and Anturan (sulphinpyrazone); and what about the fact that women on the pill are more subject to cardiovascular disorders than their more celibate sisters – could we offer them any protection in a similar way?'

I think you will agree that this quotation illustrates an extraordinary dream! Obviously the only problem remaining for Dr. de S. Pinto and Ciba-Geigy, if they achieve what they outline, will be to find a suitable indication for their prophylactic treatment in men below forty – and nuns. There is no reason to doubt that also this problem will be solved by Ciba-Geigy in a most scientific way.

However, the consumers seem to have good reasons for doubting how much of the present enthusiasm for screening for and treatment of moderate hypertension is generated by medical need and how much to sell more drugs. The same enthusiasm has not been shown by doctors in finding out how best to exploit dietary salt restriction, relaxation and exercise which are all believed to have an important effect on hypertension. In Britain a massive trial of drugs for mild hypertension by the Medical Research Council – the largest drug trial in the U.K. costing millions of pounds – has neglected to test the effect of factors other than drugs.

In Canada, there is a lawsuit at the moment against Hoffman-La Roche for giving away Valium and Librium free to Canadian hospitals in exchange for a complete monopoly of the highly lucrative tranquillizer market. 'Doctors learn their prescribing habits in the hospital...' says the prosecution counsel. The give-away policy was approved at the highest level by Etienne Junod, one of the four Hoffman-La Roche A.G. directors in Basle. M Junod is said to be a firm believer in free enterprise and the laws of the market!

However, for the consumers in the developed countries the negative consequences of the medico-industrial complex are much less than in the developing countries. The above-mentioned multinational, Hoffman-La Roche, quoted Sri Lanka a price for Valium which was 70 times higher than the price charged by an Indian company. The late Professor Senaka Bibile, former chairman of Sri Lanka's State Pharmaceuticals Corporation, said in his UNCTAD report on Sri Lanka that 'doctors often resist changes in pharmaceutical policy because many of them have been conditioned by the pharmaceutical industry'.

Couldn't cooperation between the medical establishment and the drug industry be a good thing for the customer? Yes, of course, if the cooperation is fair and open. Today this is often not the case. And, since the private drug industry is geared to the maximum sale of drugs whatever the real need, many ethical and medical problems are created. The medico-industrial complex does not make it less complicated.

Attitudes of politicians

The fourth point is the naïvity, opportunism, or cowardice on the part of the politicians towards the drug industry. The pharmaceutical industry is extremely successful. The profitability of many companies is unusually high compared with other industries. This has been the situation throughout the history of the drug industry, and these high returns have only been topped by the soap and cosmetics industry, which in many cases is linked with pharmaceuticals. This production is largely confined to a few developed countries. In 1975, West Germany, USA, Switzerland, United Kingdom and France together accounted for 71% of free-market drug exports from the developed countries. Drug production is also concentrated in the hands of a few companies. In Britain, five companies control approximately 30% of the market; in the US ten firms control over 40%. The three Swiss Firms, Hoffman-La Roche, Ciba-Geigy and Sandoz, between them account for some 15% of world sales of drugs! The drug companies are often multinationals, and they transfer their profits out of developing countries by charging their own subsidiares excessive prices. When the drug multinationals set up local manufacturing plants in the Third World, they usually produce profitable lines like cough syrups and vitamin pills, not life-saving drugs.

I admit that this simplifies the issues. In drug-exporting countries, a positive balance of payment is important to governments. Governments also want to encourage local manufacture, safeguard employment, etc. – all quite legitimate concerns, but not by exploiting the ill-health of consumers! Drug costs often represent 40–60% of the total health care expenditure in developing countries, compared with only 10–20% in the developed ones. A WHO document presented to the 1978 World Health Assembly says: ‘In recent years, many medical products have been marketed with little concern for the differing health needs and priorities of different countries. Promotional activities of the drug manufacturers have created a demand greater than the actual needs.’

Dr. Dale Console, for many years director of research at Squibb, made the famous statement that ‘the pharmaceutical industry is unique in that it can make exploitation appear a noble purpose’. The combination of ‘noble purpose’ and economic power is the benefactor of the politician – or his superior, overwhelming enemy. Where is the consumer in all this? During a cholera outbreak in 1974, the Sri Lanka government asked the local Pfizer factory to make tetracycline capsules, using raw material which the government had already purchased from Hoechst. Pfizer nobly refused!

Donations to medical schools

The fifth disturbing fact is that in some countries you can open the doors to medical schools with donations. Then, making big business out of health and illness is not very far way. This is clearly proven in countries such as Japan where the income of the doctor is dependent on the amount of drug prescribed – sometimes sold by the doctor! Being a guest in Japan, it is certainly not very polite to mention this. However, from the consumer's point of view, such a system is obviously dangerous and also unacceptable for other reasons.

Lack of independent information and research

The sixth undisputable fact is the worldwide lack of independent information on drugs and the insufficient resources for independent research. Today there is no acceptable balance between the flood of information, advertisements, and other marketing efforts from the drug companies in comparison with the few drops of independent, objective information. Not only but especially in poorer countries this situation is disastrous. The pressure from the drug companies is tremendous. In Great Britain there is one drug representative for every 30 doctors. In Tanzania there is one drug representative for every 4 doctors. 'Good drugs will always sell. Bad drugs will sell too, if heavily promoted.'

Failure of the mass media

The seventh fact is the failure of the mass media around the world to scrutinize, expose and inform about important medical matters. When President Carter had to cancel a day's schedule due to discomfort from hemorrhoids, this is of course of interest, not least – says the weekly magazine *Time* ironically – in order 'to avoid giving the stock market a heart attack', and the importance of this event is on record on more than half a page in the magazine. The SMON tragedy involving 20–30,000 people in Japan, and the continuing clioquinol scandal outside Japan, have not even been mentioned in *Time* over the years,* nor in many other important mass media.

THE THIRD WORLD

I have emphasized the situation in the Third World. The whole picture is one of 'drug colonialism', says Dr Halfdan Mahler, the Director-General of WHO. The history of contraceptive trials does not contradict Dr Mahler's statement. It has been the women of the Third World who have been used to determine whether or not contraceptives are safe and effective for the women of the developed world. 'Drug colonialism' does not always directly result in drug-induced suffering in the narrow sense of the word but it does for certain in the broad sense.

WHAT CAN BE DONE?

The friend of mine who commented on this speech said: 'I think that you say too little about doctors, because they need to change just as much as the drug companies. In some ways one can control drug companies more easily than one can control prescribers. Laws, properly enforced, may work to keep manufacturers in order, but doctors? No!' This is certainly true – and pessimistic. Let us hope, however, that it is not that doctors are actually evil, but that they behave in thoughtless and traditional ways.

The doctor is in a key position as the link between the drug consumer and the drug producer. The doctor makes the choice and recommends the treatment. In fact, a united front by doctors is the only power able to challenge the power of the drug

*In fact, a short notice was published on May 22, 1972.

industry. Unfortunately this sounds very hostile and militant. Indeed, it is. Experience is such that there is no longer room for endless discussions, solicitations, supplications or naïve wishes. When the logic of common sense and justice is constantly being insulted, then it is time to make use of the logic of economics.

One way to do this has been proven effective by Swedish doctors: that is the boycott. Another means, which I think is more effective in the long run, is *information.* Doctors will have to cooperate much more closely than at present with consumers and journalists. In such cooperation all unethical and unmedical marketing and usage of drugs should be exposed and the drug companies in question should not be allowed to wriggle out of or brush off such complaints. In perspective, to blacken its reputation is not good business for a drug company. Reputation and credibility are the Achilles' heel of the drug industry.

NEW INTERNATIONAL PHARMACEUTICAL ORDER

Senator Paul H. Douglas had the thalidomide catastrophe in mind when he asked: 'Can we learn from this lesson, or can mankind educate itself only by disaster and tragedy?' Unfortunately this question was not to be rhetorical. One of the grotesque replies to Senator Douglas is the SMON disaster.

I was asked to comment on SMON after my testimony in the Tokyo District Court in 1976. I answered that from the humanitarian point of view it is a tragedy, from the medical point of view it is a scandal, and from the moral and ethical point of view it is shameful. These words are still valid. It is time, therefore, to end the SMON disaster, to end all avoidable drug-induced sufferings, and to prevent misuse of drugs by all means given.

It is time to act! It is time to act for all of us who believe in human dignity and justice. Let us make this conference a milestone on the road to a *new pharmaceutical order* in the world!

BIBLIOGRAPHY

1. Agarwal, A. (1978): *Drugs and the Third World.* Earthscan, International Institute for Environment and Development, 10 Percy Street, London.
2. Friedrich, V., Hehn, A. and Rosenbroch, R. (1977): *Neunmal teurer als Gold. Die Arzneimittelversorgung in der Bundesrepublik.* Aus der Arbeit der Vereinigung Deutscher Wissenschaftler (VDW), Rowohlt, Hamburg.
3. Hemminki, E. and Pesonen, T. (1977): An inquiry into associations between leading physicians and the drug industry in Finland. *Soc. Sci. Med., 11,* 501.
4. Ledogar R.J. (1975): *Hungry for Profits. U.S. Food and Drug Multinationals in Latin America.* IDOC/North America, Inc., 235 East 49th Street, New York.
5. Medawar, C. (1979): *Insult or Injury? An Inquiry into Marketing and Advertising of British Food and Drug Products in the Third World.* Social Audit Ltd, 9 Poland Street, London.
6. Silverman, M. (1976): *The Drugging of the Americas. How Multinational Drug Companies Say One Thing about Their Products in the United States, and Another Thing to Physicians in Latin America.* University of California Press, Berkeley-Los Angeles, CA.

7. Silverman, M. and Lee, P.R. (1974): *Pills, Profits, and Politics.* University of California Press, Berkeley-Los Angeles, CA.
8. Sjöström, H. and Nilsson, R. (1972): *Thalidomide and the Power of the Drug Companies.* Penguin Books, London.
9. Vaughan, P. (1972): *The Pill on Trial.* Pelican Book, Penguin Books.
10. Wardell, W.M. (Ed.) (1978): *Controlling the Use of Therapeutic Drugs. An International Comparison.* American Enterprise Institute for Public Policy Research, Washington, DC.
11. Erklärung von Bern: *The Infiltration of the UN System by Multinational Corporations*, Excerpts from internal files. Vereinigung für solidarische Entwicklung, Gartenhofstr. 27, Zurich.
12. Haslemere Group (1976): *Who Needs the Drug Companies?* Haslemere Group and War on Want and Third World First, Third World Publications, 138 Stratford Road, Birmingham, U.K.
13. Interim Report of the Canadian Government's Commission on Inquiry (1971): *The Non-Medical Use of Drugs.* Penguin Books.
14. The Monopolies Commission (1973): *Chlordiazepoxide and Diazepam.* 197, Her Majesty's Stationery Office, London.
15. *Time Weekly Magazine, January 8, 1979*, p. 52.
16. WHO (1977): The Selection of essential drugs. *Wld Hlth Org. techn. Rep. Ser., 615.*

The relief of the victims

HIROSHI IZUMI

5th Floor, Yamaichi Building, 3–11 Yotsuya, Shinjuku-ku, Tokyo, Japan

Sessions I and II mainly concerned basic drug research, drug-induced suffering and side-effects and drug safety. In Session III, research papers and discussions focus on the actual state of the drug-induced suffering and relief of the victims, principally from socio-legal viewpoints.

PSYCHOLOGICAL RESTORATION TO THE ORIGINAL CONDITION

The relief of the victims is not limited to the compensation for damages. The restoration of the original psychological, physical, economic and social state must be the aim.

The Twelve Decemviral Tables in ancient Roman law state that if a man has his limbs cut off, his enemy must be treated similarly, unless peace is established between them. In the modern law, too, if restoration of the original condition is impossible, sincere and maximal efforts include financial compensation for psychological and physical damages.

In cases where large corporations are at fault, it is often possible to help the victims return to their earlier life-styles, and the approaches are sometimes associated with the prevention of subsequent drug suffering.

Regarding psychological recovery, the accounts and agreements of the thalidomide, SMON, and Niigata and Kumamoto-Minamata cases etc., regrets and apologies were expressed. In civil libel cases, a published apology is demanded by the courts.

Psychological recovery is complex, and the damage cannot be removed by such documents. Moreover it is inhuman to think that money provides the pardon.

If perpetrators of drug-induced suffering take such callous attitudes, the victims and a caring society must demand abolition of such corporations.

THE PERMANENT COUNTERPLAN

The physical and social recovery must comprise a 'permanent counterplan' or 'permanent policies'.

Diseases that cannot be cured by usual medical practices demand study by well-equipped public medical organizations.

The development of medical aid devices is essential.

A Dutch physician has raised an important matter in his book 'Medical Power and Medical Ethics' in questioning the blessing of allowing the birth of thalidomide children. What kinds of medical aids have been developed and how have the social environments been modified for those thalidomide children now growing up? How have university education and employment been prepared? Many similar problems concerning SMON and other drugs also exist.

To solve these problems individually the whole state welfare system must be galvanized into action.

THE ACTUAL STATE OF DRUG-INDUCED SUFFERINGS

The collection and critical evaluation of information on drug side-effects is difficult. When it is considered that such information concerns the drugs and not doctors, it is easy to see that plaintiffs find it difficult to gather all relevant data including prescriptional information from doctors.

In Session III research papers consider thalidomide, SMON, streptomycin, chloramphenicol and Coralgil suits. In Japan, actions are also currently pending against chloroquine, ethambutol, Myobutazolidine, Chlotaon etc.

Drug-induced diseases are sometimes overlooked by doctors and patients because confidential information is not critically evaluated. When a number of victims appear, and the damage is serious, then a social problem becomes apparent. This is why the actual number of drug-induced sufferers in Japan is incompletely known. For instance, estimates for thalidomide patients range from 700 to 1000, from 10,000 to 30,000 for SMON patients and from 100 to 1000 for chloroquine patients.

It is an important premise for the legal and administrative relief of the victims to grasp and analyze correctly the real extent of drug-induced damage.

THE MOOT POINTS OF THE MASS LITIGATION

There are several difficult problems in mass suits for the relief of the victims.

1. For instance, accumulation, control and collation of the necessary information for law suits are formidable and include the financial aspects regarding the research and collection of information.

2. In mass litigation many plaintiffs, attorneys and supporters are involved and their opinions regarding contemporary morality and sense of value vary. Unselfish and cooperative attitudes recognizing the need to relieve the victims are essential.

In one such agreement, between the Health and Welfare Ministry and SMON patients, the Government gave preferential entry into public hospitals.

The heads in the planning sections of the pharmaceutical bureau in the Health and Welfare Ministry carry out these immediate actions, but in the long term, duties owing to the patients are ill-defined. Dedication to the victims, overcoming the conflict of different opinions must be prerequisite.

3. Trials should be initiated rapidly for delay in court denies the relief. In the SMON suit, the defendants were ordered to pay part compensation before the trial ended, so that a provisional temporary payment was made.

The study of products liability is also important.

One way to expedite mass litigation is to stereotype the exhibits concerning the many hundred or thousand plaintiffs. The compensation for damages needs to be stereotyped as well, allowing for individual interests. Variation in age, profession, or residential area of the victims makes this difficult, but compared with the delays involved in proving individual damage the benefits are obvious.

In the recent suits the basic compensation has been fixed according to the severity of condition given certain allowances. The settlement of the SMON suit at the Tokyo District Court on October 19, 1977, and subsequent decisions on August 3, 1978, are notable for the plainly stated calculating standards for allowances.

For instance, rather than giving potential incomes individually, the basic settlement is supplemented by 15 to 30%, according to the severity, and by 10% or 20% for those under 30 or 50 years, taking into consideration the duration and extent of the damage caused. For dependent relatives, 10% is also added for wives with babies or school children.

Whether such standards can be generally applied or should be further divided are questions for further debate.

The manner of establishing proof should be stereotyped. Impartial and equal relief is essential in mass litigation, and providing it is not against the victims' interests, simple standards are necessary.

International legal agreements are desirable, taking into account the legal systems of each country.

THE RELIEF OF VICTIMS OF DRUG-INDUCED SUFFERING

The amendment of the Pharmaceutical Affairs Act in Japan is reported in Session II, and in Session III papers and discussions about the system for relief are given.

Concerning governmental duties to the fund, political, financial and philosophical points of view are required.

In Japan, it has become obvious that the governmental drug administration has wide responsibilities to the victims, with precedents given in the SMON suits at Kanazawa, Tokyo, Fukuoka and Hiroshima District Courts.

The system for the relief of the victims of drug-induced suffering should be discussed and applied to all cases.

For example, some SMON victims have no proof of medication; the doctor may not have written the medication or prescription on the clinical chart, or the chart was thrown away after the filing period. The district courts of Fukuoka and Hiroshima, in such cases, ordered the government to compensate in full. The government should adhere to these decisions.

THE ROLE OF THE NEWS MEDIA

The role of the television and newspapers in reporting drug-induced suffering is inestimable. The successful suits concerning environmental pollution to date owe much to the information presented and the opinions formed by the news media.

Newspapers and television widely report drug-induced suffering and, consequently, pressure is brought to solve the problems. Moreover, information which is profitable to victims may be passed on by those who have read or heard about it.

Reporting of news must be based on humanity and at the same time be impartial. A society in which a corporation is insincere in solving the problem must be condemned. The existence of corporations that cause suffering without earnestly attempting relief is questionable.

Judicature evaluates the democratic processes but it is a slow procedure not conducive to rapid relief. The guilty must respect the court decisions and rapidly, sincerely and earnestly try to relieve the victims. This is a tenet of a democratic society.

To abuse the trial system by economic means and to contest at law until the last victim dies should not be allowed.

It is absolutely right for the news 'to contribute to the happiness of the people on the basis of justice and humanity' and not simply to keep impartiality between the two extremes.

Totally neutral reporting on the intruders and the intruded, the guilty and the victims, the oppressors and the oppressed should not prevail.

THE EXCHANGE OF INTERNATIONAL INFORMATION

Mr. Sjöstrom, a Swedish attorney, says in his book: 'The thalidomide disaster can also be seen partly as a result of a lack of adequate exchange of information'. One of the results expected of this Conference is the expansion and reinforcement of the information-exchange system.

In the settlement clauses at the Tokyo District Court, it is stated: 'Pharmaceutical companies shall reflect gravely that they have encouraged the world to sell and consume drugs in bulk by their extensive propaganda; reaffirm that they pursue means towards a greater safety of drugs and make doubly sure in making and selling of drugs; try to discover any side-effects of drugs and collate information concerning these; submit all necessary data to the welfare authorities; and try their best to prevent damage from drugs by transmitting as much data as possible to the doctors, of course, and also to the users (takers) concerning so-called popular drugs, bearing in mind the known side-effects'.

It is necessary for doctors and users to assess whether pharmaceutical companies present information correctly or not, and also an organization should be established to exchange information internationally about drugs.

In reality, in the suits concerning drug-induced suffering in Japan, references to American and European countries have played an important part in proving the liability of the defendants.

The publication and exchange of information is necessary to prevent Japan exporting drug-induced suffering to countries in South-East Asia.

In conclusion, it is an earnest expectation that this Conference will produce concrete proposals for the prevention of drug-induced suffering.

SESSION I: MEDICAL AND PHARMACEUTICAL ASPECTS OF DRUG-INDUCED SUFFERINGS

The history of iatrogenic diseases in Japan

HIDERO SUZUKI

First Department of Internal Medicine, University of Environmental and Occupational Health, Kitakyushu, Japan

The term 'iatrogenic disease' has been given many definitions by a number of different authors. However, if it is defined as the undesirable consequences of all the diagnostic and therapeutic acts performed by doctors, it will include many different diseases.

Here, I would like to discuss the history of undesirable or harmful effects of drugs after World War II and the various measures undertaken in Japan to cope with this problem. This will be discussed as part of the general topic of iatrogenic diseases of this symposium.

Table 1 shows the major adverse drug reactions which have occurred since World War II and the various administrative measures taken in response to these problems.

ADVERSE REACTIONS DUE TO GUANOFRACIN

Guanofracin is an ophthalmic solution. Because of reports that eyelashes and eyelids of patients who used this drug turned white, an order was issued in 1951 to stop its manufacture and to recall all products containing guanofracin. Although this side-effect is minor, it is worth mentioning, firstly, because, it was the first drug-related incident in Japan after World War II and, secondly, because of the severity of the measures taken to stop its manufacture and to recall the products from the market.

ANAPHYLAXIS DUE TO PENICILLIN

In 1956, Professor Otaka of the Law School at Tokyo University died from penicillin anaphylaxis during treatment at a dental clinic. This is a notable incident in the sense that it warned people anew of the terrible nature of adverse drug reactions, particularly since it involved a famous law scholar. The case was treated as top news by the newspapers.

Despite the seriousness of the incident, no order was issued to stop the manufacture of penicillin because of its value as a powerful antibiotic. The Ministry of Health and Welfare merely issued a warning throughout the country for clinicians to be aware of penicillin anaphylaxis and urged them to conduct intradermal testing as a safety measure prior to penicillin administration.

TABLE 1. *Major problems of adverse drug reaction and administrative measures in response to these problems*

Year	Drug	Adverse reactions	Treatment and measures
1951	Guanofracin	Leukoderma of palpebra and cilia	Recall of product, discontinuance of manufacture
1956	Penicillins	Death due to anaphylactic shock	Warning, intradermal test
1961	Thalidomide	Teratogenicity	Recall of product, discontinuance of product distribution
			Establishment of Committee on Safety of Drugs, teratogenic studies
1963	Drug in ampule for common cold	Death due to anaphylactic shock	Recall of product, discontinuance of manufacture
			Establishment of Subcommittee on Combination Drugs, new approval system for all combination drugs
1966	Reducing drug	Psychic disorder	Prohibition of use of thyroid hormone
			Establishment of Subcommittee for Adverse Drug Reaction
1967	Chloroquine	Optic injury	Warning, discontinuance of manufacture
			Establishment of National Drug Monitoring System and Monitoring System for New Drugs
1970	Quinoform	SMON	Prohibition of use
			Meeting of Drug Efficacy Committee on Drug Efficacy Re-evaluation
1971	Coralgil	Fatty liver	Discontinuance of manufacture
			Extension of monitoring period for new drugs; obligatory report on adverse reactions to all drugs
1975	Injection drug in infants	Quadriceps contraction	Re-evaluation of injection drugs

TERATOGENICITY OF THALIDOMIDE

Thalidomide is a hypnotic developed in West Germany. The drug was used by many women in early pregnancy due to its effect on morning sickness. Because of an unusually high incidence of seal-like deformity, called phocomelia in West Germany, a detailed investigation of medications given to pregnant women was conducted and thalidomide was suspected to be the causative agent; therefore, as you know, the sale of thalidomide was prohibited in 1961.

Due to a delay in obtaining the information and taking effective measures in Japan, an order to stop its distribution and for total recall of the products was not issued until 1962, 9 months after the sale in West Germany had been stopped. Consequently, many deformed babies were born which placed the drug manufacturers and the health officials of the country under fire before the whole nation.

On account of the rather ununiform steps taken by various countries concerning this matter, WHO took up the issue and discussed the problem of insufficient international exchange of information on adverse drug effects. They passed a resolution to set up an international monitoring system for exchange of information on drug toxicities at the General Session in 1962, which became effective in 1963.

Drawing a lesson from this incident, a Special Committee on Safety of Drugs was newly established in the same year to function as a special review committee to cope with various adverse drug effects in this country. Due to this Special Committee, a regulation was established requiring all new drug applications to include teratogenic studies to confirm the safety of the drug to the fetus, which became effective in 1965.

DRUGS IN AMPULES FOR THE COMMON COLD

In 1965, a case of death from anaphylaxis due to a medicine against the common cold which was sold in ampules in large quantities over the counter, was reported in newspapers and caused great concern. The Ministry of Health and Welfare quickly called for a meeting of the Special Committee on Safety of Drugs to discuss the matter and an order was issued according to the advice of the Committee to stop the manufacture of the medicine in ampules and to recall the products from the market. This drug, of which several hundred million ampules a year had been sold, thereafter disappeared from drug stores.

These over-the-counter medicines against the common cold had their origin in the pedalling of drugs in old days, namely the so-called 'antidote sellers of Toyama' who used to cover mainly rural areas. As a matter of fact, the early prescriptions of those days used to be a fairly simple combination of 1–3 kinds of drugs including antipyretics, analgesics or expectorants. Subsequently, a manufacturer made a big hit in sales by producing a liquid preparation in ampules to be consumed with a straw. After a formal request to change the formulation, other manufacturers joined the competition, and the composition of the prescription became more and more complicated. When the manufacture of these medicines for the common cold was stopped, the best sales item contained 27 ingredients in addition to alcohol. However, how many deaths among those reported to be due to anaphylaxis were really due to these medicines is unknown. Anyhow, this is an important case in which a profound lesson was learned showing the serious consequences that can result when drugs are produced for profit making.

Based on the experiences of this incident, the current status of over-the-counter drugs has been re-evaluated and those drugs which tend to cause allergy, such as aminopyrine, have been removed from over-the-counter medicines for the common cold. At the same time, the Committee on Combination Drugs was established to place all combination drugs under a new approval system based on new guidelines.

ADVERSE DRUG EFFECTS DUE TO REDUCING DRUGS

In 1966, cases of psychic disorders were reported in patients who took a so-called 'weight-loss medicine' which was sold to those who wished to lose weight for cosmetic purposes. The true problem in these cases lies in the fact that although these 'weight-loss drugs' were effective in reducing weight because of the thyroid hormone they contained, the weight-losing effect decreased with the same dose after a certain period of time. Thus, patients increased the dose one after another and finally developed serious intoxication from the thyroid hormone. In addition, these 'weight-loss drugs' were over-the-counter items that were sold without prescription. Thyroid hormone has since been prohibited from being used as a 'weight-loss drug'.

To cope with any pharmaceutical matters which might occur in the future, the Ministry of Health and Welfare created for the first time in 1966 a Subcommittee on Adverse Drug Reactions as a substructure of the Special Committee on Safety of Drugs to specifically investigate adverse drug reactions.

VISUAL DISTURBANCES DUE TO CHLOROQUINE

In 1967, a large number of visual disturbances due to chloroquine were reported. The majority of these cases involved chronic rheumatoid arthritis and chronic glomerulonephritis patients who had been receiving chloroquine over a period of many years as a non-steroidal anti-inflammatory agent. Chloroquine was originally developed as an antimalarial agent and its side-effect on the eyes has been recognized since the time of its development. Besides, a special warning was issued describing the effect of visual disturbances when its application was extended to cover diseases other than malaria; however, caution about the visual disturbances waned when the drug came into common use. This side-effect was discussed at length and finally the maker of chloroquine voluntarily terminated its manufacture and sale based on the decision that the benefits of this drug were less than its potential serious side-effects.

Beginning in 1967, more than 400 university hospitals, national, and public hospitals across the country have been designated as monitoring hospitals under the national monitoring system in Japan as a means of collecting information on side-effects of drugs. In addition, a Monitoring System on New Drugs was implemented in the same year making it a requirement to conduct a 2-year follow-up study on the side-effects of all new drugs and subsequently the required follow-up study period was extended to 3 years.

Accordingly, in 1968, WHO established a Research Center for International Monitoring of Adverse Reactions to Drugs and called upon countries across the world to collaborate.

QUINOFORM AND SUBACUTE MYELO-OPTICONEUROPATHY (SMON)

SMON will be discussed in another section of this symposium, so I shall not describe it here. The only point I would like to mention is that quinoform, which has been suspected to be the causative agent in this pharmaceutical affair, has been regarded as a safe drug for many years and is listed in the Japanese Pharmacopeia.

Since the side-effects of drugs became a problem, the Ministry of Health and Welfare has gradually tightened the guidelines for approval of new drugs and, today, Japan is considered to have the strictest approval guidelines for new drugs in the world. But, almost no evaluation was done on those previously approved drugs; therefore, a Meeting on Drug Efficacy was called in 1970 to discuss plans for evaluating previously approved drugs and, based on the conclusions reached after several meetings, the Committee on Drug Efficacy Re-evaluation was newly initiated in 1971.

LIVER DAMAGE DUE TO 4,4′-DIETHYLAMINOETHOXYHEXESTROL

This drug, which has the brand name of Koraldil, is a coronary artery dilator and has been used mainly in patients with arteriosclerosis. Beginning about 1965, patients with many foam cells in the peripheral blood and bone marrow were recognized and reported as 'foam cell syndrome' by hematologists, but the etiology was unknown. At about the same time, patients with liver damage which was different from any of the previously known liver diseases were identified and reported under the name of 'phospholipidosis of the liver' by specialists in liver diseases in 1969, but again the etiology remained unknown.

In 1971, Professor Nishikawa et al. of Osaka University found these two diseases to be the same. Suga et al. of Tokyo Medical and Dental University who earlier had first reported the foam cell syndrome, discovered that this disease was caused by Koraldil, thereby clarifying the long-unknown ailment to be a disease caused by the side-effect of the drug. On account of these implications, the drug makers voluntarily stopped the manufacture and sale of this drug and recalled all the products from the market, hence practically putting an end to this drug-induced disease.

This incident was caused by chronic toxicity of the drug and it is worth mentioning because several years elapsed after the damage was recognized before the causative agent was identified. Using this incident, the Ministry of Health and Welfare decided to extend the monitoring period for new drugs from 2 to 3 years, and made it a requirement for manufacturers to report the important side-effects of all drugs produced.

QUADRICEPS CONTRACTURE IN INFANTS

At about 1970, the occurrence of quadriceps contracture in many infants was noted and the Ministry of Health and Welfare stepped in to investigate the matter, when the number of cases had reached 230–240. The majority of patients had received injections from doctors and the matter is still under investigation without any conclusion as to whether these cases were caused by the effect of the injected drug or by the injection technique of the doctors.

However, in a certain area when multiple cases of the disease occurred, about 90% of the cases had received injections from a single doctor; therefore, it is suspected by many that the disease may have been caused by the injection technique of the doctor. If this is true, then this represents true iatrogenic disease with the physician directly responsible. It should be remembered that among so-called drug incidents, some of them may not be caused by the drugs themselves but rather by the doctors who administered the drugs.

CONCLUSION

This concludes my statement on the major adverse drug reactions which have occurred in Japan since World War II and the measures and countermeasures taken by the country in response to these incidents. It is speculated that many of these incidents were caused by the inability of clinicians to keep pace with the rapid progress in medical science, as stated by Dr. Moser in his book *Iatrogenic Diseases*. I think it is desirable that everyone working with drugs in every field should make a coordinated effort to minimize as much as possible the menace of drugs.

DISCUSSION

Herxheimer: I would like to ask what drugs were injected intramuscularly in infants to cause the quadriceps contracture? Were many different drugs concerned or only a few?

Suzuki: Many kinds of drugs are blamed. There are patients who have been injected with many types of drugs many times, and there are also other patients injected with only 2 or 3 types of drugs. Analgesics, antipyretics and antibiotics are reported to be typical in causing the contracture.

Cabrera: Among the drugs presented by Dr. Suzuki, it would appear that the adverse effects are produced only after their prolonged use rather than by their improper use. For example, chloroquine is a good drug against malaria. In the treatment of malaria you give it for a short period of time, and the effect is not bad at all. So, in fairness to the drug, per se, or to the drug manufacturers, I think it has to be emphasized that the drug is not bad provided it is used correctly.

Hung: Apart from the contracture of the quadriceps femoris due to the intramuscular injection, are there any reported cases of contracture of the gluteal muscle due to repeated injections?

Suzuki: Yes, among the patients there are some with contracture of the gluteal muscle.

Hung: In Taiwan, in some local areas we have many patients with contracture – we call it 'frog-legs'. They develop contracture of the gluteal muscle (?). We thought this type of lesion might be due to the injection. I will take your information for a careful watch in the future.

Extrapolating from preclinical results to drug hazard in man

YASUHIRO NOGUCHI

Nagoya Pharmocology Laboratory, Pfizer Taito Co., Ltd., Aichi-ken, Japan

A drug is defined as a chemical agent possessing biological activity, and the first step of development of new therapeutic agents is the screening procedure, in which random compounds are tested for selected pharmacological activities. For example, antibacterial activity of the agents is tested in screenings against existing standard antibiotic(s) as references.

If the biological screening is encouraging, the agent is tested for animal toxicity and developed as a pharmaceutical formulation.

Before initial studies in man are permitted, the full pharmacological spectrum of a new drug must be thoroughly and extensively explored in animals, and both acute and chronic toxicity tests must be conducted on several species. Such experiments are normally prerequisite to the granting of clinical trial certificates for assessment in human volunteers prior to general release of the drug.

It has been recognized that no drug is free of side-effects. Consequently accurate prediction of the potentially harmful effects of drugs in man is essential.

Extrapolation from animals to man, however, is not easy; species differences in severity of harmful effects and time required for onset of toxicity, etc. are obvious problems. Experimental animals display considerable variations in response. Seldom is a compound uniformly active in different species. Morphine excites cats and depresses dogs. A non-steroidal anti-inflammatory drug, phenylbutazone, has a biological half-life of about 3 hours in rabbits, 5 to 8 hours in rats, guinea-pigs, dogs, monkeys, and horses, and 72 hours in man. Obviously the half-life of phenylbutazone in man cannot be predicted from the data obtained in 6 animal species.

In animal toxicity studies, excessive doses are used, compared with the therapeutic doses given in man. Direct toxicity to an organ system, drug actions, and drug or metabolite storage can be predicted from animal studies. Usually hemolytic reactions and undesirable organ or biochemical reactions, and to an extent safety, can be predicted from effects in animals.

In contrast, individual human reactivity, pre-existing pathological states producing adverse effects, iatrogenic effects, undesired effects not drug-related, interference with nutrient absorption, allergy, idiosyncrasy and others cannot be predicted from the experimental animal studies.

It is, however, rather rare to find direct toxicity to an organ system, and drug or metabolite storage although highly predictable from the animal data, the incidence being only 1 to 2%. On the other hand, allergy, idiosyncrasy and undesired effects not drug-related, which are difficult to predict from the animal studies, are fairly high in incidence, from 15 to 40%.

While the toxicity in animals is produced dose-dependently and manifested in all animals given sufficient drug, it is common to find harmful effects in only some people at the usual clinical doses.

For example, it is possible to determine a dose of carbon tetrachloride that will produce hepatic centrolobular necrosis virtually in 100% of animals or humans at risk. With drugs, the reported incidence of cholestasis reactions is less than 1%, regardless of the doses employed. While carbon tetrachloride does exhibit a dose-response relationship, chlorpromazine, for example, does not, nor do the other non-steroidal compounds associated with cholestasis. This means that predictability on the basis of therapeutic dosage is risky for those substances associated with cholestasis.

The minimal number of animals required to test toxic reaction can be calculated. If the expected frequency in man and animals were 1%, about 300 need testing to produce the cholestatic reaction in at least one animal with 95% probability of success. If the real incidence of the cholestatic reaction in man were 0.1%, the test would require about 3000 animals to produce this experimental lesion at least once with a 95% probability.

These figures demonstrate the impracticality of expecting events with a very low incidence to be picked up in laboratory animals.

The solution to this problem is not easy. One approach is to develop, accumulate and apply new techniques, data and knowledge. An injectable solvent of hydrogenated castor oil, HCO-60, caused minimal increases in blood pressure on intravenous administration at a dose of 100 mg/kg in rats, guinea-pigs, rabbits, cats and monkeys, while dogs showed dramatic decreases in blood pressure. How can the human blood pressure response be predicted? Little change in blood pressure was observed in dogs after a second intravenous injection of HCO-60. It is believed that the tachyphylaxis is related to the exhaustion of the easily releasable histamine by the first injection. Markedly elevated blood histamine levels were demonstrated by injecting HCO-60 into dogs. No increase in blood and plasma histamine levels was found in man and rabbits following intravenous injections of such agents. Thus, HCO-60 liberates mast cell histamine only in dogs and not in man. So it seems reasonable to predict that the blood pressure in man will not be lowered after intravenous injection of HCO-60.

In conclusion, there are major differences between animals and man in their responses to drugs and many inhibitory factors prevent extrapolation of data from animals to man. However, careful interpretation and insight allow certain predictions. At the same time, it must be emphasized that drugs are chemical substances possessing biological activity and none is free from adverse effects. Caution must be applied to prevent adverse reactions.

DISCUSSION

Shin: Assuming that every drug is potentially dangerous and there is a time-lag between the approval of a new drug and the re-evaluation or recalling of it due to later development of unacceptable toxicity, and also assuming that the toxicity often develops after repeated use over a long period, how do we reconcile these general discrepancies in approving a new drug?

Noguchi: We should weigh very carefully the benefits and the risks involved in introducing the new drug. The problematic point is the time when the permission is to be given. I would suggest the time is when Phase III studies are completed. At that stage, however, only a limited number of people have experience with the new drug, and nobody can assert that the drug is truly safe. Therefore, approval should never be absolute or permanent. We must be prepared for unexpected adverse effects by setting up a system for early detection and rapid reaction against this type of hazard.

Shin: Drugs may be approved if they meet certain criteria for safety and efficacy. Many of the drugs which we may not actually need can easily get marketing permission in areas where similar drugs are already competing with each other. Are there measures whereby these unnecessary drugs can be prevented from entering the market?

Noguchi: Each drug should be used and the selection of a drug and its use seems a somewhat different problem from that of new drug approval.

Predictability of drug toxicity in man from a pharmacokinetic viewpoint

RYUICHI KATO

Department of Pharmacology, School of Medicine, Keio University, Tokyo, Japan

Recent studies have indicated that serum and tissue drug levels are closely correlated with their efficacy and toxicity. Lipid soluble drugs are metabolized by the liver and other tissues and excreted as water soluble compounds. Species differences in drug pharmacokinetics reflect species differences in drug metabolism.

Most drugs are metabolized to inactive metabolites and only a few are metabolized to biologically active compounds and thence further metabolized. The latter group are termed 'pro-drugs'. On the other hand, some drugs are metabolized to chemically active intermediates which covalently bind with the nucleophilic cell macromolecules such as protein, RNA and DNA and cause cell death. In the body toxic active intermediates are detoxified to inactive metabolites, so that the balance between the rate of formation and detoxification of toxic active intermediates is the important factor in the control of drug toxicity. Drug toxicity thus results from the accumulation of either parent drugs or toxic intermediates.

This paper is primarily concerned with species differences in the formation and detoxification of toxic intermediates with a view to predicting drug toxicity in man from data obtained in animal experiments.

METABOLIC ACTIVATION AND TOXICITY OF DRUGS

Acetaminophen toxicity

Acetaminophen is mainly metabolized to glucuronide and sulfate conjugates in experimental animals and man and only a minor part is N-hydroxylated by microsomal drug-metabolizing enzymes. However, after large doses of acetaminophen, the conjugation processes become saturated and the formation of N-hydroxylated metabolites increases.

N-hydroxylated acetaminophen covalently binds with cell components. However, N-hydroxylated acetaminophen conjugates with glutathione by glutathione-S-transferase. The toxicity of acetaminophen must thus be prevented in two ways: direct sulfate or glucuronide conjugation or glutathione conjugation of the activated metabolite.

However, there are marked species differences in these metabolic pathways, especially in the N-hydroxylated pathway of cytochrome P-450 enzymes. Thus, hepatic glutathione content is markedly decreased in hamsters and mice, but only a slight decrease occurs in rats. Such data are consistent with the low toxicity and covalent binding of acetaminophen in rats and the high toxicity in hamsters and mice (1).

Hamsters are the most susceptible animals, but there is no increase in the covalent binding of acetaminophen until the dose of acetaminophen is less than 100 mg/kg. With increasing doses of acetaminophen the glutathione content decreases to less than 40% of the control level and the covalent binding rapidly increases to cause hepatonecrosis.

These results indicate that in the body are detoxification mechanisms against toxic compounds, such that small amounts of drugs do not have measurable toxicity. The doses and physiological condition of the body influence the rates of metabolic toxification and detoxification and are important factors in the development of drug toxicity.

Isoniazid and iproniazid hepatotoxicity

Isoniazid is mainly acetylated and excreted as N-acetylisoniazid in experimental animals and man, and some N-acetylisoniazid is hydrolyzed by an acid amidase to acetylhydrazine (2). The acetylhydrazine is N-hydroxylated by cytochrome P-450 enzymes and covalently bound to tissue protein. On the other hand, iproniazid is directly hydrolyzed to isopropylhydrazine and then N-hydroxylated by cytochrome P-450 enzymes and covalently bound to tissue protein (2). These systems are thought to be the most probable mechanisms of isoniazid- and iproniazid-induced hepatitis. It is well known that the rate of acetylation of isoniazid varies among individuals and is genetically controlled.

Evance divided the patients into two groups: the rapid and the slow acetylators. Among white races 60% are rapid acetylators and 40% slow; in contrast, 90% of Asians are rapid acetylators and 10% slow.

Another adverse reaction induced by isoniazid is peripheral neuritis, and this is found mainly among the slow acetylators and in white races. On the other hand, hepatitis is more common among the rapid acetylators and Asians (2).

Other typical toxic compounds

As shown for the toxicities of acetaminophen and isoniazid, recent studies indicate that most toxic compounds are metabolized by hepatic microsomal drug metabolizing enzymes (cytochrome P-450 enzymes) to toxic active intermediates. Table 1 gives some typical examples of the metabolic activation of toxic compounds.

SPECIES AND STRAIN DIFFERENCES IN METABOLIC ACTIVATION OF DRUGS

Species and strain differences in the activity and toxicity of drugs are clearly related to the rate of drug metabolism.

For example, strychnine is more toxic in guinea pigs than in rats, the former displaying a more rapid metabolism of strychnine. Moreover, the lack of carcino-

TABLE 1. *Typical examples of metabolic activation of toxic compounds*

	Parent compounds	Active metabolites	Toxicity
1.	Carbon tetrachloride	free radical	hepatonecrosis
2.	Dimethylnitrosamine	alkyldiazonium radical	hepatonecrosis, carcinogenesis
3.	Aflatoxin B_1	epoxide	hepatonecrosis, carcinogenesis
4.	Dimethylaminoazobenzene	N-hydroxy-	carcinogenesis
5.	4-Nitroquinoline N-oxide	hydroxyamino-	carcinogenesis, mutagenesis
6.	AF2	hydroxyamino-	mutagenesis carcinogenesis
7.	Acetaminophen	N-hydroxy-	hepatonecrosis
8.	Benzopyrene	epoxide	carcinogenesis
9.	Brombenzene	epoxide	hepatonecrosis
10.	Iproniazid	N-hydroxy-	hepatonecrosis

genesis of acetylaminofluorene in guinea pigs is thought to reflect an absence of N-hydroxylation of the carcinogen. Similarly, the low toxicity of acetaminophen in rats is due to a low N-hydroxylation of this drug.

As shown in Table 2 the rate of drug metabolism in man is generally slower than in other species, especially in rodents. However, there are no clear species differences in the biological half-life of indomethacin, and the biological half-life of diclofenac is shorter in man than in the rodents.

In general, therefore, the rate of drug metabolism in man is slower than in other species, but species difference varies for each drug. Therefore, species difference is unpredictable and the metabolic rate of each drug should be examined separately.

Strain differences are important factors affecting drug metabolism and drug toxicity. It has been shown that administration of methylcholanthrene increases benzopyrene hydroxylase in livers of C57BL/6N mice, but not in those of DBA/2N

TABLE 2. *The biological half-life of drugs in various species of animals and man*

Drug	Man	Rhesus monkey	Dog	Rat	Mouse
Phenylbutazone	72.0	8.0	6.0	6.0	1.5
Oxyphenbutazone	72.0	8.0	0.5	—	—
Antipyrine	12.0	1.8	1.7	2.2	0.2
Meperidine	5.5	1.2	0.9	0.5	—
Hexobarbital	6.0	—	4.3	2.2	0.4
Aniline	—	—	2.7	1.2	0.6
Indomethacin	2.0	1.5	1.5	3.0	—
Isoniazid	1.0~4.0	1.2	2.5	0.4	—
Diclofenac	1.3	2.0	3.5	4.5	—

Unit: hour

mice. Similarly, zoxazolamine hydroxylase, acetylaminofluorene N-hydroxylase and biphenyl 4-hydroxylase are not induced by methylcholanthrene in DBA/2N mice. However, all these enzyme activities are induced by polychlorinated biphenyl in both C57BL/6N and DBA/2N mice.

Thus C57BL/6N mice, 'responsive mice', are more susceptible to the toxicity induced by benzopyrene, acetylaminofluorene and zoxazolamine and to the tumor-induction by methylcholanthrene or dimethylbenzanthracene than DBA/2N mice, 'nonresponsive mice' (3).

SPECIES DIFFERENCES IN DRUG METABOLISM IN DISEASED STATES

Drugs are of course given to patients suffering from diseases, but preclinical studies on animals are usually done on healthy animals; the utilization of diseased animals is therefore recommended for the evaluation of drug efficacy and toxicity. However, drug metabolism is affected by disease and the changes in similar diseases are also species dependent (4).

A typical example may be considered. The hyperthyroidism induced by various doses of thyroxine decreases the hexobarbital hydroxylase activity in male rats, but increases the hydroxylase activity in female rats. On the other hand, the hydroxylase activity decreases in both male and female mice with similar hyperthyroidism and is unaffected in both male and female rabbits. These results further support the concept that the prediction of results in man from the results obtained in experimental animals is difficult.

SPECIES DIFFERENCES IN BILIARY EXCRETION OF DRUGS

Water soluble drugs or metabolites are excreted either via the urinary tract or via the biliary duct. In rats low molecular weight compounds, under 300, are mainly excreted in urine and compounds with a molecular weight greater than 350 are mainly excreted in bile.

There are, however, marked species differences in the biliary excretory patterns. The threshold molecular weight for biliary excretion is about 325 ± 50 in rat, 400 ± 50 in guinea pig, 475 ± 50 in rabbit, 350 ± 50 in dog, 550 ± 50 in monkey and 525 ± 50 in man (5).

Such differences in biliary excretion cause the species variation in drug toxicities, especially of those drugs subjected to the enterohepatic circulation. For example, we have found that the subacute toxicity of diclofenac is high in dogs and rats and low in monkeys and man reflecting species differences in the biliary excretion of diclofenac glucuronide (6).

Diclofenac ester glucuronide formed by the liver is mainly excreted in the bile in rats and dogs, whereas in monkeys and man it is almost exclusively excreted in the urine. Since diclofenac ester glucuronide easily hydrolyses non-enzymatically in the bile and the upper part of intestine, and free diclofenac is absorbed and subjected to the enterohepatic circulation it causes intestinal ulcer.

SIMILARITY OF DRUG METABOLISM IN VARIOUS ANIMALS AND MAN

Table 3 compares the metabolism of 31 drugs in rat, dog, monkey and man (7). The comparison considers metabolic rates and metabolic pathways of the drugs. The results show that the rat is the least similar animal and the monkey the most similar to man with the dog intermediate.

The rat differs from man in the rate of drug metabolism (in rats faster), whereas the dog differs from man in the metabolic pathways of drugs.

Usually metabolic activation of drugs to active toxic intermediates is slight, therefore undetectable species differences related to the metabolic action are also involved.

GENETIC AND ENVIRONMENTAL DIFFERENCE IN DRUG METABOLISM IN MAN

Unlike most experimental animals which are bred in closed-colonies man is not uniform genetically. There are thus marked individual differences in the rate of drug metabolism and in their metabolic pathways in man. Vesell (1968) has shown that the rates of metabolism of drugs, such as antipyrine and phenylbutazone, are identical in identical twins but differ in fraternal twins. These results indicate that the individual differences in the rate of drug metabolism in man are due to genetic differences (8). On the other hand, recent studies have shown that many environmental factors also influence the rate of drug metabolism. These factors include smoking, coffee and alcohol drinking, air pollution and medicinal drugs (8). Diets also modify the rate of drug metabolism. For example, high dietary protein intake enhances the rates of antipyrine and theophylline metabolism and some vegetables such as brussels sprouts and cabbage stimulate the rate of antipyrine metabolism.

Recently Branch et al. (9) demonstrated that Sudanese subjects living in Sudan had significantly lower average antipyrine clearances than an English group. However, there were no significant differences in antipyrine clearances between English and Sudanese subjects living in England, although the biological half-life was slightly longer in the Sudanese subjects living in England than in the English.

Thus, although the different drug metabolisms may be due to genetic factors, environmental factors are also important. There is clearly a need for comparative studies in Japanese and Europeans to elucidate racial differences in drug metabolism observed in the N-acetylation of isoniazid.

TABLE 3. *The metabolism of 31 drugs in monkey, dog and rat compared with man*

Species	Similarity		
	Good	Fair	Poor
Monkey	12	15	4
Dog	5	12	14
Rat	1	13	17

THE ROLE OF DRUG METABOLISM STUDIES IN PREDICTING AND PREVENTING DRUG TOXICITY

The species differences in drug metabolism are remarkable, especially in the metabolic pathways. Indeed, recent studies indicate that active toxic intermediates are involved in most drug toxicity, and the balance between the metabolic activation of parent drugs and the detoxification of active metabolites controls drug toxicity.

However, little is known about species differences in the metabolic activation of drugs. Such studies should be carried out to improve the predictability of drug toxicity and safety by using various species of animals. The covalent binding of radioactive drugs to tissue components is an especially useful tool to examine the metabolic activation of drugs. Based on this system, drugs which bind covalently to DNA and protein by metabolic activation have been uncovered and removed. Drug metabolism studies are also important in evaluating and interpreting drug toxicity in various species of animals and man.

Finally, extensive studies on drug metabolism in the Phase I study are essential, especially after administration of small doses. Therefore, efforts must be made to improve detection of small amounts of metabolites which may be involved in the metabolic activation processes.

CONCLUSION

1. Drug toxicities are closely correlated with the ratio of formation to detoxification of active toxic intermediates.
2. Marked species differences exist in metabolic rates and pathways of drugs. Although little is known, the metabolic study of species differences in the formation and detoxification of active toxic intermediate is essential.
3. Drug metabolism is influenced by genetic and environmental factors and pathological states; these factors vary among species and strains of animals.
4. There are large individual differences in drug metabolism in man, probably as a result of environmental and genetic variation.
5. These lines of evidence indicate that the quantitative prediction of drug toxicity in man from the toxicity data obtained in experimental animal studies is very difficult. Therefore, the safety of drugs in man is clearly established only after the administration of new drugs to many patients.
6. Metabolic and pharmacokinetic studies of new drugs are most powerful tools with which to improve the prediction of the drug toxicity in man. Such studies must be carried out intensively throughout preclinical and Phase I studies.

REFERENCES

1. Davis, D.C., Potter, W.Z., Jollows, D.J. and Mitchell, J.R. (1974): Species differences in hepatic glutathion depletion, covalent binding and hepatic necrosis after acetaminophene. *Life Sci.*, *14*, 2099.
2. Mitchell, J.R. (1976): Isoniazid liver injury: clinical spectrum, pathology, and probable pathogenesis. *Ann. intern. Med.*, *84*, 181.

3. Thorgeirsson, S.S., Felton, J.S. and Nebert, D.W. (1975): Genetic differences in the aromatic hydrocarbon-inducible N-hydroxylation of 2-acetylaminofluorene and acetaminophene-produced hepatotoxicity in mice. *Mol. Pharmacol., 11*, 159.
4. Kato, R. (1977): Drug metabolism under pathological and abnormal physiological states in animals and man. *Xenobiotica, 7*, 25.
5. Hirom, P.C., Millburn, P., Smith, R.L. and Williams, R.T. (1972): Species variations in the threshold molecular-weight factor for the biliary excretion of organic anions. *Biochem. J., 129*, 1071.
6. Kato. R. (1974): The safety of diclofenac from the point of view of pharmacokinetics (in Japanese). *Jap. J. clin. Pharmacol., 5*, 393.
7. Kato, R. (1971): Species differences in the metabolism, effect and toxicity of drugs (in Japanese). *Gendai no Rinsho, 5*, 308.
8. Vesell, E.S. (1972): Introduction: Genetic and environmental factors affecting drug response in man. *Fed. Proc., 31*, 1253.
9. Branch, R.A., Saith, S.Y. and Homeida, M. (1978): Racial differences in drug metabolizing ability: A study with antipyrine in the Sudan. *Clin. Pharmacol. Ther., 24*, 283.

DISCUSSION

Hama: The prediction of what will happen in human beings on the basis of animal findings is certainly difficult. It seems to me, however, that this has been overly stressed. It is also very important to know about factors influencing the occurrence of hazards in addition to the knowledge of racial or species difference in drug action. Dr. Kato, do you have any comment on this?

Kato: I think a very important point is this difference in the conditions. I stressed the importance of knowing the differences among animals as well as among human beings with respect to drug metabolizing activity. One of the most difficult problems concerning the quantitative prediction of human toxicity of drugs from the animal data is the difficulty in the quantitative evaluation of drug metabolism particularly in the metabolic activation and inactivation. Human beings are very heterogeneous with respect to genetic as well as environmental factors. Thus, the confirmation of the safety is only possible after many people have experienced the drug.

Hiramatsu: Drug metabolism in rats seems quite different from that of human beings. What is your opinion on the use of rats for the purpose of predicting the human toxicity of drug?

Kato: As I mentioned in my presentation, the difference in drug metabolism between rat and man is mainly the discrepancy in the rate of metabolism rather than the pathway of metabolism as in the case of the dog. Thus, if one recognizes this type of species difference in the rate of metabolism, then the rats are useful in toxicity studies. The maximum non-effective doses obtained in 3 months subacute toxicity study in rats may be quite different from the maximum safe doses in man. However, given such consideration, I think the data from the rat experiments are still useful.

Problems in preclinical assessment of drug safety

TOMOJI YANAGITA

Preclinical Research Laboratories, Central Institute for Experimental Animals, Kawasaki, Japan

Methods to assess drug safety using laboratory animals have progressed greatly in recent years, largely because of the need to prevent previous drug-induced sufferings. Today, preclinical laboratory study of drug safety is much more precise and is carried out on a larger scale, with deeper understanding and more validity for clinical prediction than previously. At the same time however, many problems have arisen. This paper considers briefly the present state of preclinical assessment, and then the problems are discussed from the theoretical and practical points of view.

TYPES OF PRECLINICAL TESTS FOR ASSESSING DRUG SAFETY

Drug toxicity is broadly classified into two categories: general and special toxicity. General toxicity concerns overall toxicity of drugs on the whole body and individual organs. Special toxicity concerns the more specific and limited toxic effects and phenomena such as teratogenicity, immunogenicity, carcinogenicity, and abuse liability.

Assessment of the general toxicity of drugs

General toxicity is usually assessed in acute, subacute, and chronic toxicity tests.

1. Acute toxicity tests Acute toxicity presupposes that toxicity can be observed from single doses of drugs. Small animals such as mice and rats are usually used but often a limited number of larger species including rabbits, dogs, and monkeys are also used. The major toxicity looked for is a functional impairment (i.e. circulatory and respiratory failures) rather than a morphological change. Toxic phenomena, mechanisms, and reactions are studied and lethal doses are also assessed in these tests.

2. Subacute and chronic toxicity tests The words ‘subacute’ and ‘chronic’ describe the drug administration period: most commonly, 2 weeks to 3 months for the former and 6 months to 2 years for the latter. Most therapeutic agents are administered once or twice daily for 6 or 7 days a week. Non-therapeutic agents (e.g. food additives, agricultural chemicals) are usually given mixed with food or drinking water. Various species of animals are used but most common are rats, dogs, and monkeys. During administration periods, detailed physiological, toxicological, hematological, and biochemical observations are made and the general health of the animals is monitored. At the end of these tests and as essential parts of them pathological examinations are done both macro- and microscopically, and often ultramicroscopically as well.

In the chronic tests, the survival test serves a double purpose as a test for carcinogenicity, which is regarded as a special type of toxicity.

Assessment of special toxicities of drugs

Preclinical assessment of drug safety has progressed and expanded to include a range of special toxicity tests, the most important being:

1. Reproduction and teratogenicity tests Drug effects on reproduction and their teratogenicity are usually tested in mice, rats, rabbits, and monkeys. In the reproduction tests, the periods of drug administration are divided into 3 phases: the pre- and early gestation periods, the organ-development period, and the peri- and post-partum periods. Reproductive capacity as well as morphological and functional abnormalities of the subsequent generations are explored.

2. Immunogenicity and allergy tests To detect immunogenic toxicity, immunologic and allergy tests are done in guinea pigs, rabbits, and a few other species of animals.

3. Local toxicity tests The local irritative effects of drugs on the eyes, mucous membranes, skin, and muscles at injection sites are examined after repeated exposure of the tissues to clinical preparations of the drugs. A variety of animal species are used.

4. Dependence and abuse liability tests Tests for drug dependence and abuse potential involve comprehensive studies of tolerance and physical dependence, while self-administration experiments examine psychological dependence. Rats, dogs and monkeys are the species of choice.

5. Mutagenicity and carcinogenicity tests The mutagenicity test is a recently developed test in which microorganisms and small animals are examined in culture, and by chromosomal damage and dominant lethal tests.

PROBLEMS IN PRECLINICAL ASSESSMENT OF DRUG SAFETY

In the progress that has been made in the preclinical assessment of drug safety, a number of problems have also come up. These are methodological and practical problems.

Methodological problems

1. Choice of animal species The correct choice of the animal species to be used is extremely important as an inappropriate one may lead to a wrong prediction of drug safety in man. In this regard, the species specificity, in terms of the pharmacological susceptibility, absorption, organ distribution, metabolism, and excretion of drugs must be compared with man. In addition the availability of particular species and experimental methods are also to be considered. Many preliminary studies have therefore to be performed, unless many extensive experiments with many species are undertaken; either approach, however, needs high budgeting and considerable research time.

2. Establishing dose regime The toxic effects of drugs are always functions of the doses, routes and periods of drug administration. The potential toxicity of any drug may not appear if the dose or period is unreasonably low or short. Thus, a rational choice to the dose regime is crucial. It is however often difficult since comparative knowledge on bioavailability and drug susceptibilities between the animals and man is lacking.

3. Observational methods of collecting clinically useful data Although the methods for assessing drug safety are well developed, much biological information is still overlooked as a result of inappropriate observational procedures. Thus methods to obtain more clinically useful data from animal experiments must be considered. For example, the lethal dose is a major concern of acute toxicity studies but treatment and specific antidotes should also be explored by investigating mechanisms of acute toxicity.

4. Criteria for evaluating toxic and non-toxic drug effects The analysis of preclinical experimental data often involves discriminating between toxic or non-toxic phenomena, both functional and morphological. This is especially difficult when the changes are adaptative and non-specific. To improve the knowledge on which to base judgements, careful follow-up of preclinical findings and feedback are essential.

5. Extrapolation of preclinical data to man The essential factors involved in extrapolating preclinical data to man are: (1) species differences, (2) dose schedule differences, and (3) differences in health and environment of the various species including man. Points 1 and 2 have already been mentioned earlier. Regarding the health and environmental aspects, the biggest difference lies in the fact that laboratory animals are usually biologically homogeneous, healthy, and similarly aged. In addition, in man, diet and life pattern vary from one individual to another. Extrapolation of animal data should take this, most subtle point, into account.

Practical problems in preclinical assessment of drug safety

1. Control of spontaneous diseases While efforts to save time during assessment are being made in some fields, in others long-term experiments are increasingly necessary, and include the testing of therapeutics for chronic diseases, chemicals contained in food, drinking water or the air and potentially carcinogenic substances. Such long-term experiments however, are often hampered by many factors including infection and spontaneous disease. In recent years animal care has improved greatly, but needs to be advanced further for long-term experiments, aiming at the control of spontaneous diseases.

2. Availability of animals, especially monkeys Ideally, all species and all disease-model animals should be available, but practically this is hardly so. Recently, a major problem has been the supply of non-human primates – particularly rhesus monkeys – which have been frequently used and about which much basic data are available. Measures to improve the supplies (e.g. domestic breeding) must be considered with a view to enhancing the predictability of drug safety in man.

3. Shortage of specialists The shortage of specialists working in this field is worldwide, but is particularly serious in Japan. There are many reasons: a lack of concern for such work delayed the establishment of the necessary training programs; a lower regard in society for such specialists compared with academic scientists, in spite of their obvious importance. These attitudes have however changed in recent years, and there is a good prospect that many more specialists will be trained and join to work in this field in the near future. Fear of an overly strict and/or unscientific regulation of the experimental design still prevails and specialists may be discouraged from this work.

4. Efficiency of preclinical assessment Specialists in this field must endeavor to eliminate useless experiments and to improve on costly and/or time-consuming approaches. Many of the current tests do not always have a scientific basis, although in some cases, validation is almost impossible since potentially teratogenic or carcinogenic substances can never be tested in man. Nevertheless, careful analysis and consideration of the relationship between man and animals may improve the efficiency of the assessment.

5. Optimal cost-benefit balance Theoretically it is desirable to carry out preclinical assessment of drug safety to the last detail, but practically, society cannot tolerate the burden of the extraordinarily high cost and wait for an excessively long time. When the benefit of outcome of the assessment is outweighed by these factors, the cost-effectiveness becomes relevant and both social and scientific viewpoints are pertinent. However, there is no clear consensus on this matter. This is at least one of the reasons for this conference. It is hoped that the meeting will be productive of outlining the broad solutions to this problem.

DISCUSSION

Kawai: When the toxicity of clioquinol, thalidomide or AF-2, a food additive, became public concern, it was reported that the toxicity had been assumed. The pharmaceutical industries will excuse themselves by saying that drugs are toxic anyway or that this agent is exceptional. I think this forms a problem in our efforts to examine toxicity. The standard toxicity tests, as mentioned by Dr. Yanagita, are significant, but in addition other tests must be applied to elucidate the problems occurring during these standard toxicity tests. Research workers must look further into the details of the doubts encountered during the standard tests.

Yanagita: The preclinical toxicity tests have recently expanded as a result of some drug mishaps as reported by Dr. Suzuki, and now more types of special toxicity tests are employed.

Kawai: Clinicians are asked to carry out the human drug study by the pharmaceutical firms and regrettably, they generally supply no detailed preclinical data. At this stage the substantial findings in the preclinical study, particularly on toxicity, should be passed on to the clinicians.

Yanagita: The concrete information obtained in the preclinical study must be passed to the clinicians who are going to perform early clinical studies. At this point I would like to emphasize that experts engaged in prediction and education are severely lacking. This is an important reason why such a bridge is generally defective.

Kawai: I was once studying a drug, and was surprised that the raw data on the drug held by the pharmaceutical firm were edited for the publication in an academic journal. Something unfavorable to the firm is often concealed upon publication. To prevent drug hazards we must ensure that the raw data are submitted to the Ministry of Health and Welfare and must be made public in full.

Yanagita: As regards the disclosure of data, the situation was unsatisfactory 2 or 3 years ago. The major safety experiments must be published and all the data obtained there must be available for those who need them. I think today that the disclosure of the preclinical data is more satisfactory. As you may know the Ministry of Health and Welfare has issued instructions and stipulated that such data should be printed, and that the pharmaceutical companies should actually publish the data for the public.

Herxheimer: Would you tell us what proportion of toxicological research in Japan is funded by pharmaceutical companies and what proportion by governmental institutions? Research that is independent of manufacturers is particularly important for the investigation in animals of toxic effects discovered in man after a drug has been marketed, and this kind of research should be officially encouraged and paid for from the public funds.

Yanagita: A major part of preclinical safety studies are conducted by the industries. The Government does not offer much funds to support such studies so far in Japan. I hope this Conference will stimulate the Japanese Government to give more research funds for the preclinical as well as post-marketing studies of drug safety.

Mutagenicity test for monitoring drugs to prevent DNA damage

TAKASHI KAWACHI

National Cancer Center Research Institute, Tokyo, Japan

Drugs often have various effects in addition to their main pharmacological actions; mutagenicity is one such side-effect. Sometimes, but not always, the mutagenicity can be separated from the main pharmacological action. With or without metabolic activation, some drugs bind covalently with DNA or intercalate into DNA, resulting in mutagenesis. In somatic cells mutagens may be carcinogens or senilogens (aging agents), while in germ cells, they may be teratogens or genotoxic substances. There are various physiological protective mechanisms, including absorption barriers and mechanisms of detoxification and excretion of mutagens, and even after mutagens have bound to DNA, damaged regions can be repaired.

Various mutagenicity tests have been developed to monitor drugs including: in vitro microbial mutation tests; *rec* assay and also mutation tests; chromosomal aberration tests; and sister chromatid exchange tests using cultured mammalian cells in vitro. Moreover, mutation tests on *Drosophila melanogaster* and the silkworm can be used to monitor the drug actions on germ cells. About 4,000 chemicals have now been tested with *Salmonella typhimurium*/microsome systems, and several compounds predicted to be carcinogenic have recently been shown to be so in vivo.

In evaluating the drug mutagenicity, specific mutagenic activities, daily dosages, and periods of administration must be considered. Furthermore, 'background' environmental mutagenicity must also be quantified.

Many environmental substances are known to cause cancer in man, and to detect them a simple method is required. The short-term mutagenicity test of Dr. Ames using *Salmonella typhimurium* is useful in this respect. We have modified and applied this method.

Pyrolizidine alkaloids require preincubation to demonstrate mutagenicity. The demonstration of mutagenicity of some azo dyes requires the presence of riboflavine. Hamster, not rat, S-9 mix is required for the phenacetin test while rutin requires hesperdinase treatment and cycasin glycosidase treatment to demonstrate mutagenicity; aniline requires the presence of norharman as comutagen. Finally dimethylnitrosamine precludes the use of dimethylsulfoxide in this area. More than 700 chemicals have been tested for mutagenicity in our laboratory and a good correlation between mutagenicity and carcinogenicity has been established. Among 167 kinds of compounds with mutagenic activity, 146 (87%) were carcinogenic. On the other hand, among 86 non-mutagenic compounds, 60 (70%) were non-carcinogenic. Of 780 compounds tested, 527 have an unknown carcinogenic activity, although 226 compounds (43%) were mutagenic.

Another short-term test is that which determines the prophage-inducing potency. Potencies are expressed as minimal inducing concentrations (MIC) in nmoles per plate. Table 1 shows that the results (with or without S-9 mix) correlate quantitatively very well with Salmonella mutagenicity tests, expressed as the concentration of the chemical in nmoles yielding 100 revertant cells. The azo dyes and arylamine are the only exceptions.

The results of the Ames test also correlate with the chromosomal aberration tests using Chinese hamster cells (Fig. 1). In Figure 1, figures at the top represent sample numbers tested in 1977, open circles show the chromosomal aberration activity of the tested sample, and closed circles the Ames test mutagenicity. The two tests largely agree. In addition, the *rec* assay correlates with the Ames mutagenicity test.

Figure 2 shows the frequency distribution of mutagenic potencies in the Ames test. Naturally occurring compounds are listed on the upper line and synthetic chemicals are cited on the lower. The mutagenic potencies range from 1 to 10 million. Three in-vitro tests – the Ames test, the inductest and the chromosomal aberration test – gave quantitatively similar results for these compounds.

TABLE 1. *Summary of mutagenic and prophage-inducing potency*

Agent	Inductest	MIC (nmol/plate)	Salmonella TA98	(nmol/100 rev.) TA100
MNNG	+	22	—	2
ENNG	+	4.0	—	1
MNU	+	1000	—	770
ENU	+	1000	—	260
MMS	+	5000	—	5000
EMS	+	10,000	—	10,000
Mitomycin C	+	0.01	—	10 (TA92)
AF-2	+	0.0035	0.08	0.01
4NQO	+	0.24	1.2	1.8

TABLE 2. *Summary of mutagenic and prophage-inducing potency*

Agent	Inductest	MIC (nmol/plate)	Salmonella TA98	(nmol/100 rev.) TA100
Sterigmatocystin	+ (± S9)	0.01	0.40	0.021
Aflatoxin B_1	+	0.0005	0.056	0.002
Benzo(*a*)pyrene	+	3.9	6.3	2.2
o-Aminoazotoluene	—		15	14
DAB	—		450	220
AAF	—		5.6	48
2-Naphthylamine	—		260	33
Trp-P-1	+	5.0	0.012	0.29
Trp-P-2	+	1.0	0.005	0.29
Glu-P-1	+	10	0.010	0.15

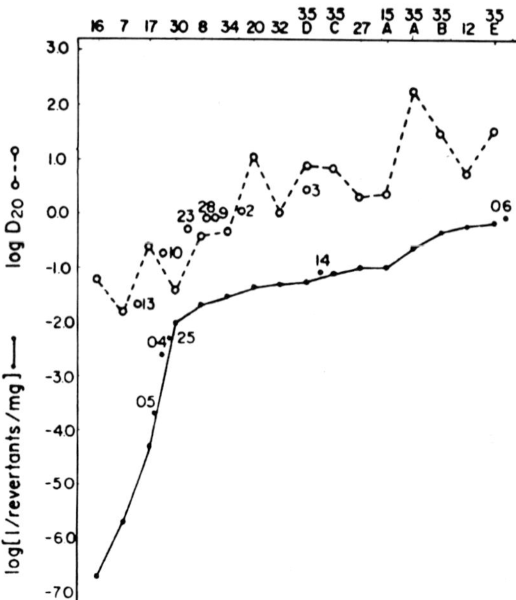

Fig. 1. Comparative activity of the Ames test and chromosomal test in samples tested in a group study by the Ministry of Health and Welfare, Japan, in 1977. For further explanation, see text.

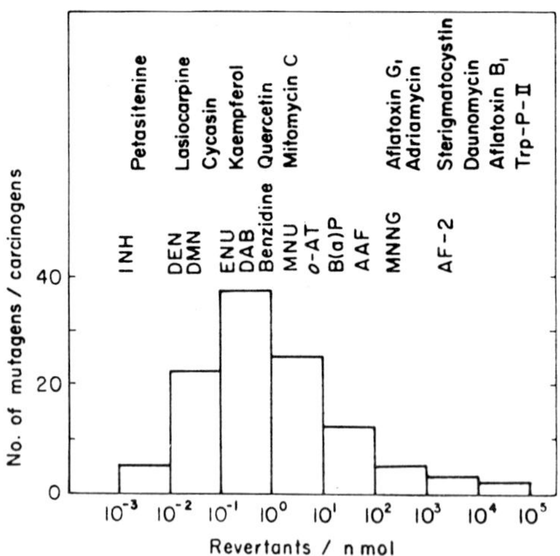

Fig. 2. Distribution of mutagenic potencies in the Ames test. For further explanation, see text.

Figure 3 shows the chronological association between carcinogens and mutagens. In 1960, only nitrogen mustard and 4-nitroquinoline-1-oxide were known to be both carcinogenic and mutagenic; in 1975, almost all carcinogens showed mutagenicity.

Recently many new mutagens have been revealed by rapid screening tests, although their carcinogenicities were largely known. It is impossibe to test the carcinogenicity of so many compounds by traditional long-term animal assay.

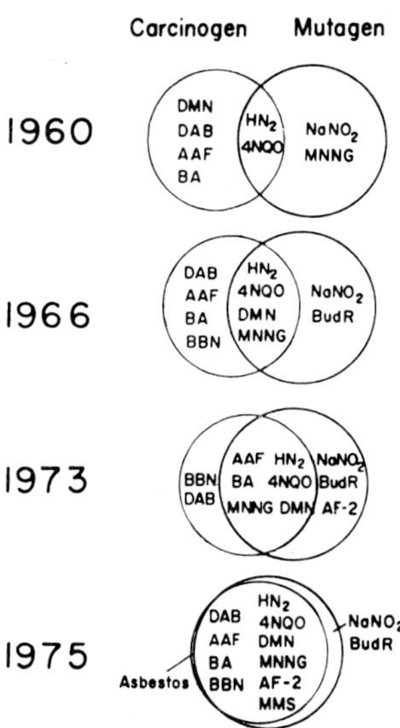

Fig. 3. Chronological association between carcinogens and mutagens.

The carcinogenicity of many compounds has already been predicted from mutagenicity data (Table 3). For example, the mutagenicity of AF-2 was found in 1973 and its carcinogenicity proved in 1974. In 1978 the carcinogenicity of many compounds was proved after earlier mutagenic studies had predicted such activity.

Thus the priority of in-vivo long-term tests should be based on results of short-term tests as follows: (1) the potency of the compound; (2) the degree of exposure to the compound; (3) other factors such as stability of the compound, route of exposure or intake etc. If the short-term potency suggests 'very strong' or 'strong' features, usage should be banned immediately, while if 'very weak', usage is acceptable (Fig. 4). Compounds with 'middle' or 'weak' potency in primary screening should be evaluated by scientific committees taking into account total activity and quantitative calculation. Social evaluation should be assessed by consumers, lawyers, statesmen, scientists and others. Of course, risks, benefits and

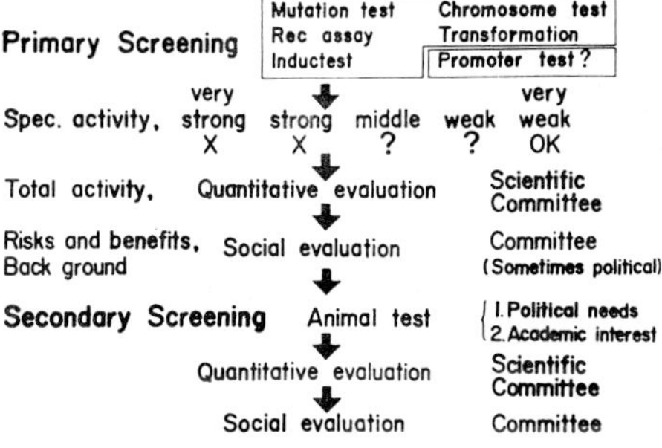

Fig. 4. Primary and secondary screening procedures for mutagens.

TABLE 3. *Mutation test predicts carcinogenicity*

	Mutagenicity		Carcinogenicity	
MNNG	Mandel	1960	Sugimura	1966
AF-2	Tonomura and other 3 laboratories	1973	Ikeda	1974
Mcthylnitrocyanamide	Endo	1973	Endo	1974
Captan	Kada	1974	NIH	1977
Phenacetin	Ishidate	1974	Isaka	1978
Barbital	Ishidate	1975	Matsuyama	1978
Hydralazine	Yahagi and other 5 laboratories	1976	Toth	1978
8-Nitroquinoline	Nagao	1977	Takahashi	1978
Tris	Ames	1977	VanDuuren	1978
	Rosenkranz	1977		
Trp-P-1	Sugimura	1977	Takayama	1978

TABLE 4. *A trial for estimation of environmental mutagenic risk*

	A (revertants per mg)	B (annual production)	A × B(f)
Tobacco (20 mg tar/cigarette)	1.0×10^3	290×10^9 cigarettes	5.8×10^{15}
AF-2	4.7×10^7	3 t	1.4×10^{17}
Captan	5.1×10^5	422 t	2.2×10^{17}
Tris-BP	2.0×10^4	200 t	4.0×10^{15}
Caramel	1.9×10^1	15,000 t	2.9×10^{14}
Broiled fish (3.9 g char/60 g fish)	8.0×10^0	9,860,000 t fish	5.1×10^{15}
Coffee	1.1×10^1	134,000 t	1.5×10^{15}
Green tea	3.9×10^1	222,000 t	7.8×10^{15}

t = tons.

background environmental mutagenicity must be considered, which will involve political decisions.

Although the animal test has been viewed here as a secondary screening procedure, the traditional long-term animal test can be independent of the primary screening, since it is impossible to test large numbers of mutagens in this way. Thus animals may be tested out for political or academic reasons, in which case scientific or other committees may pass judgement.

Table 4 summarizes data on a trial designed to estimate environmental mutagenic risk. The mutagenic risk of tobacco, a typical environmental carcinogen, can be estimated. One cigarette yields 20 mg tar and 1 mg of tar yields 1.0×10^3 revertant colonies. In 1977, 290×10^9 cigarettes were produced in Japan, so that the total production of mutagenicity from cigarette smoking should be 5.8×10^{15}. Of course, this number must be magnified by factors to assess mutagenic risks since the whole cigarette is not smoked and only 10 or 20% of the mutagenicity is inhaled.

AF-2 had been used as a food additive for 10 years in Japan. Mutagenicity of this compound was described in 1973, when its annual production was 3 metric tons, to give a total mutagenicity of 10^{17}. In 1974 its carcinogenicity was proved and usage was immediately banned.

Broiled fish, coffee and green tea have very weak mutagenicities. In spite of their weak specific activities, the extent of annual consumption, imports and production amount to about 10^{15}. If the numerical value for total mutagenicity assesses human hazard, eating broiled fish and drinking coffee and green tea are as risky as cigarette smoking!

Reactions to environmental mutagens are very complicated, and many naturally occurring compounds modify their activities. The balance between activation and detoxification of mutagens or carcinogens makes the evaluation of environmental mutagens or carcinogens very difficult.

Lastly the carcinogenicities of hormones and other materials are not readily assessed by the microbial systems. Development of other short-term tests for naturally occurring systems is necessary.

DISCUSSION

Hanano: Is there a relationship between natural mutagenic substances and diet?

Kawachi: We have only 2 years experience using our method to study environmental mutagenic or carcinogenic substances. Although many experiments have been conducted, we don't yet know much about substances causing cancer in man. Stomach cancer, a prevalent illness in Japan, is of special interest.

Yokota: Can you predict the carcinogenicity of chemical substances by your method? Could you also tell me the necessary and essential conditions for predicting carcinogenicity (and indeed mutagenicity) by the bacterial tests?

Kawachi: (1) Mutagenicity is found in 90% of carcinogenic substances, but it is difficult to give the percentage carcinogenicity of mutagenetic substances, largely because the test for carcinogenicity takes 2 to 3 years, while that for mutagenicity is simple and rapid. (2). A short-term test is not a pre-screening for a long-term test. The short-term test itself essentially checks the safety of chemical materials.

Pharmacokinetic prediction of drug distribution in the body based on physiological and anatomical principles – Studies on ethoxybenzamide

MANABU HANANO, JIUN HUEI LIN, YUICHI SUGIYAMA and SHOJI AWAZU

Faculty of Pharmaceutical Sciences, University of Tokyo, Tokyo, Japan

Ethoxybenzamide is pharmacologically more potent than salicylamide. The former is transformed to the latter by hepatic P-450 enzyme systems after ingestion. Both amides, therefore, exist simultaneously in the body. Pharmacokinetic analyses of these drugs may thus be expected to reveal information regarding pharmacological interrelationships between a parent drug and its metabolites.

The physiological model examined 11 organs or tissues (Fig. 1) on the basis that the body is divided into systemic, pulmonary and portal venous blood circulatory systems. These deliver a drug to the particular organ or tissue. The organs and tissues may be further subdivided into those which excrete or metabolize the drug and those which play a negligible role in drug elimination.

In the rat only 0.4% of a low dose of ethoxybenzamide and 3% of a high dose appears in the urine. A similarly low excretory ratio is found in the rabbit. Renal excretion may therefore be ignored in the model which is used to calculate the time course of blood concentration in relation to organ and tissue distribution: elimination of ethoxybenzamide from the body occurs almost completely by metabolic degradation.

The P-450 enzyme system which catalyzes de-ethylation of ethoxybenzamide occurs in the kidney and the lung as well as in the liver. The in-vitro metabolism of ethoxybenzamide by microsomes from those organs was examined. The hepatic enzyme activity is far higher than the others, with a larger maximal velocity (V_{max}) and smaller Michaelis-Menten dissociation constant (K_m). This activity, expressed per 1 mg microsomal protein, is much greater in the liver than the other organs; the metabolism of ethoxybenzamide in extrahepatic organs is concluded to be negligible.

The transfer of drugs from the blood to the tissues, the cellular uptake, may be investigated in studies of the drug distribution. This transfer rate varies both for the type of drug and also among the tissues. Ethoxybenzamide readily permeates the cell membrane and no special barrier to the transport of this drug has been reported, it being widely distributed in the body. The uptake rate by isolated hepatocytes as model cells was measured. Uptake rates are extremely rapid at all drug concentrations and the equilibrium of the drug concentration between the cell and

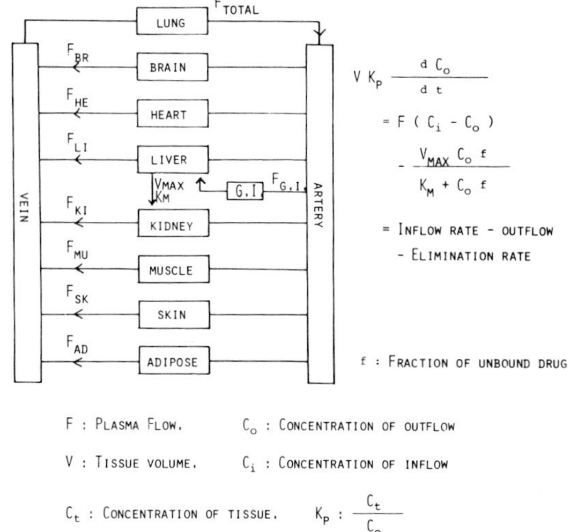

Fig. 1. Compartmental model for ethoxybenzamide and mass balance of liver.

the medium is reached within 15 sec. The liver of the rat is reported to consist of about 1.3×10^9 cells, so that the uptake clearance in the whole rat liver (the rate of the uptake related to the volume of the medium) is at least 160 ml/min. This value is much larger than the hepatic blood flow of 15 ml/min. From this calculation, the transport of ethoxybenzamide to the cells would be completed very rapidly. In addition, a passive transport process is likely since the amounts taken up are proportional to external concentrations.

Lineweaver-Burke plots of the data from microsomal suspensions are linear and a pair of K_m (0.378 mM) and V_{max} (1.17 μmol/min body) are obtained for the rat and a curve consisting of two pairs of the constants ($K_m = 0.0186$ and 1.06 mM; $V_{max} = 6.98$ and 10.984 μmol/min body) for the rabbit.

The K_m value for the rabbit is less than one-tenth that of the rat and the V_{max} value more than 5 times greater. The rabbit thus has a higher metabolic acitivity than the rat. The resultant V_{max} was converted to a value for the whole animal using the yield ratio of the microsome reported by Joly et al. by measuring the absolute spectral absorbance of P-450 with the microsomal suspension. The K_m value was corrected for non-specific microsomal binding of ethoxybenzamide, measured in the absence of the co-factor, NADPH. In the rat, the reduction in blood ethoxybenzamide concentration during passage through the liver is calculated to be about 10%, based on blood flow rate and metabolic activity. On the other hand, the reduction is about 50% in the rabbit.

Nevertheless, as will be shown below, the simulation of the drug concentration time-course in the body from in-vitro data can fit very well for the rabbit, and the discrepancy may reflect the distribution properties of the drug in blood capillaries.

The partition co-efficient (K_p) of the drug between the blood and tissue is an important factor determining drug distribution and its time-course. In-vitro and in-vivo studies on the partition of ethoxybenzamide between erythrocytes and plasma and whole blood show ethoxybenzamide to partition evenly between the plasma and the erythrocyte.

The concentration of unbound drug is thought to be the same in plasma and tissue fluid except when pH differs or an active transport process occurs. The following equations express the partition co-efficients between the blood and the tissue from the respective protein-binding data of the drug:

$$K_p = \frac{C_{\text{tissue bound}} + C_{\text{tissue free}}}{C_{\text{plasma bound}} + C_{\text{plasma free}}} \tag{1}$$

$$C_{\text{tissue free}} = C_{\text{plasma free}} \tag{2}$$

In general, the binding profile of the drug to plasma and tissue proteins shows the saturation curve at the equilibrium concentration and, therefore, the K_p values depend on drug concentrations. The protein binding of ethoxybenzamide, however, was constant in any tissue homogenate as well as plasma over the range of drug concentration expected in the body level. The K_p values are concluded to be constant and independent of the drug concentration in the respective tissues.

The K_p in vivo is measured by determining tissue drug concentrations when plasma concentrations are kept constant by constant infusion. The K_p values may also be calculated (see equations below) from the drug plasma:tissue concentration ratio determined some time after bolus injection of the drug, providing the time course in the body has linear pharmacokinetics, i.e. drug concentrations at a given time are proportional to dose:

$$C_{\text{plasma}} = \sum_{t=n}^{i=n} A_i e^{-\alpha_i t} \tag{3}$$

$$C_{\text{tissue}} = \sum_{i=1}^{i=n} B_i e^{-\alpha_i t} \tag{4}$$

$$(\alpha_n < \alpha_{n-1} \ldots < \alpha_2 < \alpha_1) \text{ if } t \gg 0$$

$$K_p = B_n/A_n \tag{5}$$

The K_p values of the respective organs and tissues obtained in vitro were compared with those calculated from in-vivo data. Although some K_p's in vitro were excessive in some organs, the consistency is reasonable.

The drug is delivered to the organ or tissue in the blood, and an equilibrium is rapidly reached between the capillary vein, the extravascular fluid and the cell. These kinetic processes are extremely rapid for ethoxybenzamide as shown in isolated hepatocytes.

The next question concerns the drug concentration profile along the capillary vein. The concentration in the tissue effluent blood must be lower than in the affluent since the drug is taken up. This distribution along the vasculature may be calculated from the local mass-balance and the geometry of the capillary and the surrounding cells. This kind of precise solution is not practical since the geometry is extremely complicated.

The assumptions generally used concerning the concentration profiles in capillary veins are as follows: (1) There is a linearly decreasing concentration along the vessel.

(2) There is a parallel arrangement of equal-diameter vessels and surrounding cells, so that the profile is an exponentially decreasing curve from input to output. (3) The concentration in the capillary is equal until it leaves the tissue. Although this assumption may seem curious, the condition may apply to the well-mixed blood in the tissue.

The third assumption was taken for our model since the calculation from this fitted the experimental data obtained from liver perfusion studies using the drug.

The tissue and organ weights were measured, but the blood flow rates were taken from the literature (rat, see ref. 1; rabbit, see ref. 2). The blood flow is known to vary with physiological state. The predicted results, therefore, may not fit very well with the experimental data, if blood flow influences the drug kinetics. The simulation was carried out by digital computer which solves numerically the differential equations of the mass balance of the model.

Figure 2 shows the simulated results and the mean values observed experimentally in the rat. The consistency of the simulation curves with the observed values are adequate for the 3 different doses (20, 50, and 100 mg /kg body weight). The fitness immediately after injection is inadequate, presumably due to the large effect of blood flow in this initial phase.

The physiological model can easily predict the drug kinetics in different species when the physiological parameters are substituted. This technique, termed 'animal scale-up', opens the possibility of predicting human effects from animal studies.

A simulation was carried out for the rabbit in which the rabbit physiological parameters were used alongside drug partition co-efficients obtained in the rat without conversion. Human physiological parameters are very precisely known. The kinetic constants for the metabolism are usually studied in vitro. The drug distribution to the organs and tissues is difficult to establish. The simulation from the rat to the rabbit was carried out to check extrapolation. The simulated results show good consistency with the observed data at the doses of 10 and 20 mg/kg body weight, but were inconsistent for 80 mg/kg. Thus the physiological kinetic model used for the rabbit study lacks an important feature.

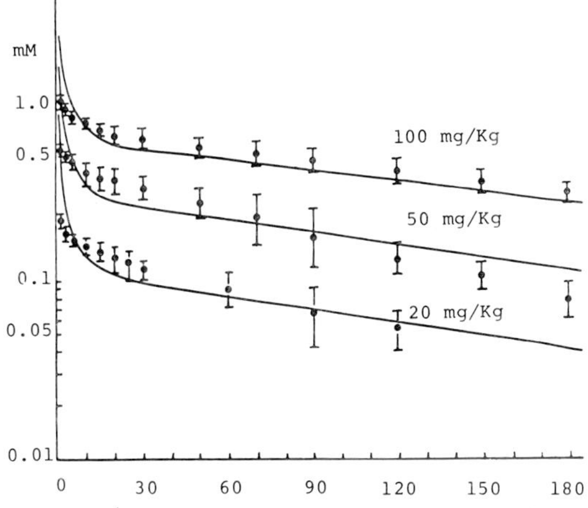

Fig. 2. Predicted and experimental concentrations of ethoxybenzamide.

There are substrate and product inhibitory actions in drug metabolism, and these are not considered in this model. Since the in-vitro study excluded substrate inhibition, the effect of the product inhibition was examined.

In the rabbit, product inhibition was found both in vitro with liver microsomes and in vivo. The experimental results confirmed the product inhibition predicted from curves using the inhibition constant (K_i) of 0.14.

The results calculated from the new model involve product inhibition on the basis of the blood concentration of salicylamide after a bolus injection of 80 mg/kg body weight ethoxybenzamide (open squares in Fig. 3). The solid and the dotted lines are the simulated results without and with the inhibition process, respectively. The dotted line closely coincides with the observed data.

Previous studies on the semi-empirical physiological model involved several parameters obtained in vivo or parameters adjusted to fit the data. The present study is the first to succeed in predicting drug disposition in the body from data based almost completely on in-vitro studies without adjustable parameters.

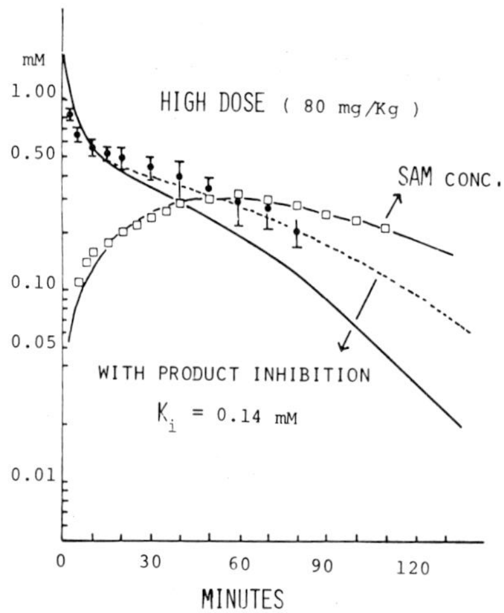

Fig. 3. Comparison of simulation curves in the presence and absence of product inhibition. For explanation, see text.

REFERENCES

1. Dedrick et al. (1973): *J. pharm. Sci.*
2. Neutz et al. (1978): *Amer. J. Physiol.*

DISCUSSION

Lunde: I would like to ask for your comments on methodology. Basically, what do you think is the relevance of performing drug-binding studies on tissue homogenates? There are several pitfalls as you certainly know, but I would like to have your comments. For example, which pH level should be chosen for equilibrium dialysis?

Hanano: It is true that there are various methods in a drug binding study and the results are different according to the method employed. We consider that the ultrafiltration method is the best to obtain a value nearest to the in-vivo data, but this method needs a large number of samples (blood and others). Accordingly, we looked for another method to give values similar to the ultrafiltration method and which would be applicable to any sample. This is an equilibrium dialysis method employing pre-dialyzed blood plasma and Toris buffer.

Nagai: Dr. Hanano, could you tell me how to proceed with studies on the prediction of toxicity before its appearance?

Hanano: There are many biochemical (in vitro) experiments which enable the prediction of various toxicities. But the results cannot simply be extrapolated to human beings. I think my presentation indicates one of the simplest methods to predict toxicity in vivo.

Individual biochemical variability and its quasi-constancy

MOTOSABURO MASUYAMA

Department of Applied Mathematics, Science University of Tokyo, Tokyo, Japan

In an industrialized area some individuals are affected and some not by the same pollutants even if sex and age are identical. Similarly the same dose of a drug is an overdose for some patients and not enough – hence non-therapeutic – for others; there is enormous individual variability. As a member of the Research Group for 'The Method of Evaluating the Safety of Metals and Chemicals' sponsored by the Science and Technology Agency, I was and still am interested in the law governing individual biochemical variabilities, to reduce the number of victims due to pollutants, food additives, overdose of drugs etc.

Most numerical results in this paper have appeared elsewhere (13–34) but some new results are added. Sources of data leading to these new results are given in the reference list with the names of quoted substances in italic.

GENERAL CONSIDERATIONS

When a drug is administered per os, the acute effect depends mainly upon the critical or effective concentration (C_e') of the drug (or its derivative) in blood (plasma or serum) at its target area, rather than the dose (D); C_e' is nearly proportional to its concentration in C_e*† in blood. Thus in computing the standard deviation (SD) of *log* C_e', C_e may be used instead of C_e' itself. Blood, plasma and serum are interchangeable except where stated. In experimental mammals the critical value of C_e' is usually about the same. There are some exceptions.

The administered drug is usually metabolized by enzyme systems and its concen-

†Individual variability of C_e is said to be small. Phenytoin may be quoted:
Adverse effects and phenytoin blood level (μg/ml) (μ_c^* denotes geometric mean)

	μ_c^*	$\sigma_x(n)$
Nystagmus on		
i. Far lateral gaze	21.61	0.102(13) #
ii. 45° deviation from midline	37.84	0.069(13)
iii. Straightforward gaze	60.62	0.038(6)
Ataxia	34.28	0.060(8)
Mental changes	50.37	0.052(10)

If one value is removed, we have $\mu_c^* = 21.61$ and $\sigma_x = 0.061(12)$. It is very likely that these SD's are overestimated, since none of these phenomena is of the all-or-none type and it is very difficult to measure the concentration exactly at the moment when it reaches its critical value C_e.

tration C_t at time t is determined by the equation of metabolic turnover:

$$dC_t = (-kC_t + a)dt \qquad (1)$$

where k (>0) is the individual decay constant of the drug and a (≥ 0) is the constant supply rate of the drug. The one-compartment model is approximately valid, if the initial absorption phase is neglected. Approaches by multi-compartment models are discussed elsewhere (23, 30).

Single administration ($a = 0$)

Given $t = 0$ at the start of administration, the solution is:

$$C_t = C_0 \exp(-kt), \text{ for } t > t_0 \geq 0, \qquad (2)$$

t_0 being the length of the initial phase. For intravenous injection, $t_0 = 0$ and hence C_0 is the initial concentration, but for oral administration the solution is valid only for $t > t_0 > 0$ so that C_0 is not the concentration at the start $t = 0$. In spite of this:

$$t_{1/2} = (\log 2)/k, \qquad (3)$$

the half-life of the drug. Thus the SD of $\log t_{1/2}$ is equal to that of $\log k$.

Since dimensionless parameters are preferable to concentrations at different units, the constant conversion factor can be neglected; the SD of $X = \log C$ (say σ_X) is used instead of the SD of C (say σ_C). We note that:

a. If the coefficient of variation of C, $\gamma_C = \sigma_C/\mu_C$, μ_C being the mean of C, is sufficiently smaller than 1, an approximate relation:

$$\sigma_X = \gamma_C \qquad (4)$$

holds with respect to the natural logarithm and $\sigma_X \neq \log \sigma_C$.

b. In most cases X, but not C, follows approximately a normal distribution when individuals in a population are grouped according to race, sex, age etc.

c. Laws governing individual biochemical variability have simpler forms in X but not in C, so that the individual biochemical variability is represented by σ_X. Hereafter, the same symbol is used for a parameter and its estimate, and the common logarithm in all numerical examples without mentioning its base is given. Thus, for example, $\sigma_X = 0.13$ in Table 1 actually means $\hat{\sigma}_X/\log_e 10 = 0.13$ (19).

Continuous (constant rate) administration

With the initial condition $C_0 = 0$, the solution is:

TABLE 1. *Decay constants of drugs ($W = \log t_{1/2}$ or $\log k$)*

Drug	$\sigma_w(n)$
Aspirine	0.13(80)
Dicoumarol	0.10(56)
Ethanol	0.10(14)
Lincomycin	0.13(58)
Novobiocin	0.17(58)
Phenylbutazone	0.14(142)

$$C_t = C_\infty[1 - exp(-kt)], \quad C_\infty = a/k, \tag{5}$$

so that for $kt \gg 1$, C_t is nearly equal to C_∞. Hence the subscript t may be omitted in C_t for sufficiently large values of t to give approximately:

$$log\, C = log\, a - log\, k. \tag{6}$$

At the start of this research, only one suggestion for *log a* was present; i.e. in the case of ethanol, a series of experiments on the alcoholic drink 'Sake' suggested that σ_X was approximately equal to $\sigma(log\, k)$,* so that at first the variability of *log a* was thought to be negligibly small and

$$\sigma_X = \sigma(log\, k) \tag{7}$$

held approximately for other substances too.

However, if we assume that $h = a/k$ is a smooth function of k, to conform to observations on the age difference among babies, children and adults, h must be a monotone increasing function of k for most normal substances in blood (32).

By either of these two hypotheses, σ_X is basically determined by the gene pool of the population and modified by the intake of wines, drugs etc., since according to twin studies, k's are almost the same for identical twins but not so for fraternal twins. Thus it can be surmised first that σ_X *is almost independent of some attributes.* This may be called the quasi-constancy of type I for σ_X.

Pollutant

For a pollutant, a and k may be assumed to be mutually independent and thus:

$$\sigma_X^2 = \sigma^2(log\, a) + \sigma^2(log\, k) > \sigma^2(log\, k). \tag{8}$$

Usually a is a monotone decreasing function of the distance R from the source of pollution and a decreases rapidly near the source and slowly with distance from the source. Thus if the population is crudely stratified by the distance R, the variability of a within the stratum will be larger near the source and smaller far from the source. Hence we may expect that σ_X would be larger for the subpopulation near the source. This is the second surmise. A similar tendency would be observed in the daily amount of a substance in urine, where the age t plays the role of the distance R, i.e. its variability would be larger for babies and children, when the class interval is excessive.

Temporal distribution

The fundamental equation for metabolic turnover (Equation 5) is:

$$log\, k + log\, t = log\,[-log\,(1 - C_t/C_\infty)]. \tag{9}$$

The time at onset (say t_e) of a physiological or pathological phenomenon is assumed to correspond to the effective concentration $C_e = C_{te}$. This is essentially the so-called first passage problem. For example, for an infectious disease, t being 0 at the time of exposure, certain toxic substances in blood increase and at t_e a certain symptom appears, where t_e is the latent period (see Table 2) (18). The SD of the term

*The same is approximately true for phenylbutazone. Note that Equation 6 holds only when the concentration is in a steady state.

on the right in Equation 9 is at most the order of magnitude of σ_x, if C_e/C_∞ is neither too small nor too large. If $Y = log\ t_e$, then:

$$\sigma_y = \sigma(log\ k) \qquad (10)$$

approximately. If so, σ_y will be almost independent of some attributes – this may again be called the quasi-constancy of type I – and Y follows a normal law, provided *log k* follows the same law. This may not be true if the value of C_e/C_∞ is extreme.

Evolution-theoretical

This is the last premise. If σ_x (or σ_y) is determined by the gene pool of the population, it must be smaller for an endogenous substance in blood (or physiological phenomenon). In other words, biological processes are very conservative and do not permit wide variations (27).

Initially the hypothesis was contrary to this, i.e. 'σ_x (or σ_y) is large for an endogenous substance in blood (or physiological phenomenon), since the divergence during the course of time is a universal phenomenon and the endogenous substance (or phenomenon) appeared at an early stage of evolution'. Accumulated data, however, were against the second hypothesis, so that the first hypothesis was applied to examine, e.g., the luteal phase of the menstrual cycle (31).

SUBSTANCES IN BODY FLUIDS AND HAIR

If n is the sample size, values of σ_x (n) of some normal constituents in blood are given in Table 3 (13–15, 18, 23, 27, 28, 31). m and f stand for male and female

TABLE 2. *Latent period of infectious disease ($Y = log\ t_e$)*

Viral	$\sigma_y(n)$	*Bacterial*	$\sigma_y(n)$	
Chickenpox	0.057(127)	Dysentery (bacterial)	0.135(97)	
	0.061(67)	Food poisoning		
Measles	0.074(199)	(bacterial)	0.170(144)	
	0.117(91)	Salmonellosis	0.181(227)	
Poliomyelitis	0.176(29)	Sore throat		
(Rhesus monkey)	0.107(107)	(streptococcal)	0.185(51)	
	0.117(75)	Typhoid fever	0.152(55)	
	0.143(229)			
	0.081(67)	*Others*	$\sigma_y(n)$	
	0.120(78)	Amebic dysentery	0.324(215)	
Serum hepatitis	0.093(5914)	Malaria	0.124(24)	
	0.104(707)			
	0.060(115)			
	0.092(105)	*Rabies (bitten part)*	μ_t *(days)*	$\sigma_y(n)$
	0.073(501)	Head or face	33.6	0.33(54)
	0.102(670)	Upper limbs	55.5	0.34(68)
	0.068(42)	Lower limbs	69.7	0.36(43)

TABLE 3. *Values of σ_X (n) of some normal constituents in blood*

ACP	Jap.	m	0.03(38)	Creatinine		m	0.11(108)
		f	0.03(15)			f	0.11(122)
	Amer.	m	0.28(20)				0.11(55)
		f	0.20(15)	Ferritin		m	0.28(174)
Albumin	Jap.	m	0.02(133)			f	0.29(152)
		f	0.03(65)			m	0.31(75)
	Amer.	m	0.03(20)			f	0.38(44)
		f	0.03(15)	Globulin		m	0.05(133)
ALP	Jap.	m	0.12(133)			f	0.04(65)
		f	0.13(65)	α_1-Globulin		m	0.05(20)
	Amer.	m	0.20(20)			f	0.03(15)
		f	0.18(15)				0.16(100)
Amylase	Jap.	m	0.12(133)	α_2-Globulin		m	0.07(20)
		f	0.13(65)			f	0.06(15)
	Amer.	m	0.12(20)				0.13(100)
		f	0.11(15)	β-Globulin		m	0.05(20)
Arsenic			$0.15(2\times10)$			f	0.05(15)
Bicarbonate		m	0.03(20)				0.11(100)
		f	0.03(15)	γ-Globulin		m	0.10(20)
Bilirubin	Jap.	m	0.14(133)			f	0.11(15)
		f	0.14(65)				0.09(100)
	Amer.	m	0.13(29)	Glucose	Jap.	m	0.05(133)
		f	0.13(15)			f	0.05(65)
Cadmium			0.11(140)		French	m	$0.06(2.5\times10^4)$
			$0.11(2\times10)$			f	$0.06(2.3\times10^4)$
Calcium			0.02(399)	G-6-PD	normal	m	0.11(184)
		m	0.02(20)	β-Glucuronidase		m	0.17(68)
		f	0.02(15)	GOT			0.13(209)
Catalase (normal)			0.06(273)				0.17(68)
Chloride			0.01(157)		Amer.	m	0.17(20)
			0.004(93)			f	0.17(15)
		m	0.004(20)		Jap.	m	0.12(133)
		f	0.003(15)			f	0.09(65)
Cholesterol	Jap.	m	0.06(133)				0.11(180)
		f	0.05(65)	GPT			0.17(120)
	Amer.	m	0.02(20)	GSH (red cell)			0.09(160)
		f	0.02(15)	GTP		m	0.20(133)
			0.07(204)			f	0.16(65)
Cholinesterase			0.33(69)	Haptoglobin			
Usual			0.12(23)	Hpl-1			0.11(60)
Intermediate			0.11(31)	Hp2-1			0.17(129)
Atypical			0.16(15)	Hp2-2			0.18(86)
Chromium			$0.09(2\times10)$	Hemoglobin		m	0.05
			$0.13(2\times10)$			f	0.05
Copper		m	0.06(120)	HBD			0.15(139)
		f	0.06(85)	Immunoglobulin		A	0.23(19)
		m	0.10(31)				0.31(18)
Corticosterone			0.16(14)			D	0.07(19)
CPK		m	0.28(20)				0.30(18)
		f	0.30(15)			E	0.54(19)

TABLE 3 *(continued)*

		—	p,p′-DDE		0.19
	G	0.12(19)	p,p′-DDT		0.20
		0.15(18)	Phospholipids		0.07(275)
	M	0.20(19)	Phosphorus Jap.	m	0.05(136)
		0.23(18)		f	0.06(260)
Insulin	m	0.21(17)	Amer.	m	0.13(20)
Iodine				f	0.13(15)
protein-bound		0.08(125)	Potassium		$0.07(3\times10^3)$
butanol-extractable	m	0.07(29)			0.05(157)
	f	0.06(52)	Total protein Jap.	m	0.02(133)
Iron		0.12(149)		f	0.02(65)
		$0.11(2\times10)$	Amer.	m	0.03(20)
		$0.13(2\times10)$		f	0.02(15)
LDH	m	0.13(20)	Wrestlers		0.03(96)
	f	0.13(15)	Control		0.02(89)
		0.13(75)			0.03(81)
		0.18(285)	Silicate		0.12(264)
LDH_1		0.21(30)	Sodium		$0.01(10^2)$
LDH_2		0.25(30)			0.009(79)
LDH_3		0.04(30)		m	0.009(20)
LDH_4		0.04(30)		f	0.007(15)
LDH_5		0.05(30)	Sphingomyelin		0.08(30)
Lead		0.13(140)	Sulphur (inorganic)		0.11(88)
Lecithin		0.06(30)	Thyroxine		0.09(70)
LAP	m	0.09(133)	Tin		$0.10(2\times10)$
	f	0.07(65)	Triglycerides		0.18(292)
Lipids		0.11(150)	Triiodothyroxine		0.05(250)
		0.10(73)	Urea nitrogen Jap.	m	0.08(133)
Lysolecithin		0.16(30)		f	0.09(65)
Magnesium	m	0.10(20)	Amer.	m	0.07(20)
	f	0.11(15)		f	0.07(15)
		0.14(140)	Athletes		0.11(114)
Manganese		$0.14(2\times10)$	Control		0.09(81)
MAO		0.09(108)	Uric acid French	m	$0.09(2.4\times10^4)$
Nickel		$0.11(2\times10)$		f	$0.09(2.2\times10^4)$
Pesticides and			Amer.	m	0.12(20)
related				f	0.13(15)
substances (n = 12)					0.10(59)
α-BHC		0.29	Zinc		0.08(126)
β-BHC		0.21			0.09(140)
γ-BHC		0.20		m	0.06(95)
Dieldrin		0.12		f	0.05(96)

respectively. Since not all reports gave the original observed data themselves and sometimes the sample size is not mentioned, 'paleostatistical' techniques were used to estimate σ_X (27).

Table 3 shows that, except for acid phosphatase (ACP), there is no appreciable race difference and no sex difference except possibly for ferritin, i.e. σ_X is quasi-

constant with respect to race and sex. From this Table it seems that:
a. σ_x lies mostly between 0.1 and 0.2,
b. σ_x is equal to 0.3 or more, when (i) the population is a mixture of subpopulations, e.g. a polymorphic case of cholinesterase, or (ii) the sample size is too small, or (iii) there are errors either in measurement or in computation, and
c. σ_x is less than 0.1 for electrolytes and some fundamental substances, e.g. total protein and glucose.
If we stratify the population in case (b,i) biologically, σ_x of a stratum lies between 0.1 and 0.2 (14). For a pollutant in body fluid, an apparent population is thought to be a mixture of many subpopulations, since its 'dose' is not fixed for the members of this population.

If we apply analysis of variance to the original data, the variance component due to 'inter-individual variation' is usually somewhat smaller than σ_x^2 obtained from the values tabulated in Table 3, except when the variance component due to the variation among replicated measurements is fairly large (27).

Pesticides and related substances are included in Table 3, since today they are common substances in industrialized countries.

The variabilities of olfactory, gustatory and skin sensitivity are given in Table 4 (13, 14, 16) as threshold values. For a drug in blood the variability of an individual dose D to reach the same critical concentration C_e can be proved to be approximately equal to σ_x obtained by the constant dose (14). The σ_x of smell sensitivity is almost constant, irrespective of the kind of smell or the chemical

TABLE 4. *Variability of olfactory, gustatory and skin sensitivity (threshold values)*

I. Olfactory			
	$\sigma_x(n)$		$\sigma_x(n)$
Acetic acid	0.40(91)	Isobutyl isobutyrate	0.39(96)
Ammonia	0.41(60)	Isobutyric acid	0.41(86)
n-Butyric acid	0.44(91)	Isocaproic acid	0.51(94)
d-Camphor	0.54(60)	Isovaleric acid	0.51(95)
n-Capric acid	0.58(94)	1-Menthol	0.42(60)
n-Caproic acid	0.50(97)	Mercaptoethanol	0.48(60)
n-Caprylic acid	0.62(96)	d-1-2-Methylbutyric acid	0.51(91)
n-Enanthic acid	0.57(95)	n-Pelargonic acid	0.53(94)
Ethylene dichloride	0.47(60)		
Formic acid	0.52(60)	Propionic acid	0.47(85)
	0.51(91)	Trimethylacetic acid	0.55(94)
Isobutyl alcohol	0.66(93)	n-Valeric acid	0.52(95)
Isobutylaldehyde	1.13(89)*		
II. Gustatory			
Quinine hydrochloride		Phenylthiocarbamide	($n = 243$)
female	0.52(52)	Normal	0.39
female retest	0.49(52)	Ageusia	0.37
III. Skin			
Mercuric chloride	0.59(36)		

*bimodal

TABLE 5. *Uric acid in sera ($X = \log C$)*

		μ_c (mg/dl)	$\sigma_x(n)$
Normal	m	3.89	0.104(1037)
	f	3.45	0.108(115)
Wrestlers		6.23	0.105(64)
Gout		9.54	0.106(200)

TABLE 6. *Free amino acids in cerebrospinal fluid ($n = 10$)*

	μ_c*	σ_x		μ_c*	σ_x		μ_c*	σ_x
Glu-NH_2	45.47	0.11	Leu	1.16	0.09	Ile	0.50	0.08
Ser	3.57	0.12	His	1.11	0.11	Met	0.32	0.13
Ala	2.79	0.15	Gly	0.85	0.13	Asp	0.29	0.34(?)
Thr	2.66	0.15	Orn	0.84	0.12	HomoCar	0.27	0.18
Lys	1.86	0.15	Tyr	0.79	0.12	α-NH_2-But	0.26	0.13
Glu	1.47	0.34(?)	Phe	0.75	0.13	Cit	0.21	0.14
Val	1.43	0.12	EtNH_2	0.67	0.20			
Arg	1.42	0.21	Tau	0.53	0.11			

*μmol/100 ml

structure, except for isobutyraldehyde where the population is bimodal. The values in Table 4 are clearly higher than those in Table 3.

As for a case where different substances (or phenomena) of a similar or related nature have approximately the same σ_x (or σ_y), one may say the quasi-constancy of type II holds. Some statistical tests are required to show the insignificance of observed differences before quasi-constancy truly applies.

Table 5 shows clearly the quasi-constancy of type I. The relatively but not absolutely weaker activity of the related enzyme is responsible for the onset of gout; 'relative' refers to the balance between input and output. If only those with absolutely weaker activity suffer from gout, σ_x must be smaller than that for normal persons (16)†.

Table 6 shows the quasi-constancy of type II. The quasi-constancy of type II holds again for amino acids and vitamins in breast milk respectively and amino acids in aqueous humor (19, 23).

The data in Table 7 were obtained from a professional group. They are to be compared with the values of σ_x's of metals in Table 3, clarifying the question mark at copper in Table 7.

At present I have no firm idea why the quasi-constancy of type II holds. Probably common regulatory genes control an enzyme system and two or more substances share most enzymes of this system, or perhaps a metabolic pathway with a matrix of decay constants is present in which a common matrix almost independent of individuals is multiplied by a scalar dependent upon individual. The existence of

† The same is true for digoxin (14):

Digoxin in plasma	μ_c(ng/ml)	$\sigma_x(n)$
toxic group	4.1	0.21(48)
non-toxic group	1.3	0.23(131)

TABLE 7. *Metals in blood ($n = 140$)*

	μ_C (μg/dl)	σ_X
Cd	0.01	0.11
Cu	1.21	0.38(?)
Fe	140.00	0.12
Mg	0.06	0.13
Pb	14.33	0.14
Zn	2.99	0.14

TABLE 8. *Excretion of VMA in urine*

Age (yr)	μ_C (mg/day)	$\sigma_X(n)$	Age (yr)	μ_C (mg/day)	σ_X
1–9	1.0	0.335(46)	<1	0.57	0.221(19)
10–29	3.6	0.215(28)	1–5	1.35	0.138(15)
30–49	4.2	0.169(33)	6–15	2.37	0.126(13)
50–69	4.1	0.154(42)			
70–99	3.2	0.170(8)			

TABLE 9. *Substances in urine which increase under stress*

	Adrenaline		Noradrenaline		VMA	
	μ_C (μg)	σ_X	μ_C (μg)	σ_X	μ_C (mg)	σ_X
Daytime (9–20 hr)	6.5	0.246	34.6	0.129	4.1	0.134
Nighttime (21–8 hr)	3.9	0.255	30.8	0.107	3.2	0.133
n	6		6		6	

C denotes the total amount.

such a matrix is plausible, since there will be a metabolic disease if the elements of this matrix are not well-balanced (see Discussion).

The quasi-constancy of σ_X is seen in the daily urinary VMA in relation to age (Table 8) (19) and in the 12-hour urinary materials which increase under stress (Table 9) (27).

A similar quasi-constancy of σ_X is observed after the instantaneous intake of alcohol (Table 10) (19). If the sample size is small, the SD is smaller (or larger) than the average and this tendency persists during the experiment. Compare the 100 ml and 300 ml groups with other groups.

For pollutants, PCB, pestides and related substances in breast milk (Tables 11 and 12) (19) are examples. These are the quasi-constancy of type I and of type II respectively.

To keep the inter-individual variability of substances in body fluids small, it is very likely that the variability of nutritional intake is also small. [See analysis in Table 13 (21).]

The last example in this section is σ_X of a pollutant in hair with respect to the distance R from the source of pollution, which shows clearly that the premise in the previous section is valid (Table 14) (19). We see again that σ_X's are almost

TABLE 10. *σ_X after intake of Sake*

Amount of intake of Sake (ml)	Size of sample	30 min	1 hr	2 hr	3 hr	Mean
100	7	0.19	0.24	0.26	—	0.23
200	83	0.09	0.11	0.15	0.27	0.16
300	7	0.07	0.07	0.08	0.10	0.08
400	40	0.15	0.11	0.08	0.10	0.11
600	14	0.13	0.08	0.05	0.06	0.08
Mean		0.13	0.12	0.13	0.13	

TABLE 11. *PCB in breast milk [$\sigma_X(n)$]*

	1972	1973	1974	1975	1976
Farm village	0.31(231)	0.34(171)	0.35(176)	0.30(93)	0.38(75)
City	0.35(291)	0.35(260)	0.31(244)	0.30(122)	0.24(123)
Around factory	0.33(51)	0.36(36)	0.34(32)	0.45(13)	0.41(18)
Fishing village	0.34(92)	0.40(125)	0.35(104)	0.34(53)	0.34(42)
Mean per year	0.035	0.032	0.028	0.027	0.025 (p.p.m.)

TABLE 12. *Pesticides and related substances in breast milk*

	Farmworkers		Non-farmworkers	
	μ_c	σ_X	μ_ϑ	σ_X
Total BHC	0.099	0.35	0.150	0.41
α-BHC	0.003	0.29	0.003	0.26
β-BHC	0.093	0.38	0.144	0.40
γ-BHC	0.002	0.41	0.003	0.47
δ-BHC	0.001	0.33	0.001	0.39
Total DDT	0.056	0.37	0.064	0.30
Dieldrin	0.003	0.40	0.004	0.37
n	213		241	

TABLE 13. *Three-day mean of intake of different substances*

	σ_X (275)
Calcium	0.124
Carbohydrates	0.109
Fat	0.105
Iron	0.096
Animal iron	0.174
Proteins	0.078
Animal protein	0.136
VA	0.145
VB_1	0.107
VB_2	0.119
VC	0.166

TABLE 14. *Mercury in hair ($X = \log C$)*

	μ_C (p.p.m.)	σ_X
American in Japan	1.9	0.23(36)
Japanese (normal subject)	4.2	0.23(120)
Inhabitant of Tokyo	5.1	0.23(101)
Dentist and employee	10.6	0.24(36)
Tuna fisherman	12.7	0.23(56)
Inhabitant of Gosyoura	35.9	0.35(485)
Inhabitant of Minimata	44.8	0.39(163)

independent of means (μ_c's) except for cases near the center of pollution, viz. Minamata and Gosyoura.

SPECIES DIFFERENCE OF σ_X

Since the molecular structures of homologous enzymes among experimental mammals do not differ greatly, one may expect that the species difference of σ_X is not large. This is true for normal substances in blood (15, 19, 32). If σ_{ij} is σ_X of the i-th substance in blood of the j-th species, let us assume an additive and a multiplicative model respectively, i.e.:

$$\sigma_{ij} = \mu + \alpha_i + \beta_j, \text{ and} \tag{11}$$

$$\sigma_{ij} = \mu (1 + A_i)(1 + B_j). \tag{12}$$

With respect to the 14 substances in Table 15 and 14 mammals (mouse, rat, hamster, guinea-pig, rabbit, cat, dog, monkey, pig, goat, sheep, cattle, horse and man) and the chicken, both models were tested (33). In the first model (Equation 11) the interaction term was significant and in the second model (Equation 12) it was not. Thus the multiplicative model is better than the additive one. This conclusion had been anticipated previously (15). The calculated values in Table 15 were obtained by the method of least squares, using the second model and taking the logarithm of σ_{ij}. Chicken is included in this analysis, since there are not many differences with respect to the variabilities – but not the means – of these substances.

Table 16 gives the variance components of σ_X's in different types of animals to show that the species difference is small (33).

TABLE 15. *Observed and calculated $\sigma_X \times 10^3$ (normal constituents in blood)*

	Observed	Calculated		Observed	Calculated
Alkaline phosphatase	197	150	Glucose	86	81
Aspartic transaminase	166	129	Lactic dehydrogenase	134	126
Bilirubin	132	138	Potassium	40	26
Calcium	49	48	Total protein	26	30
Chloride	4	4	Sodium	9	7
Cholesterol	69	118	Urea nitrogen	95	125
Creatinine	107	118	Uric acid	99	118

TABLE 16. *Variance components of σ_x in different types of animals*

Orders of vertebrates	0.00655
Species of mammals	0.00210
Genera of male monkeys	0.00231
Different breeds of dogs	0.00012
Different strains of rats	0.00017

TABLE 17. *σ_y of eruption of permanent teeth ($Y = log\ t_e$)*

		Anglo-Saxon	French		Anglo-Saxon	French
Male	I^1	0.044	0.055	I_1	0.042	0.046
	I^2	0.041	0.052	I_2	0.041	0.044
	C'	0.044	0.045	$C_{'}$	0.048	0.047
	P^1	0.059	0.061	P_1	0.054	0.057
	P^2	0.056	0.051	P_2	0.057	0.047
	M^1	0.044	0.057	M_1	0.048	0.051
	M^2	0.039	0.043	M_2	0.041	0.045
Female	I^1	0.044	0.046	I_1	0.039	0.047
	I^2	0.048	0.050	I_2	0.046	0.046
	C'	0.045	0.045	$C_{'}$	0.044	0.052
	P^1	0.053	0.053	P_1	0.054	0.058
	P^2	0.058	0.057	P_2	0.058	0.052
	M^1	0.052	0.058	M_1	0.048	0.064
	M^2	0.041	0.042	M_2	0.042	0.050

AGES AT ONSET; PHYSIOLOGICAL CYCLES

Table 17 shows the quasi-constancy of σ_y of eruption of permanent teeth with respect to two races, kind and positions of teeth (17).* This quasi-constancy holds both for man and other mammals (17).

Table 18 shows the quasi-constancy of σ_y of the menarche with respect to dwelling

*If age at eruption of the α-th permanent tooth of the i-th individual is $t_{e\alpha i}$ and its logarithm $Y_{\alpha i}$, then approximately:

$$log\ k_i + Y_{\alpha i} = log\ k_j + Y_{\alpha j} = q_\alpha, \quad (i \neq j)$$
$$log\ k_i + Y_{\beta i} = log\ k_j + Y_{\beta j} = q_\beta, \quad (\alpha \neq \beta),$$

where k and q stand for the decay constant and quasi-constant respectively.

Eliminating k's the relation becomes:

$$Y_{\alpha i} - Y_{\alpha j} = Y_{\beta i} - Y_{\beta j}.$$

Taking the mean with respect to j, the relation is:

$$Y_{\alpha i} - \mu_\alpha = Y_{\beta i} - \mu_\beta,$$

μ being the population mean of Y; i.e., if the individual observation $Y_{\alpha i}$ is plotted against μ_α, α being a variable, points lie on an approximately straight line. In cases of malnutrition, severe disease and decayed deciduous teeth, points plotted may show a large deviation from linearity.

TABLE 18. *Quasi-constancy of σ_y of the menarche*

	1961	1964	1967	1972	1977
Mean age at menarche* (yr)					
Urban	13.095	13.014	12.815	12.601	12.503
Rural	13.403	13.207	12.975	12.697	12.529
σ_y					
Urban	0.0386	0.0382	0.0388	0.0385	0.0388
Rural	0.0385	0.0384	0.0384	0.0389	0.0396

*From A. Sawada.

place and calendar years. Since the sizes of the samples taken by A. Sawada were extraordinarily large, the quasi-constancy can be vividly seen.

Since the menstrual cycle is a basic physiological phenomenon, σ_y was conjectured to be smaller than 0.1 and independent of age. This was not true (Table 19) and by dividing the cycle into two phases, σ_y of the length of the luteal phase was smaller than 0.1 and quasi-constant with respect to age. In my view the luteal phase is more fundamental than the menstrual cycle (18) and would be a basis for the Ogino method of contraception. Another basis is that the age-related change in the mean of this length of phase is also small.

As an example of the quasi-constancy of type II of σ_y only biological parameters supposed to be related to growth and sex hormones are quoted in Table 20.

With regard to pathologies analysed so far, the distribution of latent periods in an infectious disease is approximately logarithmico-normal (LN), if secondary infections are excluded. Table 2 shows that σ_y is of the order of σ_x except in the case of rabies, where vaccinated and non-vaccinated subjects are not separated. This would be one reason why we have $\sigma_y > 0.3$. The next section considers other aspects. Viral disease has, on average, a smaller σ_y than bacterial diseases, probably because the virus attacks the cell directly.

Since the genesis of autoimmune diseases has not been thoroughly clarified, an attempt was made to analyse the type of distribution of ages of patients or that of ages at onset, assuming that if the metabolic model thus far used was correct, an LN law would fit well and if the hit theory was correct, a gamma law G(a,p) would fit well.

TABLE 19. *Age-related changes in menstrual cycle*

Age	No. of cycles	Menstrual cycle	Follicular phase	Luteal phase
13–17	280	0.119	0.170	0.0568
18–19	100	0.086	0.142	0.0669
20–24	350	0.078	0.130	0.0545
25–29	1000	0.102	0.167	0.0557
30–34	750	0.079	0.131	0.0556
35–39	400	0.070	0.116	0.0555
40–52	120	0.061	0.115	0.0610

There might be other types of distribution. In a gamma distribution, the parameter p denotes either the number of foreign particles needed to modify an autogenous protein or that of damaged sites of an autogenous molecule, so as to be recognized as foreign by the immune system. Other diseases are also included in Table 21 as controls. Most immune diseases follow gamma laws rather than LN laws (18, 33).

TABLE 20. *Age at onset and duration of biological parameters related to growth and sex hormones ($Y = \log t_e$)*

		σ_Y
Eruption of permanent teeth	General	0.054
	Normal	0.040
First ejaculation		0.034
Appearance of pubic hair	m	0.036
	f	0.039
Menarche		0.038
Gestation period (rat)		0.040

TABLE 21. *Age at onset of disease ($Y = \log t_e$)*

		$\sigma_Y(n)$	Distribution
Amyloidosis (primary)		0.127(106)	Weibull
Anxiety neurosis		0.142(160)	LN
Behçet's disease			
As a whole		0.147(2261)	
Complete		0.140(852)	G(2.84,11)
Incomplete		0.145(994)	G(3.32,10)
Suspected		0.154(290)	G(3.80,9)
Possible		0.176(125)	G(4.30,8)
Colitis ulcerosa	m	0.193(465)	G(7.12,10)
	f	0.174(429)	G(6.90,14)
Depression		0.164(203)	
Hypoferric anemia		0.189(355)	LN
Mastopathy		0.096(418)	LN
Multiple sclerosis		0.175(483)	G(4.48,7)
Myasthenia gravis	m	0.553	bimodal
	f	0.505	bimodal
Myocardial infarction			
	m	0.086(1580)	Weibull
	f	0.069(338)	
Pemphigus	American	0.210(234)	
	Japanese	0.160(407)	
Prostatomegaly		0.066(478)	Weibull
Rheumatoid arthritis		0.207(407)	bimodal
Sarcoidosis	m	0.182(482)	
	f	0.204(554)	
Systemic lupus erythematosus		0.180(510)	G(4.50,7)
Systemic scleroderma		0.151(115)	G(4.53,9)

The σ_y's of cancers are given in Table 22 (18). Since the distributions of most cancers have their modes at an older age, their distributions are usually neither of LN type nor of gamma type. The σ_y's are rather small even among diseases which have distributions with negative skewness. It is of the order of that of viral infections (cf. Table 2).

σ_x AND σ_y IN CHILDHOOD

In analysing data on tooth eruption the quasi-constancy did not hold with respect to the deciduous teeth (Table 23) and the same was true for σ_x when babies and children were included in the sample (Table 24) (17, 19).

A stochastic version of the metabolic turnover was then introduced, i.e. two stochastic differential equations of the Ito type (19):

$$dC_t = (-kC_t + a)dt + (BC_t + b)dW_t \tag{13}$$

and

$$dC_t = (-kC_t + a)dt + BC_t dW_{1t} + bdW_{2t}, \tag{14}$$

where B and b are two constants and W_t, W_{1t} W_{2t} are three standard Wiener processes. W_{1t} and W_{2t} are assumed to be mutually independent.

They are derived as follows: First consider a person with two parameters as before. These parameters are modified randomly by the introduction of wines etc., corresponding to the induction and inhibition of enzymes. This view is partly supported by the comparison of normal subjects and hospital in-patients in Table 25 (22). Thus k and a in Equation 1 are replaced by $k + \xi$ and $a + \eta$ respectively. Assuming that the two random variables ξdt and ηdt are either perfectly correlated or perfectly independent, these two models are obtained.

TABLE 22. *Age distribution of cancer ($Y = \log t_e$)*

		$\sigma_y(n)$			$\sigma_y(n)$
Breast		0.105(6000)	Stomach	m	0.100(449)
Cervix		0.062(6755)		f	0.111(199)
Colon	m	0.112		m	0.084(5103)
	f	0.105		f	0.103(2514)
Gallbladder		0.094		m	0.127(5060)
Larynx		0.078(135)		f	0.135(2692)
		0.065(328)	Uterine body		0.077
Liver	m	0.129(641)	Endometrium		0.084
	f	0.128(444)	Renal adeno-		
Lung	m	0.088(582)	carcinoma		0.149(89)
		0.089(740)			
Pancreas	m	0.089(695)	Carcinoma due to		
	f	0.094(365)	ultraviolet		
Prostate		0.058(210)	ray irradiation		
Rectum	m	0.103	(albino mouse)		$0.080(10^2)$
	f	0.119			

TABLE 23. *Eruption of deciduous and permanent teeth (Y = log t_e)*

	μ_t (mth)	σ_y		μ_t (mth)	σ_y
i^1	9.9	0.110	i_1	8.3	0.135
i^2	12.2	0.112	i_2	13.1	0.111
c'	17.9	0.075	$c_{\prime}$	18.8	0.074
m^1	17.7	0.110	m_1	17.7	0.086
m^2	26.9	0.104	m_2	25.5	0.084
			$n = 43$		
I^1	89	0.043(244)	I_1	78	0.039(236)
I^2	103	0.038(231)	I_2	87	0.036(230)
C'	131	0.033(148)	$C_{\prime}$	118	0.037(184)
P^1	113	0.055(194)	P_1	118	0.051(192)
P^2	120	0.051(148)	P_2	124	0.050(108)
M^1	80	0.045(238)	M_1	76	0.048(226)
M^2	143	0.030(48)	M_2	135	0.030(97)
M^3	234	0.049(60)	M_3	228	0.042(59)

TABLE 24. *μ_c and σ_x as functions of age*

	IgG			IgE	
	μ_c (mg/100 ml)	σ_x (3 × 10)		μ_c(U/ml)	$\sigma_x(n)$
Cord blood	(maternal level)		Cord blood	2.68	0.187(33)
2–4 mth	362	0.204	<1 day	3.38	0.186(5)
5–8 mth	433	0.169	1–6 days	4.18	0.235(13)
9–14 mth	633	0.147	7 days–2 mth	7.28	0.224(8)
15–23 mth	863	0.134	3–11 mth	25.8	0.273(13)
2–3 yr	808	0.152	1 yr	67.2	0.431(11)
3½–4½ yr	963	0.099	2 yr	274	0.443(7)
5–6 yr	976	0.097	3 yr	145	0.337(8)
7–8 yr	1010	0.108	4 yr	179	0.362(8)
9–10 yr	1090	0.077	5 yr	286	0.378(10)
11–12 yr	1095	0.089	6 yr	234	0.193(9)
13–14 yr	1090	0.055	7 yr	211	0.403(10)
15–16 yr	1160	0.061	8 yr	153	0.481(7)
17–18 yr	1070	0.097	9–11 yr	220	0.427(13)
19–21 yr	964	0.084	12–14 yr	252	0.481(8)
[Adults	1044	0.084(315)]	Adults	192	0.425(15)

The explicit solutions under suitable initial conditions for both models are given in the original paper. Let us consider only the first model here.

Assuming that $E(C_0^2)$ is finite and $a \neq 0$, we obtain the exact solutions for the first and second moments, from which we get the approximate relation:

$$\gamma_c^2 = bB/a + [b^2k/(2a^2)]\,[1 + exp(-kt)]/[1 - exp(-kt)], \tag{15}$$

assuming that $k \gg B^2$. Thus the coefficient of variation of C_t, i.e. γ_c is a monotone decreasing function of t and is almost independent of t for $kt \gg 2$. Note that $\gamma_c = \sigma_x$

TABLE 25. *$\sigma_x \times 10^3$ in healthy subjects and hospital in-patients*

		Healthy, ambulant subjects						Hospital in-patients					
Age		20–	30–	40–	50–	60–	70+	20–	30–	40–	50–	60–	70+
Albumin	m	20	22	20	20	21	32	58	58	56	62	66	64
	f	20	23	21	21	24	27	59	50	53	58	62	60
Cholesterol	m	75	78	73	73	71	107	94	97	92	95	103	96
	f	76	79	71	76	63	86	88	86	92	100	101	100
Creatinine	m	72	72	72	76	76	83	72	72	75	79	81	87
	f	92	72	82	72	81	90	68	68	72	72	76	79
Glucose (non-fasting)	m	71	68	75	71	83	95	83	93	103	101	104	105
	f	68	68	75	71	80	95	85	87	99	95	104	107
Iron	m	125	118	118	128	139	139	170	187	186	183	182	182
	f	139	171	149	123	123	133	184	183	183	181	180	178
Urate (uric acid)	m	78	77	79	79	81	112	95	104	96	99	108	105
	f	89	98	95	95	89	104	100	100	105	96	107	116
Urea	m	84	73	73	76	79	90	113	106	117	111	115	119
	f	99	76	83	81	79	73	108	108	109	110	116	120

holds approximately provided that $\gamma_c \ll 1$.

This can be interpreted as follows: The stochastic equation (13) is valid for the reference individual and an individual is thought to be a reflection of the reference. Another interpretation is given elsewhere (32). The first example in Table 24 shows the expected age-related change of σ_x at least qualitatively. So far, all substances in blood show similar changes, except for IgE in the second example of Table 24. The reason why IgE is exceptional can be explained as follows: (1) normal and atopic children are not separated, (2) the half-life of IgE is very short, and (3) by introduction of an allergen the amount of IgE increases markedly to give a booster effect.

Similar reasoning states that the apparent variability is extraordinarily large for the antibody level in Table 26, where subjects are not classified by age and the con-

TABLE 26. *Variability in antibody levels*

		$\sigma_x(n)$
Influenza	Asian	0.45(119)
	B	0.43(462)
	Hong-Kong	042(345)
Parainfluenza III		0.66(15)
Respiratory syncytial virus	Children	0.62(13)
	Children	0.42(13)
	Soldiers	0.31(18)
	Soldiers	0.24(18)
Salk vaccine (for persons with no preantibody for any type)	Type I	0.51(19)
	Type II	0.57(19)
	Type III	0.38(16)

densation series of serum was not tested; a symptomless subject whose dilution series of serum gives a false-negative result is therefore classified as true negative.

BLOOD PRESSURE

If individual values of a biological parameter q are basically determined by heredity and slightly modified by chemicals etc., one may expect that the SD of q or that of its function $W(q)$ would be quasi-constant. Blood pressure (p) is a suitable example. It is well-known that p is controlled chemically and among people living in areas where the supply of sodium is scanty, no age-related increase in blood pressure is observed. Hence a function $Z = Z(p)$ is assumed such that the SD of Z is quasi-constant with respect to sex and age.

To find out the form of $Z(p)$, let us consider the species differences in blood pressure to magnify the individual differences in man. Data at hand were the ranges (L, U) for experimental mammals and man. Plotting $U = \mu_p + 2\sigma_p$ against $L = \mu_p - 2\sigma_p$, U is approximately proportional to L, irrespective of the kind of pressure (except for rat). This means that $\gamma_p = \sigma_p/\mu_p$ is quasi-constant. In other words, the variance stabilizing transformation of p is logarithmic, i.e. $Z = \log p$. The premise is true for data classified by sex and for age (Table 27). The significant deviation from constancy is observed only among the aged. This deviation may be attributable to the inclusion of pathological cases in the aged groups as will be seen in the following study.

It is well-known that excess dietary sodium causes the elevation of systolic blood pressure, so that it is interesting to see whether σ_z is quasi-constant or not with respect to the daily salt intake. As shown in Table 28, this premise is not true. However, the empirical distribution functions plotted on LN probability paper (Fig. 1) reveal that:

1. Each distribution function is a weighted sum of two distribution functions, say F_1 and F_2, one corresponding to the normotensive (N) and the other to the hypertensive (H) group respectively – this much is well-known.
2. Both functions F_1 and F_2 are normal and the H group has a larger mean and larger variance.

TABLE 27. *Diastolic blood pressure in relation to age ($Z = \log p$)*

Age (yr)	μ_p (mmHg)	$\sigma_x(n)$	μ_p(mmHg)	$\sigma_x(n)$
15 –	68.6	0.072(2681)	70.4	0.070(1966)
20 –	71.4	0.068(6393)	71.2	0.062(3161)
25 –	72.9	0.068(7466)	71.5	0.067(2396)
30 –	75.4	0.068(8022)	72.7	0.064(1337)
35 –	77.6	0.069(5873)	72.7	0.070(762)
40 –	79.9	0.070(8888)	76.6	0.067(1196)
45 –	83.2	0.073(7936)	78.6	0.073(1227)
50 –	85.7	0.072(6892)	81.8	0.072(856)
55 –	86.5	0.075(3037)	82.2	0.069(642)
60 –	88.6	0.074(1781)	84.1	0.072(354)
65 +	87.5	0.071(787)	87.4	0.066(207)

TABLE 28. *Systolic blood pressure and intake of saline food*

Misosiru (cups/day)	$\overset{*}{\mu_p}$ (mmHg)	$\sigma_z(n)$	$\overset{*}{\mu_p}$ (mmHg)	$\sigma_z(n)$	$\overset{*}{\mu_p}$ (mmHg)	$\sigma_z(n)$	
<1	129.05	0.053(87)	135.98	0.062(75)	141.46	0.0765(432)	I
1 – 2	132.25	0.057(715)	135.22	0.064(692)	144.48	0.0769(3904)	II
3 – 4	131.70	0.060(225)	138.35	0.067(191)	146.89	0.0789(1095)	III
≥5	133.07	0.066(94)	140.82	0.069(88)	147.43	0.0782(481)	IV
Age	40–44		45–49		≥50		

*Geometric mean.

3. The weight varies depending upon the daily salt intake, but variance remains almost constant for each group, i.e. the quasi-constancy holds for both groups.

The black points (S.I.) on the extreme left in Figure 1 are obtained by assuming normal laws, $\mu_1 = 2.114$ and $\sigma_1 = 0.0494$ for F_1 and $\mu_2 = 2.226$ and $\sigma_2 = 0.0731$ for F_2, the weight for F_1 being 0.70. S.I. is fairly close to Group I.

The upper and lower branches of each distribution function on LN probability paper are approximated by two straight lines, neglecting the upper and lower 5%; the 4 upper and 4 lower lines are then almost parallel (34).

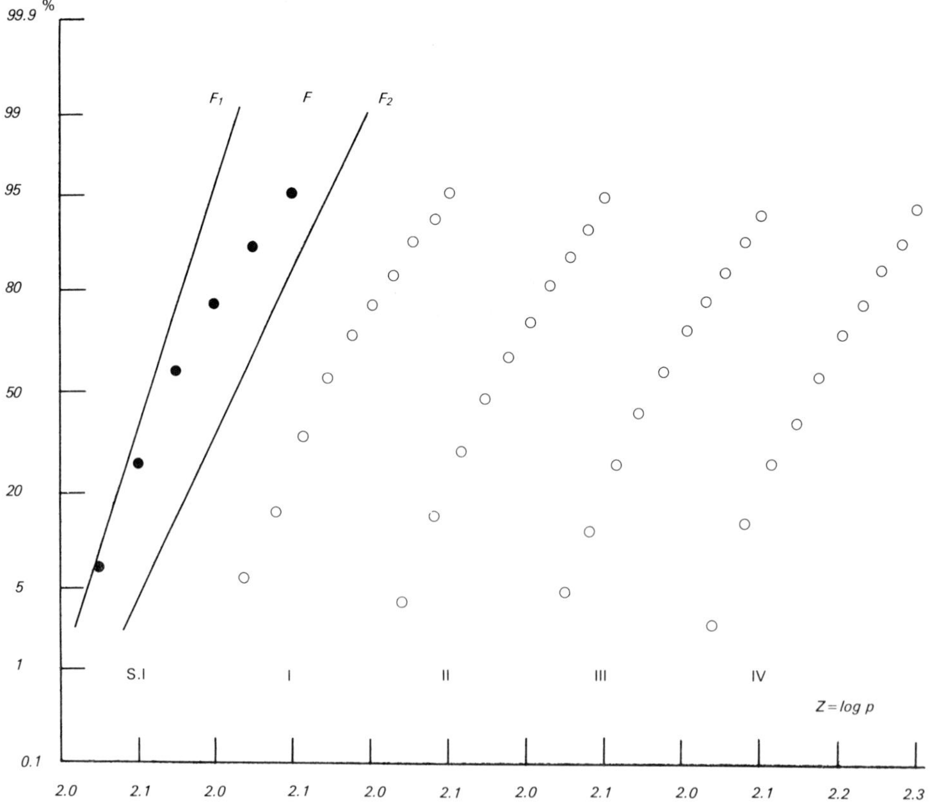

Fig. 1. Distribution function of Z.

Further analysis of similar data supporting the above is given elsewhere (34).

APPLICATIONS

To reduce the harmful effects of pollutants, drugs etc., the clear avoidance of these substances is recommended. The second method is to classify people by enzyme activities. There are indeed too many enzymes in our body but the quasi-constancy of type II suggests that all of them need not be tested. As a test substance we may use a relatively less toxic substrate. If we should use a drug itself, at first a small amount is given to establish individual values of k or $t_{1/2}$. Since k is independent of the concentration, one-tenth (or one-hundredth, if necessary) of the standard dose is used to correspond to the left-sided shift of the dose by $5\sigma_x$ through $10\sigma_x$ on the dose-response curve. Since the toxic level C_e is almost independent of individual, with this dose an adverse effect is not anticipated. Having estimated k or $t_{1/2}$, the dose may be increased to reach the individual therapeutic dose, if necessary.

To keep familial clinical pharmacology data in one place, the family doctor system rather than the open system is recommended.

ACKNOWLEDGEMENTS

I am indebted to many colleagues and friends in my past academic life in the Department of Medicine and Physical Therapy, Faculty of Medicine, Tokyo University, for collecting data and to many authors whose data were used in calculating σ_x, σ_y and σ_z. I greatly appreciate all their help.

REFERENCES

1. Allensmith, M. et al. (1968): The development of immunoglobulin levels in man. *J. Pediat., 72*, 276. [*IgG*]
2. Baba et al. (Eds.) (1976): *Syôni no Seizyôti.* Igakusyoin. [*lysolecithin, phospholipids, sphingomyelin*]
3. Bêtyet-byô Tyôsakenkyûhan (1977): *Syowa 51-nendo kenkyûgyôseki.* Ministry of Welfare. [*IgG, IgA, IgM, IgD, IgE*]
4. Diem, K. et al. (Eds.) (1970): *Documenta Geigy. Scientific Tables.* Geigy. [*chloride, copper, iodine, potassium, silicate, sulphur, zinc*]
5. Elkinton, J.R. et al. (1955): *Body Fluids.* Williams and Wilkins, Baltimore, MD. [*sodium*]
6. Fukumi, H. et al. (Eds.) (1970): *Byôgen Biseibutugaku. Wîrusu-hen.* Igakusyoin. [*para-influenza III, respiratory syncytial virus*]
7. Harris, H. (1970): *The Principle of Human Biochemical Genetics.* North-Holland Publ. Co., Amsterdam. [*cholinesterase*]
8. Kamus, H. et al. (1965): The antimode and lines of optimal separation in a genetically determined bimodal distribution, with particular reference to phenylthiocarbamide sensitivity. *Ann. hum. Genet., 29*, 127 [*phenylthiocarbamide*]
9. *Ketueki-Nyô Kagakukensa* (1976): *Nihon Rinsyô, 406, Autumnal spec. Iss.* [*ACP, corticosterone, zinc*]

10. Kokuritu Yobô-eisie Kenkyûsyo (1970): *Nihon no Wakutin.* Maruzen. [*Asian, B, and Hong-Kong influenza*]
11. Kolb, V.G. et al. (1976): *Klin. biokhim. Belorus.* [α_1*-globulin,* α_2*-globulin,* γ*-globulin*]
12. Kozakai, N. et al. (1973): *Seizyôti.* Igakusyoin. [*albumin, ALP, amylase, bilirubin, calcium, cholesterol, creatinine, globulin, glucose, GOT, GPT, GTP, hemoglobin, HBD, insulin, LDH, lipids, MAO, phosphorus, total protein, thyroxine, triglycerides, urea nitrogen*]
13. Masuyama, M. (1975): Biochemical variability of man. *Bull. int. stat. Inst., 40/4*, 476.
14. Masuyama, M. (1975): Kotaisa. In: *Rinsyô-yakuri*, pp. 225–261. Editor: Sunahara. Kôdansya.
15. Masuyama, M. (1975): Species difference of individual variability. *Rep. stat. appl. Res., 22*, 137.
16. Masuyama, M. (1975): A table of biochemical variabilities of man. *Rep. stat. appl. Res., 22*, 142.
17. Masuyama, M. (1975): Biochemical variability of a temporal variate. *Rep. stat. appl. Res., 22*, 184.
18. Masuyama, M. (1976): Individual variability of ages of onset and latent periods. *TRU Math., 12/2*, 93.
19. Masuyama, M. (1976): Stochastic models for quasi-constancy of biochemical individual variability. *Rep. stat. appl. Res., 23*, 103.
20. Masuyama, M. (1976): Quasi-constancy of individual variabilities of longevity in inbred mouse strains and of speed in human walking. *Rep. stat. appl. Res., 23*, 145.
21. Masuyama, M. et al. (1976): Quasi-constancy of individual variabilities with respect to nutritional intake. *Rep. stat. appl. Res., 23*, 147.
22. Masuyama, M. (1977): On the age-independence of biochemical individual variabilities. *TRU Math., 13/1*, 111.
23. Masuyama, M. (1977): Quasi-constancy of biochemical individual variability in a multi-compartment model. *TRU Math., 13/2*, 77.
24. Masuyama, M. (1977): Human biochemical individual variability. *Bull. int. stat. Inst., 47/4*, 326.
25. Masuyama, M. (1977): A mixture of two gamma distributions applied to rheumatoid arthritis. *Rep. stat. appl. Res., 24*, 82.
26. Masuyama, M. (1977): Individual variability of ages of onset of intractable diseases and incubation periods of infectious diseases. *Rep. stat. appl. Res., 24,* 200.
27. Masuyama, M. (1977): Seikagukuteki kotaisa no zyunkôzyôsei to sono kakuritumokei. *Ôyôtôkeigaku, 5/3*, 95.
28. Masuyama, M (1977): *Syôsûrei no Matomekata.* Takeutisyoten Sinsya.
29. Masuyama, M. (1978): Quasi-constancy of human individual variabilities of latent period of rabies and age at onset of puberty. *Rep. stat. appl. Res.,* to be published.
30. Masuyama, M. (1978): Ages at onset of a physiological or pathological phenomenon. A multi-compartment model. *TRU Math., 14/1*, 49.
31. Masuyama, M. (1978): Seikagakuteki ni mita kotaisa. *Sizen, 385*, 26.
32. Masuyama, M. (1978): Deterministic vs. stochastic model with regard to the age independency of biochemical individual variabilities. *TRU Math., 14/2*, 55.
33. Masuyama, M. (1978): Species difference of biochemical individual variabilities. Additive vs. multiplicative model. *TRU Math., 14/2*, 61.
34. Masuyama, M. (1978): Quasi-constancy of individual variability of blood pressure. *TRU Math., 14/2*, 49.
35. Mitruka, B.M. et al. (1977): *Clinical Biochemical and Hematological Reference Values in Normal Experimental Animals.* Masson et Cie., Paris. [*ACP, albumin, ALP,*

amylase, calcium, chloride, cholesterol, CPK, creatinine, α_1-globulin, α_2-globulin, γ-globulin, GOT, LDH, magnesium, total protein]

36. Nishizawa, T. et al. (1976): Some factors related to obesity in the Japanese SUMO wrestlers. *Amer. J. clin. Nutr., 29*, 1167. [*total protein*]
37. Oshima, T. et al. (Eds.) (1974): *Hito no Idenseikagaku*. Asakurasyoten. [*catalase*].
38. Salk, J.E. et al. (1954): Studies in human subjects on active immunization against poliomyelitis. II. *Amer. J. publ. Hlth, 44*, 994. [*Salk vaccine*]
39. *Sanhuzinka Deta Bukku* (1976): *Sanhuzinka no Sekai, Spec. Issue.* [*LDH_1, LDH_2, LDH_3, LDH_4, LDH_5*]
40. Siest, G. (Ed.) (1973): *Reference Values in Human Chemistry*. S. Karger, Basel [*glucose, potassium, uric acid*]
41. *SMON Hôkoku, 2.* [*pesticides*]

(All original papers written by the author in English and quoted in this paper can be found in *Human Biochemical Individual Variabilities and Their Quasi-constancy* published by the Research Institute of the Life Insurance Welfare, Yaesu 2-8-8, Tyûô-ku, Tokyo, 103.)

Note added in proof

Regarding age-dependency of σ_x, IgG is not exceptional if subjects are classified by disease. Their mean values will depend on disease, but σ_x's are almost the same and less than 0.3 (Masuyama, M., Individual variabilities of IgG in sera, *TRU Math.*, 1979, *15*, 77).

$h = a/k$ is actually a monotone increasing function of k, at least for IgG in serum and fibrinogen in plasma (Masuyama, M., Two notes on biochemical individual variabilities, *TRU Math.*, 1979, *15*, 79).

Unlike the case of smell, most elements in the correlation matrix of 17 free amino acids in serum are positive in men and in women (Masuyama, M. et al., Correlation matrix of free amino acids in serum, *TRU Math.*, 1980, *16* (to be published).

σ_x's of glycolytic enzymes of the Embden-Meyerhof pathway in red cells are almost the same and $\sigma_x<0.1$, even though the mean concentration varies markedly ($0.8\backsim2000$) (Masuyama, M., Quasi-constancy of biochemical individual variabilities of type I and II, *TRU Math.*, 1980, *16 (to be published)*.

DISCUSSION

Kato: When one pathway is fast, then the subsequent pathways are also fast. But in reality there both species differences and individual differences. In some people the second pathway may be slow. Likewise, the metabolic rate of one drug does not always parallel that of another drug in the same person. I think the difference in the pathways or in the enzyme involved causes the discrepancy in the rate of metabolism.

Masuyama: A similar discrepancy is observed for smell. Those who are sensitive to a certain type of smell may not be sensitive to another type. Thus with regard to the rate of drug metabolism, the correlations among some drugs are high, but rather low among others.

The neurotoxicity of the halogenated hydroxyquinolines*

GODFREY P. OAKLEY Jr.

Birth Defects Branch, Chronic Diseases Division,
*Bureau of Epidemiology, Center Disease Control, Atlanta, GA, U.S.A.***

An epidemic of 10,000 cases of a new gastrointestinal-neurologic syndrome – subacute myelo-optic neuropathy (SMON) – occurred in Japan between 1956 and 1970. Although the epidemic was recognized promptly and a multidisciplinary search for the etiologic agent was begun, investigators did not identify the agent for more than a decade. An astute clinical observation led to careful retrospective case-control and cohort studies that strongly implicated a halogenated hydroxyquinoline, iodochlorhydroxyquin, as the etiologic agent. These findings were announced publicly on August 7, 1970. On September 8, the Japanese government removed all the halogenated hydroxyquinolines from the market. Kono reported (1) that the epidemic had ended precipitously and, in a personal communication (June 16, 1972), reported that the epidemic had not recurred. There is little reason to doubt that the halogenated hydroxyquinolines were responsible for the epidemic of SMON.

As reported by the *Wall Street Journal* of April 11, 1972, there are those, however, who think the evidence implicating these compounds in the Japanese epidemic of SMON is 'inconclusive'. Cohn and Harun (2) suggest that the epidemic was resolving itself spontaneously before the drugs were removed from the market. If one considers the monthly incidence of new cases of SMON reported between January 1970 and January 1971 by the neurologists who were members of the SMON Research Commission (Fig. 1), there is no support for this contention (1). The monthly reported incidence rose steadily from 34 cases in February to 62 cases in July. Between January 1, 1970, and September 7, 1970, the neurologists reported 371 new cases of SMON, a monthly average of 45 new cases. Between September 8, 1970, and January 31, 1971, they reported only 19 cases, a monthly average of 4 cases. Six of these patients were known to have taken iodochlorhydroxyquin prior to the onset of the neurologic disease. The epidemic was not resolving prior to the banning of these drugs; on the contrary, the epidemic ended abruptly when these drugs were removed from the market.

Cohn and Harun (2) imply that the recent finding of a 'new' virus from a few patients with SMON means that a virus, not the drug, caused the epidemic. Even if it is shown conclusively that the newly discovered virus can cause a neurologic illness

*Reprinted by courtesy of the *Journal of the American Medical Association, July 23, 1973, Volume 225,* pp. 395–397.
**Reprint requests to 1600 Clifton Rd NE, Atlanta, GA 30333, U.S.A.

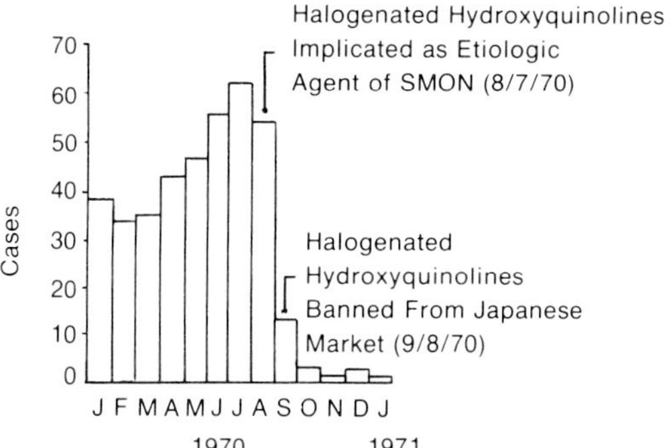

Fig. 1. Cases of subacute myelo-optic neuropathy (SMON) by month reported by 18 neurologists on the Japanese SMON Research Commission, January 1970 to January 1971. This figure was adapted after R. Kono (1).

in human beings, one cannot reason that the virus caused the epidemic of SMON. The shape of the SMON epidemic curve, with its precipitous drop, does not describe the natural course of an infectious disease epidemic. The epidemic curve of an infectious disease that is burning itself out in a community is skewed to the right with a gentle down-slope. The SMON curve is the curve of an epidemic that was suddenly ended by the introduction and widespread application of appropriate control measures. We know that the control measure was the removal of the halogenated hydroxyquinolines from the market and that there were no attempts to stop a viral epidemic.

Cohn and Harun (2) are impressed that not all cases of SMON have been associated with ingestion of iodochlorhydroxyquin prior to the onset of neurologic symptoms. They fail to note, however, that the overwhelming majority of SMON patients had taken the drug. For example, Tsubaki et al. (3) found that 96% (166 of 171) patients with SMON had taken iodochlorhydroxyquin prior to the onset of neurologic symptoms. Even proponents (4) of the viral cause hypothesis found that 79% of 113 patients with SMON had taken the drug prior to the onset of symptoms. Perhaps we should recall that although excessive oxygen to premature infants was shown to cause retrolental fibroplasia, there were some infants with the disease that had received no oxygen therapy (5). Those few cases do not invalidate the conclusion that excessive doses of oxygen caused the epidemic of retrolental fibroplasia in the 1940s. Likewise, one should not conclude that iodochlorhydroxyquin is safe merely because one cannot demonstrate that every patient with SMON ingested the drug prior to the onset of neuropathy.

WORLDWIDE DISTRIBUTION

Subacute myelo-optic neuropathy was epidemic only in Japan despite the fact that the halogenated hydroxyquinolines are marketed worldwide. The absence of epidemics in other countries, however, does not invalidate the conclusion that the halogenated hydroxyquinolines are neurotoxic. Clinicians from England (6–9), Australia (10), Switzerland (11), Sweden (12–15), Denmark (16), The Netherlands

(17) and the United States (18, 19) have described patients who developed neurologic symptoms while taking iodochlorhydroxyquin, diiodohydroxyquin, or broxyquinoline. The clinical symptoms of these patients were like the ones that characterized SMON. Moreover, the dosages and length of therapy associated with the onset of neurologic symptoms were similar to those noted in the histories of Japanese patients with SMON.

The work of McEwen and Constantinopoulos in England (8, 9) is particularly noteworthy because they observed prospectively the onset of neuropathy in 3 of 35 patients with intrinsic allergy treated for 3 months with 750 mg per day of iodochlorhydroxyquin. The first case had onset 6 weeks after starting treatment. One can conclude from this work that Englishmen are as susceptible as Japanese to the toxic effects of iodochlorhydroxyquin.

Differential susceptibility of patients to the halogenated hydroxyquinolines does not explain why the SMON epidemic was limited to Japan. Perhaps the reason for the lack of epidemics is that the drug-prescribing and drug-taking customs in other countries, fortunately, do not permit a large enough number of people to be exposed to enough of the drug for long enough to produce an epidemic. In the United States, for example, it is not sold without a prescription, so patients with chronic, non-specific gastrointestinal symptoms have not had access to the drugs over-the-counter for continued self-treatment. The only recommended reason for prescribing the drug is for the treatment of intestinal amebiasis. There are not enough patients in the United States with this disease to produce an epidemic.

TOXIC CLINICAL SYNDROME AND NEUROTOXIC DOSE-RESPONSE CURVE

Combining experience in Japan and elsewhere permits us to define the clinical neurologic syndrome associated with the use of halogenated hydroxyquinolines and to describe a neurotoxic dose-response curve for iodochlorhydroxyquin, the halogenated hydroxyquinoline most often associated with the development of neurologic symptoms. The clinical symptoms of patients taking halogenated hydroxyquinolines are primarily those of peripheral neuropathy or myelopathy, although cerebral manifestations have been noted (20). Symptoms range from minimal dysesthesia to death and include optic atrophy. Although many of the symptoms rapidly and markedly improve when the drug is discontinued, many patients have residual disease (10). Optic atrophy may progress to blindness after therapy stops (15). Some patients who have taken doses of 1,500 mg to 7,000 mg in 24 hours have had permanent retrograde amnesia (11, 16).

The neurotoxic dose-response curve for iodochlorhydroxyquin is as follows: at dosages of 750 mg per day for 4 weeks or less, there is little risk of toxic reactions (1, 8, 9, 18). Neurologic symptoms develop in approximately 1% of patients who take doses of 750 to 1,500 mg per day for less than 2 weeks (3, 21). Approximately 35% of patients who take doses of 750 to 1,500 mg per day for longer than 2 weeks develop symptoms (3, 22). A dose of as little as 1,800 mg per day can cause the onset of symptoms as early as the 5th day (21). At higher dosages, the onset of toxic reactions may occur as soon as 24 hours after beginning therapy (11, 16).

Two of the case reports are particularly enlightening because they demonstrate, in individual patients, important quantitative points of the iodochlorhydroxyquin neurotoxic dose-response curve. One of Selby's (10) patients took 500 to 750 mg of iodochlorhydroxyquin per day for more than a year without symptoms. Six weeks after he had begun to take 1,500 mg per day, neurologic symptoms developed. Kaeser and Wuthrich (11) report that neuropathy developed in a woman patient while she was taking 1,500 mg per day. The neuropathy improved when the dosage was lowered to 750 mg per day, but it became worse when the dosage was again increased to 1,500 mg per day.

DISCOVERY AND PREVENTION

The neuropathy caused by the halogenated hydroxyquinolines is preventable and at least partially reversible. We must, therefore, try to prevent new cases and to discover cases that have not been correctly diagnosed. The Japanese government met these aims by banning the sale of the drugs. The task is difficult wherever the drug is generally available.

Probably the largest group of Americans taking these drugs take it to prevent or treat traveler's diarrhea while on trips out of the country. A recent editorial (23) points out that these drugs have never been shown to be efficacious for this syndrome and warns against using them. Because the drugs are sold under a large number of different trade names, an American traveling out of the country may find it difficult to avoid being exposed to the drug if he buys any over-the-counter remedy for diarrhea.

The following partial list of tradenames is based on *The Merck Index (8th ed.,* 1968) and a report from Australia (24). The 54 names (grouped by generic name), under which the halogenated hydroxyquinolines are sold throughout the world show the difficulty one may have in avoiding one of these compounds:

Iodochlorhydroxyquin: Alchloquin, Amebil, Amoenol, Bactol, Barquinol, Budoformin, Chinoform, clioquinol, Cliquinol, Eczecidin, Enteroquinol, Enterozol, Entero-Septol, Entero-Vioform, Entrokin, Hi-Enterol, Iodoenterol, Nioform, Quinambicide, Rometin, Vioform.

Diiodohydroxyquin: Dinoleine, Diodoquin, Diodoxylin, Direxiode, Disoquin, Di-Quinol, Dyodin, Embequin, Enterosept, Floraquin, Ioquin, Moebiquin, Quinadome, Rafamebin, Searlequin, SS 578, Stanquinate, Yodoxin, Zoaquin.

Broxyquinoline (5,7-dibromo-8-quinolinol): Broxykinolin, Colepur, Colipar, Fenilor, Intestopan, Paramibe.

Chlorquinaldol (5,7-dichloro-2-methyl-8-quinolinol): Gynotherax, Gyno-Sterosan, Saprosan, Siogeno, Siosteran, Slosteran, Sterosan, Steroxin.

It seems prudent, therefore, to advise travelers to avoid buying any over-the-counter products.

Because of the risk of neurotoxicity, it is obvious that these drugs should not be used indiscriminately. Should a physician find it necessary to treat a patient with one of them, he should use as low a dose for as short a period of time as possible. There is good evidence to suggest that an oral daily dosage of 750 mg of iodochlorhydroxyquin for 2 weeks or less is relatively safe for adults. For the other halogenated hydroxyquinolines, there is less evidence on which to base recommendations as to safe doses. What data there are suggest that the toxicity of these compounds is a function of absorption. Knowing the iodochlorhydroxyquin neurotoxic dose-response curve and the absorption of the other derivatives (14), one can speculate that 750 mg of broxyquinoline, 2,250 mg of diiodohydroxyquin, or 250 mg of chlorquinaldol orally per day for less than 2 weeks would be relatively safe for an adult. Whenever these drugs are used, both patient and physician should watch for early signs and symptoms of neurotoxicity. The watch should be especially diligent should either the daily dosage or length of therapy exceed the limits described here.

Physicians in the United States should note that the Ciba Pharmaceutical Company recommends that iodochlorhydroxyquin (Entero-Vioform) be used in a dosage range (1,500 to 2,250 mg orally per day for 10 days repeated after 8 days of no therapy) that is in the neurotoxic dose-response curve (*Physicians' Desk Reference, 27th ed.*, 1972). Before prescribing doses in such high levels, physicians should recall that Yoshitake and Igata (22) observed the onset of neuropathy within 1 to 3 weeks after the onset of therapy in 44% (34 of 78) of the postoperative patients treated prophylactically with 1,350 mg per day of iodochlorhydroxyquin. None of 77 similar postoperative patients not treated with the drug had neuropathy.

The basic molecules of hydroxyquinoline and chloroquine are similar (14). Since chloroquine can cause deafness in infants prenatally exposed to it (25), one wonders if the halogenated hydroxyquinolines will subsequently be shown to be teratogenic. In any case, physicians should be cautioned against prescribing these drugs for pregnant women, since their safety in pregnancy has never been demonstrated.

Finding the undiagnosed cases of halogenated hydroxyquinoline neuropathy requires adding this neuropathy to the differential diagnosis of peripheral neuropathy and myelopathy. It is especially pertinent to look for this neuropathy in patients with chronic gastrointestinal disease who have unexplained neurologic symptoms.

REFERENCES

1. Kono, R. (1971): Subacute myelo-optico-neuropathy, a new neurological disease prevailing in Japan. *Jap. J. med. Sci. Biol., 24*, 195.
2. Cohn, H.D. and Harun, J.S. (1972): Entero-Vioform in traveler's diarrhea. *J. Amer. med. Ass. 220*, 276.
3. Tsubaki, T., Honma, Y. and Hoshi, M. (1971): Neurological syndromé associated with clioquinol. *Lancet, 1*, 696.
4. Shimada, Y. and Tsuji, T. (1971): Halogenated oxyquinoline derivatives and neurological syndromes. *Lancet, 2*, 41.
5. Silverman, W.A. (1955): Retrolental fibroplasia: role of oxygen. In: *Proceedings, 16th M & R Pediatric Research Conference, Columbus, Ohio, 1955*, p. 17. Editor: I.J. Filer Jr. M & R Laboratories, Columbus, OH.
6. Spillane, J.D. (1971): S.M.O.N. *Lancet, 2*, 1371.
7. Spillane, J.D. (1972): S.M.O.N. *Lancet, 1*, 154.
8. McEwen, L.M. (1971): Neuropathy after clioquinol. *Brit. med. J., 3*, 169.

9. McEwen, L.M. and Costantinopoulos, P. (1970): The use of a dietary and antibacterial regime in the management of intrinsic allergy. *Ann. Allergy, 28*, 256.
10. Selby, G. (1972): Subacute myelo-optic-neuropathy in Australia. *Lancet, 2*, 123.
11. Kaeser, H.E. and Wuthrich, R. (1970): Zur Frage der Neurotoxizität der Oxychinoline. *Dtsch. med. Wschr., 95*, 1685.
12. Osterman, P.O. (1971): Myelopathy after clioquinol treatment. *Lancet, 2*, 544.
13. Berggren, L. and Hansson, O. (1966): Treating acrodermatitis enteropathica. *Lancet, 1*, 52.
14. Berggren, L. and Hansson, O. (1968): Absorption of intestinal antiseptics derived from 8-hydroxyquinolines. *Clin. Pharmacol. Ther., 9*, 67.
15. Strandvik, B. and Zetterstrom, R. (1968): Amaurosis after broxyquinoline. *Lancet, 1*, 922.
16. Kjaersgaard, K. (1971): Amnesia after clioquinol. *Lancet, 2*, 1086.
17. Van Balen, A.T.M. (1971): Toxic damage to the optic nerve caused by iodochlorhydroxyquinoline (Entero-Vioform). *Ophthalmologica (Basel), 163*, 8.
18. Gholz, L.M. and Arons, W.L. (1964): Prophylaxis and therapy of amebiasis and shigellosis with iodochlorhydroxyquin. *Amer. J. trop. Med. Hyg., 13*, 396.
19. Etheridge, Jr., J.E. and Stewart, G.T. (1966): Treating acrodermatitis enteropathica. *Lancet, 1*, 261.
20. Sobue, I. et al. (1971): Myeloneuropathy with abdominal disorders in Japan. *Neurology, 21*, 168.
21. Nakae, K., Yamamoto, S. and Igata, A. (1971): Subacute myelo-optico-neuropathy (S.M.O.N.) in Japan. *Lancet, 2*, 510.
22. Yoshitake, Y. and Igata, A. cited by Kono (1).
23. Schulz, M.G. (1972): Entero-Vioform for preventing travelers' diarrhea (editorial). *J. Amer. med. Ass., 220*, 273.
24. Australian Drug Evaluation Committee (1971): Subacute myelo-optic-neuropathy and the halogenated hydroxyquinolines. *Med. J. Aust., 2*, 1090.
25. Smith, D.W. (1966): Dysmorphology. *J. Pediat., 69*, 1156.

DISCUSSION

Lunde: What do you think about the possibility of bioavailability differences between different brands of clioquinol?

Oakley: There is always a possibility, but I am impressed by the similarity as you go from country to country and not only different companies but different drugs themselves. There were 4 different halogenated hydroxyquinolines that had been reported to be toxic. And although bioavailability might be an issue, I would want to think that it wasn't until I saw some data that suggested that it was.

Mashford: The rising graphs of atrioseptal defect (ASD) and ventriculoseptal defect (VSD) and the other one, are rather alarming viewing really. Do you have any other anomalies which are pursuing a flat course or going down? It would be perhaps more convincing if you had some going up and some staying level.

Oakley: Certainly the clinicians in the United States feel that the increase in patent ductus arteriosus (PDA) is merely a function of an increase in viable low-birth-rate babies who on the average have an increased risk of having a PDA anyhow, and an increased awareness of the problem. It is a very important clinical decision in new-born nurseries in the United States to pick up babies with PDA. The VSD is not just among low-birth-rate babies and we are trying to find out whether that's ascertainment or not, but we don't have it yet.

One other point is that two birth defects are going down, namely anencephaly and spina bifida. They have been going down since the mid-30's and continue to drop slowly.

Walker: You noted that the general acceptance of the causal association is a separate stage in the process leading to the removal of a harmful agent in the environment. In your experience, do different kinds of epidemiologic studies differ in their persuasiveness for regulatory agencies?

Oakley: It varies. Data are, obviously, most persuasive when there are several case-control studies and cohort studies backed up by clinical opinion. On the other hand, a relationship can be so striking that causal inference can be made from case reports. That is the status with coumarin and lithium embryopathy. The single case-control study of 8 cases and 32 controls established the causal relationship between DES and vaginal carcinoma after in-utero exposure.

Dose-response relationships in prolonged intake of cumulative drugs

KAZUO FUKUTOMI

Department of Public Health Statistics, Institute of Public Health, Tokyo, Japan

The suspicion that a drug may cause a certain adverse effect sometimes arises after its coming on the market. In such cases epidemiological studies, as well as animal experiments, are usually conducted to reveal the causality. The first objective is to examine whether or not the association between the drug and the adverse effect is significant, the second is to test the existence of a dose-response relationship between them. The latter should make the association much stronger and will favor the causal hypothesis.

The threshold, the dose required to produce a response, varies among individuals of a population. The response rate to a given dose in the population, corresponds to the cumulative probability in the distribution of the threshold. The curve of cumulative probabilities, the dose-response curve, should be steadily increasing.

Experimentally, response rates to different doses can be estimated from some independent samples and if the dose-response curve increases steadily, a dose-response relationship is probable. If, on the other hand, the curve is not steadily increasing, the causal hypothesis is weakened.

The character of data from surveys may differ from that of experimental data and special analytical methods are required.

We take the dose-response problems associated with clioquinol (CQL) and SMON (Subacute Myelo-Optic Neuropathy) as an example.

When the clioquinol compound was extracted from the urine of SMON patients, SMON was suspected to be caused by CQL, and epidemiological data have supported this hypothesis. Various results demonstrated an association between CQL and SMON, but failed to prove a dose-response relationship between them. Because of this inconsistency some investigators criticized the hypothesis (see Meade, 1975 (1)).

Meanwhile, Nakae and the author (1974) pointed out the inappropriateness of the conventional method widely used for the estimation of dose-response curves on CQL and SMON data, and proposed a more appropriate method (2). In addition, Yamazoe et al. (1978) presented a test for the existence of dose-response relationships between CQL and SMON (3). The following section details the method and the analysis of CQL and SMON data.

METHOD AND ANALYSIS ON CQL AND SMON DATA

Studies on dose-response relations between CQL and SMON have been reported

(Nakae et al., 1974 (4); Kasai et al., 1972 (5); Yoshitake et al., 1971 (6)).

The observations comprise the total doses taken by patients prior to the onset of SMON symptoms, and total doses up to the withdrawal of treatment without any appearance of the symptoms. The total dose was termed the intensity of stimulus considering the cumulative effect of CQL. The data were classified into classes with intervals of equal length.

m_i is the number of the patients who had SMON symptoms in the total dose $t_{i-1} - t_i$, and n_i is the number of those who withdrew at the same total dose level. In the analysis of CQL and SMON data, the ratio $m_i/(m_i + n_i)$ was used to estimate the incidence rate.

Figure 1 illustrates dose-response curves obtained from the data of three hospital epidemiological surveys (4, 5, 6), showing, with one exception, a clearly decreasing effect at the highest doses. Unfortunately, this led to the conclusion that a dose-response relationship between CQL and SMON was not present.

According to epidemiological surveys, patients received a nearly constant daily dose in hospital. So we consider a model under the assumption that the daily dose is constant. This implies that the total dose up to the endpoint is proportional to the period of drug intake, and it can be considered as a survival problem with censored data.

Kaplan and Meier (1958) have proposed a bias-free approach (7), termed the life table method (see Appendix A.1). Nakae et al. (2) have analyzed the above data using the same method.

Figure 2 shows the estimated cumulative probabilities for the data in Figure 1 using the life table method. The curve obtained by this method should be always monotone increasing and, therefore, does not directly lead to the conclusion of a dose-response relationship.

The null hypothesis may also be considered. If SMON is not caused by CQL, but

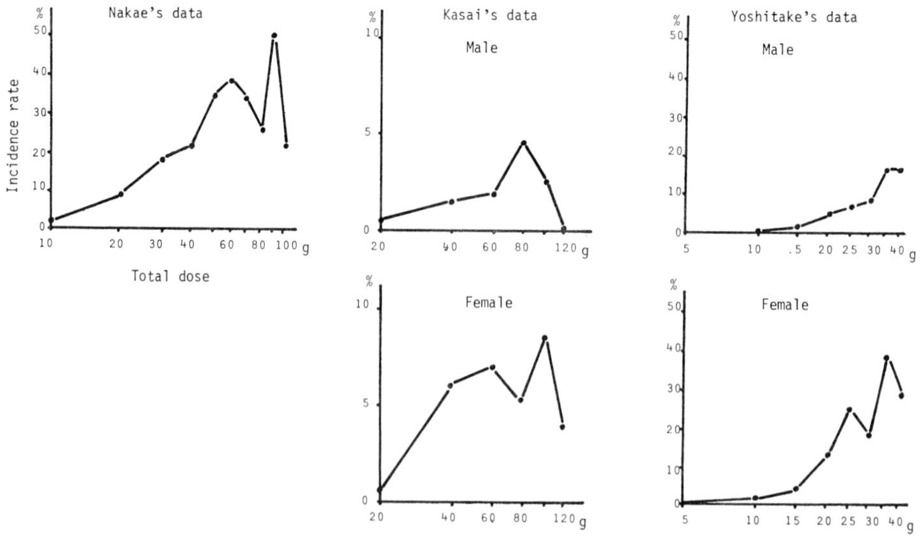

Fig. 1. Dose-response relationships between CQL and SMON for data from three epidemiological surveys.

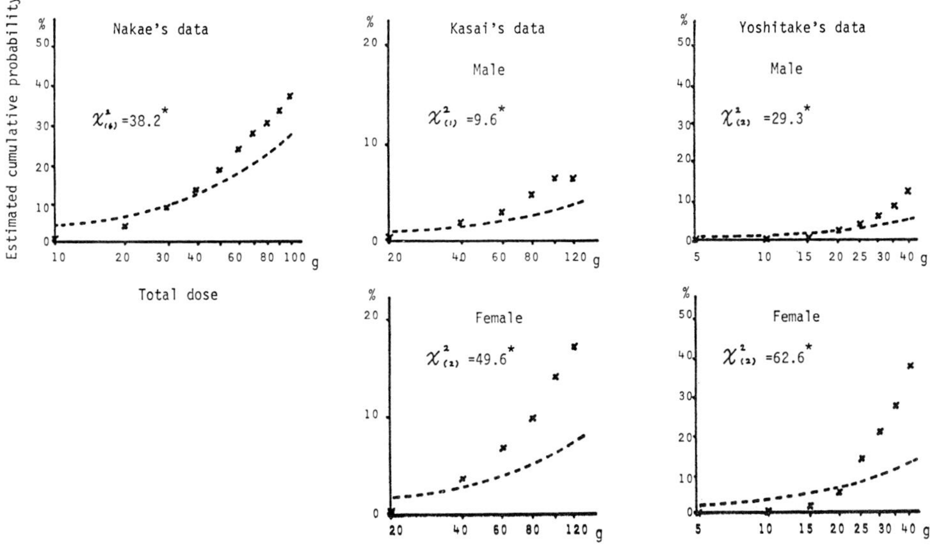

Fig. 2. Estimated cumulative probabilities from the life table method and estimated curves of cumulative probability from the exponential model (dotted line).

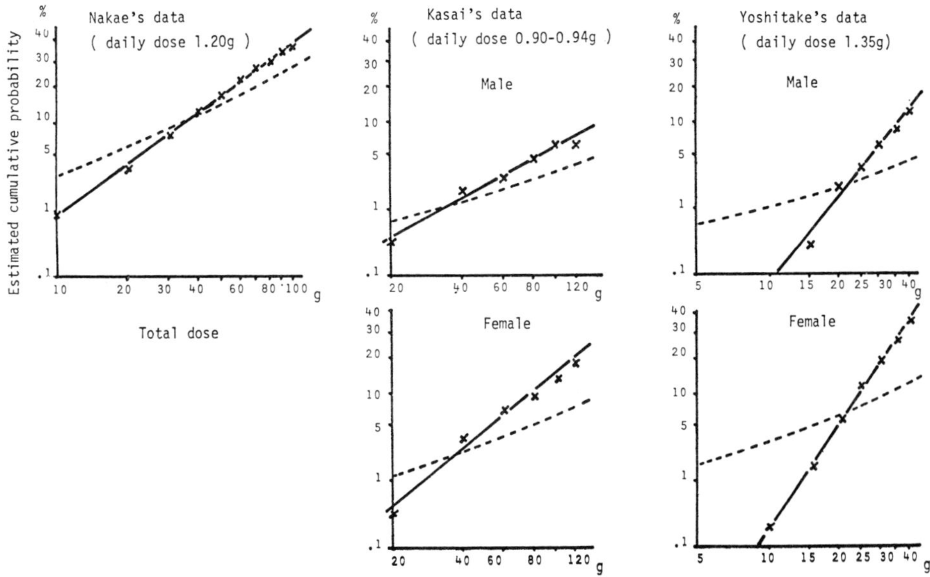

Fig. 3. Estimated cumulative probabilities of the life table method, estimated probit regression lines (solid line) and estimated curves of cumulative probability of the exponential model (dotted line) on lognormal paper.

by unknown factors affecting each patient independently of total CQL doses. It is natural to assume that the incidence of SMON only depends on the time-interval, implying that the time-interval up to the onset of symptoms is exponentially distributed.

A chi-square analysis can test the goodness-of-fit (see Appendix A.2), and the results are shown in Figure 2. The figures in parentheses with χ^2 represent the degrees of freedom for the chi-square test. The total dose level groups were assembled in such a way to make the predicted number greater than four. The null hypothesis was rejected at the 1% level of significance.

Figure 2 also shows that the estimated cumulative probabilities obtained from the exponential model do not coincide with the life table method.

In toxicological studies, the threshold dose is considered to be approximately lognormally distributed. This corresponds with the probit model. It is appropriate to examine whether the probit model applies here (see Appendix A.3). In Figure 3, the estimated cumulative probabilities of the life table method are plotted logarithmically and the probit regression lines estimated by the maximum likelihood method are drawn. The highest cumulative probability is at most 40%, and may not be high enough to allow fitting of the model. Nevertheless, it is clear that the probit model fits the data well, while the exponential model does not. The slope of probit regression lines varies from study to study. Slope variation may be explained by the daily dose.

SUMMARY

An attempt is made to describe the dose-response problem when a cumulative drug is given over a long period, using epidemiological data on CQL and SMON.

The analysis has three components: (1) estimating of cumulative probabilities by the life table method, (2) testing of the null hypothesis that an adverse effect is independent of total dose taken by patients, and (3) fitting the probit model.

These reanalyses revealed a dose-response relationship between CQL and SMON.

REFERENCES

1. Meade, T.W. (1975): Subacute myelo-optic neuropathy and clioquinol. An epidemiological case-history for diagnosis. *Brit. J. prev. soc. Med., 29*, 157.
2. Nakae, K. and Fukutomi, K. (1974): Epidemiological study on the relation between subacute myelo-optic neuropathy (SMON) and clioquinol (Report 1). A study on dose-response relationship between SMON and clioquinol. *Jap. J. publ. Hlth, 21*, 411 (in Japanese).
3. Yamazoe, S., Fukutomi, K. and Yanagimoto, T. (1978): On dose-response relationship between subacute myelo-optic neuropathy (SMON) and clioquinol. *Jap. J. publ. Hlth, 25*, 565 (in Japanese).
4. Nakae, K. and Shibata, T. (1974): Epidemiological study on the relation between subacute myelo-optic neuropathy (SMON) and clioquinol (Report 2). Relation between SMON and clioquinol in Y hospital, Okayama prefecture. *Jap. J. publ. Hlth, 21*, 607 (in Japanese).
5. Kasai, M., Kanemitsu, M. and Ito, Y. (1972): A study of dose-response relationship between doses of clioquinol and SMON incidences. Presented at Meeting of SMON Research Commission, 28th February 1972 (in Japanese).

6. Yoshitake, Y. and Ishiyama, I. (1971): On the relationship between SMON and clioquinol administration. *Igaku no Ayumi. 77*, 148 (in Japanese).
7. Kaplan, E.L. and Meier, P. (1958): Nonparametric estimation from incomplete observations. *J. Amer. Statist. Ass. 53*, 468.

APPENDIX

A.1 Estimation of cumulative probabilities by the life table method

Let T be a random variable representing the total dose required to produce the response and let k be the number of classes of total dose levels. The hazard rate π_i in the total dose $t_{i-1} - t_i$ and the cumulative probability P_i at the total dose t_i can be expressed as follows

$$\pi_i = P_r\{ t_{i-1} < T \leq t_i \mid t_{i-1} < T \}, \text{ and}$$

$$P_i = P_r\{ T \leq t_i \}, (i=1,2,\ldots,k).$$

Then,

$$P_i = 1 - \prod_{j=1}^{i} (1 - \pi_j).$$

The likelihood function of the outcome is given by

$$L = \prod_{i=1}^{k} (P_i - P_{i-1})^{m_i} (1 - P_i)^{n_i},$$

where n_k includes the number of persons exposed to the total dose over t_k.
It can be written in another form

$$L = \prod_{i=1}^{k} \pi_i^{m_i}(1 - \pi_i)^{N_i - m_i},$$

where $N_i = \sum_{j=1}^{i} (m_j + n_j)$.

From this, we can obtain the maximum likelihood estimators of π_i and P_i

$$\hat{\pi}_i = m_i/N_i, \text{ and}$$

$$\hat{P}_i = 1 - \prod_{j=1}^{i} (1 - \hat{\pi}_j), (i=1,2,\ldots,k).$$

A.2 Tests of goodness-of-fit for the exponential model

Under the hypothesis that T is exponentially distributed, the likelihood function of the outcome is given by

$$L = \prod_{i=1}^{k} (e^{-\lambda t_{i-1}} - e^{-\lambda t_i})^{m_i} (e^{-\lambda t_i})^{n_i},$$

where λ is a parameter of the exponential distribution.

The maximum likelihood estimates can be derived by an iterative method.

Suppose that the length of class interval is constant, say, h. This implies that π_i is equal to each other. Then, the likelihood function can be written by

$$L = \prod_{i=1}^{k} \pi^{m_i} (1 - \pi)^{N_i - m_i},$$

where $\pi = 1 - e^{-\lambda h}$.

In this situation, the maximum likelihood estimator of π becomes

$$\hat{\pi} = \sum_{i=1}^{k} m_i \,/ \sum_{i=1}^{k} N_i.$$

Then, we may obtain the expected number of persons with the response in the total dose $t_{i-1} - t_i$ as follows

$$e_i = N_i \pi, \; (i=1,2,\ldots,k).$$

Using this, the following χ^2 statistic for the goodness-of-fit test applies

$$\chi^2 = \sum_{i=1}^{k} (m_i - e_i)^2 / \, e_i \, (1 - e_i/N_i).$$

The statistic contains one estimator and is approximately distributed as the chi-square distribution with $k-1$ degrees of freedom under the null hypothesis.

A.3 Fitting the probit model

Under the assumption that T is lognormally distributed, the likelihood function of outcome is given by

$$L = \prod_{i=1}^{k} \{\Phi(a + b\log t_i) - \Phi(a + b\log t_{i-1})\}^{m_i} \{1 - \Phi(a + b\log t_i)\}^{n_i},$$

where $\Phi(\cdot)$ is the distribution function of the standard normal distribution and a and b are parameters to be estimated.

The maximum likelihood estimates of parameters can be obtained by the Newton-Raphson iterative method with the initial values $a_0 = b_0 = 0$.

DISCUSSION

Walker: Your data showed a very good fit to the probit regression line and there was no deviation at the lowest tail, which you suggested was the threshold. Do you see that result as in conflict with Dr. Oakley's assertion that low doses do not cause SMON?

Fukutomi: The slope of estimated probit regression line is obviously related to the amount of daily intake, so that a large amount of daily intake has a steeper probit line (see Fig. 3). If the daily intake is very low, fitness to the probit model may not be clear.

Thalidomide: Facts and inferences

W. LENZ

Institute of Human Genetics, University of Münster, Münster, Federal Republic of Germany

The marketing of thalidomide between 1957 and 1961 has raised new problems in the fields of pharmacology, pathology, teratology and medical practice. Not all of these problems can be solved by scientific and applied medicine. The drug trade, the duty of the state to protect the health of its citizens from damage, and the ethical problem of experiments on human beings necessarily connected with the introduction of any new drug had to be critically re-evaluated. Thalidomide was released for sale before carefully controlled animal and clinical experiments had been done. Large-scale human experimentation with no proper control of the results followed.

The thalidomide tragedy has led some people to form rash value judgements in defence of or against the pharmaceutical industry, often arrived at with obvious bias and without detailed knowledge and understanding. When several thousands of badly malformed babies are born as a consequence of human activities or omissions, one should not evade judgments of value. A purely legalistic evaluation may be insufficient. If the legal system of a country permits such a catastrophe to occur and to go undetected for several years, while a different system might have prevented it, then the system should be critically re-evaluated. Understandably, some pharmaceutical companies have felt excused, if the existing laws have not been violated. Any responsible and realistic discussion, however, should not only ask whether there was an offence against the legal system, but consider the possibility that the legal system itself may defend offences against basic human rights.

I am not going to discuss basic principles here, but I will try to elucidate the facts from which any evaluation should start. The first paper on thalidomide was published in August 1956 in the journal *Arzneimittelforschung*. In this paper, Kunz and co-workers described a cage invented for measuring the motor activity of mice. By comparing the summed-up whole-day activities of 3 groups of 8 mice each, they found roughly equal activities on 5 consecutive days. No comparable values for mice on thalidomide were published. There was, however, a graph showing that the motor activity of mice 10–180 min after the administration of 100 mg/kg thalidomide was less than 1/5 of a 'starting value', the meaning of which is not explained. All 6 curves showing the activity of mice on two different doses of thalidomide and on 4 other sedatives started from exactly the same point which, apparently, had only been determined for the pooled groups. No curve for animals without sedatives and only average values for an unknown number of animals were indicated. As mice have a diurnal rhythm of motor activity, as measurement was apparently not done for a constant number of mice per cage, and as they were fed by stomach tube, the results may show the tendency of mice to remain immobile after the shock, or decreased daylight activity or an influence of the number of animals in one cage, or a drug effect, or a combined effect of these factors. The authors claimed to have shown a sleep-inducing effect, though no sleep was observed. The authors apparently interpreted their results on the basis of previous experiments on human beings conducted in 1954 in which thalidomide was found to induce drowsiness and sleep. As the sleep-inducing effect of thalidomide is seen in man but not in mice, one could scarcely expect that any undesirable effects in man would be shown in animals. Kunz and co-workers administered thalidomide to rats, mice, guinea-pigs and rabbits for 30 days. They stated that they did not see morphological changes in erythrocytes or leukocytes. They do not say whether erythrocytes or leukocytes were counted. They said that the quantity and quality of urine were unchanged, but did not produce figures or define what they meant by 'quality' of urine. Body weight was said to have remained unchanged within normal variability. Again no figures were given. The authors said that the non-toxicity could not be explained by the low solubility of the substance, but that, in addition, extreme non-toxicity of the substance had to be assumed. No argument in favor of this statement was advanced. Somers, of Distillers Company, who reported similar results in 1960, attributed the relative non-toxicity of thalidomide to its low solubility.

In the same number of *Arzneimittelforschung*, a paper on 'Clinical experience with a new sedative' was published by Jung. The clinical part of the report starts with the assertion: 'In a material of more than 300 patients we satisfied ourselves of the non-toxicity of the substance.' Dosage was mostly 3 times 200, 100, 50 or 25 mg/day, but no figures of the total time or of the total dosage were given. Jung stated without supporting figures that in 20 patients with enlarged livers and pathological liver function tests no deterioration of liver function had occurred. Likewise without any figures he said that in 20 patients the 'blood picture' showed no changes after 4–6 weeks therapy and that in 5 patients the blood sugar and steroids were uninfluenced. In 50 patients with thyrotoxicosis, hyperthyroidism and vegetative dystonia an 'excellent therapeutical effect' was claimed, again with no apparent attempt at objective evaluation. Four cases without specified diagnosis from this group were mentioned as demonstrating an effect on basal metabolic rate, which was lowered from values between +25 and +68% to values between −2 and +8%. The author recommended: 'In many cases one will be able to do without thyrostatic drugs or to reduce their dosage.' In addition, thalidomide had been administered to an unknown number of patients with pulmonary tuberculosis, and a favorable impression was noted. The author said 'We create, therefore, with K 17 good conditions for the process of healing.' Jung likewise avoided quantitative data when dealing with side-effects: 'At overdosage of K 17, there may be even at daytime an undesirable sleepiness, giddiness, unrest, tremor and obstipation. The side-effects, however, subside soon after discontinuing the preparation or after reducing the doses; they can almost certainly be avoided, if dosage is not too high. Generally, it may be stated that women should be given lower doses than men, because women are more prone to undesirable side-effects.' The paper by Jung is a collection of subjective opinions which apparently were not systematically called for, carefully protocolled, counted, controlled or statistically evaluated. The question how such papers could be accepted by a journal with the title *Arzneimittelforschung*, i.e. 'Drug Research', has not been adequately discussed.

Judging from my own experience, I suppose that fear of personal and legal conflicts is one of the main obstacles to honest discussion. The lack of critical discussion on drug-promoting papers and on the editorial policy of journals which accept them is a weak point at an important junction in the system of drug marketing.

In November 1956, thalidomide was marketed for the first time in Hamburg under the name of Grippex. Neither Jung's nor Kunz's paper contains any argument for the reputed favorable effect of thalidomide on influenza. Kunz and co-workers claimed that thalidomide lowered body temperature raised by intravenous application of dead *E. coli* bacteria in rabbits. Again, neither the number of animals nor the magnitude of the effect was disclosed. In 1957, thalidomide was put on the market under the name Contergan. During the last 4 months of 1957, however, only 33 kg were sold. From 1957 to 1958 the sales figures increased 22-fold, from 1958 to 1959 again 5-fold, and from 1959 to 1960 once again 4-fold to 14,060 kg, i.e. in 3 years 440-fold.

Symptoms typical of neuropathy were reported in some of the very first clinical trials of thalidomide. Since 1959 increasing numbers of cases of severe neuropathy were reported in patients on thalidomide. Chemie Grünenthal approached Dr. Heinrich in Hamburg, an expert on vitamins, to discuss with him a research program with the aim of finding out whether thalidomide neuropathy could, as suspected on theoretical grounds, be due to an antivitamin activity of thalidomide. Chemie Grünenthal thought the costs of such a research program, estimated at 1 million DM by Heinrich, to be prohibitive and thus abandoned the idea. At that time, antivitamins were well-known experimental teratogens. Thus, the discussion of an antivitamin effect of thalidomide might have led to the suspicion that thalidomide might be teratogenic. Unfortunately, at that time the balance of decisions by pharmaceutical firms was heavily weighted in favor of promotion as compared to research on side-effects, probably because pharmaceutical firms were not generally held legally responsible for side-effects if they could produce some experimental evidence of a lack of side-effects in animals. The sum of 1 million DM does not appear to be excessive. According to a study in the USA, the costs of promotion are on average 25% of the final price of drugs. In 1960 and 1961 Chemie Grünenthal sold thalidomide for 23 million DM in Germany. In addition, almost 25% of the home consumption was exported and there was also some profit from licences. Thus, in 1960 and in 1961, the total sales figures for thalidomide were probably higher than 25 million DM. Financial arguments were possibly not decisive. At that time, the metabolism and the biochemical action of thalidomide were unknown. Thus, research might have been expected to lead not to a safer product, but to the recognition that the desired and the undesirable effect might be biochemically identical and thus inseparable.

The first patient with thalidomide embryopathy, a girl with bilateral anotia and deafness, was born on the 25th of December, 1956, at Stolberg, the site of the Grünenthal plant. Her father, who was working for the firm in 1956, got the drug from one of the firm's leading scientists and gave it to his wife who took it from March to May, 1956. Another case, in which a sample of thalidomide was handed to a pregnant woman before the drug was put on the market, was born on the 3rd of May, 1958, with bilateral aplasia of the radius and the thumbs. The drug was entered on the doctor's case-sheet on the 42nd postmenstrual day, but since the

TABLE 1

Country	Acknowledged cases of thalidomide embryopathy (no.)	Total sales of thalidomide (kg)
Ireland	32	247
Belgium	28	258
Brazil	23	?
Netherlands	14	110
Finland	10	67
Switzerland	10	113
Portugal	8	37
Syria	5	200
Austria	4	211
Spain	4	?
Mexico	2	156
Peru	2	10
Ghana	1	29
Sudan	1	60
Cyprus	1	<10
Pakistan	1	<10
Nicaragua	1	<10
Mozambique	1	27

administration of a new drug in pregnancy at that time was not understood as an experiment in human teratology, the outcome was not linked with the intake of the drug. The first case to be published was that of Weidenbach, a Munich gynecologist, who reported in 1959 on a child with phocomelia of arms and legs born on the 10th of November, 1958. Weidenbach was unable to trace an exactly similar case in the German literature or in the records of the Bavarian Institution for Crippled Children which were available back to its foundation in 1913. Six years after the birth of the child, Weidenbach found by renewed special research into the mother's history that she had been given Grippex, a thalidomide-containing drug, for a febrile condition between the 25th and 35th day after conception. In 1959, I saw my first patient, born on the 14th of August, 1959, with thalidomide phocomelia. When I suspected a thalidomide etiology two years later, a detailed history-taking and searching the family's apartment for drugs failed to trace the drug. Eventually, however, the father found the rest of the package, and even the date of prescription – October 21, 1958 – could still be seen in the doctor's notes.

At the meeting of the German Pediatric Association in Kassel from September 26 to 28, 1960, Kosenow and Pfeiffer exhibited photographs and X-rays of two cases of a new syndrome. The first case presented aplasia of both radii, shortened ulnae and humeri, absence of thumbs, hypoplastic femora, aplasia of the left tibia, deformity of the left fibula, clubfoot on the right side, duodenal stenosis and capillary hemangioma of the upper lip. The second case showed aplasia of the radii, shortened ulnae, hypoplasia of thumbs, aplasia of femora and tibiae, bilateral clubfoot, hypoplasia of the first toes, duodenal stenosis and capillary hemangioma of the upper lip. As both children had been born on consecutive days (February 28 and 29, 1960) in the same small town in Westphalia, the idea of a common exogenous cause came immediately to mind. Only a few years later, however, did an investigation disclose that one mother had been prescribed thalidomide on the 44th postmenstrual day and the other on the 46th day.

Professor Fanconi of Zürich, one of the most experienced European pediatricians and an expert in rare syndromes, commented that he had never seen anything similar before. It was unfortunate that Weicker, who up to 1960 had seen 4 similar cases, was on a trip to Japan. In early 1961 he saw 3 or 4 additional cases and felt certain that there must be an exogenous agent behind these cases.

The details of the early thalidomide story show that the suspicion and final confirmation of the teratogenicity of thalidomide came later than necessary. More attention to the potentially damaging effects on the fetus, as discussed in a great many papers up to 1959, would have prevented malformations of thousands of babies.

Even after the suspicion became known worldwide, thalidomide did not immediately disappear from all dispensaries. But for the laudable activity of the newspapers, the process of withdrawing the drug would have been still more clandestine, slow and inefficient. In April, 1962, at a press conference in Hamburg, I believed in the assertion of a representative of Grünenthal that at that time there was no more thalidomide on the market in any country. This was a big mistake, for the consequences of which I am very sorry.

DISCUSSION

Lunde: Professor Lenz, you made an important point of the fact that more or less inappropriate toxicological data were published and misinterpreted as well. I agree with you that the editors of scientific journals should be cautious in what they accept. However, I feel even more disturbed by another problem which is still relevant, usually that a number of preclinical data are never released by the producer, for the sake of confidentiality and competition. Do you see any solution to this aspect of these complex problems?

Lenz: This is a difficult legal, ethical and practical problem. My ideas on it are probably utopian. I feel that no medical doctor employed by a pharmaceutical firm should be responsible only to the salesmen of the firm, and that in case of conflict the final decision should be with the medical doctor. This, of course, would not work without some sort of outside control of the medical men working for pharmaceutical firms by some agency of the state or of an independent professional body. Independence of a state agency or of a professional body is another problem not easily solved if billions of dollars are at stake. I would not accept any system which entitles a medical doctor to withhold any relevant information from a supervising agency.

Oakley: You suggest that premarketing clinical trials of thalidomide might have decreased the number of affected babies. I wonder if that is so. For example, currently in the United States, there is a 'teratology catch 22'. Pregnant women are almost always excluded from premarketing trials, yet they become exposed soon after marketing. Do you have a solution to this dilemma?

Lenz: You certainly point to an unsolved ethical problem. If clinical trials are basically experiments on human beings, one may reach the extreme position that there is no justification whatsoever for developing new drugs. This, however, would mean that there would be no more progress and that, in the final balance, there could possibly be more human suffering. If there is, on the other hand, as I suppose it is, far more motivation by profit or by ambition than by truly humanitarian aims, then one should not embark on any new development unless there is a reasonable chance that the benefits will outweigh the risks of experiments on human beings. The difficulty is that one cannot know in advance what the chances will be. So again, while I deeply deplore the present situation, I have no solution to offer.

Oakley: Isn't it true that as soon as a drug is marketed, we actually wind up doing the experiment in pregnant women anyhow? At least we do half the experiment. We expose women or they expose themselves and yet we don't follow up systematically to find out what happens to those women. That would seem to be a partial solution to the dilemma.

Lenz: I think you are right. One solution, therefore, would be that this very experimentation really should be considered as an experiment and should be protocolled and followed, because what happened is very poor experimentation with no proper control, with no proper follow-up. Hence the story is in some way similar to what happened with Mexaform and Entrokinol which were still at the experimental stage without good follow-ups. If doctors had realized that giving drugs might be harmful, every doctor would have then realized that the SMON catastrophe might have caused less than 1% of the actual victims.

Kono: I have read a report that the intake rate of thalidomide among mothers who delivered phocomelia babies was about 80%. Is this figure correct? If so, is it possible to elevate this intake rate by a more intensive survey?

Lenz: Phocomelia is not an exact concept, so 80% has no very exact meaning. If, as has sometimes been done, phocomelia is used as a fashionable but vague word for a great variety of limb malformations, one may arrive at almost any percentage of non-thalidomide cases. If, however, phocomelia is reserved for such cases as are morphologically indistinguishable from cases with a well-documented thalidomide history, then probably less than 1 or 2% of phocomelia cases born in 1960 or 1961 were non-thalidomide cases. Such cases do occur on a genetic basis, though they are very rare, e.g. the Holt-Oram syndrome, which is an exact copy of some type of thalidomide embryopathy. Another question, of course, is that a genuine thalidomide case, for various reasons, may not show a positive thalidomide history.

Nagai: Dr. Lenz, this question might be out of touch with reality, but do you think thalidomide should be removed from the market even if it is not used by pregnant women? For instance, women who have no more possibility of pregnancy might take it. Do you think that thalidomide is too toxic to use in medical fields other than pregnancy?

Lenz: Thalidomide causes polyneuropathy, if it is taken for some time. I am not an expert on that type of side-effect, but most of my colleagues working at the neurology department felt that the neuropathy alone would have been a sufficient argument to remove thalidomide from the market. One could argue that thalidomide may still be useful if taken only on special occasions. Any soporific, however, tends to be taken chronically. In addition, there always remains some risk that the substance may inadvertently be taken by a pregnant woman. I feel that this risk, however small it may be, outweighs the potential but doubtful merits of the drug. On the other hand, thalidomide is most helpful in leprosy. Here, under strictly controlled conditions, it has won its place in therapy.

Chairman: I think you all have noticed that time is unfortunately out, and I will just close this session, together with my co-chairman, by reminding you that we are still quite blind, similar to the seven blind men who are approaching the elephant, and reaching a diagnosis which was very different depending upon where they hit the animal. Hopefully, this meeting and this session have brought us a bit further towards daylight.

Data analysis of clinical trials in Japan

SHIGEKOTO KAIHARA

Hospital Computer Center, University of Tokyo Hospital, Tokyo, Japan

Clinical trials are one of the most difficult forms of research in the field of medicine. One reason for the difficulty seems to stem from the fact that many different factors are involved, such as clinical, pharmacological, statistical and ethical. These problems in different fields are intermingled and are often confronted with each other in the study of clinical trials.

In Japan a great number of clinical trials are performed annually and articles are published in medical journals. In spite of this, strangely enough, there are few clinical pharmacologists who are supposed to undertake these clinical trials in Japan. For clinical trials, it is generally believed that three types of researchers are required, namely clinicians, clinical pharmacologists and medical statisticians. However, there are very few departments of clinical pharmacology and not a single department of medical statistics in Japanese medical schools.

In this connection, it seemed meaningful to find out who is undertaking clinical trials in Japan and how they are carried out. This study is an attempt to approach this problem using articles published in medical journals.

In the past 3 years, 120 articles on clinical trials published in 52 medical journals were analyzed. The medical journals included both professional and commercial journals. Case or uncontrolled studies were excluded so that only controlled trials were analyzed. The survey focussed on 3 items: the organizer of clinical trials and his field, the people responsible for experimental design and data analysis, and the method of data analysis.

The results revealed all the organizers of the trials (chairmen of the committees, etc.) to be clinicians in medical schools. About two-thirds of the teams were solely clinicians and one-third contained pharmacologists and/or statisticians. In teams without statisticians, clinicians with experience in this field were responsible for the experimental design and data analysis.

The number of clinics participating ranged from 1 to 55, and 6 to 10 clinics participated in about 30% of all the trials. The mean number of clinics was 13.4.

The number of cases used for the study ranged from 20 to 610 cases with a distribution as shown in Table 1.

For comparison, 40 studies used inactive placebo and 88 used drugs with similar actions. Among these, 18 studies used both placebo and active drugs.

TABLE 1. *Number of cases for study*

No. of cases	10–50	50–100	100–150	150–200	200–
Trials found	10	28	26	14	10

The fields of those responsible for data analysis (usually 'controllers') are shown in Table 2. In about 72% clinical medicine was a primary field and in 18% pharmacology or a related field was primary. No departments of medical statistics participated and all mathematicians or statisticians belonged to other schools such as engineering or sociology.

The types of design adopted are shown in Table 3. More than 90% of the designs were group comparative trials with simple randomization. Crossover trials comprised about 9% and matched pair trials were rare.

Items used for background data on patients numbered 4 to 17 and the number of items for evaluating efficacy of drugs 3 to 20. About 40% of cases measured 6 to 10 items for evaluation, half being laboratory data. Half of the evaluation items were usually clinical symptoms which included the general impression of physicians. This item was regarded as most important in assessing drug efficacy in the final stages. Some trials standardized the evaluation methods, but these were limited.

In most comparative trials, analytical procedures were similar, namely to compare all background data between groups (to prove that there is no difference); to compare each evaluating item in two groups (to prove there is some difference); to stratify evaluating data by background data and to compare evaluating items in each stratum; to compare adverse effects between two groups; and finally to compare some integrated measures of evaluation between two groups. Parametric or non-parametric tests were used depending on the nature of the scale. Data analysis by multivariate techniques was rare. In paired analysis a few studies used the sequential analysis of Armitage.

The above results characterize clinical trials in Japan as follows. Firstly, clinicians play an important role in trials including experimental design and data analysis. Since there are few medical statisticians and clinical pharmacologists, clinicians often take on these roles. Secondly, the design and method of analysis did not vary and most trials used uniform methods, usually a simple group comparison. The number of cases studied usually depends on past experience and the design of case

TABLE 2. *Persons responsible for experimental design and data analysis*

	Clinicians	Pharmacists	Researchers in				
			Pharmacology	Basic medicine	Mathematics	Engineering	Social sciences
Trials found	84	6	15	4	4	2	2

TABLE 3. *Type of design adopted*

Group comparative trial	Simple randomization	95
	Stratified randomization	2
Matched pair trial		6
Randomized block		1
Crossover trial		10

numbers based on statistical considerations is not widely used. Evaluating data are usually not analyzed intensively along with background data. The present methods in clinical trials are far from complete and new methods of design and analyses must be continuously developed; such methodological trials were very rare, a fact possibly related to the lack of medical statisticians.

In more than half of the studies, active drugs were used for comparison and the aim of the trials was only to show no differences between two drugs. However, statistically, it is insufficient in tests of efficacy simply to prove no difference between two drugs. More careful consideration is demanded in studies of this type.

There were no single Phase IV clinical trials in Japan.

In conclusion, most clinical trials in Japan are organized and executed by clinicians. Collaboration with clinical pharmacologists and medical statisticians is required in the future. There are, however, few such investigators in Japan and ways must be found to increase their numbers.

DISCUSSION

Lunde: We have recently performed almost exactly the same type of study at our 2000 bed hospital as you have described here. In Norway all clinical trials on new drugs as well as tests for new indications should be reported to the health authorities for their consideration. For the period 1974 to 1977, 146 trials were reported from our hospital and nearly half of these were never started or were interrupted mainly because of insufficient planning. At the end only about 20% of the trials resulted in publication. We feel therefore that much more attention should be given to the design and planning of clinical trials, thus avoiding at least a waste of resources and also acknowledging the need for teamwork. What was the frequency of publication in your report? Do you have any figures on that?

Kaihara: I do not have any exact figures, but I think more than 90% because most clinical trials in Japan are undertaken to obtain data for approval of drugs and for that purpose published papers are usually required. Most people who perform these clinical trials really want to have them published. I was very much interested in your comment that a very high percentage of the studies are interrupted. What is the cause of this?

Lunde: Mostly due to lack of patients, which means lack of planning.

Melmon: What do you think are the major reasons for the implied underdevelopment of clinical pharmacology in a country that uses so many drugs and is so advanced in other ways?

Kaihara: I don't think I am in a good position to answer that because I am not a clinical pharmacologist. However, my personal opinion is that pharmacologists are generally more interested in pure science than in the clinical applications of drugs. Thus in most departments of pharmacology more emphasis is given to basic than to clinical research. I think this is the general trend in various fields in Japan but I can't give you a reason for it.

Importance of clinical pharmacokinetics in the prevention of adverse drug reactions

TAKASHI ISHIZAKI

Division of Clinical Pharmacology, Clinical Research Institute, National Medical Center Hospital, Tokyo, Japan

For many drugs, the doses required for optimal therapeutic effects vary among patients; the same dose produces few effects in some patients while it is seriously toxic in others (1, 2). The frequency and severity of this phenomenon must be considered in relation to benefit-risk interrelations between the disease and drug efficacy. In general, conventional drugs can be only satisfactory when the therapeutic margins are large, and potent drug therapy becomes safer and more effective when dosage regimes are adjusted to the specific need and tolerance of a patient.

CLINICAL PHARMACOKINETICS AND MAINTENANCE OF OPTIMUM DRUG CONCENTRATION

How are optimal drug doses for individual patients determined? Pharmacokinetic principles must be applied to each patient. Clinical pharmacokinetics characterizes the time course of drug absorption, its distribution, metabolism and excretion, and relates them to the intensity and time course of therapeutic and adverse effects of drug (3–5). For many drugs, the therapeutic and toxic effects are correlated with the plasma concentrations rather than the doses (1, 2). Thus, the individual approach to drug therapy is vital to maintain both optimal therapy and prevent adverse drug reactions, the rationale being to obtain therapeutic effectiveness without adverse drug reaction(s).

PRINCIPLES OF CLINICAL PHARMACOKINETICS

Table 1 gives pharmacokinetic information concerning the monitoring of the steady-state drug concentration in the plasma or serum of patients under treatment. A simple example is that of the continuous constant intravenous infusion (R_{inf}) of a drug eliminated by apparent first-order kinetics characterized by the rate constant (K_{el}) (Fig. 1). During infusion, the plasma drug concentration gradually increases until the rate of elimination or drug clearance [volume of distribution (V_d) multiplied by the elimination rate constant (K_{el})] equals R_{inf} and the steady-state or plateau concentration is reached.

When the infusion time (T) is sufficiently long, the equation:

TABLE 1. *Determinants required to adjust optimum therapeutic drug concentrations in an individual patient*

Step I
Parameters dependent on clinical pharmacokinetics
Range of effective plasma level ($C_{min} - C_{max}$)
Volume of distribution (V_d)
Biological half-life ($t_{1/2}$) or elimination rate constant (K_{el})
Step II
Physician- and patient-dependent parameters
Dosing interval (τ)
Dose (D)
Drug handling under special clinical conditions (e.g. renal failure)

$$C = \frac{R_{inf}}{V_d \cdot K_{el}} (1 - e^{-K_{el}T})$$

can be expressed as (5 – 7):

$$C = \frac{R_{inf}}{V_d \cdot K_{el}} \quad (1)$$

Since the volume of distribution multiplied by the elimination rate constant is equal to the plasma clearance (Cl) the above equation becomes:

$$R_{inf} = C \cdot Cl \quad (2)$$

The intravenous infusion rate can be thus adjusted to produce the desired therapeutic concentration (C), if elimination rate constants, volumes of distribution or plasma clearance of drugs are known. Accordingly, the pharmacokinetics of drugs alongside their pharmacokinetics must be fully examined before any marketing proceeds. The development of new analytical methods has allowed determination of very low drug concentrations. Such techniques, including gas-liquid chromatography, high-pressure liquid chromatography, enzyme immunoassay, radioimmunoassay, and gas-chromatography mass-spectrometry, can determine nanogram amounts of serum or saliva. Since the pharmacokinetic studies of many drugs are, or have been, undertaken in clinical pharmacology laboratories, the sensitive analytical equipment should be provided with appropriate support on a nationwide basis. This approach must produce a more rational drug design and usage.

If constant doses of a drug are administered either orally, parenterally, or by other routes at regular intervals of time (τ), the plasma concentrations will fluctuate between maximal and minimal (Fig. 2). Clearly the steady-state concentrations indicated in Figure 2 will be influenced by many factors. The average steady-state concentration ($\overline{C}$) may be given as:

$$\overline{C}_{\infty} = (1.44 \cdot f \cdot D \cdot t_{1/2})/V_{d}\tau \quad (3)$$

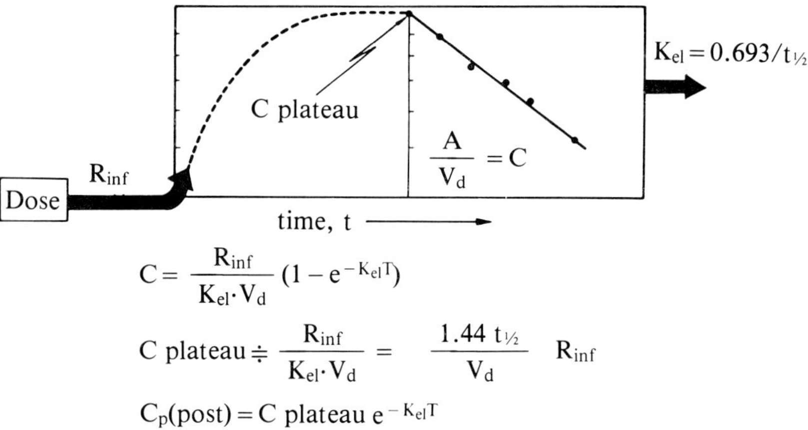

Fig. 1. Schematic illustration of plasma level profile in relation to pharmacokinetic equations. The infusion rate can be adjusted (R_{inf}) to achieve a desired maximum plasma concentration (C plateau) if clinical pharmacokinetic parameters such as K_{el} or $t_{1/2}$, and V_d are known. K_{el} = first-order rate elimination constant; $t_{1/2}$ = biological half-life; V_d = volume of distribution; t = post-infusion time; C = plasma concentration; C_p (post) = plasma concentration at post-infusion time; e = natural logarithm; T = infusion time; A = amount of drug remaining in body after infusion has ceased.

where $\bar{C}_\infty$ = steady-state plasma concentration, f = fraction absorbed, D = dose, $t_{1/2}$ = half-life of the drug, V_d = volume of distribution, and τ = dosing interval.

The plasma concentration obtained by intravenous infusion does not entail absorption as a controlling factor. In other cases the fraction delivered to the systemic circulation, the bioavailability of the drug reflecting mainly hepatic

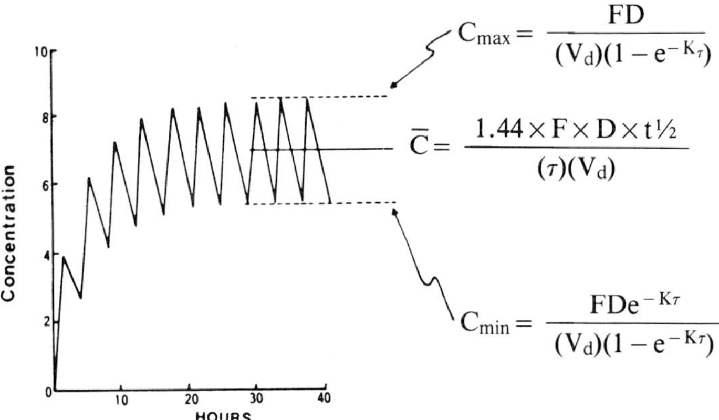

Fig. 2. Schematic illustration of plasma level profile of a drug with half-life ($t_{1/2}$) of 6 hr when this drug is administered at the dosing interval (τ) of the $t_{1/2}$. One can theoretically adjust the dosage to optimize plasma concentrations by converting equations shown. C_{max} = maximum steady-state therapeutic concentration; $\bar{C}$ = mean steady-state concentration; C_{min} = minimum steady-state concentration; F = fraction of dose (D) absorbed (= bioavailability); K = first-order rate elimination constant; V_d = volume of distribution.

metabolism, is a major and a quite variable determinant. For many drugs the relation between the amount administered orally and the resulting concentration in the body, thereby the pharmacological effect(s), is unpredictable. As shown in Figure 2, the mean steady-state concentration is influenced by the bioavailability of the dosage form used, by the completeness of gastrointestinal absorption of the dose, by body size or distribution of fluid compartments through which the drug dissolves and by the elimination half-life. All these determinants are subject to individual variations and of these the rate of elimination is quantitatively the most important.

MODIFIED PHARMACOKINETICS IN DISEASE STATES: EXAMPLE OF RENAL FAILURE

Disease-related disturbances in cardiac, hepatic, and renal function are also responsible for much variation in the biological half-life of drugs; drugs are metabolized or eliminated by hepatic or renal mechanisms and the heart supplies blood to these two major organs. In this respect, drug plasma or serum levels become useful indices for dosage adjustments when the therapeutically optimum range of serum concentrations has been defined clinically (1, 2, 7, 8). Even in cases of renal failure, certain pharmacokinetic parameters such as half-life or elimination rate constant and the fraction of the dose excreted unchanged in urine of normal patients are pertinent for adjusting dosages and preventing toxicities of drugs (9):

$$\frac{\bar{t}_{1/2}}{t_{1/2}} = \frac{1}{f_u\,(\bar{C}_{cr} / C_{cr} - 1) + 1} \tag{4}$$

where $t_{1/2}$ and $\bar{t}_{1/2}$ are the drug half-lives in patients with normal and abnormal renal function, f_u the fractions excreted unchanged in urine at normal creatinine clearances (C_{cr}), and $\bar{C}_{cr}$ the creatinine clearance in patients with impaired renal function.

To obtain a correction factor (G) for adjusting the dose ($\bar{D}$) or the dosing interval ($\bar{\tau}$) for patients with renal impairments, the following equation can be derived from equation (4) (10, 11):

$$G = \frac{\bar{K}_{el}}{K_{el}} = 1 - f_u\left(1 - \frac{\bar{C}_{cr}}{C_{cr}}\right) \tag{5}$$

$$\bar{D} = DG \tag{6}$$

$$\bar{\tau} = \tau/G \tag{7}$$

In the above equations, $\bar{K}_{el}$ is the elimination rate constant in patients with renal impairment, D and τ the usual dose and dosing interval in patients without renal abnormalities. The importance of clinical pharmacokinetic studies with monitoring of plasma drug levels is obvious if adverse drug reactions or toxicity are to be prevented and optimal drug concentrations in particular patients are to be achieved.

Other important aspects of clinical pharmacokinetics include the detection of patient compliance or non-compliance (12), of drug-drug interactions (13) and of suitable dosage regimens particularly in pediatric (14, 15) and geriatric (16) populations.

APPLICATION OF CLINICAL PHARMACOKINETICS TO OPTIMIZE DRUG THERAPY

During the past three years in our Medical Center, monitoring of drug levels in plasma has formed the pharmacokinetic basis for individualizing drug dosages to detect individual differences in rate of drug metabolism, non-compliance, bioinequivalence and abnormal protein binding of a drug. The following categories of drugs are monitored daily: (1) cardiovascular – digoxin, procainamide, N-acetyl-procainamide, lidocaine, propranolol; (2) bronchodilator – theophylline; (3) anticonvulsant – phenobarbital, diphenylhydantoin, primidone, valproic acid, carbamazepine, ethosuximide; (4) anti-inflammatory – aspirin, indomethacin; and (5) miscellaneous INH, methotrexate. These are all potent drugs with narrow therapeutic margins (1, 2, 9, 17, 18) and their pharmacokinetic behavior is relatively well described for both normal and disease states (9, 11, 19, 20). Two examples illustrate how such clinical pharmacokinetics maintain optimal drug concentration in blood (plasma) and prevent adverse drug reaction(s) (toxicity).

Optimal theophylline in asthmatic patients

The clinical pharmacokinetics of theophylline, a potent bronchodilator with a therapeutic window of 10–20 μg/ml, has been extensively investigated (21). Our division has used individual pharmacokinetic parameters as guides to the therapeutic control of acute, refractory asthmatic patients. High-pressure liquid-chromatography and enzyme immunoassay (22) allowed doses (oral or i.v. infusion rate) to be adjusted to optimal therapeutic concentrations and these reduced the toxicity and enhanced the therapeutic benefit. The influence of drug interaction and disease states on plasma theophylline levels were also studied.

Application of Michaelis-Menten pharmacokinetics of diphenylhydantoin (DPH) to dose regime adjustment in a pediatric population

The clinical pharmacokinetics of anticonvulsants for adult epileptic patients have been recently reviewed (23). DPH is one of the most useful anticonvulsants for treating grand mal and focal seizures. The pharmacokinetic characteristics, namely Michaelis-Menten kinetics, will result in a disproportionately large increase in plasma DPH concentration despite a small increment in dose (23, 24). This complexity alongside a narrow therapeutic range [10–20 μg/ml in adults (23) and

5–20 μg/ml (25) in children] makes DPH difficult to prescribe in rational dose regimes for individual patients.

Recently, several reports suggest that the rearranged forms of the classical Michaelis-Menten equation could be made to fit steady-state plasma concentration and dose data (26, 27). For example, Richens and Dunlop (26) constructed a nomogram based on this theory for adjusting DPH dosage from plasma concentration data on a known daily dose. More recently, Ludden and co-workers (27) estimated the individual Michaelis-Menten kinetic parameters from two reliable steady-state plasma concentrations. A desired steady-state plasma concentration can then be predicted from these individual parameters in the daily given dose. A dosage adjustment approach of DPH to control seizures in adults is frequently successful (26, 27). Similar approaches have not been used in pediatric convulsive disorders and a retrospective surveillance study has been carried out in my laboratory(28). Michaelis-Menten pharmacokinetic parameters were evaluated for DPH in 104 pediatric patients with seizure disorders who ranged from 0.5 to 16 years of age. The V_{max} value showed a significant inverse correlation with age ($r = -0.552$, $p < 0.001$), while K_m showed a trend towards being constant throughout the ages studied. Calculated individual kinetic parameters of DPH have not only a reasonable predictability within the same patients ($r = -0.795$, $p < 0.002$), but also therapeutic applicability to prevent plasma levels of DPH rising beyond the potentially toxic range. A preliminary nomogram was constructed for adjusting the dosage to achieve desired steady-state plasma DPH levels, given that plasma concentrations on a known daily dosage are known (28).

CONCLUSIONS

It is likely that clinical pharmacokinetic data, blood drug levels and application of pharmacokinetic principles will allow better selection of therapeutic agents, in terms of calculating the therapeutic dose, and toxicity prevention. Although the general pharmacokinetics of many drugs are known for normal subjects, these values may not directly apply to individuals with genetic differences, or with liver, cardiac, or renal disease. Finally, it is concluded that clinical pharmacokinetics may not only prevent adverse drug reaction(s) but also enhance the efficiency of human drug therapy.

REFERENCES

1. Koch-Weser, J. (1972): Serum drug concentrations as therapeutic guides. *New Engl. J. Med., 287*, 227.
2. Koch-Weser, J. (1975): The serum level approach to individualization of drug dosage. *Eur. J. clin. Pharmacol., 9*, 1.
3. Gibaldi, M. and Levy, G. (1976): Pharmacokinetics in clinical practice. I. Concepts. *J. Amer. med. Ass., 235*, 1864.
4. Greenblatt, D.J. and Koch-Weser, J. (1975): Clinical pharmacokinetics. I. *New Engl. J. Med., 293*, 702.

5. Greenblatt, D.J. and Koch-Weser, J. (1975): Clinical pharmacokinetics. II. *New Engl. J. Med., 293*, 964.
6. Gibaldi, M. and Levy, G. (1976): Pharmacokinetics in clinical practice. II. Applications. *J. Amer. med. Ass., 235*, 1987.
7. Levy, G. (1973): Pharmacokinetic control and clinical interpretation of steady-state blood levels of drugs. *Clin. Pharmacol. Ther., 16/1 (Part 2)*, 130.
8. Dvorchik, B.H. and Vesell, E.S. (1976): Pharmacokinetic interpretation of data gathered during therapeutic drug monitoring. *Clin. Chem., 22*, 868.
9. Chow, M.S.S. and Ronfeld, R.A. (1975): Pharmacokinetic data and drug monitoring. I. Antibiotics and antiarrhythmics. *J. clin. Pharmacol., 15*, 405.
10. Giusti, D.L. and Hayton, W.L. (1973): Dosage regimen adjustments in renal impairment. *Drug Intell. clin. Pharm., 7*, 382.
11. Dettli, L.C. (1974): Drug dosage in patients with renal disease. *Clin. Pharmacol. Ther., 16/1 (Part 2)*, 274.
12. Blackwell, B. (1972): The drug defaulter. *Clin. Pharmacol. Ther., 13*, 841.
13. Rowland, M. and Matin, S.B. (1973): Kinetics of drug-drug interactions. *J. Pharmacokinet. Biopharmaceut., 1*, 553.
14. Jusko, W.J. (1972): Pharmacokinetic principles in pediatric pharmacology. *Med. Clin. North Amer., 19*, 81.
15. Done, A.K., Cohen, S.N. and Strebel, L. (1977): Pediatric clinical pharmacology and the 'therapeutic orphan'. *Ann. Rev. Pharmacol. Toxicol., 17*, 561.
16. Ritschel, W.A. (1976): Pharmacokinetic approach to drug dosing in the aged. *J. Amer. Geriat. Soc., 24*, 344.
17. Baselt, R.C., Wright, J.A. and Cravey, R.H. (1975): Therapeutic and toxic concentrations of more than 100 toxicologically significant drugs in blood, plasma, or serum: a tabulation. *Clin. Chem., 21*, 44.
18. Vesell, E.S. (1974): Relationship between drug distribution and therapeutic effects in man. *Ann. Rev. Pharmacol., 14*, 249.
19. Benowitz, N.L. and Meister, W. (1976): Pharmacokinetics in patients with cardiac failure. *Clin. Pharmacokinet., 1*, 389.
20. Pagliaro, L.A. and Benet, L.Z. (1975): Critical compilation of terminal half-lives, percent excreted unchanged, and changes of half-life in renal and hepatic dysfunction for studies in humans with references. *J. Pharmacokinet. Biopharmaceut., 3*, 333.
21. Ogilvie, R.I. (1978): Clinical pharmacokinetics of theophylline. *Clin. Pharmacokinet., 3*, 267.
22. Ishizaki, T., Watanabe, M. and Morishita, N. (1979): The effects of assay methods on plasma levels and pharmacokinetics of theophylline: HPLC and EIA. *Brit. J. clin. Pharmacol., 7*, 333.
23. Hvidberg, E.F. and Dam, M. (1967): Clinical pharmacokinetics of anticonvulsants. *Clin. Pharmacokinet., 1*, 161.
24. Richens, A. and Dunlop, A. (1975): Serum-phenytoin levels in management of epilepsy. *Lancet, 2*, 247.
25. Borofsky, L.G., Louis, S., Kutt, H. and Roginski, M. (1972): Diphenylhydantoin: efficacy, toxicity and dose-serum level relationships in children. *J. Pediat., 81*, 995.
26. Richens, A. and Dunlop, A. (1975): Phenytoin dosage nomogram. *Lancet, 2*, 1305.
27. Ludden, T.M., Allen, J.P., Valutsky, W.A., Vicuna, A.V., Nappi, J.M., Hoffman, S.F., Wallace, J.E., Lalka, D. and McNay, J.L. (1977): Individualization of phenytoin dosage regimens. *Clin. Pharmacol. Ther.,21*, 287.
28. Chiba, K., Ishizaki, T., Miura, H. and Minagawa, K. (1980): Michaelis-Menten pharmacokinetics of diphenylhydantoin and application in the pediatric age patient. *J. Pediat., 96,* 479.

DISCUSSION

Yanagita: I do not wish to ask about pharmacokinetics. Rather I would like to know about costs. When you determine blood drug levels, does the cost accrue to the present social medicare system?

Ishizaki: That is a delicate question not easily answered. I work in a National Medical Center and, under the present medical regulation, you cannot charge for plasma monitoring, but in the private medical schools, you can. As you know, plasma analyses are costly involving labor, immunoassay kits etc. Therefore, ideally, we should like to make some charge. It is becoming increasingly important to monitor the therapy. I personally think that a more important thing is the assessment for individualizing drug therapy. The charge for plasma monitoring of drugs should be permitted under the social medicare system as soon as possible.

Yanagita: So you cannot charge the patient but you have research funds. Where do they come from?

Ishizaki: Some from the government.

Yanagita: Generally speaking, the support for such a study by government grant is very limited. On the other hand, we cannot charge the patient. This is one aspect of the answer to Dr. Melmon's earlier question.

Ishizaki: Dr. Melmon, would you comment on this because you know this is a significant problem.

Melmon: I can say that a major mistake that has been made in the United States is to use research funds for clinical care and then when the research funds don't become available in the future, having to compromise clinical care because of that. So I don't think that your procedure is different from that which we have experienced; but I think you may regret it if it continues. It is not terribly wise when you're trying to communicate with the public and with government to use funds for functions that are socially acceptable but not understandable to the people who issue those funds. I would be worried by it.

Predictive typing of drug-induced neurological sufferings from studies of the distribution of labelled drugs*

TOSHIAKI TAKASU

Department of Neurology, Institute of Brain Research, Faculty of Medicine, University of Tokyo, Tokyo, Japan

A drug given to an animal becomes widely distributed throughout the body, acting on the living mechanisms or structures, and is gradually excreted.

Some drugs can remain in some parts of the body for a long period. For example, ^{14}C-chloramphenicol was found to remain preferentially in the salivary gland, liver and bone-marrow of mice 24 hours after its oral administration (1). If such a drug is given repeatedly, it could possibly accumulate gradually in these organs.

Thus, when its accumulation in a particular part of the body exceeds a certain level, the living mechanism or structure may possibly be injured. The harmful effects of a drug in repeated administration are called its chronic toxicity.

I would like to discuss whether it is possible to predict the toxicity of a drug by studying its distribution in relation to time, and, if possible, the points in time. As a neurologist, I wished to study this problem especially in relation to the nervous system. This idea was conceived during my study with 8 drugs or chemicals, beginning with clioquinol in 1971.

METHODS

The method which I have employed is called freezing whole-body macro-autoradiography. It was first introduced in 1958 by Sven Ullberg of Sweden. Soon after 1960, a few Japanese investigators started to use it, but now many laboratories in Japan are equipped for it.

However, most of its use has been to collect circumstantial evidence for the beneficial effects of drugs. Only a limited number of harmful effects have been investigated and, to my knowledge, there has been no report, except my own, attempting to predict drug-induced sufferings.

In this method, the drug or chemical is labelled with a radionuclide and given to experimental animals by a certain route.

We can use not only small species, like mice and rats, but also medium-sized

*Partly supported by a Grant-in-Aid for Scientific Research (A) (1972, no. 744032) and by a Grant-in-Aid for Special Project Research (2) (1978, no. 321304) from the Ministry of Education, Science and Culture of the Japanese Government.

animals, like dogs and monkeys. The larger the animals, the greater is the scale of the necessary equipment and the consumption of human labor, time, and cost. Therefore, it is most practical first to collect as much information as possible using smaller animals, and to supplement this with data from larger ones as occasion demands.

The animals to which the labelled compound has been given are killed after a certain length of time. Their whole body is then quickly frozen and sections of about 40 μm thickness are prepared. If the frozen sections are then freeze-dried, they keep their vivid, natural color, and this greatly helps the identification of the individual organs.

In the next step, this freeze-dried section is brought into contact for a time with a high-sensitivity, industrial X-ray film, which becomes exposed to the rays emanating from the radionuclide in the section. After development of the film, a macro-autoradiogram is produced.

RESULTS

From now on, I would like to exemplify how we study and characterize the mode of drug distribution in the nervous system by using the macro-autoradiograms prepared with radioactive clioquinol. Most of this work was performed in collaboration with Dr. Osamu Matsuoka of the National Institute of Radiological Sciences, Chiba.

The whole-body macro-autoradiograms of mice killed 24 hours after intraperitoneal injection of clioquinol labelled with iodine-131 were less dense in the areas representing the brain and the spinal cord than in the areas representing the blood in the heart (2). In contrast, the density in the sciatic nerve (Fig. 1) was higher than that in the blood (2).

In a macro-autoradiogram from the eyeball of a dog which was killed 24 hours

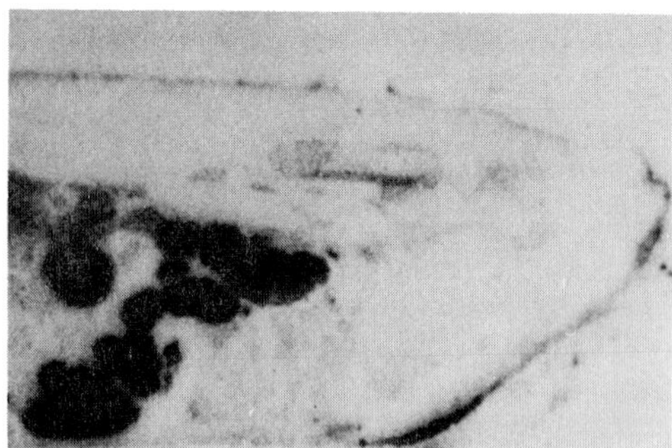

Fig. 1. A whole-body macro-autoradiogram prepared from a mouse killed 24 hours after intraperitoneal injection of clioquinol labelled with iodine-131, showing uptake by the sciatic nerve (2). In this picture, only the hind half of the body is included. The semi-dark, horizontally situated, linear structure near the center of this picture, on the upper right, represents the sciatic nerve. The dark flecks in the left half of this picture represent the bile contained in the intestinal cavity.

after intraperitoneal injection of labelled clioquinol the areas representing the cornea, anterior chamber, iris, lens, and vitreous body, as well as the bulbar tunic and optic nerve, could be recognized. It was found that the middle layer of the bulbar tunic, which was separated into 3 layers in part of one section, represented the stratum pigmenti of the retina, and the inner layer the stratum cerebrale of the retina. The density of both these layers was much higher than that of the optic nerve (3).

The distribution of clioquinol in the nervous system (Fig. 2) did not essentially differ between CRF-1 mice, mongrel and beagle dogs, and a monkey (2–7).

The distribution of labelled compounds can be determined in minute structures of small animals such as mice. For example, 1 hour after the injection of ^{14}C-5-fluoro-orotate, its concentration in the spinal dorsal root ganglia was much higher than in the spinal nerves and spinal cord.

I have studied the distribution of 8 drugs or chemicals in the nervous system of experimental animals by this method (1–13). The distribution differs between the compounds. Table 1 gives a rough estimate of the relative concentration of each drug or chemical at key sites of the peripheral and central nervous systems (12).

Clioquinol concentrated more heavily in the peripheral nervous system than in the

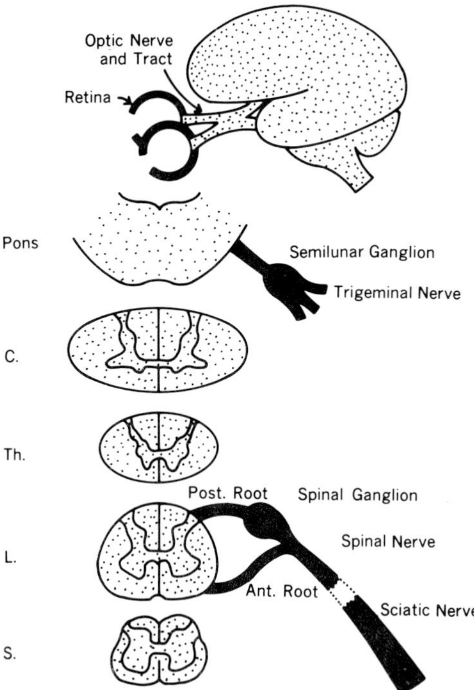

Fig. 2. A schematic illustration of the distribution of clioquinol in the nervous system about 24 hours after its administration, based on the results of the author's study (5,6). In the brain and spinal cord (the central nervous system), the concentration of clioquinol was relatively low, whereas in the trigeminal and spinal nerve roots and their ganglia, as well as the sciatic nerve (the peripheral nervous system) its concentration was much higher. The concentration of clioquinol was relatively low in the optic nerve, but much higher in the retina.

TABLE 1. *Summary of results*

	Peripheral nervous system		Central nervous system	
	Spinal ganglia	Sciatic nerve	Grey matter	White matter
Clioquinol	++	++	⊥	⊥
Chloramphenicol	++	+	+	+
5-Fluorouracil	++	+⊥	+⊥	+⊥
5-Fluoro-orotate	+++	+	⊥	⊥
TOCP	++	⊥	+	+
Methyl mercury	+⊥	+	+++	++
4-NQO	+	+	+++	+
4-HAQO	+++	+	+	⊥

Rough estimate of relative concentration of each of 8 drugs or chemicals studied by the author at key sites of the peripheral and central nervous systems showing their distributions around 24 hours after their administration (12). The results are based on studies with mice except for TOCP, where the hen was used (9). TOCP = triorthocresyl phosphate; 4-NQO = 4-nitroquinoline-1-oxide; 4-HAQO = 4-hydroxyaminoquinoline-1-oxide.

central nervous system (2–7), whereas methyl mercury concentrated somewhat more heavily in the central nervous system than in the peripheral nervous system (10). There were some drugs or chemicals such as 5-fluoro-orotate (8) and 4-hydroxyamino-quinoline-1-oxide (11, 13) which concentrated most heavily in the spinal dorsal root ganglia, and others such as 4-nitroquinoline-1-oxide (11, 13), which concentrated most heavily in the grey matter of the central nervous system.

DISCUSSION

These findings lead me to the following conclusions.

The accumulation of a drug or chemical at a site does not inevitably mean that it acts there. However, we must admit that no primary, direct action on the living mechanism or structure can occur at any site where no drug is distributed. In other words, the distribution suggests the range of its primary, direct action. If so, a difference in distribution would probably alter the range of its primary, direct action. A knowledge of distribution should make possible some *prediction* about the mode of action.

How can such predictions prevent drug-induced sufferings? Whenever we consider drug-induced sufferings in the past, the question always arises of whether they were predictable. There are at least two aspects which must be considered. One is the restriction imposed by the medical, pharmacological and scientific knowledge available at the time. The other is whether everything which could be done to prevent such sufferings was actually done and, if not, what the reasons were. This kind of scrutiny is equally relevant to the present situation. What should be done now?

I agree that toxicity studies should play a leading role.

Next, we must monitor the occurrence of drug-induced sufferings after we have started using a drug. This is not prediction in the real sense, but it is important for preventing the spread of such sufferings.

Both these approaches are most important, but it is also true that they require time, human energy, and money. It is doubtful whether as much time, energy, and money has, in the past, been alloted for demonstrating or predicting the harmful effects of a drug as for demonstrating or predicting its beneficial effects.

Therefore, efforts to raise the efficiency of these tasks are indispensable. The method I have proposed could suggest the sites of the nervous system on which we should focus our toxicity studies and the type of neurological disorders whose occurrence we should monitor. It is because the interior of the nervous system is not homogenous, like some other organs, that distribution studies may be particularly effective for predictive typing of drug-induced neurological sufferings.

CONCLUSION

Studying the distribution of a drug at the key sites of the peripheral and central nervous systems enables us to surmise the primary site of its toxicity, and to some extent predict the type and occurrence of drug-induced neurological sufferings. For this purpose, freezing whole-body macro-autoradiography is effective.

ACKNOWLEDGEMENT

The author is grateful to Professor Yasuo Toyokura for his support and comments.

REFERENCES

1. Takasu, T., Aoki, Y. and Toyokura, Y. (1976): Chloramphenicol-induced disorders of the nervous system. A macro-autoradiographic study of distribution and retention of the labelled compounds in the nervous system. *Neurol. Med., 4,* 331.
2. Takasu, T., Toyokura, Y. and Matsuoka, O. (1971): A study on the distribution of metabolism of clioquinol in mice, utilizing radionuclides. *Igaku-no-ayumi, 79,* 25.
3. Takasu, T., Toyokura, Y., Ueno, H. and Matsuoka, O. (1971): The distribution of clioquinol labelled with iodine-131 in dogs with particular reference to its uptake by the retina and the optic nerve. *Igaku-no-ayumi, 79*, 75.
4. Takasu, T., Toyokura, Y. and Matsuoka, O, (1972): Toxicity of Quinoform (5-chloro-7-iodo-8-hydroxyquinoline) for the nervous system. I. Intestinal absorption, whole body retention and distribution of ^{131}I-quinoform in mice. *Clin. Neurol. (Tokyo), 12*, 131.
5. Takasu, T., Toyokura, Y. and Matsuoka, O. (1972): The uptake of clioquinol labelled with iodine-131 by the nervous system of the dogs. *Igaku-no-ayumi, 81*, 397.
6. Takasu, T. (1974): Pathogenesis of the toxic myelo-optico-neuropathy with chinoform (5-chloro-7-iodo-8-hydroxyquinoline). A macro-autoradiographic and radiochemical study. *Clin. Neurol. (Tokyo), 14*, 232.
7. Toyokura, Y., Takasu, T. and Matsuoka, O. (1975): Experimental studies utilizing radionuclide-labelled clioquinol as tracer in vivo. *Jap. J. med. Sci. Biol., 28, Suppl.,* 79.
8. Takasu, T. and Kuzuhara, S. (1976): The distribution of RNA anti-metabolites in the nervous system. Paper presented at: XVII General Assembly of the Japanese Society of Neurology, May 19, 1976.
9. Takasu, T. and Kuzuhara, S. (1977): The distribution of tri-orthocresyl phosphate in the nervous system. Paper presented at: XVIII General Assembly of the Japanese Society of

Neurology, May 20, 1977.
10. Kuzuhara, S., Takasu, T. and Toyokura, Y. (1978): Distribution and retention of ^{203}Hg-labelled methylmercury chloride in the peripheral and central nervous system of mice. A macro-autoradiographic study. *Clin. Neurol. (Tokyo), 18*, 129.
11. Takasu, T. (1978): The distribution of 4-nitroquinoline-1-oxide and 4-hydroxyaminoquinoline-1-oxide in the nervous system. *Neurol. Med., 9*, 73.
12. Takasu, T. (1978): Distribution of toxic agents in the peripheral and central nervous system. Macro-autoradiographic studies. Paper presented at: IV International Congress of Neuromuscular Diseases, Sept. 17, 1978, Montreal.
13. Takasu, T. (1979): The distribution of carcinogens, 4-nitroquinoline-1-oxide and 4-hydroxyaminoquinoline-1-oxide, in the nervous system and its possible neurological significance. *Experientia (Basel), 35*, 668.

DISCUSSION

Yokota: (1) I have been involved with Professor Ullberg's laboratory and I have just returned from it. I think that whole-body autoradiography is quite useful in the case of the nervous system, particularly for the visual pathway. However, in addition, we must perform many other experiments, particularly those in vitro in relation to the melanin pigment, e.g. on its synthesis, its affinity to drugs, etc., in order to detect the toxicity of a drug to the visual apparatus. What you think about that?

(2) You have stated that the neurotoxicity of chloroquin and several other drugs shows no species differences between mice, dogs, and monkeys. But my experiments have demonstrated that there is a species difference in respect of the pigment in the optic fundi; e.g. in albino rats when exposed to some drugs such as ethambutol there was no change in the pigment, whereas in beagle dogs there was a definite change. Furthermore, there was an age-related factor in beagle dogs, but not in rabbits or rats. Considering these facts, I think it is very difficult for us to select one particular animal species for our experiments on the toxicity of a drug to the visual apparatus. What is your opinion about this problem?

(3) Does it not take a very long time (experimental period) before we finally observe the development of drug toxicity to the visual apparatus in banal toxicity studies? In addition, I think it is rather difficult to gauge the development of drug toxicity to the visual pathway from the clinical observation of the animal's behavior. What do you think about that? Can you suggest any points to be heeded in studying the toxicity to the visual pathway by means of in-vivo animal experiments?

Takasu: (1) I, too, am aware of the fact that the development of toxic disorders depends not only on the local concentration of the drug, but also on the susceptibility of the host, and I think that melanin pigment is related to the latter. I agree with you in saying that due attention should be paid to the affinity of clioquinol to the melanin pigment in the optic fundi and the possible occurrence of disorder of the melanin-bearing cells and their surrounding structures. However, in fact, it was not only in the stratum pigmenti of the retina but also in the stratum cerebrale that the radioactive clioquinol was most heavily concentrated in my experiments. In view of the facts that, in human SMON, the visual loss occurred during the use of clioquinol for less than a month in many cases, not long after the cessation of the drug as in many cases of the so-called melanin disorder, and that symptoms such as pigmentation of the skin, hearing loss, and extrapyramidal ones, which we also expect in such disorders, were not the typical features of SMON, it seems to me likely that it was not the melanin disorder but the direct toxicity of clioquinol to the neurons in the retina that played the leading role in the development of the visual loss.

(2) I think you may have misunderstood part of what I said. Actually I have not worked

with chloroquin, but with clioquinol, and work was not directly concerned with the neurotoxic effects of drugs, but primarily with their distribution in the nervous system. There may be certain drugs for which species differences in toxicity may be significant, just as you said, but in fact, so far as the mode of distribution of radioactive clioquinol in the nervous system is concerned, no appreciable differences were observed between a strain of mouse (CRF-1), beagle and mongrel dogs, and a species of monkey. I did not select one particular species but worked with three species.

(3) I know that melanin disorders take a long time to develop and often we see them several months or years after stopping the drug. But, in human SMON, clioquinol could cause visual loss within 2 or 3 weeks of its use. In the case of chloramphenicol, it usually takes longer for optic and other neurological disorders to develop. I think that some training in clinical neurology is useful for performing animal studies on neurotoxicity, including that to the visual pathway.

Hanano: I have been very impressed by your studies which so beautifully show a correlation between the neurotoxicity of clioquinol and its autoradiographic distribution in the nervous system. However, the autoradiographic distribution of a drug represents the distribution of its bound form (to protein or other substances). It is generally stated that the bound form has only a weak drug action, while the unbound has a strong one, and that in the unbound form the drug shows the same concentration throughout the whole body, unlike your finding with clioquinol. Thus the main and side actions (disordering effect) on a particular tissue depend on the susceptibility of the tissue. What do you think about this notion?

Takasu: I have mentioned the example of chloramphenicol and I have shown you a slide on this. If you look, you will see that, within the brain and spinal cord, the concentration of ^{14}C-chloramphenicol was high after 5 hours, but it had decreased to a much lower level after 24 hours. In the bone marrow, on the other hand, the rate of decrease during the same period was only very low. This difference suggests that there are at least two different kinds of binding between this drug and the tissues. The rapid decrease in the brain and spinal cord may indicate one and the very small decrease in the bone marrow another, and there may possibly be more. In my experience, though limited, the mode of development of chronic toxicity after repeated administration of a drug seems to correlate better with its distribution at 24 hours after a single administration than with that at early intervals. I assume that at least some of the chronic toxicity of a drug depends on its binding with a certain receptor, which is stronger and more long-standing than that which mediates the more acute pharmacological actions, main or side. I admit that this assumption needs further scrutiny.

I suppose that there must also be a role played by the susceptibility of nerve cells (neurons), for, in the case of clioquinol, its concentration within the brain and spinal cord was fairly homogenous and, on the whole, unexpectedly low compared with that in the spinal ganglia and sciatic nerve. We must assume that the susceptibility to clioquinol of the primary motor neuron originating in the cerebral cortex is relatively high because it was constantly affected in SMON, selectively among the neurons in the brain and spinal cord, and equally with the primary sensory neuron originating in the spinal ganglia. I think the discrepancy between the distribution of a drug and that of the disorder induced by it may suggest local susceptibilities to the drug.

Melmon: Could you tell us the known limitations of your method? I am concerned with the proven sensitivity. Could you get false negatives? How many drugs that are known to cause optic neuropathy in clinical settings would not be concentrated and detected in the optic nerve by your method? Conversely, what proportion of drugs with high partition coefficients would concentrate in the optic nerve and be detected there, but produce no noticeable adverse effects in the eye?

Takasu: I can say that my method is very sensitive and there is theoretically no limit to the detection of small amounts of radioactivity because it is generally said that the correlation of the film density with the amount of exposure to β-, X-, or γ-rays is expressed by a straight line running through the origin, and this has been reconfirmed in my preliminary experiments. Therefore, I think there is no false-negative in this sense. The limitation of my method comes about when the exposure of the film has exceeded a certain high level, above which the increments in the density gradually abate to a plateau, so that any quantitative assessments become difficult.

Of the 8 compounds I used, it was only for clioquinol in dogs and TOCP in the hen that the distribution of the radioactivity in the optic nerve could be studied; mice were too small for us to examine this structure macroscopically. As for TOCP, only a very limited amount of the radioactivity was detected in the optic nerve of the hen after 24 hours. However, the level in the wall of the eyeball looked somewhat higher than that in the optic nerve. Acute retrobulbar optic neuritis was described in some outbreaks of TOCP poisoning. As for clioquinol, a relatively low but definitely positive level of radioactivity was detected in the optic nerve of the dogs after 24 hours, and a much higher level was detected both in the stratum pigmenti of the retina and in the stratum cerebrale. In human SMON, about 20–30% of the cases suffered visual loss, and about 5% became totally blind.

Apart from the optic nerve and turning to the entire nervous system, it was again only with clioquinol and TOCP that the level in the brain and spinal cord was unexpectedly low compared with that in the spinal ganglia. Both the compounds are well known for their ability to induce marked degeneration of the primary motor neurons originating in the cerebral cortex. Therefore, I assume that the latter neurons must be more susceptible to these drugs than the primary sensory neurons originating in the spinal ganglia.

My overall impression from the results of my own studies is that severe disorders can arise where a heavy concentration has been achieved, but that such disorders may also arise where only a relatively low concentration has been achieved if the susceptibility of the structure at that site is high enough.

Drug and product selection – an essential part of the therapeutic benefit/risk ratio strategy?

P.K.M. LUNDE

Division of Clinical Pharmacology and Toxicology, Central Laboratory, Ullevål Hospital, University of Oslo, Oslo, Norway

Basic human needs include fresh air for breathing, water and adequate food to satisfy thirst and hunger, heating or clothing to counteract frost and in the widest sense, appropriate hygienic measures to limit dirt and pollution. The priorities to be set as regards *drugs*, which are secondary to those mentioned – as well as to several other elements of human wellbeing – varies according to the benefit/risk and benefit/cost ratios, depending upon how real needs versus demands are defined in relation to local conditions.

Today's models in market mechanisms are based, at least in developed countries, mainly upon product offer as balanced by existing product control, the latter being intended to safeguard the public. Again, demands versus needs should be considered and related to the varying cultural, economic, political and professional factors and criteria present. The field of drugs can be considered as a relevant example in this context.

At this stage it is necessary to state that drugs are not necessarily as bad – or good – as our mode of using them. In terms of safeguarding the public as well as of preventing disease and restoring health, both the risks and benefits of drugs have, in general, been considerably overestimated. Accordingly, the drug explosion in the 1950's and 1960's gradually became a hindrance to rational drug utilization. In many countries, drugs became an inappropriate compensation for an inadequate or unsuccessful health strategy. When recalling the WHO definition of *drug utilization* (1) – 'the marketing, distribution, prescription and use of drugs in a society, with special emphasis on the resulting medical, social and economic consequences' – one should not unanimously blame the drug industry, but rather look critically at our way of prescribing and using drugs.

Consequently the establishment of a national drug policy (strategy), aimed at safeguarding the public, should include: (1) a control system ensuring the appropriate quality, efficacy and safety of the approved (selected) drug products, as well as (2) a wider strategy for the establishment of rational drug utilization at all levels of the therapeutic chain. These goals can only be achieved if sufficient education and unbiased information are given to professionals as well as to the public (2, 3).

The necessity of reducing the free flow of drugs in our societies, by adopting appropriate selection criteria, is not only a matter of comparative *product* quality as guaranteed by the producers and health authorities, but also includes the quality of *drug utilization* as reflected in the prescribers' and the public's behavior. Thus it has never been proven that an infinite number of drugs provides any greater benefits for public health than a more reasonable product offer. On the contrary, a large number of drugs may result in confusion at all levels of the therapeutic chain, and represent a waste of manpower and money. Moreover, experience in drug committee work in Scandinavian countries and Italy has shown that *routine* drug treatment works well with a selection of 200 to 500 drugs (2, 4).

Whereas drugs alone are insufficient to provide adequate health care, the last 10–15 years of clinical pharmacological research have repeatedly shown that drugs are not used to their full potential (5). The wide geographical variations in overall drug therapy profiles (6, 7), as illustrated in Figure 1 for hypotensives, also add to the complex question – What is really rational and optimal drug therapy? In this context, a drug economy should be considered which includes the identification of real patients, the basic question of whether to treat or not, the choice between drugs and other alternatives, dosage adjustment and evaluation of effect.

Despite the widely varying attitudes to drugs in our international society, many developing countries felt unanimously that as the drug control measures in many developed countries were improved or became more restrictive, increasing pressure from drug marketing interests was put on them. This again gradually forced the WHO to participate more actively, as stated in the Resolution from the 28th WHA in 1975 to the Director General of WHO Geneva, '... to develop means by which the organization can be of greater direct assistance to member states in advising on the selection and procurement, at reasonable cost, of essential drugs of established quality corresponding to the national health needs' (8).

The criteria involved were partly professional, partly economic and administrative, including such key phrases as 'health needs', 'established quality', 'reasonable cost' and 'procurement'. The strategy should be to select drugs for the treatment of the dominant diseases affecting the majority of the population.

Accordingly, the WHO procedure for the selection of so-called essential drugs, which might better have been named 'basic', can be outlined by the following 10 stages:

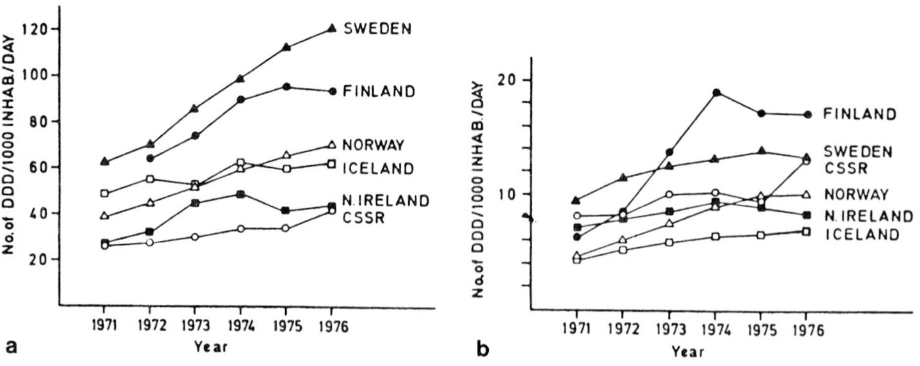

Fig. 1. (a) Sales of hypotensives, including beta-blockers, diuretics and Rauwolfia preparations in 6 European countries 1971–1976. For information on the unit of comparison (Defined Daily Doses) used, see refs 6 and 7. (b) Sales of synthetic hypotensives (hydralazine, α-methyldopa, guanethidine etc.) in 6 European countries 1971–1976. From Baksaas 1979 (7).

1. WHA resolution, May, 1975, to the Director General.
2. Reorganization, including the establishment of 'The Drug Policy and Management Division' of WHO HQ, collection of material from Member States, Autumn 1975–Spring 1976.
3. First working documents prepared May–June 1976 (background and criteria for drug selection, administrative aspects etc.).
4. Working documents circulated to WHO Regional Offices for comments Summer 1976.
5. Internal revision before the first *informal* expert consultation, October 1976. Informal report DPM/76.1 prepared containing background and a *model* list of essential drugs.
6. DPM/76.1 circulated to all Member States for comments, Winter–Spring 1977. Drug industry informed and reacts by initial protests (9).
7. Additional internal revision upon the comments. The first *formal* expert consultation held in Geneva, October 1977. *WHO Technical Report Series No. 615* printed and distributed from December 1977 (1).
8. Drug industry goes into dialog with WHO; increasingly positive comments from professionals within or outside health authorities. Many countries start or continue work on drug selection, and ask WHO for assistance.
9. WHO Executive Board passes resolution EB 61/SR/17 on essential drugs, January 1978. The 31st WHA approves 'Action Program on Essential Drugs', May 1978 (see below).
10. Future revision and supplements: (a) The model list will be regularly and continuously updated, whenever necessary. (b) Relevant, independent information (master sheets) related to the drugs on the model list *and their alternatives* will be produced within the frame of WHO and its expert panels. (c) Special attention will be paid to defining and procuring the optimal dosage and administration forms for the relevant drug products (see ref. 12).

The following is the present author's unauthorized translation of the WHO 'Action Program on Essential Drugs':

I. The *Member States* should establish *national* drug lists according to the *criteria* given in *Technical Report Series No. 615*, including the distributional and legal (registration) apparatus necessary. Independent drug information should be provided, and international collaboration on drug price policy, production and other strategic aspects should be strengthened. As a rule, generic drug names should be preferred.

II. *The Director General of WHO* should continue efforts to identify the scientifically best-documented drugs and to collaborate with the Member States according to *their* conditions: (a) to ensure a supply of knowhow and resources through collaboration with UNICEF, UNIDO, The World Bank and other Developmental Banks and Funds; (b) to stimulate reasonable local production of drugs; (c) to study price-setting for drugs and mechanisms for their marketing; (d) to exchange information and experience and to give feedback to WHO, among others.

During the continuous work on the selection of essential drugs it was felt that the *criteria* adopted for drug selection, including appropriate and unbiased information, formed the most important contribution on the part of WHO. The selection itself is clearly a national or local task, based upon these criteria. In brief, they refer to the *scientific* documentation on drug efficacy and safety, pharmaceutically, pharmacologically and clinically, the cost/effectiveness, the possibilities for adequate stocking and distribution, the acceptability and accessibility for the user, as adjusted to the local morbidity pattern, manpower and other resources available for correct diagnosis and appropriate drug utilization. Accordingly the resulting essential drugs chosen will vary depending on these factors.

Despite this, the various WHO expert committees involved in this program found it necessary to illustrate the application of the criteria by establishing a *model list* of essential drugs. This list, being first of all an example of a basic national list, contains some 210–220 substances, including vaccines, infusion fluids, vitamins, some diagnostics and relevant antidotes. Of about 160 drugs left when subtracting those mentioned, some 55 are antimicrobials, 20 cardiovascular and only 6 are psychotropic drugs. In the first official report (1), the safety aspects were especially questioned for drugs such as chloramphenicol, phenylbutazone, aminopyrine-like drugs and for clioquinol, all still widely used. These discussions will continue during the continuous work of revising the criteria and their adoption. Special attention will be paid to improving communication of drug information, and regulatory experiences, between WHO and the Member States, not least in relation to drug innovations.

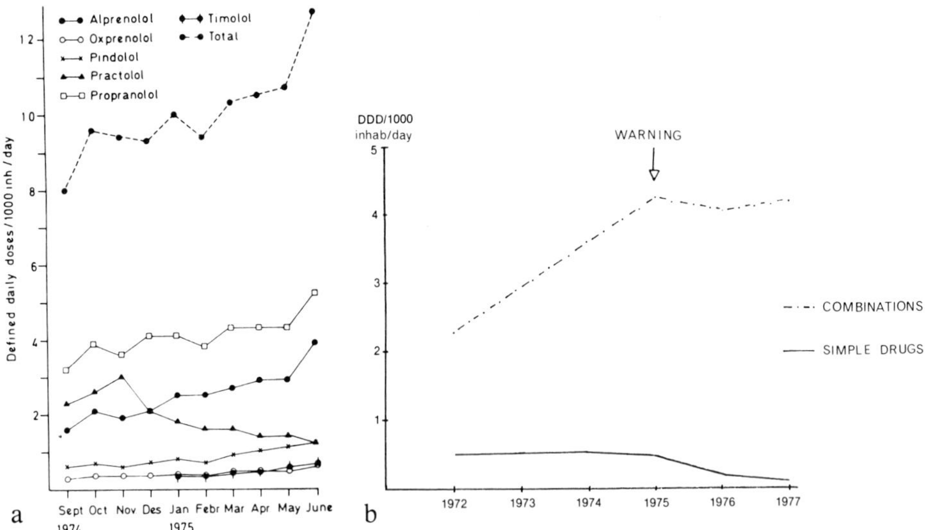

Fig. 2. Effect of drug control and information measures on two separate occasions in 1974–1975. (a) Decreased sales of practolol in Norway following informational efforts on serious practolol-induced eye, skin and peritoneal complications, during late Autumn 1974, as given in dose statistics. Also note the on-going overall increase with regard to other beta-blockers. Practolol, except for a parenteral preparation, was banned from September 1975. For unit of comparison (Defined Daily Doses), see refs. 6 and 7. (b) The effect of official warnings on the indiscriminate use of dextropropoxyphene, after its narrow therapeutic range, in terms of even lethal respiratory depression, especially when combined with ethanol, was known.

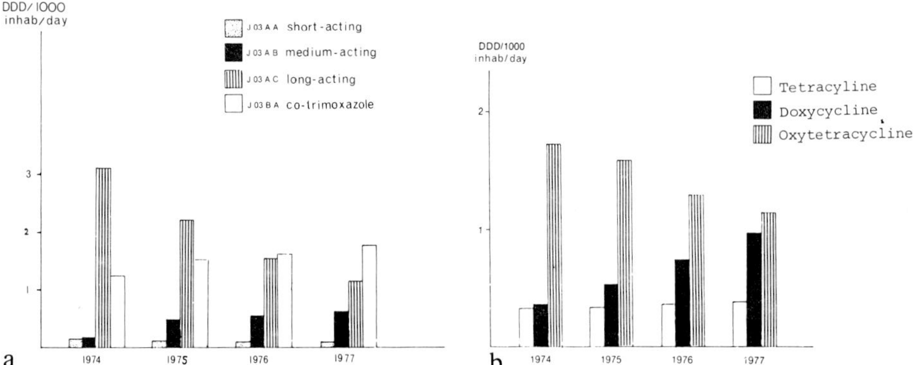

Fig. 3. Gradual changes in the sales profiles of sulfonamides (a) and tetracyclines (b) in Norway, 1974–1977. From various independent information sources, including local drug committees and health authorities it was repeatedly stressed that long-acting sulfonamides were less justified than was previously claimed by the producers, because of the risk of prolonged adverse reactions. Accordingly, doxycycline, despite its relatively high price, is recommended as the tetracycline of choice because of its non-renal clearance and its somewhat (?) lesser proneness to cause tooth discoloration.

As an example, some aspects of drug regulatory and information measures taken in Norway during recent years are shown in Figures 2 and 3. For explanation and comments, see the figure legends.

In conclusion, appropriate drug and product selection, with the resulting simplification of the product range, may become an important part of the procedure for improving drug utilization, in terms of enhanced efficacy as well as safety. Accordingly, such a selection procedure, involving thorough scrutiny of other therapeutic as well as diagnostic measures in the various fields of health care – and elsewhere in our societies – should be adopted.

REFERENCES

1. WHO Expert Committee (1977): The selection of essential drugs. *WHO techn. Rep. Ser., 615.*
2. Halse, M. and Lunde, P.K.M. (1978): In: *Controlling the Use of Therapeutic Drugs. An International Comparison*, Chapter 9, pp. 187–210. Editor: W.M. Wardell. American Enterprise Institute for Public Policy Research, Washington, DC.
3. Herxheimer, A. and Lionel, N.D.W. (1978): Minimum information needed by prescribers. *Brit. med. J., 2*, 1129.
4. Tognoni, G. (1978): A therapeutic formulary for Italian general practitioners. *Lancet, 1*, 1352.
5. Averij, G.S. and Adis, S. (Eds.) (1976): *Drug Treatment. Principles and Practice of Clinical Pharmacology and Therapeutics.* Churchill Livingstone, Edinburgh-London.
6. Lunde, P.K.M. (1976): Differences in national drug-prescribing patterns. In: *Report from Symposium 'Clinical Pharmacological Evaluation in Drug Control', Deidesheim 1975*, pp. 19–47. WHO Regional Office for Europe, Copenhagen.
7. Lunde, P.K.M., Levy, M. et al. (1979): Drug utilization: geographical differences and clinical implications. In: *Advances in Pharmacology and Therapeutics, Vol. 6, Clinical*

Pharmacology, pp. 77–170. Editor: P. Duchène-Marullaz. Pergamon Press, Oxford – New York – Toronto – Sydney – Paris – Frankfurt.
8. *Off. Rec. Wld Hlth Org., 1975, No. 226*, pp. 35–36; *Annex 13*, pp. 96–110.
9. Tiefenbacher, M. (1977): In: *WHO's Essential Drug List Now Being Studied.* Script 1977, June 11, pp. 22–23.
10. WHO and the pharmaceutical industry (guest editorial). (1978): *J. Wld med. Ass.* 25.
11. WHO on essential drugs (editorial). (1978) *Lancet, 2*, 977.
12. WHO Expert Committee (1979): The selection of essential drugs. 2nd Report. *WHO techn. Rep. Ser., 641.*

DISCUSSION

Dukes: I have always understood that even in countries with a large number of drugs on the market, only a small proportion of these are in fact of significance as regards their sale and general use, and that the number of drugs which the individual general practitioner uses is very limited indeed. A lot of noise is made when the drug list is reduced, but it does not in fact meet with much opposition from the practitioner. Are there any figures on this and can Dr. Lunde say anything about this?

Lunde: I can't give you any hard figures and thus I would never dramatize the harmful effects of having a high number of drugs in a society. However, I would rather turn it in a positive way and question the benefit of having such a huge number of products as that seen marketed in many countries. In relation to the general practitioners, I agree with you that they may routinely tend to stick to a limited number of some 50–70 drugs each. In an open and sometimes quite complicated society, allowing free choice of drugs and physicians, it can't be avoided that physicians are also regularly faced with drugs with which they have no experience of their own. This problem certainly arises for most of us, when asked to reiterate a drug previously prescribed by another physician. This dilemma is felt especially by the general practitioners, which may explain why they often have a positive attitude towards 'limited drug lists'.

Melmon: I think your question is a very interesting one and I will say, at least for the United States, that physicians don't have any information about the epidemiology of drug use. The only people who do have that information are those who pay an awful lot of money to get it. And they are the drug houses. It's of interest when you examine the data that factors which are quite unconnected with medical decisions can greatly influence the way in which a drug is available and will be used and some of these are very difficult to understand. For instance, the sale of phenformin in the United States went up after there was a threat that the drug would be withdrawn from the market.

Lunde: Sorry to say, Dr. Melmon, but I think this is a matter of confidence, a confidence that must exist between the health authorities/drug regulatory bodies and the medical profession. I can tell you that in the early 60's our health authorities in Norway were warning about the risks of using chloramphenicol in banal infections. These warnings did not become effective until a number of specialists also started to argue about the potential misuse of this drug, which was efficiently promoted by the producers and also sold at a very low price. In a small country like ours I think it is now quite easy to establish the confidence necessary and also to communicate efficiently as I showed you for practolol and sulfonamides, among others (for review, see Halse and Lunde, 1978).

Melmon: I think that's an extraordinarily good point, that if you have an organization which you do feel confident about and it provides you with feedback information on drug effects, the chances of getting information on a drug and the inappropriate effects associated with it, may be much greater than if there is no confidence in either the regulatory or investigative group.

Kono: I understand that clioquinol was withdrawn from the WHO list of essential drugs. I heard that a WHO official explained that the Japanese SMON incidence was not a reason for the withdrawal of clioquinol. Is that right?

Lunde: Dr. Kono, I happened to be a participant in this WHO program from the very beginning, that is since the first working documents on drug selection were prepared in 1976. Initially we discussed leaving out clioquinol, partly because of insufficient documentation on its effect in all the claimed indications, partly because of the potential risks, especially when used without sufficient diagnostic facilities and when sold without prescription. But yes, it is correct that clioquinol, after consulting previous WHO expert recommendations, was tentatively listed in the first *informal* report (DPM/76.1) prepared upon the first expert consultation in October 1976. However, it was stressed that its use should be limited to the treatment of amebic dysentery. Upon reconsideration in 1977, clioquinol was deleted even for this very limited indication, for which better and safer alternative drugs can be used. Some of the confusion is, I believe, due to a misinterpretation by the drug industry, and others, of the whole concept of essential drugs.

Mashford: Would you like to comment on the 10-fold disparity between the number of drugs available in Norway and that in the essential list and perhaps in particular say how much the increased number in Norway is due to duplication of agents which have similar properties and how much to the presence of drugs which wouldn't be covered in the basic list.

Lunde: Thank you, Dr. Mashford, for giving me this opportunity to make myself completely clear. The 1850 drug products marketed in Norway involve about 700 substances. Thus, there is a 3-fold difference between the number of substances in the WHO model list of essential drugs and those on the Norwegian market. Although Norway does have a long historical tradition in practicing a 'restrictive' drug policy, based upon a so-called 'clause of need' in our drug legislation (for details, see Halse and Lunde, 1978), the concept of drug selection as outlined under the WHO program on essential drugs has not been strictly adopted. However, a major reason for the limited number of drug products on our market is that very few combination drugs have been accepted. We have no special rules as to how many synonyms should be allowed, but 'the clause of need' can be, and is, used here depending upon the assumed importance of the drugs in relation to alternative drugs available and the dimension of the medical problem in question. Accordingly, cardiovascular drugs and psychotropics are quite broadly available. In my personal opinion, our national drug range ought to be somewhat revised and reduced, based upon thorough professional scrutiny of each therapeutic class of drugs. Because of the traditions already existing, such a revision would occur over a certain period of time.

Kaihara: I have two questions. The first concerns the response of clinical physicians. Are they all in favor of restricting the number of drugs available to them? The second question is: What is the attitude of other European countries to the concept of 'essential drugs'? If you have any information, would you please tell us?

Lunde: I will try, but I do not pretend to give you more than generalized answers. First of all, it should be emphasized that the hospital drug committees that started in Scandinavian countries in the 1960's were basically a result of informal initiatives by clinicians, pharmacologists, and pharmacists. These committees are still working on a more or less informal professional base, although somewhat linked to *local* or *regional* (but not national) health authorities. The recommendations made are considered as guidelines and advice to the medical profession. After more than 10 years of experience it is clear that this procedure is quite fruitful, because it activates a great number of physicians and others during the discussions which form the basis for the recommendations. The basic principles, being simplification in order to improve drug efficacy and safety, are accepted by the broad majority of those involved. Although professional disagreements occur in questions of detail, it has become possible to conduct discussions based upon real arguments rather than 'opinions' only.

As to the European countries and their reactions to the concept of essential drugs, one should of course be even more cautious regarding generalization. I have the feeling though that after some initial frustration about the relevance of this program, which was partly due to misunderstandings basically on the part of several drug producers and some key professionals, the philosophy is now better understood and accepted. However, there is still some concern that such an assumed restrictive line would tend to suppress research and drug innovation. Personally I would not exclude the possibility that this program, which points to the necessity of identifying basic health needs, could just as well lead to a better drug research and development policy. Again, personally, I strongly believe that the philosophy behind this program is valid in developed as well as in developing countries. The adoption of the program will, and should, vary depending on the available resources and the local therapeutic traditions. Of course, there is no fixed number of drugs that is magically relevant in all countries, but the idea of selection, thus ending up with a *reasonable* product range, is a general one. Finally, it should be mentioned that the discussions around the WHO program on essential drugs have also brought WHO into direct dialog with the drug industry. This may result in improved programs for providing drugs which are either missing or not available where needed.

Melmon: The list you have helped to create clearly has some major assets in the third-world countries and perhaps in more developed areas. Does it have a potential for decreasing economic incentive for development of new drugs by the industry?

Lunde: To the best of my judgement the basic ideas and criteria for the selection of 'essential' (or better 'basic') drugs, as given in *WHO Technical Report Series No. 615*, should be valid for all countries, irrespective of their state of development. However, the adoption and practical application of the selection procedures will vary depending on local conditions, as outlined in my paper. Some countries may have to give special priority to the most basic needs and demands, reflecting the limitations in terms of funds and manpower resources for health care in general.

The second part of your question is still somewhat hypothetical, although already raised from the very beginning by the drug producers and some scientists with special concern for the future of innovative drug research and development. First of all, I should like to state that this has never been the intention of this work. The basis is that some simplification is necessary if we wish to solve a reasonable number of the problems related to drug efficacy and safety, in view of the limited possibilities of performing Phase IV (epidemiological) studies to the extent necessary. So far, the increased interest and will to identify the health problems and needs which up to now have been of low priority for those allocating resources for drug development (such as a number of 'tropical infections'), could rather produce improved possibilities for future research. This obviously *must* be a joint effort between the appropriate international organizations and the traditional drug producers. As part of this it is necessary to build up sufficient research competence on the spot, that is to improve local competence for an appropriate diagnostic, epidemiological and therapeutic apparatus.

As to the present flow of unjustified 'me too' drugs and ill-documented drug combinations etc., I would personally not regret their disappearance. To my mind, this type of drug does not contribute to progress – if anything, they hamper development of medicine as a whole.

Drug safety in regard to manufacturing processes and utilization

TSUNEJI NAGAI

Department of Pharmaceutics, Hoshi Institute of Pharmaceutical Sciences, Hoshi College of Pharmacy, Tokyo, Japan

Drug safety is usually investigated from the pharmacological or toxicological viewpoint. However, even if such investigations are exhaustive, safety is not assured if there is any deficiency in the manufacture or use of the drug.

DRUG SAFETY IN MANUFACTURE

From the manufacturing angle, drug safety depends primarily on correct formulation and proper quality control. 'Bioavailability', that is the amount absorbed and the rate of absorption of drug, is one of the most important factors. There have been several cases of poisoning caused by variations in the bioavailability of a drug in different products.

Such variations usually depend on the formulation. The cases of poisoning by phenytoin in Australia and digoxin in England are famous examples.

In 1968 in Australia, a number of patients who had been treated with antispasmotics for epilepsy suffered poisoning. Following an investigation, it was revealed that all the phenytoin sodium 100 mg capsules administered to these patients were from the same company and that the diluent used had been changed from calcium sulfate dihydrate to lactose in November, 1967. The two kinds of capsules were therefore compared in an absorption study in patients (1). The result showed that the bioavailability from the capsules with lactose was very high compared with those with calcium sulfate dihydrate. Thus the poisoning had resulted because a product of low bioavailability had been changed suddenly to one of high bioavailability.

Poisoning by digoxin was reported in the *Lancet* in 1972 (2). Of 19 patients who were on a stable treatment with a certain kind of digoxin 0.25 mg tablets, 3 suffered from poisoning and in 15 the blood concentration increased when they changed to tablets produced by a different company. On returning to the original tablets, the blood concentration reverted to the previous state after 6 days. Following this discovery, the blood concentrations of digoxin were determined after administration of various preparations supplied by different companies (3). The result showed that there were differences of between 4 and 7 times between companies and about 5 times between different lots made by the same company. Generic equivalents do not, therefore, always have the same therapeutic effect. Such variations in bioavailability usually result from differences in the dissolution behavior of the drug according to the method of formulation.

Some drugs, which are safe when produced, are apt to develop some toxicity because of decomposition during storage. Therefore, the safety of decomposition products of the drugs should be investigated in detail, and strict evaluation of stability and control of formulation are absolutely necessary. In regard to stability, manufacturers have devoted attention to decreases in content of the effective component. For example, in the past they have often, in the case of an easily decomposing drug, formulated the component at over 100% of the described content. Thus the product might pass scrutiny even if the principal component suffered considerable decomposition. Such overconcentrated preparations should not be allowed, so long as the safety of the decomposed products is not assured.

Some preparations for external use may produce irritation by very small amounts of decomposition products, from the principal component, the base, or additives. Therefore, it is important for pharmaceutical manufacturers to establish suitable methods for testing the stability of drugs.

Moreover, it is important that there shall be 'no mistake' and 'no contamination' during the manufacture of drugs. A simple mistake in labeling may cause serious suffering. For example – and this is a true story – a bottle labelled 'sodium chloride' which, in fact, contained potassium bromide, was supplied for preparation of physiological sodium chloride solution in a hospital in Tokyo. The two substances are similar in appearance. Fortunately, an able pharmacist discovered the mistake, otherwise a serious accident might have taken place. Mislabeled products are much worse than decomposed ones. Good manufacturing practice (GMP) should function to prevent any such defects, for complete protection of the patients.

DRUG SAFETY IN REGARD TO USE

As mentioned above, GMP functions to ensure rationally indicated drugs of quality throughout the whole process from raw materials to the administration of the finished products to patients. This approach should be expanded to cover all the people concerned with hospital pharmacies. Drug safety depends not only on technological facilities for quality assurance and rational indications, but also on the ethics of medical specialists.

If medical doctors or pharmacists are inexperienced or misunderstand the use of drugs, serious suffering may result. For example, phenobarbital, a hypnotic and a powerful drug, is often prescribed under the name 'Phenobal' which in Japanese pronunciation in similar to 'Phenovalin', a laxative. If the former were administered in the usual dose of the latter, a patient would suffer danger. Barium sulfate, used as an X-ray contrast medium, is usually called 'barium'. When, about 20 years ago, a thoughtless medical doctor used barium chloride instead, a patient died. Reflecting on these examples, the education in pharmacology of medical doctors and pharmacists should clearly be strengthened, in respect of side-effects or adverse reactions as well as of the principal effects on the drugs.

There are many problems regarding the use of drugs. In Kanagawa Prefecture last summer, many patients visited ophthalmologists for treatment of an inflammation of the eyes which had been caused by misuse of an aqueous preparation for eczema instead of eye drops. It has long been customary to apply the eczema preparation with a small brush. Just recently, however, a new one was marketed in a bottle similar to that of eye drops and for use in a similar fashion. Moreover, the indications were not clear, which led to the accident.

As even adults sometimes make such mistakes, special care should be taken of children. Sugar-coated tablets, which look like some kind of chocolate candies, sometimes cause accidents. It is important to develop 'child-proof' methods of dosage. For example, as an inhalation for childhood asthma may be used until the container is empty, poisoning is possible if the container is too large.

At present, so many kinds and such amounts of drugs are used in Japan that it is said to be 'pickling in drugs'. In particular, many kinds of drugs are too often prescribed together. We should seriously consider whether combinations of more than two kinds of drugs influence their effectiveness and safety. It is difficult enough to be sure about the interaction even when only two drugs are combined. For development of new combinations, pharmaceutical manufacturers have to prove the clinical merit by precise investigations of the effectiveness and the safety. The enormous necessary efforts may explain why only a few new combination drugs are currently being born. On the other hand, many kinds of drugs are often combined in medical practice. It is by no means rare for more than 10 kinds of drugs to be mixed in intravenous infusions. Nobody knows the resulting toxicity. Even physico-chemical interactions are not investigated in detail, which should be a prelude to toxicological or biological investigations. Such is the situation, that drugs combined without any precise information about drug safety, but solely on the basis of the doctor's right to prescribe, carry the risk of drug-induced sufferings.

Interactions can arise not only between drugs in a single prescription but also between those in different prescriptions for the same patient. Recently, clinical departments have become increasingly specialized with the progress of medical care and thus many patients receive different prescriptions from several departments at the same time or within a short period. For example, one patient was treated in 5 departments during one month in a hospital in Tokyo. In such a case, if all the prescriptions are followed, sufferings may be induced both by overmedication due to overlapping and by side-effects due to interaction. To protect patients, computer systems are being introduced in hospitals to check the prescriptions, giving pharmacists diverse information so that they can advise doctors. However, such a system is not yet established to ensure co-ordination between different hospitals.

Drug abuse or overmedication may also be induced by social, economic or legal factors. For example, an excessively competitive or dazzling advertisement to promote the purchase of drugs may have such results. This problem is not solved even if proper cautions and warnings are given in the package insert.

DRUG SAFETY IN RELATION TO THE ABILITY OF PHARMACISTS AND PHARMACEUTICAL EDUCATION

It is regrettable that pharmacists in Japan lack the ability and the chance to play a proper role in the assurance of safety in the manufacture and use of drugs. This situation arises because of the present failure to complete 'iyakubungyo' (professional specialization of pharmacists). Moreover, it must be said that pharmaceutical education in Japan is not drug-oriented but chemistry-oriented.

In the manufacturing process, a pharmacist is not so important legally regarding the responsibility in in-process control in an integrated quality assurance system. Although GMP has come into effect, a pharmaceutical factory of any size can be formed if only one pharmacist is employed. Moreover, many managers are not pharmacists. For a pharmaceutical company, a 'pharmacist' is not important for selling; only the 'actual results' are important. A pharmacist may not always achieve satisfactory results, especially in selling to practising doctors who are not interested in listening to explanations about drugs.

In the practice of medical care, a pharmacist has no part in such important work as the mixing of intravenous infusions, which may be one of the most risky procedures. A nurse usually takes care of it, and drug safety depends on his or her ability. In this connection, it is jokingly said that the experts on drugs are, in order, the nurse, the doctor, the patient and, lastly, the pharmacist.

Following the frequent cases of drug-induced sufferings in the past, there has been an increasing need for pharmacists to work in medical care as specialists in drugs. A new field named 'clinical pharmacy' has already been established in the United States. We also have a similar movement in Japan. However, it is too slow, probably for two reasons. First, though everybody recognizes the importance of clinical pharmacy, there are various difficulties which prevent pharmacists from entering the existing system, and also pharmacists do not have the ability to join medical-care teams. The second reason relates to pharmaceutical education. Everybody recognizes the importance of training in clinical pharmacy, but there are many difficulties in amending current pharmaceutical education. For example, there is a shortage of suitable staff. At present in Japan, the curriculum for pharmaceutical education lasts for 4 years, and this includes both general education and special education. Moreover, no practical training or internship is required before the national examination is taken. From the legal point of view, therefore, pharmaceutical education is poorest amongst the developed countries. This system of pharmaceutical education has been established on the basis of the special situation of pharmaceutical affairs in Japan in comparison with European and American countries. In Japan, the professional specialization of pharmacists is not complete, as mentioned already, and the important place of pharmacists in medical care is occupied by medical doctors. Therefore, a large number of graduates in pharmacy, especially those from the leading schools, have worked for pharmaceutical companies, taking part in research, development or production. Pharmaceutical education has, therefore, inclined towards science and engineering rather than medical care. In other words, the education of pharmacists to play an important role in assuring the safety of drugs in manufacturing and use has been ignored. Unfortunately, even teachers in pharmacy schools usually have no appreciation of the responsibility of pharmacists for drug safety.

COMMON SENSE AMONGST THE PUBLIC IN MATTERS OF DRUG SAFETY

Finally, it should be added that many Japanese are not sensible about using drugs, in spite of the spread of education about them. For example, we like drugs so much that we do not value highly any medical advice against using them. It is difficult to find a method to promote scientific understanding of drugs. Therefore, many of us accept a drug blindly or underestimate its effects. It seems very necessary to educate the public, so that very safe drugs are manufactured and safely used in practice.

REFERENCES

1. Bochner, F. (1972): Factors involved in outbreak of phenytoin intoxication. *J. neurol. Sci., 16*, 481.
2. Editorial (1972): Bioavailability of digoxin. *Lancet, 2*, 90.
3. Lindenbaum. J., Mellow, M.H., Blackstone, M.O. and Butler, V.P. (1971): Variation in biologic availability of digoxin from four preparations. *New Engl. J. Med., 285*, 1344.

DISCUSSION

Shin: In connection with the use of drugs, such terms as 'abuse', 'misuse', 'addiction', 'habit-forming', 'tolerance' and 'dependence', which are often used interchangeably, should be properly defined. In 1957, WHO officially adopted the following usages: abuse – drug use without medical supervision; misuse – wrong use of drug under medical supervision; addiction – specific side- or adverse effects of drugs caused by prolonged use. In the case of addiction, WHO recommended the use of the term 'dependence', subdivided into psychological or physical. Further, such terms as 'habit-forming' and 'tolerance' should also be properly defined in advance of dealing with the problems of drug use.

Nagai: I appreciate Dr. Shin's comment. It is most enlightening. In Japan, GMP (articles of good manufacturing practice) has been introduced to cover the whole manufacturing process starting from the raw materials. Next to be introduced are GLP (good laboratory practice) and then GPSP (good promotion and supply practice), and with regard to the latter, Dr. Shin's view is most instructive.

Transmission of drug information to physicians and drug-induced suffering

ROKURO HAMA

Department of Internal Medicine, Hannan Central Hospital, Osaka, Japan

Safe drug utilization requires reliable and accurate information about both the benefits and the demerits of drugs. Such information by itself is meaningless unless it is properly handled by practising physicians. Ironically enough, little that is really useful is available in spite of the rash of new drugs and the excessive information in recent years. It is very difficult for a physician himself to collect, select and utilize truly useful information in daily practice. Thus, it is increasingly important to organize the collection, evaluation, rearrangement and transmission of information about drugs.

The occurrence of several disasters indicates that these activities are insufficient in Japan. Although some lessons have been learned, many problems remain unresolved.

This report briefly reviews the history of transmission of information to physicians, discusses current problems, including the malfunctioning of the official communication media, and makes some proposals.

A BRIEF HISTORY OF TRANSMISSION OF DRUG INFORMATION TO PHYSICIANS

The transmission of drug information, especially that concerning adverse drug reactions, is a fairly recent development. It can be divided into four periods. In the first, prior to the issue of the circular notice, 'Principles for the Approval of New Drug Production', or 'Kihontsuchi' ('Circular Notice on Principles') in September 1967, the Government rarely played any part. The only important exception was the circular notice on penicillins. Neither pyrazolone-induced shock nor the thalidomide disaster directly affected the system for transmission of information to physicians, though they facilitated the regulation of over-the-counter drug advertisements and fetal toxicity tests, respectively. The effectiveness and the benefits of drugs have often been exaggerated in advertisements and promotional pamphlets. This is also true of drug inserts. In Japanese a drug insert is called 'Nogaki'. Literally this means 'proof of effectiveness', but sometimes 'unreliable statements'. Physicians' distrust, and neglect, of drug inserts might well have been established in this period.

For example, Coralgil, a coronary vasodilator, was banned in 1970 because of toxicity, including systemic lipidosis (1,2) and fatal liver damage (3,4). Information provided by the drug firm was misleading in several ways:

1. A high dosage rarely prescribed in other countries was introduced and recommended in the drug insert as a normal dosage in Japan.

2. In other countries periodical suspension was called for in the instruction for prolonged treatment, but this instruction was neglected in Japan. 'Coralgil is well tolerated' and 'Coralgil is suitable for a long period of treatment' were statements made by the drug firm.
3. Data which demonstrated hypercholesterolemia (5–8) were neglected. Unapproved claims such as 'hypocholesterolemic action' or 'lipostatic ation' were widely disseminated by advertisements and promotional pamphlets.
4. There were several findings which clearly pointed to possible hepatotoxicity (6,9), but they were not referred to either in the drug inserts or in the promotional literature.

On the other hand, drug information activities were organized by medical people. Medical meetings, journals and personal communications were available, though even these tended to emphasize only the benefits of the drugs.

The second period lasted from the issue of the 'Circular Notice on Principles' until 1971. The national adverse drug reaction monitoring system started just before the beginning of this period. The 'Circular Notice on Principles' imposed upon the drug firms the duty of describing adverse reactions to new drugs in the reports and literature submitted for approval. Cautions about the use of chloramphenicol and other antibiotics were instituted in accordance with the 'Circular Notice on Principles'. Subsequently, cautions for the use of some other antibiotics, chloroquines etc. were also compiled and printed in the drug inserts. Most of the drug inserts, however, were no different from those in the first period. Extravagant promotional materials became so numerous that another circular notice was required to call attention to the fact that 'most of the drug inserts were inaccurate because they exaggerated the safety of the drugs and the rarity of adverse effects'. Consumption of prescription drugs was intentionally promoted by drug firms. Towards the end of this period, sufferings induced by such drugs as clioquinol, Coralgil and chloroquines were brought to public attention. The information on 'chloroquine retinopathy' was finally included in the drug insert, but this was no guarantee that it would be transmitted to physicians (10). This seems to have been one of the important reasons why the suffering continued. The information that Coralgil might be the cause of 'foam cell syndrome', presented both at a meeting and in a paper, was not adequately conveyed to physicians (11). The promotion of Coralgil as 'suitable for a long period of treatment' continued.

Effective education for safe drug use was not organized by the medical circle, although The Japanese Medical Association (JMA) began to issue 'Drug Information Cards' to its members.

The third period lasted until the circular notice 'On the Standardization of Drug Insert Forms' in February 1976. During this period, revision of drug inserts was promoted by the occurrence of drug-induced sufferings.

'MHW Adverse Reactions Information News' and 'MHW Drug Information' were first issued in 1973 and 1975, respectively. Statements such as 'No side-effects' or 'Safe for a prolonged treatment' gradually disappeared from advertisements in medical journals. Instead, 'Please read the cautions respecting use in the drug insert' or a full statement of the caution appeared. The number of special editions devoted to 'adverse reactions to drugs' increased, reflecting the growing interest of physicians. But no effective media for information were systematically organized by the JMA and other medical societies. Many severe cases of hypoglycemic reactions induced by oral hypoglycemic agents, as well as cases of 'quadriceps contracture' induced by injections, indicated clearly the deficiency in organized activities by medical persons. Drug information services by pharmacists were initiated.

In the fourth period, the media for information have remained essentially the same as in the third period, except that the drug inserts are required to be more standardized and detailed.

TRANSMISSION OF NEW INFORMATION ON ADVERSE REACTIONS TO PHYSICIANS

Cautions respecting the use of 306 drug components were published in circular notices issued by the Director General of the Drug Administration MHW.

A survey by questionnaire was carried out in 1973 to investigate the success of this venture. The subjects of the survey were 243 physicians who worked mainly in wards at Osaka University Hospital; 126 responded. Of 106 physicians who had prescribed indomethacin, 29% answered 'I know' that 'indomethacin is contraindicated in aspirin-sensitive asthma patients' (Fig. 1). Of 117 physicians who had prescribed metoclopramide, an antiemetic, 52% answered 'I know' that 'metoclopramide may induce extrapyramidal symptoms including dystonic reactions', and 22% that 'this adverse reaction is precipitated by phenothiazines when used in combination'. To an enquiry about the statement: 'This adverse reaction and the drug interaction have been newly described after the revision of the drug inserts', only 7% answered 'I know because I have read the drug insert'. To the question 'How well do you think new information on adverse reactions has been transmitted to you?', 65% answered 'not well' or 'not at all' (Table 1a). 48 physicians answered the question about the media for new information. Medical media were used most frequently (25 physicians), in contrast with the two official media (circular notices and drug inserts) which were each used by one physician (Table 1b). 91 physicians answered the question about the information source

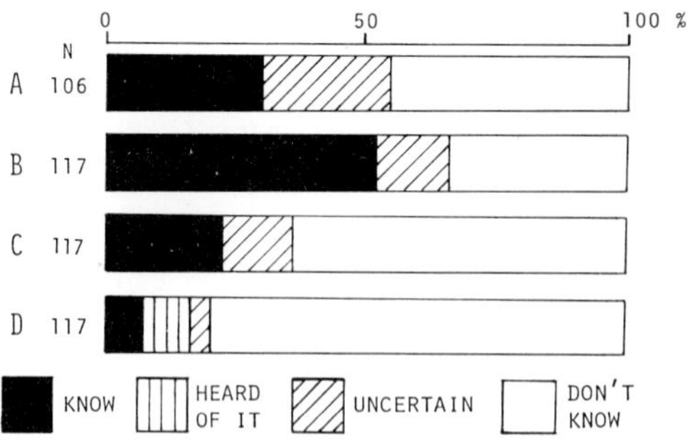

Fig. 1. Physicians' knowledge about newly described adverse drug reactions in drug inserts. A = Indomethacin is contraindicated in aspirin-sensitive asthma. B = Metoclopramide may induce extrapyramidal symptoms including dystonia. C = B is precipitated by phenothiazines. D = B and C are stated in the drug insert.

TABLE 1. *Results of survey by questionnaire to physicians on information regarding adverse drug reactions (ADR)*

a. How well do you think new ADR information, provided by MHW and/or drug firms, has been transmitted to you?

	%	%
Sufficiently	0.0	9.5
Fairly well	9.5	
Intermediate	21.4	
Not well	53.2	65.1
Not at all	11.9	
No answer	4.0	
	100.0	

b. Through what media is new ADR information transmitted to you?

	(%)
Medical media (meetings, journals, colleagues)	25 (37.9)
Drug firms	14 (21.2)
Mass media	12 (18.2)
Pharmacists, DI section at Hospital	12 (18.2)
Circular notice by MHW	1 (1.5)
Drug inserts	1 (1.5)
Others	1 (1.5)
N = 48	66(137.5)

c. Information sources through which doctors first learned of 'chloroquine retinopathy'

Medical media	48.4%
Mass media	36.8
Pharmacists etc.	5.5
Drug inserts	4.9
Drug firms	0.0
Others	4.4
N = 91	100.0

through which they first learned of 'chloroquine retinopathy' (Table 1c); 49% selected medical media, 37% mass media, 5% drug inserts, and none selected drug firms.

These data suggest: (1) information about safe drug use was not well communicated to practising physicians; (2) official measures such as circular notices and drug inserts had little effect. Physicians mostly relied on medical media. Although these private channels of communication are professional and certainly important, they take place at random and are not systematically organized.

The deficiency in systematically organized activities concerning the safety of drugs in Japan is indicated by the small number of reports of adverse reactions to the national monitoring system (10). The proportion of physicians who knew that 'Osaka University Hospital is one of the monitor hospitals of the national adverse reaction monitoring system', was only 9% in the survey of 1973. But it increased to 20% in a similar survey carried out in 1975 (subjects: 736 physicians, respondents: 421) (12). The survey of 1973 (with 126 physicians responding) revealed that no single case of an adverse reaction had been reported in the preceding year. In the survey of 1975, however, there were 18 cases reported to Osaka Prefecture and 8 cases to the national system. When asked to mention, in a simplified form, the cases of adverse reactions which they remembered from the preceding year, 317 cases were elicited from 150 physicians out of a total of 421 respondents. After the survey, 64 cases of adverse reactions were officially reported to Osaka Prefecture in the following 2 months. At Hannan Central Hospital adverse drug reactions observed in the medical clinic are registered in the Ambulatory Disease Registration System (13,14) which started 2 years ago, and drugs dispensed have been registered for the past 5 years. 208 adverse reactions were registered in 186 patients during 1978, representing 2.2% of 8633 patients seen in the same period (15).

Thus, with effort, these systems can be made to function efficiently, not only at large institutions like university hospitals but also at a community hospital.

CURRENT PROBLEMS AND SOME PROPOSALS

Current problems involved in the communication of drug information to physicians are as follows. First, the drug insert, which is the only mechanism regulated by governmental acts, does not function well because of its limited reliability, limited usefulness, inconvenience, lack of speed and insufficiency of supplementary information.

Standardization and reinforcement of the contents of drug inserts have been carried out since the circular notice in 1976. This represents some progress, but the drug insert is still too general, insufficiently specific, and ambiguous. For example, 'Use cautiously with the following patients: patients with liver dysfunction and kidney dysfunction, etc.' is sometimes stated without giving any reasons. The insert provides no answers to clinically important questions, such as whether laboratory examinations are necessary because of the possibility of liver and/or kidney toxicity, or a reduction of dosage is necessary because of impaired metabolism and/or excretion. Similar expressions are used even in drug inserts for aminoglycosides. Clinically useful information is listed in Table 2. Unless the listed information is included in a readable form, physicians will continue to be reluctant to use drug inserts.

Drug inserts are inconvenient, especially in a hospital, where physicians have to fetch them from the pharmacy. The inserts so obtained are not always the latest. The time interval between the revision of an insert and its recognition by physicians depends upon the amounts of the drug purchased and the frequency of its dispensation. At our hospital, the pharmacist reponsible for the monthly check of drug inserts found that the interval averaged 9 months and ranged from 3 to 23 months. More than 10 hours of work is necessary every month to compare the old and new inserts. The drug firms should be required to send promptly any new inserts with a list of the revised points, giving the reasons for revisions.

TABLE 2. *Information useful and necessary for safe drug use*

For indication decision
- a. Indications
  - Degree of effectiveness (effective or possibly effective)
  - First choice or second choice
  - If second choice, what drug is the first choice?
- b. Contraindications
  - Absolute contraindications and their reasons, and signs and symptoms when administered by mistake
  - Conditions in which precautions should be given and their reasons
- c. Warnings

For prevention, early detection and treatment of adverse drug reactions (ADRs)
- a. Severe or important ADRs
- b. Frequently observed ADRs
- c. ADR listed by organ/system, with frequency
- d. Important ADRs of related drugs
- e. Drug interactions
- f. Overdosage or exaggerated responses
- g. Names of substitutes and the precautions

For appropriate dosage and administration
- a. Standard dosage and administration for adults and children, without complications
- b. Adjustment of dosage and administration in patients with complications, e.g. renal or heart failure, liver diseases, in newborn infants, and in pregnant or nursing mothers

Other useful information
- a. Ingredients, generic names, chemical and structural formula
- b. Clinical pharmacology
  - Principal actions, absorption, therapeutic plasma concentration, plasma half-life, principal metabolizing organ, excretion by kidney
- c. Animal pharmacology and toxicology
  - Toxic manifestations and findings in animal tests, maximum safety dose (MSD), MSD/therapeutic dose
- d. How supplied, precautions in management
- e. Date revision, details of revision, list of particulars before and after revision, reasons for revision
- f. References
- g. Others

A compendium making the drug inserts readily available should be delivered to physicians, free of charge, by drug firms.

The second point is that the information on safe drug use is small and insignificant compared with the impressive and huge amount of promotional information. Promotional material is clear, to the point, beautifully printed, and uses various emphases and expressions appropriate to its purpose. It is sent repeatedly to physicians. In contrast, information about safe drug use is tedious, too general, stereotyped, and in small print. It has the same message as the drug insert. Often, 'Please read cautions on use in the drug insert' is the only statement included. Promotional information should be regulated more strictly. In the United States, expressions used in brochures were subjected to regulation (16) in 1960, well before the Kefauver Harris Amendment Act of 1962. There is much for us to learn from this lesson.

I would like to propose a plan to regulate promotional information. This starts with a definition of the grades of preciseness for the indications and cautions of a drug insert. In promotions, the drug firm should be required to use the same degree of preciseness, and allowed only the same amount of space.

For example, the grades of preciseness would be as follows:

1. Important warnings, contraindications, indications substantially confirmed.
2. In addition to (1), the list of the diseases and conditions which require special precautions, important adverse reactions, and indications other than (1).
3. Full statement of the drug insert.
4. In addition to (3), a summary of the data which prove the statements in (1) and (2), and references.
5. Details of (4) and/or the original papers; data in support of (3).

Other points worth mentioning are as follows. The use of multiple brand names for a single compound is troublesome. Brand names are familiar to physicians in daily practice, but generic names are usually used in reports about adverse reactions. This may be one reason why knowledge of adverse reactions is not effectively conveyed to physicians.

It also seems important that the lack of any clinical pharmacology and therapeutics in present medical education and the inadequacy of any organized activity about drug information by the Medical Association and societies, leave many physicians at the mercy of a flood of promotional information. Evaluation of drugs should be carried out independently of drug firms and administration. The establishment of information media organized by the medical professions is much desired.

Concerted efforts by physicians, clinical pharmacologists, pharmacists, government officials and drug firms are necessary. Specifically, a counterbalance must be struck between the excessive energy applied to promotion of sales and the insufficient energy devoted to the scientific and safe use of drugs.

REFERENCES

1. Adachi, S., Yamamoto, A. et al. (1970): Studies on drug-induced lipidosis. I. Report of clinical cases. *Arch. J. Soc. intern. Med., 60*, 224 (in Japanese).
2. Yamamoto, A. et al. (1971): Drug-induced lipidosis in human cases and animal experiments: Accumulation of an acidic glycerophospholipid. *J. Biochem. (Tokyo), 69*, 613.
3. Oda, T., Shidata, T. et al. (1970): Phospholipid fatty liver: A report of three cases with a new type of fatty liver. *Jap. J. exp. Med., 40*, 127.
4. Committee for the study of 'DH' (1971): A peculiar syndrome induced by diethylaminoethoxy hexestrol (DH). *Saishin-igaku, 28*, 2205 (in Japanese).

5. Kishikawa, M. (1964): Clinical experience with 'Coralgil'. *Shinryo, 17*, 1232 (in Japanese).
6. Katsu, M. et al. (1965): Clinical experience wth 'Coralgil'. *Shinyaku-To-Rinsho, 14*, 531 (in Japanese).
7. Nakamura, H. (1967): Effect of 4,4′-diethylaminoethoxy hexestrol on the synthesis of cholesterol. *Acta hepat. Jap., 8*, 37 (in Japanese).
8. Nakamura, H. et al. (1971): Hypercholesterolemia induced with 4,4′-diethylamino-ethoxy hexestrol in the rabbit. *Med. Biol., 83*, 167 (in Japanese).
9. Urasawa, K. et al. (1965): Effect of Coralgil on serum lipid level and the mechanism of action. *Diagn. Treatm., 53*, 2066 (in Japanese).
10. Hama, R. et al. (1973): Questionnaire survey on drug information transmission to physicians. *Igaku-no-Ayumi, 86*, 403 (in Japanese).
11. Hama, R. (1974): Systemic lipidosis induced by 4,4′-diethylaminoethoxy hexestrol. *Med. Drug J., 10*, 52 (in Japanese).
12. Hama, R. et al. (1976): On the method for promoting adverse drug reaction monitoring. In: *Annual Report of the Study Group for Adverse Drug Reactions of Osaka Prefecture*, pp. 57–93 (in Japanese).
13. Hama, R., Hashimoto, N. et al. (1978): Monitoring adverse reactions to drugs in outpatients. I. An application of the Ambulatory Disease Registration System. In: *Annual Report of the Study Group for Adverse Drug Reactions of Osaka Prefecture*, pp. 53–63 (in Japanese).
14. Hashimoto, N., Hama, R. et al. (1979): Ambulatory Disease Registration System at a community hospital. In: *Proceedings, MEDIS '78*, pp. 169–172. The Medical Information System Development Center and Kansai Institute of Information Systems.
15. Hama, R. et al. (1979): Monitoring adverse reactions to drugs in outpatients. II. Statistical analysis of 1978's data. In: *Annual Report of the Study Group for Adverse Drug Reactions of Osaka Prefecture.*
16. Kessenich, W.H. (1960): Safe new drugs and their control under law. *Clin. Pharmacol. Ther., 1*, 53.

DISCUSSION

Yanagita: Although there is certainly a problem about the provision and transmission of information to doctors, the final solution depends on whether the doctors themselves make the effort to read it. What is your opinion about this, Dr. Hama?

Hama: It is very difficult for doctors to change already adopted practices. Information must be repeatedly presented to them. Only then will doctors break their customary habits.

Herxheimer: I wonder whether we could hear something about graduate medical education in Japan and about the extent to which it is concerned with therapeutics.

Hama: Japanese graduate medical education on therapeutics traditionally depended on experience, emulation of the senior doctors and learning from them. Of course, things have been changing, and although we are getting away from this, a new form of education has not yet truly been established. At the postgraduate stage, information from the pharmaceutical companies predominates, without much information in any other form.

Herxheimer: Are there no postgraduate courses in diagnosis and in general medicine after doctors have qualified, for example, as general practitioners? Do they stop learning once they have left medical school?

Hama: There is a 2-year intern system, a kind of voluntary training through affiliation with hospitals or other facilities, but there is no legal stipulation for on-going lifetime education and training.

Darmansjah: I have just returned from a discussion in another room on 'Doctors' responsibility for SMON'. There, a question was asked why there was such a great difference between Japan and other countries regarding the employment of clioquinol in high doses over long periods. No satisfactory answer was given, but I would like to ask here whether the difference arose from what was taught about clioquinol in the Japanese medical schools. Does anyone remember what was taught in pharmacology about the drug in the pre-SMON period?

Takasu: Clioquinol first became widely marketed in Japan around 1955. I graduated from college in 1958, but in my college days I did not receive any detailed information.

Regarding Dr. Hama's response to Dr. Herxheimer's question about postgraduate education in therapeutics: probably each doctor should respond individually, describing his own background. But I would like to add that there are also some well-known books which provide influential guidelines on therapeutic matters.

Further, in Japan, postgraduate courses in clinical medicine do exist, though the instruction in therapeutics is not the most sufficient. Postgraduate courses in clinical medicine more resemble day-to-day clinical practice than systematic education providing basic knowledge and information.

It should also be mentioned that at the regional doctors' association level, some kinds of training seminars corresponding to postgraduate courses are provided.

Patient information, an opportunity for preventing unwanted effects

FREYA HERMANN[1] and ANDREW HERXHEIMER[2]

[1] *School of Pharmacy, Oregon State University Corvallis, OR, USA and*
[2] *Charing Cross Hospital Medical School, London, U.K.*

In many countries of Western Europe, medications are dispensed in unit-of-use packages which contain package inserts as a matter of common practice. The inserts have not always been regarded as vehicles for information to patients, but for some time now they have been considered widely for that purpose. Although one might hesitate to inform a patient of unwanted effects, fearing the power which such a suggestion may have, one must accept the right of a patient to know the hazards of therapy. A close look at package inserts which are currently used in Europe shows, however, that patients are not always adequately informed about the unwanted effects that may occur if they take their medication.

Some package inserts do not list side-effects at all. The French insert for allopurinol, for example, has only information on ingredients, indications, contraindications, dose, need for adequate intake of liquids, and number of tablets per package.

Some inserts list side-effects but do not draw attention to them with a subheading or other technique of layout, and rather include them with other information for the reader. The Austrian insert for phenylbutazone lists several side-effects under the heading 'Attention'. Included in the same section is a mixed bag of cautions, some directed to patients, others to physicians: take only under the supervision of the physician, prescribe with caution for elderly patients, observe contraindications and drug interactions. There are instructions on how to dose if hypersensitivity is suspected, to do blood tests periodically, prescribe one to two treatment-free days per week during long-term therapy, and there is an admonition to store the medication out of reach of children. Side-effects are mentioned – allergic skin reactions, decrease of leukocytes and/or thrombocytes – but they are difficult to find among all the other cautions and directions.

Other inserts list side-effects and also designate a separate section for them. But they may do it in technical language, unintelligible to many patients. The Belgian insert for allopurinol lists some side-effects as 'pruritic exanthema', 'changed hepatic function test', and 'idiosyncratic reactions'. How can patients be expected to understand?

Even if unwanted effects are listed, designated as side-effects and described in plain language, the terms used may still make the information unusable for patients. The German insert for hydrochlorothiazide states that 'in exceptional cases, hypersensitivity reactions of the skin have been observed', and what are patients to do if they read that?

Finally, inserts, though listing and designating side-effects, describing them in plain language and usable terms, may fall short of the ideal because they do not include follow-up advice to patients. The German insert for propranolol lists 'occasionally occurring diarrhea', 'constipation' and 'nausea', and goes on to say that 'a few cases of dizziness, tingling, numbness of hands, reddening of skin have been observed'. Patients are left on their own to decide what to do if any of these problems occur.

Package inserts can be a vehicle for the complex information on unwanted effects because patients will have them and can refer to them at once whenever they need that information. Written information can help those patients who have not been informed by the physician or pharmacist, those patients who had been told but had not understood the instruction, and also those patients who had been told and had understood, but have forgotten.

In general, written information should not replace spoken instruction, but information on side-effects is often extremely detailed and therefore may very well be the exception. Although not much is known about the impact of such information, it seems reasonable to assume that complex information of this type will be most useful if it is available for reference at the time when it is needed. A study of the effects of spoken and written instructions showed that patients who had received only written instructions reported more adverse effects, although they had not experienced more adverse effects, than those who had received only spoken instructions (1).

The message of the insert must be intelligible, concise, and comprehensive. Firstly, then, to be intelligible, information must be in plain language so that patients can understand it. Attempts by governmental agencies to regulate this kind of communication have emphasized the need for simple language (2, 3). The need for increasing readability by decreasing complexity of sentences and the use of abstract concepts has been discussed in the literature (4). What has been said for inserts in general must certainly be true for adverse effects. The adverse effect must be conveyed in terms which the patient can use. It must be described not only in words which the patient can understand, but described in a useful way, i.e. in terms of symptoms which the patient can observe. It is not useful to talk of 'hypersensitivity reactions of the skin', but much better to talk about 'itching and skin rash'. A patient cannot observe hypokalemia as such but can notice abdominal discomfort and muscle weakness, which may be due to hypokalemia.

An adverse effect which causes no symptoms by which the patient can observe it, need not be described in the package insert but must be dealt with by describing how this effect can be detected. For example, the patient may have to be told to see the physician periodically for that purpose.

Secondly, the information must be concise, or patients will find it too difficult to handle. Extraneous information can be confusing or misleading. Long sentences and unfamiliar words will increase the difficulty of written material. It has been shown that more information is recalled when the material is summarized and reorganized (5).

Thirdly, while information has to be concise, it must cover all aspects of a problem, it must be comprehensive. The adverse effect itself must be described and patients must also be told what they should do when the effect occurs. Even though patients are told how to recognize an effect, they still cannot be expected to judge its meaning or importance, nor can they be expected to think of all ways for coping with the effect, let alone to select the best way. The same symptoms may have a different significance and may call for different measures, depending on the drug which causes it and the circumstances. Nausea is not nausea, is not nausea – if one is caused by tetracycline, the other by nitrofurantoin, the other by digitalis.

If one expects patients to do something about an adverse effect, then they must somehow be given the relevant information. Patients may be able to do something to prevent an unwanted effect or, if that is not possible, to recognize it when it occurs. If they recognize it, they may do something to cope with it: tell the physician immediately, or do so the next day, tell the physician during the next office visit, call the pharmacist, stop the drug, change its dose, or change the manner of taking the drug. Patients can do many things to minimize unwanted effects.

While it has been suggested that the most dramatic effect of package insert information will be an increased compliance, it has also been argued that compliance may not always be the most appropriate behavior (6). If adverse effects occur, in fact, non-compliance may be preferable. In a broader sense, then, it is the cooperative patient and not the compliant patient who has the best chance for safe and effective therapy. Of course, only adequately informed patients can be expected to be cooperative.

Although it is difficult to inform patients well, it is by no means impossible. The German insert for allopurinol can serve as an illustration. It states side-effects, in a separate section, in plain language, in terms of symptoms that patients can recognize, and also adds follow-up directions. The message is intelligible, concise, and comprehensive.

Patients can be given the responsibility for making their own therapy as safe as possible. We must show them clearly that we expect them to cooperate. What better way than by giving them the appropriate information?

REFERENCES

1. Newcomer, D.R. and Anderson, R.W. (1974): Effectiveness of a combined drug and patient teaching program. *Drug Intell. clin. Pharm., 8*, 374.
2. Anon. (1976): Gesetz zur Neuordnung des Arzneimittelrechtes. II. Anforderungen an die Arzneimittel. *Pharm. Ind., 38*, 5.
3. Messer, O.A.L. (1978): Empfehlungen des Europarates an die Regierungen seiner Mitgliedstaaten zur Harmonisierung des nationalen pharmazeutischen Rechts. *Dtsch. Apoth. Z., 118*, 481.
4. Pyrczak, F. (1978): *Application of Some Principles of Readability Research in the Preparation of Patient Package Inserts*. Publication Series, The Center for the Study of Drug Development, University of Rochester Medical Center, School of Medicine and Dentistry, Rochester, NY.
5. Ley, P. (1976): In: *Communication between Doctors and Patients*, pp. 86–89. Editor: A.E. Bennett. Oxford University Press, London.
6. Sharpe, T.R. (1977): Potential effects on the patient. II. *Drug Inf. J., 11*, 58S.

DISCUSSION

Johnson: Miss Hermann pointed out some deficiencies in some European patient package inserts. I would like to point out for the record that in the United States, as a general rule, patients receive no printed information on prescription drugs. Patient package inserts are distributed in only three cases: oral contraceptives, intrauterine devices and postmenopausal estrogens. For the last, the drug industry and the American College of Obstetrics and Gynecology have gone to court to block distribution of information on postmenopausal estrogens. For over-the-counter drugs, patients do receive this kind of information, so although the European inserts frequently fall below the desired standards, Europe is far ahead of the United States on this score.

Hermann: Indeed, package inserts are used in the Unites States, but they are not at this time as clear, concise, and comprehensive as one would want them to be.

Oakley: Is it true that in Europe, for every drug with every prescription, there is a package insert for the patient? Could you say a little more about that?

Hermann: This is not true for all countries, but it is in all countries where unit-of-use distribution of medication is practised.

Oakley: What does that mean?

Hermann: It means that the physician prescribes a predetermined package and does not individually decide the quantity of medication to be dispensed as is done in the States. These fixed quantities are prepackaged by the manufacturer and supplied with a package insert. Let me repeat, this is not true of all European countries, but for example in France, Germany, Switzerland, Austria and Belgium, this is very much the case.

Oakley: What proportion of drugs are sold in prepackaged units?

Hermann: Well, you may be aware that we also have some unit-of-use packaging – we have oral contraceptives, we have corticosteroids where the manufacturer has felt that in the interests of increasing compliance etc. it is advantageous to have unit-of-use packages. We have one pharmaceutical manufacturer marketing a sulfa drug in this way. It does not leave room for the physician to underprescribe, but it may settle the patient with extra medication in his medicine cabinet.

Westerholm: In Sweden, package inserts were abandoned many years ago because they contained advertising and overstatements about the positive effects of drug. Now, however, we feel a strong need for the inserts, and therefore we have tested inserts produced by the industry as well as by a government agency. These inserts contain information about what the patients should know about the drug, written in a simple way. So far, our experience has been that the patients who obtained the package inserts knew more about their drug, but the question of whether compliance was achieved is left open.

Hama: I agree that we need package inserts. However, looking at the medicare system in Japan, the biggest obstacle to their use would be in the case of the anti-cancer drugs. How do you deal with package inserts for anti-cancer drugs in Europe? What type of inserts are packaged with them?

Hermann: I do not know of any special approach for anti-cancer drugs. Ways must be found to state the information in an unemotional way. These patients need information as much as any other; the patients themselves have expressed such interest, since patients are now more enlightened, have 'come of age', so to speak.

Shin: Commenting on Dr. Herxheimer's presentation, questions may be asked by patients to their doctors, but improving the content of the package inserts with regard to adverse effects does seem to be an ideal means of avoiding unwanted drug effects. Still, the doubt remains that if the patients don't ask the questions and the doctors don't or can't answer them, or if the patients don't read the inserts – and such is commonly the case for the majority of patients – we won't be any better off than we are now in terms of reducing unwanted drug hazards.

Herxheimer: I agree that questions from the patient about drugs are an important way of stimulating the doctor to find out the details that he *should* know.

Yanagita: In comment to Dr. Hermann: if we present information on side-effects to patients too precisely, or vividly, one might say that the possibility may be opened for the patient to become nervous and preoccupied with it, and develop psychosomatic responses. Therefore, it seems to me that the extent to which such information is to be released is a critical point.

Hermann: It is not easy to write good patient information; I can only repeat that I am in agreement with you. But ways of doing so must be found – we cannot afford to do otherwise. Would not printed information describing the symptoms that signalled SMON have helped some of the victims perhaps to assert themselves in the face of their physicians' suggestions to continue the therapy?

Dukes: I would simply add the comment that, whether or not a patient reads a package folder the *first* time he receives a drug, he probably does *not* re-read it if he gets the drug again later – consequently, he does not notice any changes or additions, for example with respect to newly discovered adverse reactions. One has to find some other way of drawing his attention to these. There was such a problem which we faced in The Netherlands with respect to SMON: the addition of such a warning would have simply gone unnoticed, and we had to take supplementary measures.

Balanced and complete drug information can help doctors to use medicines well

A. HERXHEIMER and N.D.W. LIONEL

Charing Cross Hospital Medical School, London, U.K. and Faculty of Medicine, University of Sri Lanka, Colombo, Sri Lanka

Modern medicines may still be magic to patients, but they should now be much less magic to doctors because our abilities to diagnose disease and to analyse health problems have given us the opportunity to use medicines rationally. We also now know a lot about what durgs can do, how they can help and how they can do harm, and this detailed knowledge is increasing all the time. We must use this knowledge with care and precision to ensure that a drug produces the intended benefit and that we minimize any risk of harm from it. To be used effectively, the requisite information must be well organized in the prescriber's mind. The prescriber needs it for two purposes – first, to help him choose the most appropriate drug for his patient from all those that might be used, and second, to use the chosen drug in the best way.

The choice of the most appropriate drug for a medical problem is a matter of judgement in which there is room for differences of opinion. Often the choice has to be made from a number of drugs with fairly similar properties, made by manufacturers competing for the same market. A good choice can be made only by comparing the efficacy and safety of the drugs that are worth considering in the circumstances that apply to the patient who is to be treated. When the drugs are similar in efficacy and safety, their convenience and cost become deciding factors. In general, the longer a drug has been in use the more is known about it, and information about it is more trustworthy than information about new drugs. The prescriber's familiarity and experience with a particular drug is also important in his choice. If he is familiar with it, he will use it better than a drug that is new to him. We think that a prescriber should not choose a new drug unless he can give clear and objective reasons for preferring it to a long-established drug.

The promotional claims made by manufacturers usually exaggerate the advantages and play down the disadvantages of their products, and the prescriber should not accept such claims uncritically. If he has little experience in the critical assessment of claims, he needs help from more experienced professional colleagues, among them clinical pharmacologists, whether through publications or more directly through consultations, medical meetings, hospital committees, and so on. Published assessments in independent general medical journals, such as the *New England Journal of Medicine*, the *British Medical Journal* and the corresponding journals in other countries are valuable, but not enough. The *Medical Letter* in the U.S.A and *Drug and Therapeutics Bulletin* in Britain were among the first specialized journals founded to publish evaluations of drugs. Now others exist in The Netherlands, Federal Republic of Germany, Australia, India, Sri Lanka,

Switzerland and elsewhere. The scope and distribution of such journals needs to be extended until doctors everywhere can get prompt and critical evaluations of new products and new methods of treatment.

When the physician has decided what drug to use, he must know how it is best given and for how long, what benefit to expect, and what to do if the desired effect does not occur as and when it should. He must also know in what circumstances it may be dangerous to use the drug, and what possible ill effects it may cause. He should know how to prevent these ill effects, and when they do occur how to detect and treat them. Most prescribers can remember all this information for only a few of the drugs that they prescribe. The information must therefore be immediately accessible to the prescriber in a formulary or compendium that he can keep in his pocket or on his desk. It must be presented clearly in a standard way that makes it easy to find a particular item of information quickly. Such a format has been proposed by the World Health Organization's expert committee on the selection of essential drugs (5) and elaborated by us in the *British Medical Journal* last year (4). The main headings under which the information is arranged are: the names of the drug, non-proprietary and proprietary; pharmacological effects and mechanism of action; pharmacokinetics; indications (that is, the conditions in which the drug is worth using); contraindications, warnings, precautions and adverse effects, including interactions; dosage and manner of administration; pharmaceutical information on dosage form, composition, appearance (these details will of course vary from country to country); storage conditions; and the names and addresses of the manufacturers. As Dr. Lunde has said, WHO is now planning to prepare such sets of information for all the 200 drugs in the model list of essential drugs.

In our title we stress balanced and complete information, because at present much drug information is neither balanced nor complete. The provision of balanced and complete information is in our view the most effective way of preventing drug-induced suffering. It is unrealistic to expect a manufacturer's information to be balanced, because he feels very enthusiastic about his drug and also wishes it to be used as widely as possible. So, as we have already said, manufacturers tend to overstate the virtues of their products and to minimize their disadvantages. Balanced information can be obtained only from an impartial and critical review of the data about a drug. In the U.S.A., the FDA requires manufacturers to provide balanced information, but the resulting package inserts have not been very satisfactory. They represent a bureaucratic compromise between the regulators and the manufacturers, with insufficient regard for the practical needs of prescribers. In our opinion, practising clinicians and clinical pharmacologists who are independent, both of regulators and of industry, should play a major part in the preparation of drug information for prescribers. The drafts should be edited critically and sent for comment to manufacturers and to expert professional groups, before the final version is prepared. A procedure of this kind is now used in Australia, and the results are promising.

So much for balance. Completeness is a separate problem. At present we lack important items of information for many drugs, for example on the value of loading doses, on the best dosage intervals, and on the optimum duration of treatment. Recommendations about these aspects of use are therefore often arbitrary, or omitted entirely. For instance, the optimum duration of treatment of otitis media with ampicillin is not known. Should a child with otitis media be given ampicillin for 3 days, or for 10 days, or until the symptoms and signs have disappeared? We don't know, and need to find out, by doing clinical trials.

Likewise, we frequently know far too little about the incidence of various unwanted effects, or on how to prevent them or minimize their intensity. Information that is known for many drugs, but rarely stated, concerns the likely benefits and risks of increasing the dose beyond the usual level. With some drugs it is completely pointless to increase the dose if the desired effect is not achieved, while with other drugs it may be worth increasing the dose to a higher, sometimes much higher level. We think that whoever compiles the information about a drug should note in it what important items are missing. Often research will be needed to fill the gap. This type of research must be encouraged and paid for from public funds. It cannot be regarded as the responsibility of the manufacturers, though they may sometimes wish to sponsor research that is of medical rather than commercial importance.

Once doctors have balanced and complete information about the drugs they use, it must of course be kept up to date. Changes are most likely to be needed for relatively new drugs, but even old drugs like aspirin and digoxin need review when new data about their use become available. Revision of the drug information should be considered whenever important data appear that affect the use of the drug.

Finally, how can doctors be persuaded to use the balanced and complete information that we want to provide? The biggest obstacle is that prescribers feel that they know all about the drugs that they have long been using in their practice. Where new drugs are concerned, doctors are more likely to be aware of their ignorance, and therefore more likely to look up the information. Doctors need to become aware of important aspects of drug therapy that they are used to neglecting. We need to make it easy and natural for them to discuss therapeutic methods and problems with their colleagues. Medical students and doctors in training must learn to think about treatment as methodically and as clearly as they are taught to think about diagnosis and investigation. They should learn whenever they prescribe a drug, to define their aim, to decide how they will assess the therapeutic effect, and after what intervals. They must recall how the drug is inactivated in the body, and how this is affected by impaired kidney and liver function. And they must recall and take all the other appropriate precautions to prevent harm or at least minimize the risks for the patient (2).

Practising doctors can benefit from informal group discussions of the treatment of individual cases, with help, when necessary, from a clinical pharmacologist or other appropriate specialist. Doctors can also become more aware of their information needs through their patients. The patient can often make an important contribution to the effective and safe use of medicines, but he can do so only if he has the necessary information (1). Doctors must therefore do their best to give patients the information, or to see that they get it from others working with them, e.g. the pharmacist or the nurse. Doctors should encourage their patients to ask about important aspects of their medication, for example how it is expected to help, how important it is to take the treatment, and whether there are side effects (3). A doctor who tells his patients that such questions are worth asking will of course have to know the answers, but that will help him to use the drugs well.

In conclusion, we believe that it is the responsibility of the medical profession through its professional organizations, of the drug regulatory authorities, and of the pharmaceutical industry, to provide balanced, complete, relevant and up-to-date information about all the medicines in use. The provision of such information would probably do much more to prevent drug-induced harm than new laws or regulations. Doctors must be helped to get into the habit of using this information effectively and efficiently. They may well find that this is easiest to achieve if they use a relatively small number of drugs with which they are familiar. We believe, with Dr. Lunde and Dr. Tognoni (This Volume), that more thought and self-discipline in the choice of drugs, as well as in their use, will benefit the patient and will also ease the work of doctors, nurses and pharmacists, not to mention lawyers.

REFERENCES

1. Hermann, F., Herxheimer, A. and Lionel, N.D.W. (1978): Package inserts for prescribed medicines: What minimum information do patients need? *Brit. med. J., 2*, 1132.
2. Herxheimer, A. (1976): Towards parity for therapeutics in clinical teaching. *Lancet, 2*, 1194.
3. Herxheimer, A. (1976): Sharing the responsibility for treatment: How can the doctor help the patient? *Lancet, 2*, 1276.
4. Herxheimer, A. and Lionel, N.D.W. (1978): Minimum information for prescribers. *Brit. med. J., 2*, 1129.
5. World Health Organization (1977): The selection of essential drugs. *Wld Hlth Org. tech. Rep. Ser., 615*.

DISCUSSION

Westerholm: I think your questions for doctors and patients constitute a very good educational tool and should be tried internationally. I am participating in a study in which doctors have to write down why they prescribe a drug, and preliminary results indicate that this simple action reduces prescribing in some instances.

Yokota: I have read Dr. Herxheimer's paper, but in the case of Japanese patients, I feel we are dealing with a rather special mentality. If the Japanese patient received anti-cancer medicine with his knowledge, in most cases we could expect him to lose hope and perhaps become suicidal. Therefore, I cannot agree with your opinion but wonder if you have any further views.

Herxheimer: I did not want to suggest that patients should always ask such questions about their treatment, but *only when* they wish to do so. Many cancer patients do not want to be informed of their disease, and they would have no desire to ask questions that would give them such unwelcome information. But if the patient *does* want to know and asks, I don't think that the doctor has the right to deny him the information he wants.

Mashford: I am impressed by doctors' ability to learn what is necessary for them to function, and I should like to return to the proverb earlier mentioned. One way to get the horse to drink is to make it thirsty. Could Dr. Herxheimer comment on the possibility of raising the patient's logical curiosity by making his 'questions the patient should ask' available in doctors' waiting rooms? The patients could read them if they liked but would not be forced to do so. I don't think that this would cause distress to patients regarding a disease like cancer – the patient does not ask because he does not want to know.

Herxheimer: I agree completely with Dr. Mashford, but it is not as easy as it appears, because doctors may become too anxious if patients ask questions to which they do not have certain answers. First we need to identify such anxieties and to relieve them with good information; then the doctors will be more willing to discuss these questions with their patients (Julian, P. and Herxheimer, A. (1977): Doctor's anxieties in prescribing. *J. roy. Coll. gen. Pract., 27,* 662).

Post-marketing follow-up

HERSHEL JICK and ALEXANDER M. WALKER

Boston Collaborative Drug Surveillance Program, Boston University Medical Center, Waltham, MS, U.S.A.

There is a general but strongly held view that, after drugs are marketed, additional epidemiological information is needed on their clinical effects, particularly adverse effects. This notion is soundly based on the fact that the clinical experience with a drug prior to marketing is limited in size and scope. Recently, considerable interest has been evident in this area and has focused on the term 'post-marketing surveillance' (PMS). That the interest is widespread and intense is reflected in the many meetings which have taken place, articles which have been written, and committees which have been formed to consider the designing of large formal systems of PMS (1–15). Given the diffuse nature of the subject, it is essential to take an objective and informed look at the real needs in this area and to consider practical means of satisfying these needs. Without a clear understanding of the nature of the problems that can be addressed epidemiologically after a drug is marketed, much of the current discussion may be of little utility. Without a realistic appraisal of the mechanisms for solving these problems, such discussion can even be counterproductive.

BACKGROUND

To begin to define in more specific terms the most important objectives of a large systematic effort to obtain additional epidemiological information on drugs after marketing, it is instructive to consider those events that appear to have stimulated the current interest. In Europe in general, and the United Kingdom in particular, there is little doubt that the experience with the beta-adrenergic blocking drug practolol was the major stimulus. Practolol had been marketed and used extensively in the United Kingdom (and elsewhere) for a number of years before serious and potentially lethal adverse effects – entirely unanticipated – were recognized (16). It is estimated that hundreds of instances of serious practolol toxicity had occurred prior to the recognition of the oculomucocutaneous syndrome. The obvious need for systems to detect such problems earlier was immediately recognized and has led to the intense interest in Europe in the matter of post-marketing follow-up. In Japan, the experience with a serious neurological disease – subacute myelo-opticoneuropathy (SMON) – induced by the drug iodochlorhydroxyquin (clioquinol) (17) has led to major concern about preventing such a disaster in the future. It is estimated that thousands of cases of SMON occurred prior to the recognition of its drug etiology and a recurrence of this experience would be intolerable.

Until recently, no disaster approaching the size of that resulting from practolol or clioquinol has been recognized in the United States. Perhaps the most recent experience of this general kind here has been with lincomycin and clindamycin which produced an unanticipated syndrome, pseudomembranous colitis. This syndrome, however, occurs less frequently than those associated with practolol and clioquinol; it is more often reversible and the frequency of serious or lethal consequences has been much smaller. Whereas practolol has been removed from the market in Britain and clioquinol in Japan, lincomycin and clindamycin remain marketed in the United States (and elsewhere). Despite the relative absence of a major particular incident, interest in PMS in the United States is, nevertheless, quite strong. This interest appears to have been stimulated largely by Senator Edward Kennedy, Chairman of the Senate Health Subcommittee. At a press conference held on November 30, 1976, Senator Kennedy stated that, judging from the testimony before his committee, 'a consensus exists that ... drugs are not optimally used ... We simply don't know how different kinds of doctors use different categories of drugs; we don't know the true incidence of adverse effects nor do we appreciate the very real benefits of appropriate drug usage.' Senator Kennedy went on to announce that, as a result of these concerns, he, together with a broad spectrum of the medical and pharmaceutical community, had formed the Joint Commission on Prescription Drug Use. The purpose of the Commission was to develop data-collecting systems to collect 'reliable information' on 'how drugs are being used' and to systematically collect data on adverse drug reactions. The Commission was given a three-year charter and a $750,000 budget to carry out its charge.

The current interest in post-marketing surveillance in the United States covers a broader range of activities than it does in Europe and Japan. It encompasses matters of drug utilization as well as adverse and beneficial drug effects, and Senator Kennedy implies that his concern is with older drugs already marketed as well as those recently or newly marketed drugs.

The initial investigation of the Joint Commission revealed that there is more information on drug utilization patterns in the United States than might be surmised from Senator Kennedy's statement. IMS America, a multinational information gathering organization, obtains information and prepares regular reports on the patterns of drug use and physician prescribing practice in the United States. In addition, information on drug utilization patterns may be obtained from organizations which use computers to process claims for programs such as Medicare and Medicaid. There appear, therefore, to be adequate systems for investigating drug use patterns and the need for additional systems or centers to perform this function is questionable.

As to the issue of drug efficacy, the primary research technique which can be used to evaluate the usefulness of drugs is the randomized clinical trial. Large-scale systems of non-experimental data collection are likely to contribute relatively little to our knowledge of drug efficacy.

It seems then that the major objective of new, large-scale formal systems to obtain additional information on drug effects after marketing should be directed toward increasing knowledge of the adverse effects of drugs.

TYPES OF ADVERSE DRUG EFFECTS

To understand the needs for systems to obtain additional information on adverse drug effects after marketing, it is necessary to perceive that these effects may be (1) recognized or unrecognized, (2) common or uncommon, and (3) acute or long term.

Recognized adverse effects

If an adverse drug effect is known, i.e. recognized to be inducible by a particular drug, the task to be performed is to quantify its frequency in terms of severity and factors which modify the rate. This task is generally straightforward and techniques to accomplish it have been tested and found to be quite satisfactory.

If the recognized adverse effect is acute and reasonably common, substantial data should already be available from pre-marketing testing. Should the accumulation of additional data in the usual clinical setting be deemed desirable, this can be accomplished efficiently by a follow-up study of the drug for acute effects. Many such studies have been carried out satisfactorily for drugs in general (18) and for specific drugs (19–24). If the adverse effect is acute but uncommon, further quantification beyond the documentation that the event is 'uncommon' can often be accomplished by use of vital statistics or registry data, national voluntary reporting systems or formal case-control studies of the particular illness which the drug is inducing. Numerous studies, directed to the more precise quantitation of the magnitude of risk of relatively acute adverse drug effects known to be rare, have come from Sweden (25,26) and the Boston Collaborative Drug Surveillance Program (BCDSP).

Adverse drug effects may occur after prolonged drug exposure. The quantitation of such effects, once recognized, is again a straightforward matter whose key is an efficient case-finding mechanism. In the United States, we have found that the Commission on Professional and Hospital Activities – Professional Activity Study (CPHA-PAS), which records some 35% of all hospital discharges, is an excellent resource in this regard. The BCDSP and CPHA-PAS have cooperated, for example, in estimating the actual number of cases of benign liver tumors attributable to oral contraceptive use in the United States (27). Together, we have been able to estimate the contribution of oral contraceptives to the risk of another rare disease, myocardial infarction in young women (28). Each of these studies was carried out in less than a year at relatively little expense.

From the viewpoint of public policy, the low cost of these studies is very important. Projects to quantify recognized adverse drug effects *can* be inexpensive. They should be carried out on an *ad hoc* basis with the study design tailored to the particular drug and adverse effect of interest. In the case of exceedingly rare drug-induced illness, such as aplastic anemia, case-history studies encompassing a series of consecutive cases can provide reasonable quantitation of its drug etiology. Case-control studies can be employed when there is remaining doubt about the validity of an association. *The establishment of additional elaborate and expensive ongoing comprehensive 'systems' are not indicated for the study of recognized adverse effects.*

Unrecognized adverse drug effects

Conceptually, a strategy for the study of unrecognized adverse drug effects is exceedingly complex. Hundreds of illnesses may be appropriate candidates for close scrutiny. Indeed, one may even have to deal with an illness which is virtually unique to the drug causing it, e.g. clioquinol-induced SMON, diethylstilbestrol (DES)-induced vaginal carcinoma in very young women, practolol-induced oculo-mucocutaneous syndrome. The illness may be induced shortly after the drug is first taken, e.g. SMON, pseudomembranous colitis; it may be induced many years later, e.g. DES-induced vaginal carcinoma, estrogen-induced endometrial cancer, methysergide-induced retroperitoneal fibrosis; or it may be induced at variable intervals after the first exposure, e.g. oral-contraceptive-induced venous thromboembolism. It may be induced reasonably often, e.g. thalidomide-induced phocomelia, practolol-induced oculo-mucocutaneous syndrome, or very rarely, e.g. chloramphenicol-induced aplastic anemia.

In the absence of even a hint as to the possible illness or illnesses a particular drug many induce, the emphasis in formal methods for discovery must be the follow-up approach for particular drugs because such an approach encompasses all possible outcomes. An illogical and even dangerous alternative would be to limit inquiry to conditions known to have been drug-induced in the past. When there is good pharmacological reason to believe that a new drug may share with other drugs some known adverse effects, those effects can be pursued by the methods indicated above. However, under no circumstances can this justify a failure to pursue previously unrecognized complications of drug therapy by means of appropriate follow-up study.

In the past, the primary source of discovery of drug-induced illness has been serendipitous suggestion on the part of clinicians or clinical investigators. When this informal approach has been successful, its major inadequacy has been the time lag between the first occurrence of cases and the discovery of the drug etiology. Nevertheless, in considering future research needs, it should be noted that informal clinical observation is likely eventually to uncover many unrecognized drug effects. The discovery of the toxicity of thalidomide, practolol, and chloramphenicol was accomplished within 5 years of widespread use. It seems likely that relatively little serious acute toxicity remains undiscovered for drugs that have been marketed for many years. The major concern then is with drugs that have recently been marketed and those to be marketed.

From the above, we conclude that:

1. The primary objective of further large-scale data-gathering programs in the field of drug-induced illness related to unrecognized serious drug effects.
2. The major concern is with recently or newly marketed drugs where clinical experience may be insufficient for the early discovery of serious unanticipated adverse drug effects.
3. In the absence of any clue as to the illness or illnesses one is concerned about, the methodological approach required is the follow-up study.
4. Because uncommon effects are a major concern, large cohorts are required for each drug of interest.
5. Since long-term or delayed side-effects are of concern, long-term follow-up is necessary.

RESEARCH STRATEGY

Having determined the objectives in some detail, one must decide on practical means of achieving these objectives. In this regard, it is crucial to recognize that long-term follow-up studies of large numbers of people are exceedingly expensive and difficult to manage. It should, therefore, be obvious that any system (or systems) that is designed to accomplish the stated objectives must be simple and clearly defined so as to be as efficient as possible. Otherwise, it will surely fail.

The two essential ingredients in a follow-up study whose objective is to discover unrecognized serious drug-induced illness are, first, the identification of a large cohort of users of the drug of interest and, second, the follow-up of the cohort to identify episodes of serious unanticipated illness.

Identification of the cohort

Since the size of each cohort must be in the thousands, it is essential that its identification be rapid and inexpensive. This requires that the identification procedures be automatic or at least semiautomatic. The use of computer files which register people who fill a prescription for the drug of interest is the ideal mechanism of identifying users. Unfortunately, relatively few such files exist and most that do are of limited size. Nevertheless, the potential utility of the use of computerized prescription data has been demonstrated in the United States in very large group medical practices. For example, among the 250,000 members of Group Health Cooperative of Puget Sound in Seattle, Washington, the BCDSP has used such files to identify the number of women taking replacement estrogens (29). To a small but growing extent, such facilities are appearing elsewhere.

An alternative method of identifying a large cohort would involve the cooperation of vast numbers of community pharmacists who would send the names of individuals using the drug of interest to a central registry. (Such a scheme has been jointly proposed by the BCDSP and the American Pharmaceutical Association.) In the Oxford area, this concept has been used successfully.

Still another method utilizes pharmaceutical representatives who enlist the cooperation of large numbers of physicians to identify patients who are receiving the drug of interest. This method has been tried with excellent success by Smith Kline & French, but would only be applicable to drug firms that have large numbers of field representatives.

In summary, the identification of a large cohort of users for each drug of interest must be simple and inexpensive in order for the entire scheme to be feasible. It appears that this task can be accomplished by one or more of the techniques mentioned above.

Follow-up for serious illness

The achievement of the second goal – the long-term follow-up of the identified cohort – is far more difficult to accomplish. Once a cohort of, say, 20,000 has been identified, how does one carry out follow-up for years at reasonable cost? Without national health systems, such as those in Scandinavia, that have computerized information on hospitalizations, the task would appear at first glance to be hopelessly difficult and expensive – particularly if a number of drug cohorts were to be followed simultaneously. However, there are three potential sources for information on serious illness, all of which have been used in the past for large follow-up studies: (1) computer records of diagnoses, (2) physician follow-up, (3) patient follow-up.

Computer records

Computer recording of hospital discharges is now ubiquitous. In the United States, most hospitals maintain such files either on their own or through some agency such as CPHA-PAS of Ann Arbor, Michigan, which has computer files on about 35% of all hospitalized patients in the United States. In Scotland, the Stockholm county region, and many other defined areas, all hospital diagnoses are recorded in computerized files.

In terms of a post-marketing follow-up program, it is essential that one is able to identify automatically hospitalizations in the cohort of people one has identified for follow-up. In the United States, certain large group medical practices such as those mentioned earlier provide such an opportunity. Our experience is with Group Health Cooperative of Puget Sound which computerized its pharmacies in 1975 and has had its discharge diagnoses computerized since 1972. The patient identification number for the two files is the same and it is, therefore, possible to identify users of any drug from the pharmacy computer files and obtain diagnosis information automatically from the discharge diagnosis file.

The Group Health system is, in principle, virtually ideal for the follow-up of patients exposed to particular drugs. It is extremely inexpensive and the information on exposure and outcomes can be obtained automatically for long periods of time. The major limitation of the Group Health resource is the size of the population itself. Unless a drug were commonly prescribed, one would not be able to accrue rapidly a cohort of many thousands of users. Another limitation is that, at least until now, illnesses that are primarily treated in the outpatient setting would likely be missed. However, since we are concerned primarily with serious problems, this latter limitation need not be considered terribly important.

Another example of such follow-up potential comes from a pilot study in Oxford (30). Prescriptions filled in a large pharmacy area of Oxford have been computerized by researchers at Oxford University with the cooperation of the local Prescription Pricing Authority. Patient-identifying numbers on the prescription are the same as those present in the routinely computerized records of hospital discharges for the Oxford area. This system has been tested for some 40,000 people and found to be feasible. Conceptually, it is identical to that described for Group Health Cooperative. It is ideal for follow-up studies of serious drug-induced illness. Although it covers only a small population at present, the system could, in principle, be expanded to cover large parts of Great Britain.

Both the Group Health system and the Oxford system depend on unique patient-identifying numbers. An alternative, used when such identifiers are lacking, has been employed by the Scottish Hospital In-Patient Statistics (SHIPS) system, in which patients admitted to Scottish hospitals can be identified on the basis of surname, initials, date of birth, and sex. The identification is not perfect, but seems adequate for follow-up of large cohorts (31). Cohorts of drug recipients would need to be identified by a separate program with follow-up in the SHIPS system.

Physician follow-up

A second method of obtaining information on the continuing health status of a cohort of people is periodic review of patient medical histories by attending physicians. The feasibility of this means of obtaining important medical information has been demonstrated in the Royal College of General Practitioners study which has been ongoing for over 10 years (32). The cohort is some 46,000 young women. Over 1000 physicians have provided information on the occurrence of medical events in this cohort. The information has apparently been of satisfactory quality and this investigation represents one of the classic drug follow-up studies. The limitation of this method is cost. Obviously periodic physician review of thousands of patient histories is far more expensive than reviewing computer files. Nevertheless, this method has promise and, if the reporting of illnesses is restricted to a few illnesses which are serious and unanticipated, the utilization of attending physicians to provide critical information on a large cohort of their patients may prove to be feasible for achieving the goals of drug follow-up. The Smith Kline & French study on cimetidine mentioned above utilizes this technique and results of this study will be followed with interest in terms of the cost and quality of the information obtained.

Patient follow-up

In the absence of computer information, the patient himself/herself may be the most economical and valid source of information on the development of serious medical problems. Since each patient is likely to be very familiar with his/her medical history, this means of obtaining medical information may be more satisfactory than review of physician records. The feasibility of this approach has been demonstrated in the long-term follow-up study by Vessey et al. of some 25,000 young women (33). Here, information on hospitalizations is obtained directly from the women who participate in the study, with subsequent review of the hospital record where indicated. The experience of the BCDSP is that, in general, patients themselves are excellent sources of information about important aspects of their own medical histories.

A limitation of this method is the potential cost of repeated periodic contacting of the many people who comprise the cohort being followed. This might be accomplished economically by use of the mail.

In considering the various possibilities for follow-up studies to discover unrecognized effects, it is critical to remember that the primary objective is qualitative and not quantitative. That is, the overriding objective is to find the first clue which identifies an illness which appears to be connected with a drug. This means that absolute completeness of data acquisition is not essential. Once the particular illness is identified qualitatively, the objective of verification and quantitation is relatively straightforward as outlined above in the section on recognized effects of drugs. Furthermore, it should be accepted that if a side-effect is exceedingly rare – say, 1:50,000 – no formal system is sufficiently cost-effective to discover it and we must continue to rely on serendipity to uncover such problems.

CONCLUSIONS

In view of the above, we believe the formal large-scale research strategy which is now called for is the systematic follow-up of cohorts of about 20,000 users of selected recently or newly marketed drugs for serious unanticipated adverse effects. The ideal mechanism for identification and follow-up would be the use of computer files of users that can be linked to computerized files of hospitalizations and, where feasible, outpatient events. If current facilities are insufficiently large to satisfy the needs, we recommend that additional funding be provided to computerize pharmacies of fixed population groups which are able to identify hospitalizations in their populations and link these to prior drug use.

Failing this, we recommend careful evaluation of other systems for achieving the desired goal such as that being used by Smith Kline & French which utilizes company representatives to accrue a large cohort and to assure valid follow-up, and that proposed by the BCDSP and the American Pharmaceutical Association which proposes to use pharmacists to identify large cohorts and patient follow-up to identify the occurrence of serious illness.

Whatever systems are suggested, it is evident that they must be simple and inexpensive and designed primarily for the rapid identification of unrecognized serious adverse drug effects.

REFERENCES

1. Report (1977) of a European Workshop held in Sestri Levante, Italy, September 28-30, 1976. Towards a more rational regulation of the development of new medicines. *Europ. J. clin. Pharmacol., 11*, 233.
2. Gross, F.H. and Inman, W.H.W. (1977): *Drug Monitoring. Proceedings of an International Workshop held in Honolulu, 1977.* Academic Press, London.
3. *Post-Marketing Surveillance of Adverse Reactions to New Medicines.* Report of a meeting, 1977. Publication No. 7, Medico-Pharmaceutical Forum, London.
4. Harris E.L. (1975): Surveillance des médicaments mis sur le marché. Distribution contrôlée. In: *Contrôle des médicaments: évaluation clinique.* Symposium organisé par le Bureau Régional de l'Europe de l'O.M.S. Heidelberg, 1973. Bureau régional de l'Europe, O.M.S., Copenhague.
5. N.N. (1976): The proposed U.S. drug and devices administration. *Int. Drug Ther. Newslett., 11*, 13.
6. N.N. (1976): Towards better prescribing. *Lancet, 1*, 1249.
7. Walden, R.J. and Prichard, B.N.C. (1978): Post-marketing drug surveillance. *Brit. J. clin. Pharmacol., 6*, 191.
8. Dollery, C.T. and Rawlins, M.D. (1977): Monitoring adverse reactions to drugs. *Brit. med. J., 1*, 96.
9. Remington, R.D. (1978): *Post-Marketing Surveillance: A Comparison of Methods*, p.1. Publication Series No. 7811, The Center for the Study of Drug Development, University of Rochester, New York.
10. Lawson, D.H. and Henry, D.A. (1977): Monitoring adverse reactions to new drugs: 'restricted release' or 'monitored release.' *Brit. med. J., 1*, 691.
11. Wilson, A.B. (1977): Post-marketing surveillance of adverse reactions to new medicines. *Brit. med. J., 2*, 1001.

12. Jick, H. (1977): The discovery of drug-induced illness. *New. Engl. J. Med., 296*, 481.
13. N.N. (1977): Intensified adverse drug reaction reporting scheme. *N.Z. med. J., 85*, 157.
14. Howie, J.G.R. (1977): Drug monitoring and adverse reactions. *Brit. med. J., 1*, 1467.
15. Drury, M. (1977): Monitoring adverse reactions to drugs. *Brit. med. J., 1*, 439.
16. Brown, P., Baddeley, H., Read, A.E., Davies, J.D. and McGarry, J. (1974): Sclerosing peritonitis, an unusual reaction to a β-adrenergic-blocking drug (practolol). *Lancet, 2*, 1477.
17. Oakley Jr, G.P. (1973): The neurotoxicity of the halogenated hydroxyquinolines. *J. Amer. med. Ass., 255*, 395.
18. Jick, H., Miettinen, O.S., Shapiro, S. et al. (1970): Comprehensive drug surveillance. *J. Amer. med. Ass., 213*, 1455.
19. Jick, H., Slone, D., Borda, I.T. and Shapiro, S. (1968): Efficacy and toxicity of heparin in relation to age and sex. *N. Engl. J. Med., 279*, 284.
20. Boston Collaborative Drug Surveillance Program (1973): Oral contraceptives and venous thromboembolic disease, surgically confirmed gallbladder disease, and breast tumours. *Lancet, 1*, 1399.
21. Wood, A.J.J., Moir, D.C., Campbell, C. et al. (1974): Medicines evaluation and monitoring group: Central nervous sytem effects of pentazocine. *Brit. med. J., 1*, 305.
22. Paddock, R., Beer, E.G., Bellville, J.W. et al. (1969): Analgesic and side effects of pentazocine and morphine in a large population of postoperative patients. *Clin. Pharmacol. Ther., 10*, 355.
23. Koch-Weser, J., Sidel, V.W., Dexter, M. et al. (1971): Adverse reactions to sulfisoxazole, sulfamethoxazole, and nitrofurantoin. *Arch. intern. Med., 128*, 399.
24. Koch-Weser, J., Sidel, V.W., Federman E.B. et al. (1970): Adverse effects of sodium colistimethate: Manifestations and specific reaction rates during 317 courses of therapy. *Ann. intern. Med., 72*, 857.
25. Böttiger, L.E. and Westerholm, B. (1973): Drug induced blood dyscrasias in Sweden. *Brit. med. J., 3*, 339.
26. Böttiger, L.E., Strandberg, I. and Westerholm, B. (1975): Drug induced febrile mucocutaneous syndrome. *Acta med. scand., 198*, 22.
27. Jick, H. and Herman, R. (1978): Oral-contraceptive-induced benign liver tumors; the magnitude of the problem. *J. Amer. med. Ass., 240*, 828.
28. Jick, H., Dinan, B., Herman, R. and Rothman, K.J. (1978): Myocardial infarction and other vascular diseases in young women. *J. Amer. med. Ass., 240*, 2548.
29. Jick, H., Watkins, R.N., Hunter, J.R. et al. (1979): Replacement estrogens and endometrial cancer. *New Engl. J. Med., 300*, 218.
30. Skegg, D.C.G. (1978): Use of record linkage for drug surveillance. In: *Computer Aid to Drug Therapy and to Drug Monitoring*, pp. 77–83. Editors: H. Ducrot, M. Goldberg and R. Hoigne. North-Holland Publ. Co., Amsterdam.
31. Goldacre, M.J., Clarke, J.A., Heasman, M.A. and Vessey, M.P. (1978): Follow-up of vasectomy using medical record linkage. *Amer. J. Epidemiol., 108*, 176.
32. Royal College of General Practitioners' Oral Contraception Study (1977): Mortality among oral-contraceptive users. *Lancet, 2*, 727.
33. Vessey, M.P., McPherson, K. and Johnson, B. (1977): Mortality among women participating in the Oxford/Family Planning Association Contraceptive Study. *Lancet, 2*, 731.

DISCUSSION

Inman: Dr. Walker commented on the probability that most acute problems become apparent within a few years of first marketing a new drug, and I agree that this is true when the reactions are of the kind that doctors commonly associate with drugs. But quite common and serious conditions such as coronary thrombosis could occur without their being recognized as adverse reactions. In the case of practolol, only 1 case of conjunctivitis was reported in 4 years (100,000 patients exposed). We suspect now that perhaps 2000 eye reactions had occurred by the time the problem was recognized.

Walker: I certainly agree with you that there are some classes of adverse drug effects which cannot be discerned by any practical means, even though they may be serious, acute, and relatively common. These effects are those conditions which have a very high rate of occurrence even in the absence of drug exposure. The conjunctivitis resulting from practolol would have gone undiscovered but for the occurrence of oculo-mucocutaneous syndrome to draw attention to it. The milder peripheral neuropathies associated with clioquinol would probably have remained a mystery had there not been the Japanese tragedy of SMON.

Oakley: I would like to thank the speakers and the audience; it's been a good session. We have looked at a wide range of problems that can be weak links in the chain in the effective and safe use of drugs. One sort of feeling that stays with me as I've listened to these papers this morning is that some solutions have been proposed. I hope that as we work on implementing some of them, we will be as critical of whether they work or not as we are of clinical trials, *before* we get involved in rather complex, expensive systems the efficacy of which, as it were, has not been demonstrated.

SESSION II: ADMINISTRATIVE ASPECTS OF DRUG-INDUCED SUFFERINGS

Administrative policies for safety of drugs in Japan

NOBUO MOTOHASHI

Pharmaceutical Affairs Bureau, Ministry of Health and Welfare, Tokyo, Japan

Even if a drug is administered at the proper dosage and in a suitable form, noxious or unexpected reactions sometimes occur. Therefore, when the drug is evaluated we have to take adverse reactions as well as its efficacy into consideration. Such evaluation should be made not only in the pre-marketing stage, but also after it is marketed. It must be continuously updated. Care is needed, not only to detect adverse drug reactions and to evaluate the usefulness of drugs, but also to establish measures for safety in use.

The administrative measures can be divided into two categories: those at the pre-marketing stage and those at the post-marketing stage.

ADMINISTRATIVE MEASURES DURING THE PRE-MARKETING STAGE

In accordance with the Pharmaceutical Affairs Law, we have established approval and licensing systems for the manufacture of drugs. The advisory committee to the Minister of Health and Welfare, 'The Central Pharmaceutical Affairs Council', carefully evaluates data from animal tests and clinical trials. However, at the time of licensing, it is impossible to get all the necessary information to ensure complete safety. Usually, animal data are available, but these cannot predict certain safety for man, because of species differences. The same can be said of clinical trials because they are strictly limited to a small group of patients. Once the drug has been marketed, it will be administered to various patients in different stages of disease and under different conditions. For example, the method of administration, combinations with other treatments or drugs, dosage and term of medication will vary considerably. Consequently, adverse drug reactions which were unknown at the time of granting will be discovered. Therefore, the investigation of adverse drug reactions in the post-marketing phase is very important. MHW is taking the following measures.

ADMINISTRATIVE MEASURES IN THE POST-MARKETING STAGE

1. Obligation of manufacturers to investigate adverse drug reactions

Manufacturers have been required to report all adverse drug reactions of newly approved drugs to MHW by Circular 645 issued on September 30, 1967, by the

Director General of the Pharmaceutical Affairs Bureau entitled 'Basic Policy Concerning Drug Manufacturing (Importation) Approval', and the manufacturers have to investigate adverse reactions to drugs for a period of at least 3 years after they are placed on the market. For drugs already marketed, according to Circular 1059 issued by the Director General of the Pharmaceutical Affairs Bureau, on November 15, 1971, entitled 'Reporting Drug Adverse Reactions', the manufacturers must conduct their own investigations upon receiving reports about adverse reactions from medical institutes, pharmacies or pharmaceutical distributors. Adverse drug reactions which manufacturers must report to MHW are the following: (1) unknown reactions, (2) serious reactions, and (3) known reactions which show drastic changes in frequency, severity or symptoms.

2. *National drug monitoring system*

a. The national drug monitoring system in Japan was inaugurated in March, 1967. A total of 817 hospitals were designated as monitoring hospitals (95 national hospitals, 125 university hospitals, 264 prefectural or municipal hospitals and 333 hospitals owned by medical cooperations), which includes almost all the major general hospitals in Japan. Information concerning adverse drug reactions is now collected rapidly and efficiently from these hospitals.

b. In addition to this drug monitoring system, MHW is also making an effort to collect information from foreign countries. The thalidomide episode evoked worldwide attention. In 1963, WHO recommended member countries to set up the machinery for collecting information about adverse drug reactions. WHO inaugurated the international drug monitoring system in 1968, corresponding to the starting of the national drug monitoring systems of member countries. Japan started to participate in the international drug monitoring system in 1972, and established a system for exchange and collection of information. In addition, MHW has been exchanging information on administrative measures for drug safety with some foreign countries.

EVALUATION OF ADVERSE DRUG REACTIONS

First of all, it is necessary to examine the causal relationship between the adverse reactions and the suspected drug. Often, it is very difficult to distinguish the adverse drug reaction from the symptoms of the original disease or from reactions due to other drugs. Moreover, every adverse drug reaction has its own particular characteristics. Generally, to evaluate the adverse drug reaction, we have to take into consideration the following points: (1) difficulty of discovery, (2) reversible or irreversible, serious or mild, (3) frequency, (4) balance between effectiveness and adverse reactions, and (5) connection with the original disease. Specialized knowledge is required to evaluate such information, and MHW therefore has the Committee on Safety of Drugs and a Subcommittee for Adverse Drug Reactions, both belonging to the Central Pharmaceutical Affairs Council, and composed of a number of specialists in basic or clinical medicine.

ADMINISTRATIVE MEASURES

After careful evaluation of information, MHW may take appropriate administrative measures as follows: (1) Revision of cautions and warnings on the package insert. (2) Modification of dosage, mode of use or indications. (3) Designation of an over-the-counter drug as a prescription drug or powerful drug in order to restrict its distribution. (4) Banning of the manufacture or distribution of a drug if its continued existence is questioned because of serious adverse reactions.

In addition to the above, MHW has made efforts to regulate precautions on package inserts. The Pharmaceutical Affairs Law, Article 52–1, stipulates that the package insert of a drug must contain precautions concerning handling and use. Therefore, it is basically the responsibility of pharmaceutical manufacturers to provide adequate precautions. However, MHW is also collecting its own information and this is evaluated by the Subcommittee on Adverse Drug Reactions and the Committee on the Safety of Drugs of the Central Pharmaceutical Affairs Council. The minimum requirements of the contents of precautions have thus been defined in turn for each pharmacological group of drugs. These revised precautions are notified to all the manufacturers through the prefectural governments.

FEEDBACK OF INFORMATION

For feedback of information from the manufacturers, changing the instructions on the package insert or sending letters to doctors and pharmacists are normal methods. MHW also has made efforts in this direction by instituting two information letter systems. One is 'Information on Adverse Drug Reactions', a bimonthly information letter inaugurated in 1973. At first, it was intended only for monitor hospitals, but recently MHW have tried to deliver it to all hospitals and doctors. Many medical publications and journals now reproduce the letter. The other medium is the MHW Drug Bulletin, which was inaugurated in March, 1975. It is published two to three times a year, contains the more important information on adverse drug reactions, and is distributed to all doctors in Japan. This system is similar to the FDA's 'Drug Bulletin'.

RE-EVALUATION OF DRUGS

The approval of any drug as safe and effective is based on the standard of pharmaceutical and medical sciences at the time. But such sciences progress, so the original conclusion needs periodic re-examination. We have promoted such work since 1973, and the results of re-evaluation have been announced 15 times. So far, for single component drugs, 670 components (11,350 products) have already been re-evaluated, which is 74.4% of the total requiring re-evaluation. Up to 448 products, 4% of the total, were judged as useless, their manufacture and distribution were banned, and they were recalled from the market. For combination products which number 2,500, re-evaluation was started in 1975 and 139 products have been examined to date. Re-evaluation of over-the-counter drugs began in 1978.

REVISION OF THE PHARMACEUTICAL AFFAIRS LAW

Since the thalidomide episode in 1961, drug safety has become a worldwide issue. As the present Pharmaceutical Affairs Law was enacted before this episode, the necessary procedures to ensure the safety of drugs, e.g. the collection of information on drug safety, re-evaluation or good manufacturing practice, have been enforced by means of administrative guidance. To strengthen and consolidate such measures, revision of the Law will include the following points:

1. Drugs listed in the Japanese Pharmacopeia can now be manufactured on licence; for each product, approval must also be obtained under the new law.
2. Clarification of standards for approval.
3. Provisions on drug re-evaluation; for new drugs, re-evaluation is to be made within 6 years from the time of approval and for existing drugs, systematic re-evaluation must be made.
4. Establishment of an obligatory period for investigation of adverse drug reactions; manufacturers must look into adverse drug reactions of newly approved drugs for 6 years from approval. (At present, the term is 3 years, fixed by administrative guidance.)
5. Obligatory indication of the expiry date on pharmaceutical products.
6. Giving power to MHW to withdraw approval as an emergency measure.
7. Giving a legal basis for good manufacturing practice.

DISCUSSION

Kimbel: Dr. Motohashi, I wonder how adverse effects from drugs used in general practice are investigated in Japan. Are there any organizational measures to obtain reports from general practitioners? Are the representatives of the pharmaceutical houses obliged to collect reports and give them to the pharmaceutical houses and, in turn, to your Ministry?

My second question concerns the follow-up of adverse reactions by prospective or retrospective studies as to causability and frequency and in circumscribed patient populations. Is there any activity from your Ministry to organize and to finance studies similar to those done in the United States and in England on the hormonal treatment of postmenopausal complaints?

Motohashi: As regards your first question, we do have a system. We collect information from out-patient and in-patient hospital departments in cases where the adverse reactions are seen and can be suspected to be from certain drugs. We also receive reports from pharmaceutical companies and from the medical associations, and the Ministry of Health and Welfare also conducts its own investigations. All this information is assessed by the Subcommittee on Drug Reactions and the Committee for the Safety of Drugs of the Central Pharmaceutical Affairs Council.

In answer to your second question, we do not do this on a large scale, but we have allocated some part of our budget to study the frequency of the adverse effects of certain drugs.

Darmansjah: The Japanese drug industry has been expanded quite considerably and has made exports to other countries. Indonesia is one of the countries that receives and uses Japanese medicines. Are there any requirements by your authorities that these exported drugs should also comply with the requirements that you request in your own country?

Motohashi: We have no special regulations for drugs to be exported. Once a drug has been given approval by the Japanese Government, then it can be exported.

Nagano: Dr. Motohashi, you have 817 monitor hospitals. How many reports did you receive from them in 1978?

Motohashi: In 1978, we received 530 from all the hospitals, and the number is increasing.

Drug registration and the foreseeability of drug-induced injury

M.N.G. DUKES

Editor, 'Side Effects of Drugs Annual', Excerpta Medica, Amsterdam, The Netherlands

The pursuit of truth is one of the most challenging, and at the same time one of the most frustrating, exercises in which as human beings we choose to engage. What is truth? The Christian Bible, in one of its most poignant passages, provides us with the question, and leaves us to ponder on it, but does not deliver the answer. Certainly when one takes as one's field of endeavour the study of adverse reactions to drugs one soon finds that truth is elusive, fragile, and amoeboid in its ability to change its form. I was trained in medicine a quarter of a century ago. Like all other medical people who had their schooling at that period, I was taught about the side-effects of drugs, but I was not taught very much. Side-effects were troublesome rather than tragic. The older drugs presented no problem: one knew that morphine must be treated with healthy respect, and that atropine could make the patient somnolent. Herbs did little good, but certainly no harm. Of the synthetic drugs which had been with us since the turn of the century little ill could be said; phenacetin was a blessing for the patient with a headache and oxyphenisatin for the constipated. Then there were the new wonder drugs – the antihistamines, the antibiotics, the sulphonamides; their adverse reactions were few and far between. I remember, too, that all this knowledge, such as it was, was neatly set down in tables, which confirmed the certainty of all these truths.

All this happened before the drama of thalidomide and before MER-29 ran its brief and disastrous course. It was these two dramas, in the early 1960's, which did more than anything else to spur the legislators into action, to bring new drug registration laws onto the statute book, and to ensure that existing pharmaceutical laws were revised in the public interest. Yet one wonders, in retrospect, whether these two events did not at the same time mislead legislators, and many physicians as well, as to the true nature of the adverse reaction problem, and as to the instruments required to cope with it. Both the thalidomide drama and the grave complications with MER-29 could in part have been anticipated by appropriate preclinical and human pharmacological studies, prevented by appropriate cautions in packaging folders or at the very least have been rapidly detected even by the most primitive systems for adverse reaction monitoring in the field. Consequently, these were the solutions which the legislators adopted for all drugs. The laws which were created at that time, and which still prevail in the great majority of countries, would not have sufficed, and did not suffice, to detect and arrest the more subtle processes of injury which we today associate with many a drug thought to be harmless at the time of its introduction, such as oxyphenisatin, phenacetin or even clioquinol.

Some 4 years ago, when I engaged with a large group of colleagues from many countries to establish a system for thorough and critical analysis of the adverse reaction literature throughout the world, we engaged in a series of discussions as to why the adverse reaction problem presents such difficulties in practice (1). Some of the answers are self-evident, but it may be useful to recall them very briefly.

Firstly, as we all know, there is no model for a sick human being except another sick human being. Animal models and healthy human models have grave limitations. Where a side-effect only occurs in patients, or where it is rare (and many a drug causing agranulocytosis does so only once in every 10,000 cases), it will not emerge from clinical pharmacological studies prior to marketing, and may well fail to appear even in well-documented clinical trials. It follows that unless pre-marketing requirements are to be inflated to an impossible degree, many types of drug-induced injury will only emerge after marketing, and it is vital to create optimal systems to detect them rapidly at that time.

Secondly, and this is often not realized, even where animal studies might provide some evidence as to the adverse reactions to be anticipated, this evidence very rarely gets into print. It is in my view astonishing that the bulk of the pharmacological and toxicological work which a pharmaceutical firm undertakes before a product is introduced, much of it excellent work, gets buried in the archives of the drug registration authorities and is labelled there as 'confidential' (3). I have every faith in the critical abilities of these authorities, but this information should surely be filed in a public place and accessible to the medical and scientific world as a whole. The reason, of course, is that any medical researcher who has grounds to suspect that a drug on the market is causing a particular adverse reaction should be able to go back to the animal evidence and see if there are findings which would tend to support or refute his hypothesis.

A third problem is that at the time when information on the effects produced by a drug in practice does begin to become available in the literature, it is buried among a mass of irrelevant or misleading data. You will notice that I make a distinction between information and data. Data, you will recall, is a Latin word which simply means 'that which is given'. Well, much of what is given is not true, not useful, not clear, not information at all. This situation has several causes. One is naturally the fact that we shall never find the true facts at all unless we are prepared to record every suspicion of an adverse reaction, and most of these suspicions will ultimately, and fortunately, prove to be unfounded. How are we to separate the corn from the chaff? How necessary it is to do so is illustrated by a rather typical product label imposed by the United States Federal Food and Drug Administration on sodium cromoglycate, surely one of the safest drugs ever developed, so far as we can currently see. The label lists no less than 33 adverse reactions, including haemoptysis, peripheral neuritis and nephrosis, and though it attempts to separate the sheep from the goats it does obscure the fact that, in practice, adverse reactions to this drug are virtually unknown (2). One way of avoiding this additive effect is certainly to ensure that the literature is continuously and critically analyzed, not by computers or documentalists, but by expert physicians and clinical pharmacologists, in a long-term effort to identify well-documented reports at the earliest possible stage, an international project in which we are currently engaged and which is proving highly rewarding. If this project had been in operation in the mid-1930's, when SMON was first described in South America, it would have been picked up instead of disappearing into the files of a Spanish-language journal.

However, there is also another problem as regards the flow of irrelevant information. For every one impartial and serious report from a physician recording his observations conscientiously and in a useful manner there are in the literature some 10 or 20 papers of merely promotional character, written, it is true, by physicians, but commonly ghost-edited and sponsored by the promotional departments of drug companies and published largely (but not exclusively) in second-rank journals. Such papers as these are characterized, to say the least, by a certain optimism as regards the infrequency of adverse reactions to the drug concerned. They can utterly mislead many a reader; one must regard this form of pseudoscientific drug promotion, involving misuse of the medical literature, as one of the bad habits into which the industry has got itself entangled and which it would do well to abandon in the interests of its own reputation.

This leads me on to my fourth problem, and that relates to the whole attitude of industry to adverse reactions. There are some instances where a drug company has behaved impeccably on this score – I do not think, for example, that any rebuke is called for when one looks at the policy adopted by the manufacturers of practolol, megestrol acetate, or more recently clofibrate, when problems arose with respect to these compounds. Many other larger and small manufacturers, unhappily, are a great deal less conscientious in handling their own information, or that available from other parties, with respect to adverse reactions. Perhaps it is not even fair to expect a firm to be entirely objective in its approach; there is something to be said for the view that if the truth about an adverse reaction is to be determined fairly and quickly, it can best be done in the same way as that in which a court of law seeks to determine the truth, in other words by argument between the counsel for the plaintiff and counsel for the defendant, neither of whom is expected to be entirely impartial. However, in a court of law there must also be a judge to decide the case, and in the present situation the registration authorities tend to find themselves in these instances acting both as plaintiff and judge, which is not the happiest of situations. Perhaps it is a matter to which our legislators should give a little more thought.

Now, in the light of what I have said so far – and of course much more could be said about the problem of detecting adverse reactions at an early stage – it is more than evident that many an adverse reaction will be detected only after a drug has entered the market. How well adapted is present-day drug legislation to deal with this problem? The answer, as I implied a little earlier in this paper, is that it is in most countries not well adapted at all. To take an example from my own country, The Netherlands: the Medicines Act of 1958 set as criteria for registration of a new drug that the product must have been 'reasonably well shown' to be effective and safe when used according to the printed instructions, and that the printed information supplied must be full and reliable. The Act indeed allowed for registration to be suspended or withdrawn at a later phase if new information became available which would justify this step, but the procedure involved is a harsh one and the public interest must be at stake to put it into motion; there is no simple and rapid procedure for obliging a manufacturer to revise his information or alter his product as knowledge about it develops. What is more, no provision was introduced for the revision of the licence by the authorities at intervals – for example after a period of some years, by which time a clearer view of the drug is likely to have been formed. Finally, and this is most important, the Medicines Act, like the corresponding laws in many other countries, gives the drug control agency absolutely no authority to require at the time of marketing that a system of post-marketing surveillance is set up to study the drug's performance in the field.

As I have said, these relative shortcomings of the Netherlands Medicines Act, which one can fairly and reasonably criticize after 20 years, are to be found in many other national laws as well. It is particularly worrying to find a similar failing in the newly created norms for the European Community. Here, too, drug registration is a black and white process of absolute acceptance or absolute rejection of a new pharmaceutical product, with no provision for the imposition of conditions or for post-marketing surveillance and regular revision of the licensing conditions as needed. It is understandable that a Community concerned primarily with economic interests should have taken this course, but the interests of public health demand that future regulations be more attuned to the realities of drug investigation.

In viewing these problems as a whole, I would think that in the further development of drug registration procedures throughout the world, and particularly as these are unified or harmonized over large areas, 5 principles should be borne in mind in order to meet the problem of dealing with the new knowledge which becomes available on a drug in the course of the years:

1. I would suggest that *drug licences in every country should be issued for a limited period only*, perhaps 5 years. At the end of that time, all the information which has become available on that drug as regards its efficacy and its side-effects should be rescrutinized and then the licence revised (and perhaps even withdrawn) if the data justify such a step. It is entirely understandable that the pharmaceutical industry favours licences of unlimited duration, but the interests of public health run counter to this approach.
2. *It should be possible in every country to attach appropriate conditions to the issuing of a drug licence*, for example as regards the physicians who are to use it, the places where it can be used, or the way in which it is to be distributed; such conditions should be appropriate to what is known about the drug's properties and dangers, and they can be revised as knowledge expands.
3. It should be possible *to render obligatory the reporting of adverse reactions in certain circumstances*, for example for particular new drugs where the animal pharmacological studies or the early clinical work suggest the existence of risks which are still poorly defined, but which do not seem to prohibit marketing. The obligations would involve both the physicians prescribing these drugs and the firms selling them, and they would be maintained until the problem in question had been cleared up and the licence revised as necessary.
4. *The drug firm marketing a new drug should surely be obliged to pass on to the registration authorities all the information which it has received itself, worldwide, on adverse reactions to the drug in question.* I say 'worldwide' because the division of the world into national compartments is, medically viewed, an absurdity. There may indeed be genetic or other differences between the nations, but the majority of adverse reactions occur universally.
5. I would plead for a more regular *channel of communication from the drug*

registration authority to the physician on new or suspected adverse reactions. For most physicians, the pharmaceutical industry, in the form of the medical visitor, is a much more tangible entity than the drug registration authority, which very commonly fails to communicate to physicians at all, and in some countries is not even authorized to do so. Only by enlisting the help (and firing the enthusiasm) of the bulk of physicians to solve these problems will the drug registration authority be able to fulfil optimally its task in the interests of the public health.

Some of the remarks which I have made may well be construed as being highly critical of the pharmaceutical industry. They are certainly not intended to be destructive. The trouble, I believe, is that a certain part of the drug industry still fails to realize the gravity of the problem of long-term adverse reactions. I do not believe that the industry is basically dishonest, but the conscience of many a company is difficult to localize, and there is sometimes within a company a feeling, engendered by loyalty and mutual indoctrination, that the drug which has been created with such expense and effort cannot possibly be as harmful as some would say. There is also a reluctance to abandon patterns of promotion which have been practiced for such a long time, though they may obstruct and retard one's quest for the truth. It is, I sincerely believe, better that the drug industry seek to put these things right before public opinion and medical opinion oblige it to do so; if it does not, drug-induced injury may prove most injurious to industry itself.

REFERENCES

1. Dukes, M.N.G. (Ed.) (1977): The moments of truth. In: *Side Effects of Drugs Annual 1, 1977,* pp. V–IX. Excerpta Medica, Amsterdam-Oxford.
2. Nelemans, F.A. (1979): Drugs used in bronchial asthma and cough. In: *Side Effects of Drugs Annual 3, 1979,* pp. 148–150. Editor: M.N.G. Dukes. Excerpta Medica, Amsterdam-Oxford.
3. Kennedy, D. (1978): Letter to Hon. Edward M. Kennedy dated May 5th, 1978, relating to the release of safety and effectiveness data.

DISCUSSION

Böttiger: Dr. Dukes, you mentioned that adverse drug reactions may indeed be detected later. Therefore, it is dangerous to have a 3-year limit of the type mentioned by Dr. Motohashi because that will mean that drug manufacturers as well as physicians will get less observant after that time. Secondly, I would like to inform you that in Sweden now the Government has proposed an amendment to the Drug Law stating that approval can be given with conditions. I think that is extremely important in giving authorities a much better opportunity to see what is happening, especially in the period immediately after marketing of the drug.

Westerholm: Dr. Dukes, you mentioned the need for regular communication between drug agencies and physicians on available data. Do you have any such regular publication and how effective is it?

Dukes: Well, our own Drug Authority in The Netherlands is not authorized to communicate directly with physicians at all. We get around the problem by establishing a government-sponsored foundation which does write to physicians and send a regular bulletin every two weeks on drug matters, but it would have advantages if this communication was direct from the Drug Authority. As to the efficacy of such a communication method, I shall come back on the fact that a Court of Law has actually doubted the physician's ability to read all this information, even though it is only a small 4-page document sent twice a month. There might be some advantage in a communication direct from the Drug Authority to the physician rather than from an independent organization.

Inman: I believe that the methods of monitoring short-term effects of drugs are improving quite rapidly, but I would like to ask Dr. Dukes about the prospects of very long-term effects such as carcinogenicity and mutagenicity. Does he think that the existing arrangements are in any way adequate?

Dukes: No, I am very concerned about it. Regarding the carcinogenic effect of the 'pill', it may require studies lasting 15–20 years. WHO's report on the induction of tumors by the contraceptive pill shows how pathetically little has been undertaken on this problem. Drug firms are no longer themselves primarily interested in doing this work on the preparations which are largely out of patent. Here is surely a role for an international organization to play. I don't see any other way of ensuring that one will monitor large numbers of women taking the 'pill' over a period of 20–25 years, which is in fact the only way of getting answers to problems like that. The same, of course, may apply to many other drugs used for long periods.

Mashford: Dr. Dukes, do you envisage the implementation of compulsory reporting of drug reactions? It is very difficult to compel physicians to recognize an adverse drug effect if they don't particularly want to.

Dukes: My impression is that this should be used restrictively. One will tend to do it for a particular drug looking to a particular problem which is already suspected at the time when a drug is introduced on the market. I don't see how on a large scale one can effectively oblige all physicians to report all their suspicions about adverse reactions to drugs. We are rather concerned about the limited interest of physicians in this type of information. The other point is that one can impose an obligation on the drug industry to pass on the information which is received from its detail men worldwide and through other channels. It is obvious that at the moment much of this information remains within the national organization of a particular drug company and does not cross national frontiers.

Major challenges to effective post-marketing surveillance*

BRIAN L. STROM[1] and KENNETH L. MELMON[2]

[1]*Division of Clinical Pharmacology, Department of Medicine, University of California, San Francisco and* [2]*Division of Clinical Pharmacology, Department of Medicine, Stanford University Medical Center, Stanford, CA, U.S.A.*

Useful post-marketing surveillance (PMS) should detect and quantitate effects of drugs and patterns of drug use after drug marketing. This approach is required to allow a useful product to reach the patient in a timely manner because all clinically important drug effects cannot be detected or quantified prior to marketing an effective drug. Methods of post-marketing detection of drug effects have been enumerated (1–4), but how to assemble these methods into a systematic system of surveillance is debated. Equally debatable, though not widely discussed, is how we should obtain information about the rates of intended efficacy of a marketed product. Without this information we will have difficulty making appropriate decisions about the societal and medical importance of many adverse reactions to the same drug. In this paper we will emphasize the areas where methodology is insufficient or insufficiently tested to allow us to determine whether an optimal PMS system can be set up today.

TECHNIQUES TO DEMONSTRATE CAUSAL ASSOCIATIONS

The measurement of drug effects can be viewed as a problem in establishing causality: Does drug A cause event B? To answer this question, one must first demonstrate an association between drug A and event B. Once an association has been established, the next tasks are to determine whether it is artifactual, indirect, or causal. An artifactual association, also known as a spurious or false association, is one that is due either to chance or to bias. Chance can effectively be ruled out by using statistical analysis. Bias can be minimized by appropriate design of the study. An indirect association, in contrast, cannot be excluded as readily. An indirect association, in contrast, is a real but non-causal association due to both factors (in this case, drug A and event B) being associated with some common, causally related underlying condition. These underlying factors have been called confounding variables (5). Effect modifiers are non-causally related underlying conditions which can mask or accentuate an apparent causal effect (6). Any study of causality must control these potential confounders or effect-modifiers, either through study design or

*This work was supported by NIH Training Grant GM 07546 and by funds from the Joint Commission on Prescription Drug Use.

through appropriate analysis. As an example, the association between nitroglycerin and myocardial infarctions is not causal: both the choice of therapy with nitroglycerin and the occurrence of myocardial infarction are related to underlying coronary artery disease, a confounding variable. Thus, it must be controlled in order to imply a *causal* association. Similarly, though age is not causally related to hepatitis or therapy with isoniazid, it is related to isoniazid-induced hepatitis in a way which could mask or emphasize a causal relationship: if all patients in the isoniazid-treated group were children, the resulting relationship would appear very much weaker than if all were over 70. Thus, age is an effect-modifier in the relationship between isoniazid and hepatitis and needs to be controlled for.

There are 3 basic techniques to demonstrate association: experimental trials, non-experimental trials, and uncontrolled observations. The most powerful tools for demonstrating causal association are experimental trials, also called intervention trials. In these, subjects are randomly allocated by the investigator to treatment and control groups. Thus, all potential confounding variables (even if they are not identified) are assumed to be randomly distributed between the two groups.

The next most powerful technique is a non-experimental trial. This also is known as a quasi-experimental trial. These studies approximate experimental trials, but the assignment of therapy is not within the control of the investigator. Included in this category are cohort studies (also called prospective trials or follow-up studies) and case-control studies (also called retrospective, case-history, case-referent, and trohoc studies).

The last technique of demonstrating association is that of uncontrolled observations. This method is clearly the weakest of the three in establishing causal associations. The likelihood of the effect occurring spontaneously, rather than as a result of a drug, cannot be determined.

Each of these techniques has its advantages and disadvantages, as can be seen in Table 1. An association between a drug and its purported effects that is demonstrated by an experimental trial is most likely to be causal. However, the power of a research design is not the only determinant of its utility. Experimental trials are frequently logistically difficult. They require the investigator to control therapy, introducing clinical artificiality into therapeutic decision-making. In addition, economic and ethical restrictions often preclude this type of study. Cohort and case-control studies are more feasible and economical to carry out than experimental approaches; but the associations they generate are less certain to be causal. Cohort studies are most useful for studying the multiple effects that may result from a single drug and for estimating their incidence rates. Case-control studies are most useful for studying the multiple possible causes of a rare event. It can be useful, thereby, as a hypothesis-generating technique.

APPLICATION OF THE TECHNIQUES OF DEMONSTRATING ASSOCIATION TO MEASUREMENT OF DRUG EFFECTS

For the purposes of surveillance, drug effects can be classified into 4 types: unanticipated adverse effects, anticipated adverse effects, unanticipated beneficial effects, and anticipated beneficial effects. Unanticipated adverse effects are those

TABLE 1. *Potential problems of techniques of studying post-marketing drug effects*

	Design			
		Quasi-experimental		
Potential problems	Experimental	Cohort	Case control	Uncontrolled observations
Lack of power*	+	+ +	+ + +	+ + + +
Logistically difficult	+ + + +	+ + +	+ +	+
Requires investigator control of therapy	+ + + +			
Artificial	+ + + +			
Ethical restrictions	+ + + +			
Random allocation impossible		+ + + +	+ + + +	+ + + +
Bias in observation of drug effects		+ + + +	+ +	+ + +
Long follow-up required	+ + + +	+ + + +		
Loss of patients during follow-up	+ + +	+ + + +		
Changes in criteria and methods over time	+ + +	+ + + +	+ +	
Only one drug per study	+ + + +	+ + + +		
Only one effect per study			+ + + +	
Cannot study rare effects	+ + + +	+ + + +	+	
Bias in obtaining exposure history			+ + + +	+ + +
Incomplete data			+ + +	+ + + +
Incidence rates impossible			+ + + +	+ + + +
Bias in selection of controls			+ + + +	

*Power is defined as the ability of a research design to discriminate between causal and indirect associations.

undesirable effects previously unknown and, thereby, unexpected. The primary task of surveillance is to suspect or discover the association between the drug and the unanticipated event. The secondary task of surveillance is to confirm the association as causal. Usually hypotheses arise out of preclinical experiences or out of uncontrolled observations once a drug is on the market (7–9). Alternatively, they can be systematically sought by using a case-control surveillance procedure. In such an instance a systematic study is made of preselected biological events, looking for preferential exposure of the subjects exhibiting these effects to a drug (10). In either case, these hypotheses become increasingly more difficult to generate as the incidence of the event increases in the non-drug exposed population. Once generated, these hypotheses can then be confirmed or denied by case-control studies (11) and, if felt necessary, prospective studies (12).

Anticipated adverse effects are those undesirable effects expected at the time of study. The question posed for surveillance to answer is: What is their incidence? Through voluntary reports or use of case-control surveillance, a very approximate estimate of whether a toxic effect is rare or common can be made. However, 'denominator data', i.e. data on the size of the population put at risk of the adverse effect through use of the drug, is absent in both approaches. These data can only be obtained from a prospective approach, whether experimental or non-experimental (cohort). A successful example of such a study is the 'Phase IV' study of prazosin. The manufacturer studied a cohort of 23,000 patients treated with the drug finding that the incidence of syncope caused by the drug was 0.1% (13).

Unanticipated beneficial effects become new indications for the drug. They are discovered after marketing. Methodologically, they are sought in exactly the same way as unanticipated adverse effects. The only difference between studies of beneficial and unwanted side-effects is the inevitably larger number of patients required to find the former. Studies of 'toxic effects' need sufficient subjects to achieve a statistical power adequate to demonstrate some relative risks (risk relative to placebo) greater than 1. The actual relative risk can often be 5 to 10 or even greater, with a large arithmetical difference between incidence rates in the treated and untreated groups. In contrast, studies of unanticipated beneficial effects often are studies of prevention of events. Therefore relative riks of less than 1 must be detected. The resultant arithmetical difference between incidence rates of the prevented effect in the treated group and in the untreated group is necessarily small. Thus large numbers of patients are required to achieve statistical significance.

Mathematically, $n = (Z_{(1-\alpha)} + Z_{(1-\beta)})^2\sigma^2/\Delta^2$, where n is the required number of subjects needed to detect a clinically significant arithmetical difference in outcome Δ, using a technique with variance σ^2, considering acceptable a probability α of Type I error and a probability β of Type II error. $Z_{(1-\alpha)}$ and $Z_{(1-\beta)}$ are the cumulative areas under the standard normal frequency distribution curves (mean = 0, standard deviation = 1) corresponding to probabilities $(1 - \alpha)$ and $(1 - \beta)$, respectively. As is apparent from the formula, assuming constant α, β and σ, a smaller Δ would require a substantially larger n. As an example, with the same α, β, and σ, a study designed to detect a relative risk of 0.5, a successful protective therapeutic effect, would require 16 times the number of patients as one designed to detect a relative risk of 2.0, a not-uncommon toxic effect. Thus, studies of beneficial effects must be considerably larger than studies of toxic effects.

The last and perhaps the most vexing type of drug effect (from the perspective of effective PMS) is assessing the drug's anticipated beneficial effect, or efficacy. Strictly, efficacy is the *ability* of a drug to achieve its intended beneficial effect. This presents a unique methodological problem. In non-experimental studies, *the drug's indication becomes a confounder*. The indication for use of a drug will inevitably be present more frequently in any treated group of patients than it would in any group that did not receive treatment. The presence of the indication per se also inevitably will have a bearing on the outcome of the group that has the indication. Non-causal indirect associations are created *a priori*. For example, if one were to ask whether propranolol is associated with sudden death, a non-experimental assessment would *a priori* indicate a positive association between the two events that could be mistaken as a causal association. The association between angina pectoris and therapy with propranolol on the one hand, and angina pectoris and sudden death on the other, automatically creates a treated group with a higher underlying incidence of sudden death than would be expected from an untreated group without the same indication for treatment. Thus, the presence of the indication for therapy, angina pectoris, produces the appearance that propranolol is *causing* sudden death (presumably fallacious). New non-experimental techniques must be developed if such techniques are ever to be used in studying the success in achieving the intended benefit from a marketed drug. The remainder of this paper will deal with the issues raised by our interest in determining whether non-experimental techniques can be used to define the efficacy of marketed drugs.

NEED FOR POST-MARKETING STUDIES OF DRUG EFFICACY

Of the 4 types of drug effects, anticipated beneficial effects are the most straightforward to study using experimental techniques but the most difficult to study using non-experimental techniques. Nevertheless, there are many settings in which only non-experimental studies of efficacy are likely to be possible in post-marketing settings (see Table 2). Phase III studies of drug efficacy are necessarily incomplete for optimal clinical use of the drug. Of necessity, they are greatly limited in time. Thus, long-term efficacy cannot be studied in Phase III. For many drugs, their intended effects are short-term and, so, such a deficiency is inconsequential. However, for other drugs the whole purpose of use is long-term prevention of an undesirable outcome. These drugs often must be approved for marketing on the basis of their intermediate, short-term effects. Ultimate efficacy for the long-term intended effect then remains to be proven. An example of drug marketing on the basis of proven intermediate efficacy is the antihypertensive drugs. These are approved on the basis of their ability to decrease blood pressure. However, they are

TABLE 2. *Need for post-marketing studies of drug efficacy*

1. To study long-term efficacy
2. To study efficacy in settings not subject to the artificiality of Phase III experimental trials
3. To study efficacy in settings subject to ethical restrictions of experimental studies
4. To study the efficacy of a drug used for indications other than the one originally approved
5. To study efficacy where biology is changing
6. To study relative efficacy
7. To study efficacy of drugs used in combination for the same indications
8. To place toxicity information in proper perspective, allowing risk/benefit decisions

really prescribed for their presumed effect of decreasing undesirable morbid or mortal cardiovascular abnormalities. Other examples are the use of lipid-lowering drugs or hypoglycemic drugs. In both instances the drugs' intermediate effects may not be accompanied by long-term positive effects on atherosclerosis or diabetic vascular disease, respectively. In both, despite experimental post-marketing studies performed at considerable expense and with considerable difficulty, unequivocal long-term efficacy remains to be proven (14, 15).

Phase III studies of drug efficacy are also incomplete because they require contrived clinical settings. The patients selected to participate in Phase III randomized experimental trials are usually highly atypical (willing to undergo experimentation, selected by entrance criteria which usually include that they take no other drugs and have no other complicating illness, etc.). Once selected, they often are given atypical regimens (usually constant dose, regardless of the patient's response) in atypical settings (very close follow-up in a center capable of carrying out research). Phase III's artificiality could also be postulated to affect a patient's compliance to a regimen. All of these circumstances affect the ultimate drug effects. For example, diuretics augment both efficacy and toxicity of digoxin (16). Thus, once a drug's efficacy is proven in the highly skewed setting of a pre-marketing experimental trial, it still remains to be determined whether it persists in the 'real world' of routine practice.

Phase III studies can be limited by ethical considerations. In some cases random allocation of therapy can be considered unethical (17, 18). In others, it is considered unethical to administer an unproven therapy and just as unethical to prove it (e.g. in pregnant patients, children and unconscious patients). Yet, each of these groups consumes large amounts of drugs (19) and their special conditions can affect the pharmacokinetics and pharmacodynamics of those drugs (20, 21).

Studies of the efficacy of a marketed drug are also needed to obtain information that was not sought in Phase III. One example is the efficacy of an indication other than the one originally approved. Currently in the U.S., studies of efficacy for a new indication only need to be performed if a manufacturer wants to advertise the drug for that indication. As another example, post-marketing studies of efficacy are needed in clinical settings which can change. Examples would be infectious organisms developing resistance to an antibiotic (e.g. the gonococcus), or immunity changing over time in subjects given vaccine. Other post-marketing studies of drug efficacy which could potentially be clinically useful include studies of the relative efficacy of drugs used for the same indication and studies of the efficacy of drugs used in combination for the same indication. Note that under current U.S. FDA regulations, if a combination product is to be marketed, each component of the combination must be shown to add efficacy to the others. Finally, and most basically, post-marketing information on drug efficacy is needed in order to properly place the incidence of toxicity into practical perspective. In order to make accurate medical and legal risk/benefit decisions, data on drug toxicity must be accompanied by data on drug efficacy obtained without the artificial constraints of randomized experimental trials. Until now, however, obtaining data in scientifically sound yet economically feasible ways has been thought to be near impossible. Use of non-experimental techniques has been considered infeasible because the problem of confounding seemed insurmountable (22).

TECHNIQUES FOR POST-MARKETING STUDIES OF DRUG EFFICACY

Studies of drug efficacy need not always be formal research. Research is only necessary as an approximation of truth. When the truth is known for the patient at hand, formal research is superfluous. In such a setting, a study of drug efficacy would simply be an aggregation of these individual truths (a series of uncontrolled observations). For example, there is no need to incur the expense or inconvenience of formal research in determining the post-marketing efficacy of intravenous naloxone in reversing the effects of methadone. Every doctor who uses the drug knows that within minutes after administration, a patient who is comatose from an overdose of methadone will totally awaken. One to two hours later the patient again becomes comatose and again promptly responds to naloxone (23). This repeatable cycle proves the efficacy of naloxone beyond any doubt. No more need be done. Thus a simple collection of 'cases' is all that is needed to prove the point. Additional expense or time would be a waste of a precious commodity. Note that the same pragmatic philosophy has been expressed by Japan's Special Subcommittee for Drug Re-evaluation. In contrast to the analogous U.S. National Academy of Sciences in its 1969 Drug Efficacy Study which was restricted to the legal definition of demonstrated 'substantial evidence of effectiveness' (24), the Japanese committee has included in its category of drugs considered 'effective (proven)' the following two types of definitions:

> 'i. Drugs which are judged as effective on the basis of results of well planned and thoroughly controlled comparative tests.
> ii. Drugs which have been shown clearly and without exception to alleviate symptoms or shorten the course of a disease known previously.' (25).

Thus, for most drugs post-marketing studies of efficacy are needed. However, only a subset of these studies need to be performed by using formal research methodology. A further subset is not subject to confounding by the indication and so can be studied by quasi-experimental methods. For example, diagnostic agents, such as contrast agents, drugs used for skin tests, and drugs used in provocative tests, are not used because they cause or modify an outcome but, rather, because they predict an outcome. Thus, inasmuch as 'diagnostic agents' are not causally related to the outcome, they cannot be confounders. In addition, some agents given for prophylactic purposes are usually given regardless of the risk of a particular patient developing the outcome that is being prevented. For example, there is no reason to think that patients who receive poliomyelitis immunization differ from those who do not get the drug in ways which would meaningfully predict the likelihood of contracting the disease. Any differences between the two groups is more likely to be economic, social or philosophical. Since the indication is not an underlying factor related to both drug (vaccine) and outcome (contraction of poliomyelitis), it will not be a confounder.

Yet, as previously demonstrated, many indications for drug use are confounding factors that can limit the usefulness of quasi-experimental studies. In some cases innovative selection and manipulation of subsets of the data potentially available in a PMS system can circumvent this. For example, when a readily quantitated measure of the severity of illness is available (e.g. the blood pressure), groups can be matched for their initial severity of illness, despite what therapy they may be receiving. When therapies of comparable potency are to be compared (e.g. antacids and cimetidine), if physicians who use only one and others who use only the other can be found, their patients can be compared. In such a setting, any initial systematic difference between the two groups is then related to differences between the physicians rather than differences among the patients. The differences between the physicians probably would be unlikely to be related to the ultimate outcome or response to the drugs.

Nevertheless, there will be situations post-marketing when confounding by the indication cannot be circumvented non-experimentally. In these, randomized experiments need to be performed in clinical settings which do not re-introduce all the artificiality of Phase III trials. For example, the Boston Collaborative Drug Surveillance Program conducted a study where a prescription written for an 'hypnotic study drug' would be filled with a drug selected randomly from those under study. Observation for efficacy and toxicity, dosage adjustment etc. continued under the care of the prescribing physician. This introduced minimal artificiality (26). Another method of introducing randomization into post-marketing trials would be to match physicians in a group practice setting and ask each to use a single drug randomly selected from among the study drugs in each of his next x patients who have the appropriate indication. Again, care would otherwise remain undisturbed. Other similar variations are possible.

Thus, in post-marketing evaluation of efficacy, some drug indications need no formal research, some can be studied using non-experimental techniques and some require randomized experiments, though these can be performed in more natural settings than Phase III trials. At present, the fraction of indications that fall into each of these categories is unknown. Inasmuch as this knowledge is key to a proper design of a post-marketing surveillance system, the U.S. Joint Commission on Prescription Drug Use has undertaken a study to determine the proportion of drugs whose efficacy might be studied by non-experimental techniques. The 100 most commonly prescribed drugs in the U.S. approved since the 1962 law requiring pre-marketing studies of efficacy will be identified. They will then be classified into the above categories of study according to their originally approved indications, all currently approved indications, and all indications for which the drug is currently used, whether or not the indication is approved by the FDA. The study is currently underway.

LONG-TERM EFFICACY

Studies of long-term efficacy present methodological problems in addition to those already mentioned. One problem is the poor reliability of the historical data related to drug taking. If a drug is given for only a short time and a study is attempted of its delayed effects many years later, any historically obtained data on drug exposure must be assumed to be nearly worthless: we must surmise that a patient would be extremely unlikely to accurately recall his exposure to the drug. Thus the investigation would be limited to what could be found in old records of the patient. Any association between a drug given for a week or two and a delayed effect 20 years later is even less likely to be made spontaneously by either the patient or the physician. Even if the drug is used for a long term, retrospective studies on delayed effects of drugs would be questionable because of the unreliability of the information. Prospective studies could circumvent this problem. However, these studies have their own logistical problems. First, the expense and the organizational difficulties of a 20-year study are untold (see Table 1). In addition, the therapy of a chronic disease would not be likely to remain constant for such a long period.

Another problem of studying long-term effects of drugs used for long-term therapy is determination of the effect of compliance to the regimen as an effect-modifier. Those patients who experience success with therapy are probably more likely to comply with their regimen than those who do not. This would occur regardless of whether success was caused by the drug or by spontaneous variation in the disease. Thus, a group of patients who have remained on long-term therapy will include a disproportionate number of patients whose disease has spontaneously resolved, giving falsely successful apparent efficacy. Similarly, those who experience toxic effects are more likely to have their therapy discontinued. Thus, retrospectively created treatment groups might have an excess of patients with mild or responsive disease and a minimum of patients with adverse effects. In contrast, a retrospectively created untreated group might have an excess of patients with severe disease or treatment failures. These factors would bias the study toward falsely positive impressions of apparent drug efficacy and falsely low apparent toxicity. The longer the therapy, allowing more time for changes in therapy on the basis of the results of therapy, the worse this problem would become. Thus, a good study would need to compare patients on the basis of their initial therapy. This requirement presents a major problem when a disease like hypertension is considered, however, where therapy is changed often in the same patient. How could a delayed effect be assigned to a specific agent?

The final major problem with long-term studies is the frequent inconsistency of the severity of the underlying disease. Though one might assume that patients with comparable blood pressures are comparable today, how can we assume they would still be comparable 20 years later? How could we tell what factors other than therapy might have accounted for apparent success or failure? We do not know if baseline blood pressure alone would be predictive of the natural history of hypertensive disease, and we cannot assume that the natural history of untreated disease would remain stable under different and changing therapies. Thus, how would we match patients for severity of illness when they are under long-term therapy?

CONCLUSIONS

Techniques are available to study anticipated and unanticipated adverse drug effects and unanticipated beneficial drug effects that are produced by marketed drugs. Methodology to study the intended beneficial effects of those drugs has been presented. The effectiveness of some drugs can be studied by uncontrolled observation, others by quasi-experimental techniques. Because the indication *per se* can be a confounding factor, some drug efficacy studies will need to be performed using experimental techniques. Study of long-term efficacy presents additional problems that we have summarized. Yet we do not know whether a substantial number of settings of drug efficacy could be studied with 'non-experimental' techniques or whether additional solutions must be sought to the problem of confounding caused by the indication. The Joint Commission on Prescription Drug Use has sponsored a study which will classify the 100 most commonly used drugs in the U.S. into categories related to the methodology necessary to study their efficacy. The study is currently underway. Its results should help us to both plan the approach to a complete PMS system and estimate the relative costs of study of drugs used for definable indications.

ACKNOWLEDGMENTS

The authors express thanks to Sally Mixer and Millie Kong for aid in the preparation of the manuscript.

REFERENCES

1. Gross, F.H. and Inman, W.H.W. (Eds.) (1977): *Drug Monitoring*. Academic Press, New York.
2. Stewart, R.B., Cluff, L.E. and Philp, J.R. (Eds.) (1977): *Drug Monitoring: A Requirement for Responsible Drug Use*. Williams and Wilkins, New York.
3. IMS America Ltd. Health Care Services Research Group (1978): *Final Report – Task A: An Experiment in Early Post-Marketing Surveillance of Drugs*. IMS America, Ambler, PA.
4. Strom, B.L. and Melmon, K.L. (1979): Can post-marketing surveillance help to effect optimal drug therapy? *J. Amer. med. Ass., 242,* 2420.
5. Miettinen, O. (1970): Matching and design efficiency in retrospective studies. *Amer. J. Epidemiol., 91*, 111.
6. Miettinen, O. (1974): Confounding and effect modification. *Amer. J. Epidemiol., 100*, 350.
7. Lee, B. and Turner, W.M. (1978): Food and Drug Administration's Adverse Drug Monitoring Program. *Amer. J. Hosp. Pharm., 35*, 929.
8. Inman, W.H.W. and Price Evans, D.A. (1972): Evaluation of spontaneous reports of adverse reactions to drugs. *Brit. med. J., 3*, 746.
9. McBride, W.G. (1961): Thalidomide and congenital abnormalities. *Lancet, 2*, 1358.
10. Slone, D., Jick, H., Lewis, G.P., Shapiro, S. and Miettinen, O.S. (1969): Intravenously given ethacrynic acid and gastrointestinal bleeding. *J. Amer. med. Ass., 209*, 1668.
11. Lenz, W. and Knapp, K. (1962): Thalidomide embryopathy. *Arch. environ. Hlth, 5,* 100.
12. Taussig, H.B. (1962): A study of the German outbreak of phocomelia. *J. Amer. med. Ass., 180*, 1106.
13. IMS America Ltd., Health Care Services Research Group (1978): *Final Report – Task A: An Experiment in Early Post-Marketing Surveillance of Drugs – Appendix*, pp. 261–275. IMS America, Ambler, PA.
14. The Coronary Drug Project Research Group (1975): Clofibrate and niacin in coronary heart disease. *J. Amer. med. Ass., 231*, 360.

15. The University Group Diabetes Program (1970): A study of the effects of hypoglycemic agents on vascular complications in patients with adult-onset diabetes. *Diabetes, 19, Suppl. 2*, 747.
16. Shapiro, S., Slone, D., Lewis, G.P. and Jick, H. (1969): The epidemiology of digoxin. *J. chron. Dis., 22*, 361.
17. Gehan, E.A. and Freireich, E.J. (1974): Non-randomized controls in cancer clinical trials. *N.Engl. J. Med., 290*, 198.
18. Weinstein. M.C. (1974): Allocation of subjects in medical experiments. *N. Engl. J. Med., 291*, 1278.
19. Doering, P.L. and Stewart, R.B. (1978): The extent and character of drug consumption during pregnancy. *J. Amer. med. Ass., 239*, 843.
20. Morgan, D., Moore, G., Thomas, J. and Triggs, E. (1978): Disposition of meperidine in pregnancy. *Clin. Pharmacol. Ther., 23*, 288.
21. Mirkin, B.L. (1978): Pharmacodynamics and drug disposition in pregnant women, in neonates, and in children. In: *Clinical Pharmacology, 2nd ed.,* Chapter 5, pp. 127–152. Editors: K.L. Melmon and H.F. Morrelli. Macmillan, New York.
22. Slone, D., Shapiro, S., Miettinen, O.S., Finkle, W.D. and Stolley, P.D. (1979): Drug evaluation after marketing. *Ann. intern. Med., 90*, 257.
23. Becker, C.E. and Morrelli, H.F. (1978): Alcohol and drug abuse. In: *Clinical Pharmacology, 2nd ed.*, Chapter 22, pp. 1018–1019. Editors: K.L. Melmon and H.F. Morrelli. Macmillan, New York.
24. National Academy of Sciences – National Research Council (1969): *Drug Efficacy Study – Final Report to the Commissioner of Food and Drugs*, pp. 1–9. NAS, Washington, DC.
25. Pharmaceutical Affairs Bureau, Ministry of Health and Welfare, Japanese Government (1977): *Pharmaceutical Administration in Japan*, pp. 324–331. Yakuji-Nepo, Tokyo.
26. Shapiro, S., Slone, D., Lewis, G.P. and Jick, H. (1969): Clinical effects of hypnotics. II. An epidemiologic study. *J. Amer. med. Ass., 209*, 2016.

DISCUSSION

Nagano: In the report made by Dr. Melmon, he referred to the re-evaluation of drugs conducted in Japan. In the United States, the drug efficacy study showed certain drugs to be possibly effective. The same drugs, in Japan, were classified as having substantial effects, e.g. dipyridamol. However, when only uncontrolled studies are conducted as is currently done in Japan, it entails a great danger.

Melmon: The rule itself seems admirable to me. It is senseless to waste money and human resources on the answer to a question which has already been easily and unequivocally settled. I am unsure of the way that the rule is being applied. If it allows the use of a new antianginal agent without experimental proof that it works, then I would fear the rule is being misused. As we all know, proof of the efficacy of an antianginal agent is almost certain to require experimentation.

The Swedish Adverse Drug Reaction Committee: 13 years of experience

LARS ERIK BÖTTIGER

Department of Internal Medicine, Karolinska Institute and Hospital, Stockholm, Sweden

The thalidomide disaster at the beginning of the 1960's may be said to have set the zero-point for modern work on drug development and drug control. However, large outbreaks of severe adverse drug reactions have, in fact, occurred *before* as well as *after* the thalidomide disaster. From the pre-thalidomide era an early unfortunate vaccination in France with strongly virulent BCG vaccine may be mentioned, and from the 1950's the Cutter episode in the U.S.A. with inadvertently live polio vaccine, and the 'grey syndrome' caused by the prophylactic use of chloramphenicol in the newborn who have immature enzyme systems incapable of detoxifying the drug. From the post-thalidomide period there is, of course, the SMON disaster in Japan, the very reason why this Conference has been organized.

All of us hope that such disasters can be avoided in the future – without the demand for safety tests, of which it is difficult to tell whether they are relevant for the use of drugs in man, becoming so high, so time-consuming and so costly that the development of new drugs is virtually slowed down or totally arrested. There are those who affirm that valuable drugs are being kept from patients who need them because of the fact that bureaucratic and formal tests are in progress.

It is important to realize that modern pharmacotherapy is a young discipline going back only to the 1940's, i.e. one generation. It was born with the introduction of penicillin during the Second World War. Before that time, drug therapy – with few exceptions – was symptomatic and of short duration, was often rather ineffective and in most instances was also without serious adverse effects. The physician of today has a large number of very effective drugs at his disposal. Many of them have a very narrow therapeutic range, many are given simultaneously with other drugs, many are prescribed for long periods of time, perhaps for life. The patient is likely to be elderly. These facts, and many others, make adverse drug reactions a serious part of our everyday drug therapy.

There can be no doubt that it was thalidomide that awakened medical authorities as well as public opinion to an awareness of a drug problem, previously unheard of. All over the world this led to increased efforts for drug control, in many instances with new and more effective organizations and new legislation – and also, to a slow and gradual growth of interest in work on adverse drug reactions.

Many, even today, adopt a very negative attitude towards active work on adverse drug reactions. To mention only a few examples, Ingelfinger wrote in a recent editorial (1) that 'the total number of adverse reactions per given population per year may be a figure for the record books, but in itself is hardly of any pragmatic importance'. The American Medical Association started a registry for adverse drug reactions but had to abandon it due to lack of cooperation from physicians.

Many countries, however, now have national systems for collecting reports of adverse drug reactions. This is the case in the Scandinavian countries, in the U.K., The Netherlands, New Zealand and others, most of which also report to the WHO monitoring centre, now located in Uppsala, Sweden. In other parts of the world, great emphasis has been put on localized intensive projects, the best known being the Boston Cooperative Drug Surveillance Program.

In Sweden, we take a positive view and are proud of the results of our Adverse Drug Reaction Committee. I intend to describe the Swedish Committee, tell you how it works and present a selection of the results that have been obtained by analyzing its material, results that in some instances have had an active influence on the Swedish drug market. At the end of the presentation I would like to stress some of the points we have found particularly important and suggest how future work should be conducted, nationally as well as internationally.

THE SWEDISH ADVERSE DRUG REACTION COMMITTEE

The Swedish Committee started its work late in 1965. It has 11 members, all M.D.'s, who represent pharmacology, clinical pharmacology and clinical specialities such as internal medicine, pediatrics, psychiatry and anesthesiology. The joint associations of pharmaceutical industries in Sweden also have one member on the Committee, intended to act as a spokesman for general aspects on behalf of the drug manufacturers. The Committee meets in full approximately 4 times a year.

Much of the everyday work is done by a full-time medical officer who performs a preliminary cause-and-effect classification of all incoming reports. These classifications are further discussed by a working party of 3–4 medical officers and finally reported to and discussed by the Committee itself. The Committee has been working with the following categories of *causal relationship,* viz. (a) 'probable', (b) 'not excluded', (c) 'unlikely', (d) 'frequency registration only' (accepting probable relationship) and (e) 'information insufficient for classification'. The difference between the two categories (a) 'probable' and (b) 'not excluded' is in fact very small – both carry a high degree of causal relationship and together comprise approximately 40% of the reports. Another 40% falls into category (d) 'frequency registration only'. Into this class are put all reports of well-known and accepted mild adverse reactions. Very few reports are put into group (c) 'causal relationship unlikely' – only 2–3%. A somewhat larger number (10–15%) has to be labeled (e) 'information insufficient for classification'. This applies mainly to cases of polypharmacy in which it is impossible, even with complete information at hand, to evaluate the individual importance of the numerous drugs prescribed and taken.

It should be mentioned that the Committee in all fatal cases, as well as in all more severe ones, always asks for additional information and generally works with the complete medical record from one or several physicians and/or hospitals.

The present regulations for reporting adverse reactions state that *all* physicians have to report *all fatalities* suspected of being caused by the intake of therapeutic drugs, as well as *all severe adverse reactions*, which although not causing death nevertheless have had a considerable influence on the general condition of the patient, the course of the disease, the time of hospitalization etc. Further, *all new, unexpected or otherwise remarkable reactions* should be reported. Finally, so as not to discourage anybody who wants to report, it is stated that every physician is free to report any reaction that he wants to bring to the attention of the Committee, even if it does not fall into the above-mentioned categories. Also, it is added that it is especially important to report those adverse reactions that seem to be increasing in frequency, be they severe or mild in character. It is also of interest to note that the regulations state that a reaction should be reported on the suspicion of a causal relation between a drug and the reaction. The reporting physican does not have to perform an analysis of the case; that is the task of the Committee. These regulations have been valid since January 1, 1975 – the previous ones in all essentials were the same, but had turned out to be somewhat difficult to interpret.

RESULTS ACHIEVED BY THE COMMITTEE

During the years 1965–1978 a total 18,000 reports were received and classified by the Committee. The annual number of reports has increased from 600 in the beginning to over 2200 in 1978 (Fig. 1). There have been stepwise increments in the number of reports. At least for some of these, probable explanations can be found, but the important fact is that there is an overall, gradual increase. It is difficult to tell whether this is due to an increase in the number of reactions occurring or to better reporting. There is, however, nothing to indicate that the number of adverse drug reactions should increase in this fashion. Therefore, most of the increase is probably due to better reporting. A recent study (2) found that the number of

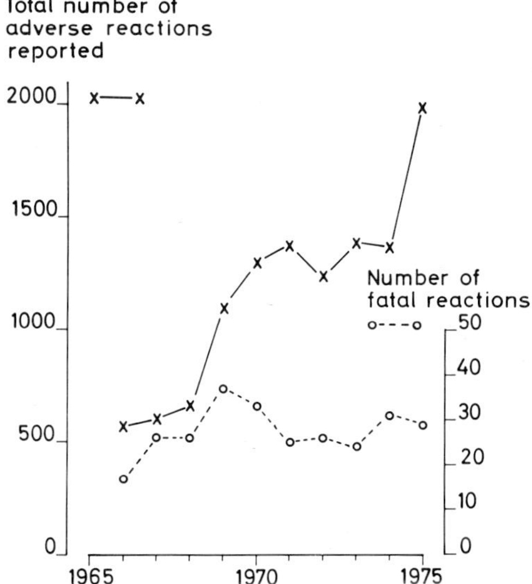

Fig. 1. The total number of adverse drug reactions reported to the Swedish Committee and the total number of fatal cases, 1966–1975.

reports per active physician, although low, had doubled in 10 years time. The same analysis also was able to demonstrate that the reporting frequency was very similar all over the country with a constant ratio between the size of the population and the number of reports from the different counties in Sweden.

Previously, it had been shown in several independent studies that the frequency with which severe drug-induced blood disorders were reported – 4 types of cytopenias – was on average 31% (3). These results could be arrived at through an analysis of total morbidity in one of Sweden's health-care regions, with 15% of the total population, in which all hospital discharge diagnoses are registered and analyzed in a computer.

A reporting frequency of 30% may seem low. There is, however, reason to believe that the more severe the reaction, the more often it is reported. This is supported by the fact that the number of reported fatal cases has remained remarkably constant through the years, with 25–30 cases annually. This could indicate that almost 100% of such cases have been reported.

The Committee twice yearly publishes a report that is distributed free of charge to all physicians in Sweden, and is also published in the *Journal of the Swedish Medical Association.* To date, 29 such reports have been issued, each of them discussing a number of new or especially important adverse reactions. Some have contained warnings against the use of certain drugs or advice on precautions.

Also, a large number (~70) of studies on the material of the Committee has been published. They have dealt with various aspects of the panorama of adverse drug reactions, e.g. the composition of the *total material* and of the material of *fatal cases* (age and sex distribution, offending drugs, types of reactions etc.), reactions from *specific drugs* (e.g. oral contraceptives, halothane) or drugs causing *specific reactions* (drug-induced blood dyscrasias, febrile mucocutaneous syndromes). I would like to present here a few results from these studies.

The age and sex composition of the total material is important (Fig. 2) (4). *Women* predominate in the material. This is at least partly due to the fact that women consume more drugs than men (1.5/1), but there are indications that women are more likely to develop some types of adverse reactions to drugs. More studies are needed in this field.

Age is a very important factor. The prevalence of adverse drug reactions increases very markedly with age. This is clearly visible in the whole material, but even more so if one looks at the fatal cases (5). There are many reasons for this increase with age – elderly (60–75) and old (above 75 years of age) people have *many simultaneous diseases* and ailments, they get *many drugs* – but they also may have alterations in their *drug metabolic capacity*, they do have *impaired renal function* and there are indications that they have *increased sensitivity at the receptor level.*

Further analysis of the fatal cases clearly showed that in this, the most severe group of adverse reactions, the majority of the cases were due to damage to the blood and bone marrow. This finding initiated a series of studies of drug-induced blood disorders (3, 6). These studies have been performed on two different occasions at an interval of 5 years, making it possible not only to demonstrate which drugs were responsible for most of the drug-induced blood disorders, but also the changes that have taken place in the last few years.

The yearly incidence of drug-induced cytopenias has been calculated for two

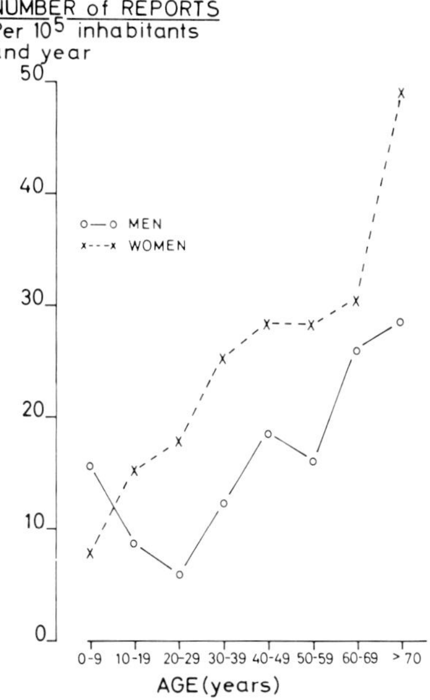

Fig. 2. Age and sex composition of the material of adverse drug reactions reported to the Swedish Committee, 1972.

consecutive 5-year periods and shows a possible slight increase in the number of drug-induced cases of hemolytic anemia, but virtually no changes for the other cytopenias. This could be taken as an indication that individual susceptibility plays an important role, more important perhaps than the offending drug. In other words, at least at a low degree of exposure to 'toxic' or 'sensitizing' drugs, a number of susceptible individuals will have negative reactions to a variety of different drugs.

Rapid changes occur in the spectrum of adverse reactions, especially due to shifts among the drugs commonly prescribed. This is well illustrated, e.g., by drugs causing blood disorders. Of 12 drugs, or group of drugs, responsible for drug-induced cytopenias, only *one* (methyldopa) remained in the same position on the list during two consecutive 5-year periods. All others had appeared, disappeared or changed position on the list.

Other examples of rapid changes are the oral contraceptives which 10 years ago made up 40% of all reports to the Swedish Committee – to-day the figure is 5%. Antibiotics and sulfonamides have increased from 9% in the late 1960's to 30–35% at the present time.

CHANGES IN THE SWEDISH DRUG MARKET

As already mentioned, the results and actions of the Adverse Drug Reaction Committee in some instances have changed the drug market in Sweden, in as much as drug manufacturers have had to withdraw drugs or change their composition.

Dipyrone (noramidopyrine), used mainly as an antipyretic, caused a significant number of cases of agranulocytosis in Sweden, including a number with fatal outcome. The drug is a derivative of, and is chemically closely related to, amidopyrine, a drug well known to cause agranulocytosis, in fact one of the first drugs for which a relationship between drug and agranulocytosis could be established. The Committee issued several warnings against the use of dipyrone. Only the third warning had effect – but a remarkable one (3) (Fig. 3) – such that sales figures dropped dramatically, as did the number of cases of agranulocytosis. The sales figures stayed low, but the number of patients with agranulocytosis showed a tendency to increase – and in 1973 the drug was taken off the market.

Chloramphenicol-induced aplastic anemia is a disorder of special interest in Japan and other countries of the Far East. Aplastic anemia is so common in Japan that a special Research Group on Aplastic Anemia has been established, sponsored by the Government. A study of aplastic anemia with comparisons between the Far East and the western world showed that much, if not all, of the difference could be explained by external toxic factors, such as the use of *insecticides* of the organic phosphorus type or the widespread use of *chloramphenicol* in eastern countries (7). It is of great importance to note that the study by Yoshimatsu et al. (8) showed that only a retrospective study of the drug record of the patients with aplastic anemia could demonstrate that a large group of them had been treated with chloramphenicol, a drug intake not suspected or listed in the primary hospital records, and probably not known by the patients.

In Sweden, the Committee gave an early warning against the indiscriminate use of chloramphenicol, a warning that helped bring down the already decreasing sales figures and led to the virtual disappearance of chloramphenicol-induced aplastic anemia in Sweden. Later the same disappearance has been registered elsewhere, as in Australia and in the central files of the WHO monitoring center (9). Chloramphenicol was first replaced by the antiphlogistic drugs oxyphenbutazone and phenylbutazone as the cause of drug-induced aplasia, a place now taken instead by sulfonamides – in fact, a remarkable shift in 10 years!

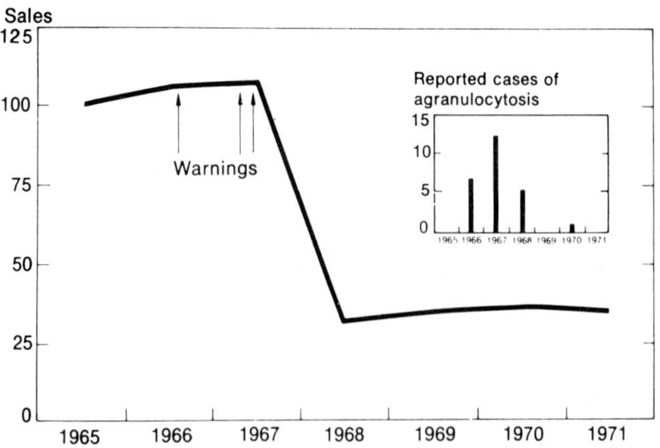

Fig. 3. Dipyrone tablet sales before and after warnings and corresponding incidence of dipyrone-induced agranulocytosis (1965 = 100).

Chloramphenicol can teach us another lesson (7). The risks of a new drug are always grossly underestimated in the beginning. Four separate studies of the risk of developing chloramphenicol-induced aplastic anemia have been summarized in Figure 4. It shows that the estimated risk has gone up from 1:200,000 to 1:20,000 – a 10-fold increase in 10 years!

The *'halothane* controversy' was a very heated discussion, especially in the U.S.A. and the U.K., about whether halothane could cause liver damage or not. Swedish studies (10) demonstrated not only a totally different *age pattern* from that of infectious hepatitis, which had been thought responsible for the jaundice reported, and from that of surgery in general in a large university hospital, but more important, they were able to establish a form of cause-and-effect curve – the more exposures to halothane, the more severe the liver damage, measured e.g. by serum bilirubin levels. This led to discussions with surgeons and anesthesiologists in Sweden, and special precautions were formulated to minimize the risk of liver damage by halothane.

Recently, *thenalidine*, an antihistamine that caused a number of cases of agranulocytosis, has in the same way been taken off the market. In fields other than blood disorders, it is worth mentioning that the Committee was active in banning oral contraceptives with a high estrogen content.

Another important aspect is to relate the number of adverse reactions to the consumption pattern, i.e. to the number of doses sold – and used – of the drug in question. A study of adverse reactions during treatment of urinary tract infections (11) demonstrated that, whereas reactions to sulfonamides stayed at a comparatively low and constant level, the number of reactions to *nitrofurantoin* not only increased in absolute numbers but, more importantly, in relation to the amount sold of the drug. This problem is now under discussion in Sweden, but so far no official steps have been taken. Severe adverse reactions with lactic acidosis and death have been reported after the use of biguanide preparations in diabetes. Initially, *phenformin* was the major biguanide in Sweden, and almost all reactions were reported after the use of this drug. This led to warnings against phenformin, which in their turn had the effect that in 1976 metformin became the most common

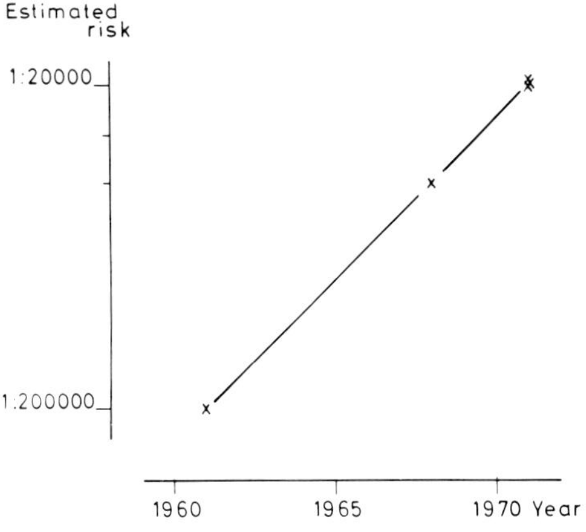

Fig. 4. Change in estimate of risk of developing chloramphenicol-induced aplastic anemia.

biguanide – and a number of negative reactions were reported also after the use of that drug. A study performed by Bergman et al. (12) showed, by comparing sales and prescription figures for phenformin and metformin, that the total number of reports of adverse reactions did not differ between the two drugs. However, if only the cases of lactic acidosis and death were calculated, there was a highly significant difference in favor of metformin. This study led to the withdrawal of phenformin from the Swedish market.

CONCLUSIONS

It is important not only to *collect* reports on adverse drug reactions but also to *evaluate* them in order that only reports with a reasonable positive connection between drug intake and the ensuing reaction are used for further analyses.

It is essential *continually to analyze* the material – rapid changes do occur – with regard to the drugs used as to the reactions found.

The *number of adverse reactions* should be related to the *pattern of drug consumption.* More studies on how and why drugs are used are urgently necessary.

It is important *continuously to inform the prescribing physicians* – and to *a large extent also the public* – about adverse drug reactions. This is a difficult and delicate problem! Press and TV tend grossly to exaggerate and overdramatize the risks and dangers, without mentioning the positive effects of the drugs in question. This prevents a realistic attitude and is overtly harmful to those patients who are afraid to take the drugs that they really need.

REFERENCES

1. Ingelfinger, F.J. (1976): Counting adverse drug reactions that count. *New Engl. J. Med., 294*, 1003.
2. Böttiger, L.E., Hast, R. and Holmberg, L. (1979): Vem anmäler läkemedelsbiverkningar? (Who reports adverse drug reactions?) *Läkartidningen., 76,* 860.
3. Böttiger, L.E. and Westerholm, B. (1973): Drug-induced cytopenias in Sweden. *Brit. med. J., 3,* 339.
4. Böttiger, L.E. (1973): Adverse drug reactions: An analysis of 310 consecutive reports to the Swedish Adverse Drug Reaction Committee. *J. clin. Pharm., 13*, 373.
5. Böttiger, L.E., Furhoff, A.-K. and Holmberg, L. (1979): Fatal reactions to drugs. *Acta med. scand., 205,* 451.
6. Böttiger, L.E., Furhoff, A.-K. and Holmberg, L. (1979): Drug-induced blood dyscrasias. *Acta med. scand., 205,* 457.
7. Böttiger, L.E. (1978): Prevalence and etiology of aplastic anemia in Sweden. In: *Aplastic Anemia*, pp. 171–180. Editors: Japan Medical Research Foundation. University of Tokyo Press, Tokyo.
8. Yoshimatsu, H., Uetake, S., Miyao, S. et al. (1978): A retrospective survey of drugs and chemicals associated with the development of aplastic anemia. In: *Aplastic Anemia*, pp. 189–193. Editors: Japan Medical Research Foundation. University of Tokyo Press, Tokyo.
9. De Gruchy, C. (1975): *Drug-Induced Blood Disorders*, p. 39. Blackwell Scientific Publications, Oxford.

10. Böttiger, L.E., Dalén, E. and Hallén, B. (1976): Halothane-induced liver damage. *Acta anaesth. scand., 20*, 40.
11. Böttiger, L.E. and Westerholm, B. (1977): Adverse drug reactions during treatment of urinary tract infections. *Europ. J. clin. Pharm., 11*, 439.
12. Bergman, U., Boman, G. and Wiholm, B.-E. (1978): Epidemiology of adverse drug reactions to phenformin and metformin. *Brit. med. J., 2*, 464.

DISCUSSION

Darmansjah: In your monitoring system, you described 5 classes of causal relations. In the WHO system we have about 10 or 12 classes. I wonder whether this discrepancy in classification will not cause problems of interpretation with the WHO system?

Böttiger: It is, as a matter of fact, better to work with few classification categories. We are in the process in Sweden of abandoning our 4–5 categories in favor of only 2, i.e. 'probable causal relationship' or 'unlikely', the latter group including also those reports that cannot be classified due to lack of pertinent information. We do not use the term 'definite' causal relationship. Our task is to collect statistical evidence on the frequency etc. of adverse drug reactions, not to investigate individual cases in detail. A statement of a 'definite' causal relationship might indicate a more thorough investigation of the individual case, possible for use, e.g., in court procedures.

Tognoni: You quoted the example of noramidopyrine which was excluded from the market. As you know, many countries still widely use noramidopyrine as the preferred drug. About a causal relationship or the possibility, I believe that it is necessary to extend international communication at least to discuss internationally these issues in order to see whether the provisions taken in one country could avoid the damage caused in other countries. I would like to hear your comments, especially with regard to Dr. Dukes's presentation about the importance of international cooperation. I think the same could be true for phenformin, which is still widely used. It must also be the role of the medical profession to hold international discussion forums so as to educate both the medical profession and public opinion and in order to avoid long-term effects in more vulnerable populations as in Italy.

Böttiger: I can only emphasize the importance of increased international cooperation in the field of drug control. Of course, when drugs are taken off the market etc., Sweden reports to the WHO, but it turns out that those reports have very little effect on conditions in other countries. However, when the manufacturer himself withdraws a drug after negotiations with and pressure from the control authorities, we are by law not allowed to report to the WHO. This law will, however, be changed in the near future.

Inman: We have heard rumors, as yet unconfirmed, of cases of SMON in Sweden. Could Dr. Böttiger please tell us how many of these have been reported to the Swedish Committee who are now supposedly receiving reports which doctors are obliged to send in. If they have not been reported, who is making the diagnosis of SMON?

Böttiger: I think Dr. Hansson can answer that question because he has many of the cases who were not initially reported to the Committee. That is due to the fact that they were not related to the intake of the drug at all. I don't have the information on how many of the approximately 20 or 30 cases that are now under discussion actually were initially reported to our Committee.

Westerholm: With regard to the WHO reporting system, there is a possibility of giving a number of levels to the cause-effect relationship, but this is used very differently by the different participating countries and the information is really very pliable and difficult to use. I think the information on whether re-challenge has taken place or whether there was no cause-effect relationship at all because the dates didn't fit or the drug wasn't taken is useful, but all other reports have to be handled as one category.

Liljestrand: May I add that dipyrone was not reported to the WHO, but that the manufacturer himself withdrew the drug on the condition that we did not report. We will have a change, as Dr. Böttiger said, in our legislation so that we will report even such things in the future.

The barriers to effective post-marketing surveillance

WILLIAM H.W. INMAN

Committee on Safety of Medicines, Finsbury Square House, London, U.K.

I have been working in post-marketing surveillance (PMS) for the past 15 years and I am sure that similar problems are encountered in most of the countries which currently conduct this type of work. At present we depend almost entirely on voluntary reporting systems (1). They have had some successes, but have sometimes failed to detect serious hazards, not because they are a bad method, but because doctors are often unable to appreciate the significance of the events they observe during treatment or because they fail to report them

We must look for new methods of surveillance which will allow us to compare benefits and risks and which will enable us to link records of drug treatment with both short-term and long-term adverse effects, and we must do this without interfering with essential treatment (2). Our duty to identify drugs which are safe and effective is just as important as our duty to identify those which are dangerous to a minority of individuals who receive them.

THE INCIDENCE OF TOXIC EFFECTS

Before designing new systems we must be clear about the relationship between the size of populations which may be available for study and the incidence of adverse reactions which we can hope to detect in them using various methods. Clinical trials, for example, should detect events which occur in more than 1% of patients. Voluntary reporting may bring to light very rare effects, for example those with an incidence of 1 in 10,000 or less. We need to look for realistic methods which will bridge the gap between these two extremes, and which will detect events occurring perhaps in 1 in every 1,000 patients.

BARRIERS TO POST-MARKETING SURVEILLANCE

There are many difficulties to be overcome and I shall attempt to review some of them under 5 general headings: (1) need for confidentiality, (2) popular misconceptions about drugs, (3) compensation and litigation, (4) technical problems, and (5) cost.

Confidentiality

The doctor/patient relationship depends on the confidential exchange of information between two individuals. It is essential for the practice of medicine. Paradoxically, it also creates a major barrier to the epidemiological research which is intended to help the whole community.

Many doctors are concerned about the use which might be made of information which identifies them and their patients. This barrier has been created at least partly by the public itself, by the news media and by increasing cases of litigation.

Information collected for epidemiological research must be protected for as long as may be necessary to complete each investigation. Not only must the records remain confidential, but pressures to analyse or publish them prematurely must be resisted.

Popular misconceptions

The public does not yet appreciate that all effective treatment carries some risk and that even when risks are known it is usually impossible to identify, in advance, which individuals will suffer. Patients demand total efficacy and complete safety. They must be educated to accept that neither of these will ever be achieved and that the existence of safety committees does not guarantee protection from injury.

The greatest danger in essential therapy is not the deaths or serious injury that may result from drug toxicity, but the risk that patients will not comply with treatment or that doctors will not prescribe it. PMS must not interfere with compliance. This is a strong argument for a retrospective approach (3) in which case-histories are examined, perhaps as long as a year after the drug was first prescribed, rather than a prospective approach in which the patient may be aware that he has been 'monitored' from the start of treatment (2, 4).

Compensation and litigation

Having accepted that some risk is inevitable, it is obvious that patients should be insured as they are when travelling in a motor car. The unfortunate minority who suffer serious effects should receive the same high standard of care that can be expected by any patient who has been injured by accident or disease. But there is no reason, just because the illness has been caused by a drug, why the victim or his relatives should be specially favoured with disproportionately large sums of money when no one has acted improperly. We must not create an 'elite' of drug-disabled people. Compensation should be reserved for the victims of medical, pharmaceutical or administrative malpractice. In all other circumstances some form of social security insurance should take care of them. The state may have to make additional funds available to deal with large-scale accidents.

Because the public expects compensation for almost any injury, it has become interested in PMS. Once it is known that a new drug is being monitored, patient 'action groups' and the press may try to persuade researchers to release the results of their work prematurely. Stories about alleged or unconfirmed adverse effects become exaggerated and bias is introduced. Patients may stop taking the drug because of unjustified fears of toxicity and doctors may stop prescribing it because of fear of involvement in litigation. If this happens, realistic PMS ceases.

There is no easy answer. A partial solution may be to conduct as much PMS as possible on records that are routinely available for any patient. If prescription data are stored routinely on a computer, it can be used to identify patients treated with a particular drug. If events such as new diagnoses or causes of death are also stored on the computer, careful study of their incidence in groups of patients treated with different drugs can 'signal' possible hazards.

We require medical record-linkage on a scale which is large enough to reveal comparatively rare events, and for the records to be immune to access by people who are not authorized to conduct research.

Technical problems

Obviously it is not possible to review all the methods that have been suggested in this article. I shall simply assume that by one means or another, any PMS system will identify populations of patients who have been treated with drugs and will examine their progress in order to determine what beneficial or harmful effects subsequently occur.

The technical difficulties include: (1) measurement of background incidence, (2) effects of 'noise', (3) effect of concurrent drug-treatment, (4) data-capture, (5) data-processing, and (6) motivation.

We must record adverse 'events' and not only suspected drug reactions. If I may repeat an example I have often quoted, a broken leg is an adverse event which may have resulted purely by accident, may have been caused by drug-induced dizziness, or because of some metabolic effect which has softened the bones. The important principle is that it is an event which must be recorded. If we found that broken legs were significantly more common during treatment with drug X than with drug Y, we have identified a problem requiring further study. Similarly when considering the effects of concurrent therapy, an adverse event may be found to be more common in patients receiving drugs A + B + C than those receiving drugs A + B + D.

Nearly all patients, whether they need it or not, receive a prescription when they visit their doctor and it is usually impossible to find large populations of untreated cases in which to determine the background incidence of disease. The key to detection of new hazards will lie in our ability to perform 'between-drug' comparisons and to detect disease trends which may be related to the time of introduction and the volume of sales of new drugs.

We must learn how to recognize unusual patterns of signs and symptoms. The practolol syndrome should have been identified much earlier by the unusually high frequency with which patients were affected simultaneously by more than one of the following conditions: dry eyes or corneal ulceration, rashes, which sometimes resembled psoriasis, hyperkeratosis, visceral symptoms, deafness. Combinations of two or more of these symptoms or signs rarely occur among patients receiving other drugs, although most of the individual symptoms or signs are not uncommon.

There are a number of moments of contact between a patient and those who care for him when the chances of entering useful data into the medical record are greatest. They include, for example, the moment of first diagnosis or prescription of a drug, the moment at which the patient complains to a doctor or a nurse of a new symptom, the moment of admission to or discharge from hospital, the moment of death certification or the moment of entry on to a special registry such as a cancer registry. Each moment must be exploited to the full and the appropriate data entered in a simple way on to the patient's record.

We also have to consider the problem of maintaining the enthusiasm and collaboration of those who observe and record the information. Most monitoring schemes encounter difficulty. Three years ago, a colleague started to collect data in the X-ray departments of 182 hospitals, but today only 82 (45%) are still submitting data. Possibly my friend asked for too much detail. I am sure that the most important factors are simplicity of method and feedback of information. The extra work involved in recording data must be small and those who provide it must be continuously stimulated by evidence that their effort is worthwhile.

The technical problems may not be as great as we think and their solution may lie in the micro-processor. The next 10 years may see a computer terminal in every practitioner's office and every hospital records department. Medical record-linkage, which has for so long seemed out of reach, may quite soon become a reality.

Cost

I will not dwell on the question of cost. Obviously, improved PMS will be expensive, but if the methods for recording information are simple and accepting that the micro-processor will vastly reduce the cost of collecting and analysing the data, more effective PMS should be possible at only a fraction of the total cost of developing new drugs.

SUMMARY

The success or failure of new methods of PMS depends on preserving the confidentiality of epidemiological data; educating the public to accept that some risk has to be taken in order to benefit from treatment; providing, through social security insurance, the means for caring for the occasional victims of drug toxicity; removing pressures on research workers which could lead to premature release of unconfirmed or misleading results; and on the introduction of more sophisticated and less expensive methods of medical record-linkage. Of the barriers that I have described, I believe the medicolegal and educational ones will prove to be more difficult to overcome than the purely technical or financial barriers.

REFERENCES

1. Inman, W.H.W. (Ed.) (1980): *Monitoring for Drug Safety*. MTP Ltd. In press.
2. Gross, F.H. and Inman, W.H.W. (Eds.) (1977): *Drug Monitoring*. Academic Press, London.
3. Wilson, A.B. (1977): *Brit. med. J., 2*, 1001.
4. Dollery, C.T. and Rawlins, M.D. (1977): *Brit. med. J., 1*, 691.

DISCUSSION

Westerholm: I have two questions. Do you have a drug insurance system in your country and if so, do you get more reports on serious known adverse reactions than the monitoring center? The other thing is that if you register prescriptions for a large number of patients and want to link them with their medical record linkage scheme do you at the same time put the records in order so that it is easy to find out what events have happened to the patients?

Inman: The answer is negative to both questions. We do not to have systems for drug insurance. But I would like to emphasize that I would not distinguish drug insurance from any other form of insurance and that all disabled people should receive the same high standard of care. In my view, I would not artificially separate those who would be unfortunate enough to suffer drug reactions. We have in our country through the National Health Service the ability to identify patients through prescriptions because all National Health prescriptions are handled in a common manner. If we could persuade doctors to add a thing called the 'registration number' which everybody has or may have forgotten, to the prescription when it is written, it will at least be possible to identify when that patient died and the cause of death because these are processed using the same numbers. It will also be possible to pick patients up on the cancer register or one or two other special registers. So there is at least this possibility of developing the National Health Service procedure of drug monitoring.

Tognoni: I would like to ask two questions. I am in agreement with the idea of not having special compensation for patients, but I just want to ask about compensation when malpractice is demonstrated. What chance does the public have to bring a malpractice suit against for instance advertising institutes? Second, what is the experience you have had in collaborating with industry in PMS? What is the feasibility of your proposals in the real world, for instance, in Europe?

Inman: First of all, I should say that malpractice suits in the case of drugs are extremely rare in our country. With regard to excessive advertising, presumably this could be handled if it is demanded, but such a case has not yet arisen. We do have in the Department of Health an Advertising Inspection Group which is looking for excessive claims, but it hasn't actually come to a court case yet as far as I am aware.

With regard to the feasibility of restricted or monitored release conducted by industry, the industry has the same sort of difficulty as we do. We have many drugs which have been released through a procedure which we call 'monitored release' where company doctors indeed produce huge numbers of reports but mostly of very trivial reactions. We have enormous difficulty maintaining the enthusiasm of the reporters. The first month you might get 1000 reports, the second month you might get 200, the third month you might get one. This has been fairly typical of the difficulty, even, I may say, when the companies have paid for the reports.

Monitoring by industry has been a help and I can think of several occasions where it has actually been able to identify a problem for the first time, but I think we need something more than that on an international scale, using a standardized technique.

Nagano: I am in charge of SMON litigation cases in Japan. The victims are really angry about the pharmaceutical companies because they sold clioquinol, claiming it was effective and safe. Therefore, these victims are demanding the punishment of the pharmaceutical companies. I think this attitude is a correct one to be maintained by the victims.

In Japan, many drug-induced sufferings could have been avoided. The solution to these problems through social insurance, I believe, will be faced with a very great resistance by the general public. I would like to invite Dr. Inman's comment on this vis-à-vis the present situation in Great Britain.

Inman: It's very difficult to answer this question. I would like to look forward rather than backward. I think the SMON incident has certainly reinforced public opinion. Nevertheless I disagree that the courts are the right place to fight these things out, for one reason, and one reason only perhaps, that patients must receive help immediately. In court cases it takes a long time. They need some sort of instant care which can only be provided by some form of social security insurance.

Activities of the Australian Adverse Drug Reactions Advisory Committee

M.L. MASHFORD

Adverse Drug Reactions Advisory Committee, Department of Medicine, St. Vincent's Hospital, Fitzroy, Victoria, Australia

Australia set up a voluntary reporting scheme for the registration of adverse drug reactions in 1964. Since that time about 20,000 reports have been received. The system has undergone gradual change and improvement during that period and at present we consider it to be the cornerstone of our efforts to minimize suffering induced by these agents used to bring assuagement.

The Australian Registry of Adverse Drug Reactions is administered by the Australian Department of Health in Canberra, which is a government ministry, but the direction of activities in this field is lodged with an independent committee. In 1963 it was appreciated that the system then in operation gave no assured protection against adverse drug effects and an independent expert committee was established to advise the Minister of Health on matters of drug safety. This was termed the Australian Drug Evaluation Committee (ADEC). Later under new legislation the scope of its activities was widened to include matters of drug efficacy. This widening of scope caused the parent body to set up in 1971 a subcommittee known as the Adverse Drug Reactions Advisory Committee (ADRAC) and this is now responsible for supervision of all matters related to drug-induced suffering but acting still through the parent committee, ADEC. It is thus in close touch with the main organ of decision relating to drug regulation.

Another feature of drug control in Australia which is important in the overall system is that there is a Pharmaceutical Benefits Scheme whereby the State pays for all drugs on a specified list, provided that they have been legally prescribed. The list is extensive but not all-embracing and its composition is determined by another separate committee. There are obvious financial advantages flowing to a drug firm from inclusion of one of its products on the approved list and it is reasonable to say that only an exceptional agent, i.e. one both demonstrably valuable and without listed competitors, can flourish outside that charmed circle. Decisions to include a particular drug are based on complex considerations, but important elements are its efficacy and safety. This then permits a graded release of a drug. One with a limited and justifiable special use, but a potential for over-prescription or pregnant with danger if improperly used, can be accepted in the list only for specified conditions or a drug about whose overall value, doubts are entertained can be released for marketing and allowed the opportunity to make its way without subsidy. If it proves its value and safety, it can then be accepted for listing; this occurred for instance with cimetidine. Needless to say, this only occurs with agents which show a clean bill of health in animal and preliminary clinical studies. This two-tiered system is bitterly resented by the drug industry, but it gives considerable flexibility in dealing with the thorny problems of drug registration.

The voluntary reporting system for adverse drug reactions which was established in 1964 is similar to that in many countries. Medical practitioners, dentists and pharmacists are invited to report adverse events which are suspected of being drug-related. They can do so by telephone or letter but they are regularly supplied with brief forms on which the report can conveniently be made and which when folded is a pre-paid and addressed envelope ready for mailing. Hospitals are also encouraged to submit summaries of inpatients who suffered an adverse reaction during their hospital course. Upon receipt by the secretariat these reports are classified in various ways and these assigned categories and the actual clinical information are coded for storage. Further information is requested by phone or mail from about 10% of reporters. The reports are submitted to ADRAC in the business papers of its regular meetings. Batches are allocated to each Committee member so that every report is scrutinized to ensure that recorded details are free from obvious errors and that only reasonable reports are accepted. Those which are doubtful or particularly interesting are discussed by the Committee. The classifications referred to above are concerned with the source, the body system involved, the type of reaction and most importantly the probability of a causal relationship between drug and event. A decision on this score must be arbitrary but is undertaken using standard criteria. The hierarchy adopted ranges from *definite* through *probable* and *possible* to *unlikely*. Each report is classified on its merits and previous knowledge of the relation of drug and event is not considered. This is done to avoid the 'band-wagon effect' which is likely to occur if the event is common in the absence of drug. For instance, a drug suspected of hepatotoxicity could in this way be further incriminated by any case of viral hepatitis not pinned down by laboratory study, which fortuitously occurred in patients taking the drug.

To be classified as *definite* a drug/event association must be confirmed by rechallenge, or the temporal or spatial relationship should leave no doubt: e.g. 'end of the needle' or injection-site responses or objective evidence such as in-vitro studies, should demonstrate the reality of the causal role of the drug. The nexus is considered *probable* if there is a convincing temporal relationship and no obvious alternative explanation of the event. Treatment for the adverse effect which may have led to its disappearance concomitant with cessation of the drug would invalidate this classification. Most reports, however, cannot attain either of these levels of acceptance and are placed in the category *possible*; this will always be so if two or more drugs are being given concurrently unless there is subsequent negative rechallenge to all but one, thus eliminating them as sole cause. By these criteria about 7% are judged *definite*, 21% *probable* and most of the rest *possible*. A few are regarded as *unlikely* but kept in the file since a possible connection cannot be absolutely excluded.

The stored data are reviewed with the aid of a variety of tabulations which are examined at each Committee meeting but also, of course, regularly by the secretariat. The displays include comparisons of numbers of reports implicating each drug in a given month with the number in the previous 3 months and 12 months and a similar listing for reactions, tables linking drug and reaction, and summaries of data stored on any particular category of reactions. The entire data-base can be accessed in various ways which are used from time to time. For instance, certain drugs are kept under surveillance and a listing of associated reports is prepared and examined quarterly. On several occasions a cumulative listing of reactions by drug has been prepared and this is now to be undertaken at intervals of 12–18 months. The drugs are listed by trade name if given in the report and the numbers of reactions summed under the categories of the WHO reaction dictionary. The probability ratings are also included. This compendium is distributed to all medical and dental practitioners and to pharmacists.

A voluntary reporting system has only a limited possible yield and expectations must be realistic. ADRAC accepts that the system which it supervises cannot give valid estimates of incidence of reactions; low, variable and often biassed reporting makes the numerator conjectural or sometimes misleading and only indirect estimates of exposure are available. The information can at best be regarded as semiquantitative. Nonetheless, vigorous support leads to several considerable benefits. These functions for the system may be described as (1) the clearing house role, (2) 'testing the water' and (3) the educational resource centre.

By the term 'clearing house' I mean the ability to put together pieces of information from various sources and then promote further action to clarify a particular issue. An example of this is the delineation of a new syndrome of bismuth toxicity in 1972 following the receipt of 12 reports from a lay association of patients with colostomies or ileostomies. Many members of this group used bismuth subgallate as an effective means to firm and deodorize bowel contents, but in the 12 of which we were notified there had been progressive mental deterioration which was attributed to the therapy. The part played by the drug was uncertain since most of the patients were old and in several the bowel resection had been for carcinoma, but the cases were followed up and the involvement of the drug as a cause of the condition was confirmed. Several neurologists contacted had also encountered cases and thus a hitherto unrecognized toxic action of bismuth was documented and has since been confirmed in France and the German Federal Republic. The next year, 1973, was marked by the accumulation of a number of reports suggestive of SMON occurring after exposure to clioquinol. While the syndrome was of course already notorious, its occurrence outside Japan was at that time hotly contested.

The function which I think of as 'testing the water' regards the voluntary system as a comparatively rapid-response probe to determine what is going on out there in the community when a possible problem has been suggested. We have been impressed by the prompt response to news of the hepatotoxicity of oxyphenisatin, the practolol syndrome and the occurrence of infected mid-term abortions with the Dalkon Shield. This last instance is instructive; the subject was first raised in July, 1974 and in October, 1974 an alerting letter was sent to all medical practitioners. By the end of 1974 67 reports had confirmed the occurrence of this problem in the country but also that it was occurring with most other intrauterine devices as well. The effectiveness of this mechanism cannot be tested since a planned false alarm is not to be considered. Perhaps the nearest to this was the similar alerting letter also sent in October, 1974 concerning reserpine and breast cancer, which produced a negligible response in the way of reports.

The third function is as an educational resource centre. The majority of adverse effects due to drug use are well-known associations yet there is still frequently a delay in diagnosis and institution of appropriate management. The place of the voluntary reporting system must be viewed in this context. Whatever its merits in detecting new drug/event associations the impact of the whole operation on the relevant professional groups can be considerable. This works in several ways. Most doctors find adverse drug reactions interesting if they recognize them, but the lack of precise diagnostic criteria and the difficulty in attributing the problem to a specific drug are frustrating. It is the rare individuals who have the time and energy to publish their experience, but the minor commitment of effort to report the reaction can often be summoned. We send by return mail an acknowledgement but, in many instances, also the summary entered into the data store is included for checking together with a printout of the data-base concerning the suspected drugs. It is planned to make this response in all cases as soon as resources permit, although a filter will be interposed to prevent an assiduous reporter from receiving masses of repetitive material. About 5% of reports include specific questions and these are responded to as promptly as possible. The scheme leads to the accumulation of a large amount of interesting clinical material which can be used to exemplify the problems of drug-induced suffering. This is published regularly. Brief case histories drawn from this source together with appended comment are published in suitable wide-circulation periodicals. These are easy to read and we are optimistic about their educational value. We have some evidence that such exposure is effective. During the 8 months from November, 1974 to June, 1975 ADRAC published a monthly *Adverse Drug Reaction Bulletin* which consisted of a single folded sheet in which 4–6 articles dealing with timely subjects were briefly abstracted and related to Australian experience. The reporting rate from individual doctors quadrupled over this period and subsided again when circumstances enforced cessation of the enterprise. Increased reporting of previously known reactions may not be a particularly useful end to pursue, but it reflects an heightened suspicion of adverse drug effects among clinicians and this is a prerequisite for better diagnosis of recognized problems and the swifter detection of new ones.

This last point deserves to be stressed. Detection of an adverse effect by any but an intensive monitoring system, depends upon the intuition of an alert clinician recognizing the possibility. This is so, no matter what feasible method is used for registration and aggregation of data. The educational role of the voluntary reporting system thus becomes one of its most important products and contributes indirectly to any other mechanism which is operating to detect new drug-related adverse effects.

A variety of efforts to gather data in a more formal fashion have been attempted in Australia by individuals but they have not attracted funding. These include attempts to establish an intensive monitoring program in several teaching hospitals using a common form of data acquisition. A large measure of co-operation was achieved but funds have not been forthcoming for data-processing. In addition, a plan for monitored release of drugs in which the responsibility for data acquisition was placed on the drug companies involved, has been applied to 3 drugs, metoprolol, timolol and dantrolene. This has not been judged to have been effective in its present form.

In Australia, as elsewhere, there is great dissatisfaction and anxiety at our inability to deal confidently with drug-induced suffering which is always present like a spectre at our *agape*. It seems unlikely that there can be a definitive solution to these problems.

Pound could perhaps have been describing the art and science of adverse drug reactions rather than an Edwardian lady:

> 'Trophies fished up; some curious suggestion;
> Facts that lead nowhere; and a tale or two,
> Pregnant with Mandrakes, or with something else
> That might prove useful and yet never proves,
> That never fits a corner or shows a use,
> Or finds its hour upon the loom of days'.
>
> (Pound – *Portrait d'une femme*)

But just as he acknowledges that the orts and scraps from other people's minds finally fuse to produce a distinctive personality in the woman whose portrait he gives –

> 'Yes you richly pay
> you are a person of some interest,
> one comes to you
> and takes strange gain away'.

So something worthwhile does come of the fusion of the various imperfect and derivative parts that go to make up the body of developing knowledge of drug-induced suffering.

DISCUSSION

Yamashita: You said that in 1973 30 cases of SMON were reported in Australia. The first question I would like to raise is: How many patients have been reported as SMON cases? The second question is: What government action was taken against these SMON questions?

Mashford: In 1973 we had approximately 30 cases of suspected SMON. Some of these were written up by George Selby, a Sydney neurologist.

The action taken by the Federal Committee was to recommed to the various States that clioquinol and similar drugs should be made prescription-only items and this was subsequently done, more rapidly in some States than others. Since that time there has been a fair bit of publicity about SMON; the prescription rate is very low indeed. So the use of the drug in Australia is now very low and we haven 't had any further reports, but I am not saying that no further cases have occurred since that time.

Hermann: I would appreciate your comment on the participation of pharmacists in your program. I wonder especially whether this is restricted to hospital practitioners or whether community practitioners are also involved.

Mashford: Pharmacists in hospitals make a large contribution because they are frequently involved in systems of what I call extensive monitoring. They are responsible for many of the hospital-based reports. Community pharmacists do not contribute very extensively; I would say that only about one-fifth of our reports are from pharmacists. They are particularly asked to contribute reports on over-the-counter remedies.

Takano: I would like to put a question to Dr. Mashford. I believe that more accurate reports can be obtained when the information from the manufacturing company is correctly disseminated to the doctors. Therefore, it might be necessary to obligate the manufacturers to submit all the known information regarding the drug hazard even if it is in a suspected form. The information should be disseminated to doctors so that they will look out for these suspected drug hazards. I am sure that this would be a very difficult thing to implement, but it might help a great deal if we obligate the manufacturer to submit information. What is your opinion on this subject?

Mashford: We have an obligation placed on the drug industry to report adverse reactions. They do, by and large, cooperate as far as we know. Many useful reports come from them and many doctors will report to the drug firm but not to the Committee, so that we get the input from the drug industry which goes into our ordinary processing.

World Health Organization drug control support in Latin America

MORRIS L. YAKOWITZ*

4133 E. Pima Street, Tucson, AZ, U.S.A.

Many recent advances in medical treatment involve new synthetic chemicals and purified substances from herbs and animal glands. These medical successes have led to an enormous increase in drug production. It is estimated that 1975 global drug sales reached 37 billion dollars at the manufacturers' price level. Using the generally accepted figure of 15% growth per year, global drug sales at manufacturers' prices will total 65 billion dollars in the current year.

The flood of new drugs and the great increase in drug use have produced a number of complex problems that have overwhelmed the drug control agencies of many countries. The problems may be summarized as follows:

1. What proof of efficacy and safety must be required before a new drug is allowed to enter the market?
2. How can a drug be monitored after it has entered the market in order to determine whether it causes adverse effects that were not observed previously?
3. What standards are needed to insure that each lot of drug has the proper strength and purity?
4. How can we insure that the claims made for a drug in its advertising are accurate and expressed with scientific objectivity?
5. Which drugs should be restricted to dispensing on the prescription of a licensed physician?
6. How can we minimize the abuse of habit-forming drugs?

The Health Ministers of the nations assemble each year at Geneva to guide the activities of the World Health Organization. Many of their Resolutions in recent years have related to the drug problems enumerated here. The WHO secretariat has been directed by the Health Ministers to act on a broad front to solve these drug problems. Thus, WHO has responsibility for publishing the International Pharmacopoeia (a book of drug standards), for distributing pure chemicals used as reference standards in drug testing procedures, establishing standards for vaccines and other biological substances, establishing international non-proprietary names for drugs, monitoring adverse reactions caused by drugs, and establishing a system for certifying the quality of drugs in international commerce.

WHO operates in the field through 6 regional bodies. One of these covers North and South America and is designated as the WHO American Regional Office. It is combined in Washington with the Pan-American Sanitary Bureau (the health arm

*Former drug control official at the United States Food and Drug Administration and drug control advisor at the American Regional Office of the World Health Organization.

of the Organization of American States) to form the Pan-American Health Organization (PAHO).

For a number of years, PAHO has devoted a portion of its funds to support drug control activities in the countries of the Americas. In order to obtain advice regarding solutions to the existing problems of the region, PAHO convened a seminar at Maracay, Venezuela in 1970. This seminar was attended by 29 senior drug control officials representing 24 American countries.

A PAHO official attending the 1970 seminar provided comment as follows:

'To the extent that available resources have permitted, the Pan-American Health Organization has assisted countries in achieving good drug control.

General advisory services have been furnished to the governments and adoption of the following principles has been recommended.

a. Each country should enact a comprehensive drug law. The laws of the various countries should be uniform to facilitate international commerce and to guarantee the preparation of drugs of high quality.
b. Each country should have a well-coordinated agency to administer its drug laws. This agency should form part of the national health services.
c. The agencies' inspectors, analysts, and administrators should have specialized training.
d. The governments should support the drug control agencies with sufficient funds to enable them to carry out high-level control activities.

In addition to providing general advisory services, PAHO has provided technical advice on special aspects of drug control. During 1960–1970, PAHO sent technical advisors for this purpose to Argentina, Brazil, Chile, Costa Rica, Mexico, Panama, Peru, Uruguay, and Venezuela, and to the English-speaking countries of the Caribbean. These experts remained in the countries from 1 week to 3 months. In each case, PAHO provided the government with a report of the expert's findings. It is interesting to note that although various specialists participated in these studies, their opinions and recommendations were uniform and consistent. In general, the reports pointed out the need to improve the organization of the national drug agencies, supplement the training of the personnel, and increase the funds available for control activities.

On numerous occasions, PAHO has provided the government agencies with reagents, laboratory texts, and other similar items. To the extent that its resources permit, PAHO responds to technical assistance requests from the countries.

Since personnel constitute the most important element in any organization, PAHO has devoted a large part of its funds to training government health officials. Over the years, PAHO has sponsored the award of fellowships for the training of numerous analysts and other drug control officials.

In 1970, an intensive 5-week training course by the Food and Drug Administration in Washington was arranged by PAHO for drug analysts from 9 Latin American countries and the Caribbean area. This was PAHO's first attempt at sponsoring a group training program.

PAHO's special concern with the need for training drug control officials has led it to sponsor the establishment of an American Regional Institute for Drug Quality. The Institute would serve the following purposes:

a. It would provide advanced training for drug analysts in Latin America.
b. It would serve as a training center for senior drug control administrators and inspectors and as a forum for the exchange of ideas among the officials charged with applying the drug laws.
c. It would improve the professional prestige of drug analysts, drug control administrators, and inspectors and thereby increase their effectiveness in verifying the quality of drugs in each country.

d. It would prompt each Latin American drug firm to make sure that its analysts are as well-trained as the government's analysts, thus improving drug quality at the production point.
e. It would act as an information center to provide national laboratories with reliable analytical procedures obtained from a world-wide array of scientific publications.
f. It would aid the countries in solving unusual analytical problems.
g. It would carry out research to establish examination procedures applicable to new drugs introduced in Latin America.
h. By fostering uniformity of analytical procedures and standards, the Institute would have a beneficial effect in facilitating uninterrupted trade between countries.
i. It would improve the governments' ability to examine drugs and guarantee their quality. This, in turn, would increase the confidence of government administrators who make large-scale drug purchases based on the relative prices offered by competing suppliers.

It should be pointed out that the Institute will not act as a control laboratory for any country, nor will it have legal powers of any kind. Its purpose will be simply to facilitate the tasks of the national drug control agencies; all its activities will therefore be aimed at supporting and strengthening the national authorities.'

The full text of the PAHO statement at the 1970 seminar plus all of the working documents and the recommendations of the seminar participants are contained in a pamphlet designated PAHO Scientific Publication No. 225, titled *Drug Control in the Americas*. Copies of the pamphlet are still available by writing to the Pan American Health Organization, 525 23rd Street, N.W., Washington, DC 20037, U.S.A. The working documents in the pamphlet deal with such topics as 'Modern Drug Control Legislation', 'Health Registration Procedures for New Drug Pharmaceuticals', 'Efficacy and Safety: Elements of Drug Registration' and 'International Aspects of Drug Monitoring'.

The pamphlet contains a model of a national drug control law which sets forth the points that should be dealt with by a modern drug law.

Although PAHO Scientific Publication No. 225 is now almost 10 years old, its contents are still of considerable interest to anyone dealing with drug control problems.

Under the guidance of PAHO's Dr. Pedro Acha, PAHO has continued its drug control support along the lines described at the 1970 seminar. As to the drug quality Institute, it now exists in embryonic form at Sao Paulo, Brazil, where it is supported financially by the Government of Brazil, the United Nations' Development Programme, and PAHO. The Institute has already conducted courses in pharmaceutical analysis, especially by means of biological testing procedures. Although all of the students thus far have been Brazilians, the Institute already has an international aspect. Its chief technical advisor, a PAHO staff member, is Dr. Marcelo J. Vernengo, who was formerly director of Argentina's National Food and Drug Testing Laboratory. Instructors at the Institute have included specialists from Argentina, Brazil, Chile, England, and the U.S.A.

PAHO recently published a new pamphlet titled *Guidelines for the Development of a National Drug Control Program*. This pamphlet contains detailed comments and recommendations concerning the principal aspects of drug control.

Since the main subject considered at this Conference is the serious problem of injury caused by drugs, I would like to quote the following from the new PAHO pamphlet:

'The National Drug Control Agency should be assigned full responsibility for insuring that drugs meet all of the requirements of the drug control act and regulations. This should include a requirement that drugs have been adequately tested and evaluated for quality, safety and efficacy before they are released for marketing. This is not an easy task since no drug can be considered to be without risk. Furthermore, the Agency will always be faced with the problem of assessing the risk versus the benefit, and determining the importance of the drug to national health needs.

At the point at which a drug is registered, a great deal of time and effort has already been expended by the Drug Control Agency to insure its quality, safety and efficacy. The data on the chemical and pharmaceutical aspects have been reviewed, the pre-clinical and clinical studies evaluated, the manufacturing facilities and controls employed in its production have been inspected, a sample of the final dosage form analyzed or assayed in the laboratory and the labeling and promotional material scrutinized. But the task of the Drug Control Agency is not finished by any means.

An inspection of the manufacturing plant must be conducted at regular intervals, or as required, to ensure that good practice in the manufacture and quality control are being maintained. Samples must be taken and submitted to the laboratory for analysis. The labeling and advertising of the drug must continue to be reviewed. A system of collecting information on adverse reactions should be established and the data obtained collated and evaluated.

It is obvious that national governments and, in particular, the National Drug Control Agency should be involved in the monitoring of adverse reactions to drugs. WHO has published two reports by a group of experts on the subject of international drug monitoring: one on the role of the hospital, and the second on the role of national centers. The prime objective of drug monitoring for adverse reactions is to diminish the time necessary to recognize that a drug produces an adverse reaction and to determine the importance of the reaction in relation to the therapeutic use of the drug.

Copies of this new PAHO pamphlet may be obtained by writing to PAHO, 525 23rd Street, N.W., Washington, DC 20037, U.S.A.

In concluding, I wish to refer to PAHO's strong program for improving the training of medical students in Latin America. Under this program PAHO encourages the teaching of pharmacology as part of the medical curriculum. The student who receives good training in the action of drugs in animals and humans will be a more scientific and careful prescriber of medicaments when he becomes a physician. Also, he will be better able to evaluate the claims made for their products by drug manufacturers.

DISCUSSION

Shin: Some countries do not follow or are not willing to accept certain international standards established by such organizations as WHO. In these cases, how do we possibly recommend or ask those countries to comply with such standards?

Yakowitz: By training the national drug control officers, they can convince their national political leaders of the value and benefit of an active drug control program.

Yamashita: Are the other WHO Regional Offices as active in improving drug control activities as the WHO American Regional Office?

Yakowitz: The European Regional Office of WHO is as active in drug control work support as the American Regional Office! The Western Pacific Office also has good programs in drug control. I do not know about the other WHO Regional Offices.

Liljestrand: In the Middle-East region of WHO, great efforts have been made to organize drug control with the aid of two eminent consultants, Dr. Lunde and Dr. Dukes.

Yakowitz: I would agree that these consultants provide excellent assistance in that part of the world. Perhaps there is someone present from another region of WHO of which there are 6 covering the entire globe, to tell us something about the WHO drug control work in his area.

Peculiarities of drug side-effects and countermeasures

RENZO MATSUSHITA

The Green Cross Corporation, Osaka, Japan

DAMAGE TO HEALTH CAUSED BY DRUGS

The following types of damage to health caused by drugs can be considered:

1. Those which are caused by defects in product quality (including defective labeling).

2. Those which are caused by inadequate use of drugs. These can be further classified into two subtypes: those which are due to inadequate use of drugs by the medical profession (physicians, pharmacists and nurses) and those which are due to inadequate use of drugs by patients themselves, or members of their family or others nursing the patients. Damage to health as a result of the combination of points (1) and (2) due to the defective labeling of a drug is also possible.

3. Those which are caused by side-effects of drugs. 'Side-effect' here can be understood to mean, as defined in the 'Bill for Relief Fund for Drug Side-Effect Victims' currently under deliberation in the Japanese Diet, the harmful action which occurs in man even when the drug is used for a definite purpose in an adequate manner. This definition of a side-effect of a drug presupposes that the quality of the product is satisfactory.

Side-effects can be classified into 3 subtypes as follows: (a) those which are not discovered during the stages of development but only after the drugs have been put on sale for reasons such as that the incidence is small, relevant testing methods were not available, the side-effects are of the type that requires a fairly long time before appearance etc., e.g. allergic reactions to antibiotics such as penicillin, teratogenetic effects such as that caused by thalidomide etc.; (b) side-effects which were known but which, after the start of the actual clinical use of the drugs, have proved to be more serious or higher in incidence than had been estimated previously; (c) side-effects, the possibility, course, incidence etc. of which are known but which are considered to have to be tolerated, because the effectiveness of the drugs outweighs the risks from the side-effects, e.g. slight fever, skin eruptions, nausea etc. The acceptable range of side-effects as described under (c) above differs according to the purposes for which the drugs are intended to be used. In the case of anticancer drugs, it is considered that their side-effects should be tolerated to a considerably serious extent.

MEASURES FOR PREVENTION OF DAMAGE TO HEALTH CAUSED BY DEFECTIVE PRODUCT QUALITY OR LABELING, OR BY INADEQUATE DRUG USE

Measures against these two types of damage to health are peculiar in that it is difficult for general consumers to assess the adequacy of the measures, or that the patients who are the end-consumers can have little option about these measures in the case of ethical drugs since these drugs are handled by professionals like physicians and pharmacists. But, fundamentally they can be included in the general measures for the protection of consumers. The quality of each product is specified by the Japanese Pharmacopoeia, or by the standards established for specific drugs designated by the Minister of Health and Welfare, or by the quality specifications established at the time of manufacturing approval. In order to guarantee that manufactured products conform with these quality standards or specifications, the authorities have established Standards for Manufacture and Quality Control, the so-called GMP, as an administrative guide, requiring manufacturers of drugs to observe the standards in carrying out manufacturing operations. Furthermore, all lots of some types of drugs are required to be submitted to governmental tests. Regarding labeling, by which is meant statements on package leaflets or containers/packages, the Pharmaceutical Affairs Law gives detailed provisions. Prevention of inadequate use of drugs should be realized by continuous professional education of physicians etc., by dissemination of knowledge on drugs among the general public through general health education, by improvement of advertisements and of package leaflets etc. to ensure accuracy of information, etc.

In the draft Amendment of the 'Pharmaceutical Affairs Law', the manufacturers and sellers of drugs will be obliged to give the necessary information to physicians and pharmacists in order to strengthen this part.

PECULIARITIES OF SIDE-EFFECTS OF DRUGS

The problem of side-effects of drugs is slightly different in nature from the above-mentioned general problems for consumers. This is because the safety of consumers is the fundamental requirement for general merchandise and if its use involves some risk, it can directly be considered to be defective, while 'drugs inevitably and invariably reveal adverse side-effects, if the degrees may be different among individual drugs, together with revelation of certain degrees of therapeutic effects on diseases' (quoted from a report by the Council for Deliberation of Drug Efficacy). Therefore, in evaluating the usefulness of each drug with regard to effectiveness and safety, the various steps taken to minimize the side-effects of drugs while letting them exert the maximum effect, can be said to be measures against side-effects.

These steps can be presented roughly as follows, when they are considered from the relation between the administration and industry, with classification into each stage of drug development and marketing.

STAGES OF DEVELOPMENT

The process of drug development from the start of basic research to application for manufacturing approval is complicated but can roughly be presented as follows: basic research → study for substance creation → determination of physicochemical properties and structure → screening tests → preclinical trials → Phase I clinical trial → Phase II clinical trial → Phase III clinical trial. Confirmation of safety of the drug is made at and after the preclinical trial stage performed on animals. Needless to say, these tests are carried out by the pharmaceutical company trying to develop the drug. Data requirements for application for manufacturing approval were set forth in the notification, 'Basic Policy concerning Approval for Manufacture or Import of Drugs' issued by the Director General of the Pharmaceutical Affairs Bureau of the Ministry of Health and Welfare (MHW) in 1967. The requirements include voluminous data on safety such as those on acute toxicity, subacute toxicity, chronic toxicity, special toxicity, general pharmacology, absorption/excretion, distribution/metabolism, and results of clinical trials. Regarding clinical trials, the Phase I trial is performed on healthy persons primarily for the purpose of confirming the safety of the drug, but needless to say, the confirmation of safety is as important as the confirmation of effectiveness in the ensuing clinical trials, i.e. the Phase II trial which is carried out with a small number of patients as subjects and the Phase III trial carried out with a considerable number of patients.

The Pharmaceutical Affairs Law currently in force provides no regulations concerning the performance of clinical trials. The only regulations applicable at present are notifications by the Director General of the said Bureau of MHW, requiring pharmaceutical companies to submit in advance to the MHW plans for clinical trials when they are going to undertake clinical trials on drugs such as biological preparations, anticancer agents, antibiotics etc. However, the planned revision of the Pharmaceutical Affairs Law contains regulations in this field such as the specification of standards to be observed in conducting clinical trials, submission of plans for clinical trials, and measures for prevention of damage to health in clinical trials. After the new Law is enacted, it is considered that more detailed administrative measures will be laid down and enforced.

MANUFACTURING APPROVAL AND LICENSE FROM THE ADMINISTRATIVE POINT OF VIEW

Under the present Pharmaceutical Affairs Law, as is well known, governmental approval and license have to be obtained for each drug when drugs other than those recognized in the Pharmacopoeia of Japan are going to be manufactured. 'Approval' here is the recognition that the drug applied for possesses adequacy or qualification as a drug with regard to its usefulness by evaluation of its effectiveness and safety, while 'license' is the recognition of the physical adequacy or qualification of the specific manufacturing facilities for manufacture of the drug.

That individual approval is not required for drugs recognized in the Pharmacopoeia of Japan is interpreted in such a way that there is considerable experience with those drugs in actual clinical practice and, consequently, their usefulness has been verified. But there has been debate about this point because even pharmacopoeial drugs are subjected to re-evaluation and the usefulness of some of them has in fact been denied as a result of re-evaluation, e.g. quinoform. Thus, the draft for the new Pharmaceutical Affairs Law provides that even pharmacopoeial drugs will require approval in principle.

As stated above, data requirements for application for manufacturing approval are prescribed in the notification of Basic Policy from the said bureau director. There are differences in the scope and severity of data required according to the novelty of the drugs, degree of difficulty of evaluation etc., but considerably voluminous data are required for application of new drugs. It should be noted also that the main data have to be those which were presented at authoritative academic congresses or published in authoritative scientific journals.

A new drug application submitted to the MHW is referred to the Central Pharmaceutical Affairs Council for examination, and based on the recommendation from this Council approval or disapproval is granted. The Council is composed of three stages, the Investigation Committees, the Special Sectional Committees and the Standing Committee. The following investigation committees are concerned with the examination of applications for new drugs: the First and the Second Investigation Committees on New Drugs, and the Investigation Committees on Combination Drugs, on Antimitotic Drugs, on Radioactive Preparations, on Drugs for Dental Uses, on Insecticides, on Drug Nomenclature, on Antibiotic Preparations, on Blood Preparations and on Biological Preparations. As special sectional committees, there are the Special Sectional Committee on Drugs, which deals collectively with matters handled by the above-mentioned investigation committees from the first investigation committee on new drugs up to that on drug nomenclature, and the Special Sectional Committees on Antibiotic Preparations, on Blood Preparations, and on Biological Preparations respectively.

The Law does not give a clear provision on standards for examination of new drug applications. Consequently, the adequacy for approval has to be judged from the purport underlying the whole part of the Law. But it is known, as the authorities have explained time and again, that the examination is done by assessing the usefulness of the drug which is the total of effectiveness and safety.

The new Pharmaceutical Affairs Law is going to provide that the data required for new drug application will be prescribed separately in a ministerial ordinance, and it is also going to provide in writing the following cases where approval will not be granted: (a) where the applied effectiveness of the drug is not substantiated; (b) where the drug is suspected of producing harmful side-effects compared with its effectiveness; and (c) where the drug is suspected to be inadequate as a drug. In other words, under the new Law a new drug will be approved only when its effectiveness has been substantiated, and its side-effects are within acceptable limits.

COLLECTION OF DATA ON SIDE-EFFECTS AND EFFECTIVENESS AFTER LAUNCHING A DRUG ON THE MARKET, AND MEASURES

It may be impossible to discover every side-effect of a new drug at all stages from the start of development till manufacturing approval. As stated above, there is the case, which is not rare, where a side-effect of low incidence or a side-effect which takes a long time before its appearance is discovered after the drug has been put on sale and used widely. Another point to be noted concerning side-effects in this context is that a certain side-effect of a new drug is at first considered to be within acceptable limits with regard to its effectiveness, but later its relative usefuless is questioned because of a change in disease structure, an increase in bacteria resistant to the drug, the development of a more safe and yet equally effective drug etc. For these reasons the collection of side-effects and effectiveness to be compared thereto are indispensable for the safety assurance of drugs, and these activities are carried out by pharmaceutical companies as well as the administration.

Voluntary efforts

Distribution of ethical drugs in this country occurs through scientific-information propagandists, generally called simply 'propagandists', of pharmaceutical manufacturers who visit medical institutes to convey scientific information on the drugs of their companies and recommend their use. When the medical institutes accept the drugs, they are delivered through wholesalers who have agent contracts with the manufacturers. These distribution routes, i.e. propagandists and wholesalers, are at the same time the main routes by which information on side-effects experienced by physicians is collected. Each pharmaceutical manufacturer has a department to deal with safety problems of drugs at its head office, where the information collected on side-effects is analyzed and evaluated. When necessary, a report is made to the MHW and also some measures are taken such as revising the package leaflet, informing physicians of the side-effect etc. Furthermore, if necessary, the company may voluntarily withdraw the product from the market.

Collection of information by the administration

a. Reports by the manufacturer

The manufacturer of a new ethical drug has to collect and report to the MHW information on the side-effects of a new drug for 3 years after the date of its manufacturing approval (or the date of its inclusion in the Drug-Price Standard List of the Medical Insurance System if the drug is included in the List). This obligation should not be regarded as a general administrative guide but as a legally-binding obligation or a condition which is added to manufacturing approval based on the provision of the Pharmaceutical Affairs Law Article 79.

The new Pharmaceutical Affairs Law is going to provide that the manufacturer of a new drug will report the results of usage of the drug, including its effectiveness and side-effects, for 6 years from its approval and will receive the review made by the Minister of Health and Welfare in order to be authorized as suitable according to the standards of approval at that time. This is the so-called Phase IV system.

b. Side-effect monitoring system (domestic)

The MHW started the side-effect monitoring system in Japan in 1967 with participation of major hospitals across the country. Currently there are 817 monitor hospitals which report side-effects to the MHW.

c. Side-effect monitoring system (WHO)
There is an international monitoring system of side-effects under the WHO, in which major countries (23 countries at present) are participating. Japan joined it in 1972 to exchange side-effects information internationally.

d. Administrative measures against side-effects
When information on a side-effect is obtained through system (a), (b), or (c) or from some other general source, which has been unknown until then, or which has been known but the severity or incidence of which is found to be considerably stronger or higher than was thought, or which is suspected of being unacceptable when the risks are compared with the effectiveness of the drug, the MHW refers the information to the Side-Effects Investigation Committee under the Central Pharmaceutical Affairs Council and, based on the report by the Committee, directs the manufacturer of the drug to take the necessary measure or measures such as revision of package leaflets, information to clinicians (letters to doctors), discontinuation of manufacture and sale and withdrawal of the product from the market, partial alteration of administration/dosage, indications etc., or designation of the drug to the category of powerful drugs or drugs requiring direction, annulment of manufacturing approval (generally called 'liquidation of approval'), or others deemed necessary. None of them is prescribed in writing under the present Pharmaceutical Affairs Law but takes the form of administrative guidance. The revised Law will give written provisions concerning the measures which the administrative office can order on the occurrence of serious damage or for other definite reasons, such as emergency measures of sales discontinuation etc. or annulment of approval or alteration of approved matters, or the order for withdrawal of the product from the market, or other necessary measures. In this way, the new Law will provide a legal basis for the above-mentioned measures which have so far taken the form of administrative guidance.

Drug re-evaluation

Evaluation of the adequacy of a drug is done in terms of usefulness which is the total of effectiveness and safety or the balance between them. This method of evaluation will remain unchanged at all times. As a practical problem, however, some of the drugs which were judged to be useful and consequently approved (or permitted under the old law) in the past may be judged not to be useful if evaluated today in the light of current progress in the medical and pharmaceutical sciences, current disease structure, availability of other drugs for use for the same or similar indications, etc. So far, disposal of this kind of drugs had been left to the 'natural weeding out' which takes place mainly through the experience of clinicians. However, the tightening of the standards of approval in 1967 gave rise to the opinion that drugs that had been permitted or approved before 1967 should be subjected to review. Since the Council for Deliberation of Drug Efficacy in 1971, drug re-evaluation has been performed in the form of administrative guidance. It is carried out gradually for the respective therapeutic groups of drugs in the following way: an announcement is made about the therapeutic group of drugs to be subjected to re-evaluation, and the manufacturer of the drug in this therapeutic group has to submit scientific documents on the safety and effectiveness of the drug; the documents submitted are brought to the Central Pharmaceutical Affairs Council where they are examined in 3 steps: by the Investigation Committee for that particular therapeutic group of drugs, by the Special Sectional Committee for Drug Re-evaluation and finally by the Standing Committee; after examination, the results are announced publicly in 3 ratings – Useful, Partly Useful (useful for some of the indications heretofore approved), or No Ground to Support Usefulness – and administrative steps are taken according to the respective ratings. Re-evaluation has now been carried out on about 65% of all target drugs.

According to the new Pharmaceutical Affairs Law, re-evaluation is to be carried out on drugs designated by the Minister of Health and Welfare after consultation with the Central Pharmaceutical Affairs Council, in order to confirm whether the standards for approval of the drugs at that time are suitable or not.

RELIEF OF VICTIMS IN THE CASE OF OCCURRENCE OF UNAVOIDABLE SIDE-EFFECTS

As indicated in the foregoing section, it is almost impossible to avoid side-effects of drugs completely, unlike the case of other merchandise, however hard we may try with whatever measures. A minimum incidence of side-effects cannot be avoided at present. Relief of the victims will comprise restoration of the original situation in principle, but actually we cannot find any method in many cases other than economical ones. There are no legal measures for relief of victims of side-effects at present except for those caused by preventive inoculations enforced by the State. Therefore, the victims have no means of claiming relief except for claims for compensation under civil law or the general social insurance schemes. However, the recent series of side-effect problems such as thalidomide and SMON provoked much social concern about the side-effects of drugs, and public opinion rapidly called for social or legal relief for the victims. Under the mounting public opinion, and also under the influence of the legal institution of an insurance system for relief of such victims in the Federal Republic of Germany, the Japanese MHW has proposed after several years of deliberation a relief plan called the 'Bill for Relief Fund for Drug Side-Effect Victims' which is presently being debated by the Diet. According to the plan, the relief fund is to be financed by endowment from pharmaceutical companies and by government subsidy. There is a body of opinion calling for the adoption of the concept of product liability or liability without fault in the relief system, but when the peculiarities of the drugs are considered, ideas on the present relief plan are considered to be almost adequate, even if the content of individual articles may not be completely adequate.

CONCLUSIONS

There is growing concern about the safety of drugs, and measures to ensure safety have been gradually strengthened as indicated above in this report. The planned revision of the Pharmaceutical Affairs Law is also, as the authorities concerned have declared, intended mainly to strengthen the safety assurance of drugs. However, total evaluation with regard to both effectiveness and safety will be influenced by diverse factors: (a) it is difficult to apply only one standard for evaluation of drugs of differing type, lethality, severity etc. of target diseases; (b) in some drugs, the discovery of side-effects is delayed considerably when compared with ascertainment of effectiveness; (c) when a side-effect occurs in patients of special physical constitution or in persons with special physical conditions such as pregnancy, diagnosis of such physical constitution or condition is mandatory; (d) availability of preventive methods of side-effects; (e) availability of other drugs indicated for the same or similar diseases and which have greater safety. Therefore, evaluation of drugs cannot but be flexible to some extent, being influenced partly by advances in the medical and pharmaceutical sciences and partly by the prevailing public opinion.

It should be kept in mind at the same time that drugs are indispensable for life and for maintenance and improvement of health and that too much emphasis on safety may hinder the development of new drugs more useful than the existing ones. Therefore, for the total evaluation of drugs from the point of view of effectiveness and safety, it is necessary to collate the wisdom of mankind and form an impartial and rational judgement, on the assumption that most data on safety will be collected.

DISCUSSION

Chairman: It is very important to preserve human life and to maintain and improve human health, but I think it is also important to incorporate safety with efficacy. Together with this morning's presentation by Dr. Motohashi, I am sure that those who have come from abroad will have been able to grasp what the pharmaceutical affairs situation is in Japan.

Takano: For the industry it is quite important and quite necessary for its survival to develop drugs which can be mass-produced. In such a situation, voluntary efforts by industry to produce only safe drugs cannot be expected. The present proposed amendment only concerns what to do after something has happened. I feel that something is missing on the part of the manufacturers as well as on the part of the Government.

Matsushita: I do not know whether I am in the position to answer your comment. Whether there is mass administration or not, it is not a question of the manufacturing company. We do try our best, so that good drugs are developed and we have always asked the patients to use them in an appropriate way.

Katahira: I believe that the treatment given to those who have suffered damage should be looked at from a broader point of view. In the case of SMON, not only medical treatment but also the establishment of a system for permanent social rehabilitation is urgently required.

Matsushita: I don't think I am in the position to answer that question.

The dilemma of adverse drug reactions

JOHN C. BALLIN

Department of Drugs, American Medical Association, Chicago, IL, U.S.A.

> '...I firmly believe that if the whole materia medica, as now used, could be sunk to the bottom of the sea, it would be all the better for mankind – and all the worse for the fishes.'
>
> Oliver Wendell Holmes, 1860

When this familiar expression of therapeutic nihilism was uttered over a century ago, it was probably more a reflection on the lack of efficacy of the few simple medicinal agents then in vogue than concern over excess toxicity. Since the time of Holmes, and particularly in the last 40 years, the advances in pharmacology and therapeutics have been spectacular. Today, the physician has available to him a vast armamentarium of highly effective drugs which has revolutionized medical practice. The profession has had to pay a price for these spectacular successes, however: modern drug therapy, while offering greater specificity for the amelioration or cure of disease, carries with it a much greater potential for iatrogenic illness – suffering brought about by the drugs themselves.

Modern drugs are generally potent chemical entities that are capable of producing a wide variety of unintended adverse drug reactions (ADRs). It should not be implied, however, that the problem of ADRs is strictly a modern phenomenon. Physicians have *always* known that iatrogenic disease is an accepted hazard of medical practice. The aim of rational therapy, today as in antiquity, is to choose the course of treatment that will achieve the desired therapeutic results with the least amount of drug-associated toxicity.

There is another medical maxim deserving of comment – the ancient Latin guideline for physicians, *primum non nocere* ('above all, do no harm'). It is doubtful that modern physicians could literally ascribe to this axiom. If a physician wants to be absolutely certain of doing no harm, he will do nothing, thereby leaving the patient free from risk but also deprived of any possible benefits. If Holmes were alive today, his absolute therapeutic nihilism would probably be modified by an admonition for physicians to *weigh the benefits versus the risks each time a therapeutic decision is made.*

How can physicians be assisted in making wise benefit-versus-risk assessments? Clearly, the answer must involve better physician education, not only during the undergraduate years but throughout a lifetime of practice. Although formal training in pharmacology has been part of the medical school curriculum throughout this century, the emphasis has traditionally been on such aspects as pharmacokinetics, mode of action, metabolism, and excretion. Even though it is important, this kind of knowledge does not enable the physician in training to appreciate fully the actions and uses of drugs in sick patients. Classical pharmacologists have always maintained that the clinical aspects of drug use can be learned at the bedside during later training and in practice. These traditional educational concepts are now being challenged. Today, more and more medical educators are realizing the importance of early clinical orientation in the teaching of pharmacology and therapeutics. As a consequence, departments or divisions of clinical pharmacology have been established in many American medical schools and, in fact, efforts are now under way to provide recognized medical specialty status to the discipline of clinical pharmacology. These salutary efforts are certainly a step in the right direction.

In addition to these efforts at the undergraduate level, the physician in practice now has available a vast array of educational tools to enable him to make wise benefit-versus-risk assessments. His problem in utilizing this material is one of quantity – the information explosion in therapeutics has made it utterly impossible for any physician to evaluate the enormous amount of drug literature. Therefore, the physician needs sources or reliable drug information that he can assimilate quickly and conveniently. Without such assistance, he cannot be expected to exercise rational choices in selecting the most effective drug for his patient. In the United States, many such educational resources are available. These emanate from the pharmaceutical industry, the federal government, and the medical profession itself. The organized medical profession, as represented by the American Medical Association, has a long history of commitment to better therapeutics. I am particularly proud of our encyclopedic reference source, *AMA Drug Evaluations*, now entering its fourth edition. This book, in the hands of some 250,000 American physicians, is widely recognized as one of the most authoritative and current compilations of drug information available today. Its judicious use, in conjunction with other valuable reference sources, can be of great assistance in improving the quality of therapeutics.

Although the key to improved therapeutic practice is better physician education, the unpredictable nature of drug response precludes any foolproof method for early detection of *all* serious ADRs. Thus, therapeutic misadventures are bound to occur no matter how judiciously drugs are administered. The goal of therapeutics, therefore, is to decrease the number of such episodes to the irreducible minimum. In particular, physicians should strive to reduce the incidence of what have been called 'preventable' ADRs.

One of the major problems in attacking the dilemma of ADRs is the confusion about their incidence. How serious a problem are ADR's? Unfortunately, the public in the United States has been subjected to a macabre 'numbers game' about fatal ADRs that is as alarming as it is sensational. Thus, we have been told that anywhere from 30,000 to 160,000 deaths occur each year as the result of therapeutic misadventures. Although it has been conceded that perhaps 20% of fatal ADRs are unavoidable, the clear implication from this publicity has been that most of these fatalities are due to physician error. An analysis of the data used to estimate the purported fatality figures led Karch and Lasagna (1) to conclude that 'the data on ADRs are incomplete, unrepresentative, uncontrolled, and lacking in operational criteria for identifying ADRs.' They further observe that 'no quantitative conclusions can be drawn from the reported data in regard to morbidity, mortality, or the underlying causes of ADRs, and attempts to extrapolate the available data to the general population would be invalid and perhaps misleading.'

Many of the studies used to document inappropriate drug use have relied on retrospective value judgments by other physicians following review of patient records. This kind of medical 'second guessing' can yield conclusions of dubious validity. Even when all the laboratory data are available and the course of an illness known, experts sometimes disagree on the best course of therapy for an individual patient. How much more difficult are therapeutic decisions for the attending physician when the course of the illness is uncertain. When confronted with a sick patient, the physician must make a rapid decision based on the available data and his own clinical judgment. Retrospectively, that decision may prove to be wrong. But it should not necessarily be labeled as irrational or inappropriate prescribing.

There is no question that the problem of preventable ADRs exists. How extensive it may be is unknown. Regardless of the magnitude of the problem, however, there is agreement that better methods for early detection of serious ADRs are needed.

In the United States, as in most countries, governmental clearance is required before a drug can be marketed. The regulatory procedure involves examination of the animal data and the results of clinical trials to support the efficacy and relative safety of a drug. The rigorousness of these pre-marketing requirements varies from country to country, but in no nation is a drug permitted to be marketed without evidence that it will exert beneficial pharmacological effects in human patients.

The proof of efficacy is generally not difficult. Controlled trials in a relatively small number of patients usually are adequate to demonstrate a beneficial therapeutic response. The proof of safety, however, can be elusive, time-consuming, and difficult. Frequent side-effects or unwanted reactions that are an extension of a drug's pharmacological action are relatively easy to identify. But proof of safety becomes very complex when one is dealing with serious adverse reactions that occur infrequently and that cannot be predicted on the basis of known pharmacological actions. Examples of such serious drug misadventures abound: phocomelia following use of thalidomide, vaginal adenosis in the daughters of women given diethylstilbestrol during pregnancy, blindness and sclerosing peritonitis following administration of practolol, and here in Japan, SMON allegedly due to clioquinol. These serious ADRs were unsuspected when the drugs were approved and could not have been expected to be detected within any reasonable period of pre-marketing trials. Therefore, because it is unrealistic to expect complete safety, and because valuable therapeutic agents might be denied to the public if pre-marketing trials were further lengthened, regulatory agencies have always predicated approval decisions on the expectation that benefits will outweigh risks. As we have observed with the foregoing drugs, these decisions are not always vindicated.

If, as seems obvious, the marketing of a drug is always a calculated risk, what can be done to detect these unsuspected, serious ADRs earlier? It is unfortunately true that, once a drug is in general distribution, gathering of additional information regarding its toxicity is at best sporadic, unstructured, and haphazard. The association of adverse effects with drug administration is often difficult, and determining the cause of toxicity is further complicated when multiple drug therapy is employed. When the incidence of serious ADRs is quite low, there is a natural tendency by the attending physician to attribute the patient's problems to factors unrelated to drugs. For example, chloramphenicol was in widespread use for almost a decade before it was recognized that approximately 1 of every 20,000 patients developed aplastic anemia as a result of its administration. It is abundantly clear, therefore, that early detection of serious ADRs requires more than surveying the medical literature for reports by particularly astute physicians. What is needed is an organized effort to collect, evaluate, and tabulate information on suspected ADRs.

The first such organized effort was begun in 1954 by the American Medical Association. Because chloramphenicol was then beginning to come under suspicion, this initial program was restricted to hematological disorders and was known as the AMA Registry on Blood Dyscrasias. The Registry was based on a system of voluntary reporting by physicians of suspected drug-induced blood dyscrasias. With a potential information source of over 7,000 hospitals and almost 300,000 physicians, the Registry was launched with high hopes that it could provide a mechanism for early ADR detection.

After an early flurry of activity, it became obvious, even to the most ardent enthusiasts, that the project was in trouble. The average busy practitioner regarded ADRs with ambivalence. He was anxious to learn about such things but not to fill out another report form. As a result, reports were sporadic and those received were often sketchy, inaccurate, incomplete, and frequently illegible. Nevertheless, the Registry persevered and the data were gathered, evaluated, and tabulated; semiannual reports were sent out to the profession. Despite the inadequacies, some important information was gleaned. For example, knowledge of the toxicity of dipyrone and chloramphenicol was documented. There were even some early enthusiasts who thought that the idea of a Registry might be 'catching on'.

In 1961, the Registry on Blood Dycrasias was expanded to the more comprehensive Registry on Adverse Drug Reactions and expert panels were appointed to evaluate the information being submitted.

About this time, the U.S. Food and Drug Administration launched an ADR reporting system of its own, and the AMA entered into a cooperative agreement with the FDA: The FDA would gather information from university-based, government, and teaching hospitals of 350 beds or more, and the AMA Registry would concentrate on smaller hospitals and individual physicians. Unfortunately, this cooperative venture never came to fruition. Problems concerning confidentiality of the reports developed and it was estimated that only 1 to 2% of all ADRs were being reported.

In the intervening years, both organizations used various techniques in an attempt to infuse enthusiasm into their programs, but the effort was largely futile. Finally, in 1967, the AMA embarked upon one last effort to salvage the program. Because of concern that the length and complexity of the report form inhibited voluntary reporting by physicians, the AMA entered into a grant contract with the Boston Collaborative Drug Surveillance Program (1) to devise a simple report form that physicians would be willing to complete, and (2) to determine what kind of in-hospital surveillance would be successful in gathering meaningful ADR information. The results of the Boston study were discouraging. They indicated that it seemed impossible to devise a report form simple enough to garner the cooperation of significant numbers of physicians, and that intensive monitoring of hospitalized patients by paid monitors was the only reliable method of gathering useful ADR information. Clearly, the cost of such intensive monitoring precluded its application on a national scale. Therefore, in 1971, the AMA reluctantly abolished its Registry on Adverse Drug Reactions.

Although the AMA program for the voluntary reporting of serious ADRs did not succeed, this does not mean that the principles involved were without merit. As more public attention has focused on the subject of ADRs, pressures have increased to develop a systematized method for the earlier detection of serious reactions. There is now unanimous agreement that some type of national system for post-marketing surveillance is needed. This concept has been written into proposed new drug laws in the United States and was the basis for the formation of the Joint Commission on Prescription Drug Use. The chairman of that Commission, Dr. Kenneth Melmon, is on the program of this Conference and will discuss in some detail the work of the Commission. Suffice it to say that a workable program for monitoring drug experience on a national scale appears to offer the only hope of identifying serious ADRs earlier. The kind of national system for post-marketing surveillance that will eventually evolve remains to be seen. On the basis of AMA's earlier experience, however, certain basic principles of such a system seem apparent: (1) the cooperation of practicing physicians in reporting suspected ADRs is necessary; (2) physician cooperation can best be gained with a voluntary reporting system rather than mandatory requirements; (3) the system should have built-in protection for the confidentiality of patient records; (4) physicians must be protected from legal liability as the result of voluntary reporting; (5) the reporting mechanism should be simple and not time-consuming; (6) a national agency independent of the federal government should be set up to administer the program; and (7) prior to the establishment of the program, these must be a major educational effort to persuade physicians that voluntary reporting will benefit the public health and will not interfere with the integrity of the physician-patient relationship.

Some of the more extremist elements of society have implied that the ADR program would disappear if a governmentally controlled system of mandatory surveillance of therapeutics was established. We know, of course, that this is utter nonsense. We are convinced, however, that a system of post-marketing surveillance employing the principles enumerated above could go a long way to help resolve the dilemma of ADRs.

REFERENCE

1. Karsh, F.E. and Lasagna, L. (1975): Adverse drug reactions: a critical review. *J. Amer. med. Ass., 234*, 1236.

DISCUSSION

Liljestrand: I agree with most of what Dr. Ballin said, but why would the reporting become worse if it becomes mandatory and not voluntary? Our experience is the opposite.

Ballin (J.): I can only respond to that by conveying to you the attitudes, as I perceived them, of physicians in the United States. I think the physicians in our country have become very concerned about what they perceive as intrusions of the Federal Government into the practice of medicine and into the control of therapeutics. I would suspect that a mandatory system, initially at least, would be resisted as another such governmental effort to control how they practice medicine. I would have to say, however, that if a voluntary effort didn't do any better than the one I earlier described, it might be necessary to go to a mandatory system. But I would suggest that, at least in the United States, we start off with a voluntary system.

Westerholm: After listening to the descriptions from various countries, it's obvious that a system which works in one country might not be the ideal one in another country, and the description of the United States' situation may not at all be comparable to that in smaller countries where you can reach your physician population much more easily. But I think what one should do is to look around in one's own country and look at the various hospital routines to see whether monitoring could be built in as an easy part of this routine. For instance, in the WHO classification of diagnosis of diseases, there is an instruction how you should record adverse reactions to drugs as a discharge diagnosis and doctors always write discharge diagnoses. This is one way to try to get a better idea of the number of cases to use. There is a possibility to write in the adverse reaction as an adverse reaction discharge diagnosis.

Melmon: I bet that was a comment more than a question. I think that there is a problem in mixing up the issue of voluntary or mandatory contributions of a spontaneous nature with the systematic surveillance system that doesn't have anything to do with voluntary reporting. At least in the United States, the voluntary reports don't account for more than 40–50% of new information for post-marketed drugs. Increasing the amount of reporting doesn't necessarily lead to better or more information and it may not be one of the objectives of a surveillance programme. In fact, although I am sure it is unofficial, the comments that Dr. Inman has made from time to time have indicated that as the report numbers fall, the value increases. Because there is a tendency of feeding back to people who are very helpful in their screening procedures, information encourages them to report subsequently. So it may not be that a system should concentrate on gathering as much information as it can in terms of quantity.

When it comes to being systematic about surveillance, the voluntary effort may have no value, and what we might have to do is require that selected people help us. I think that's the area where Dr. Liljestrand was beginning to focus on. We have to be very careful in separating voluntary reports of an *ad hoc* nature from mandatory participation in a systematic surveillance system.

Ballin (J.): I agree with what Dr. Melmon says. Those of you who are familiar with efforts to revise the American drug law will realize that this was in mind when it was suggested that certain drugs be put into what was called 'limited distribution' on their first commercial appearance which has had the mandatory requirement of adverse drug reaction reporting. Certainly that's a very favorable kind of way of approaching a problem.

Laetrile – the case of a disputed drug

BORIS VELIMIROVIC*

*Field Office U.S.-Mexico Border, Pan American Sanitary Bureau, World Health Organization, El Paso, TX, U.S.A.***

This Conference is dealing with drug-induced suffering, whereby as drugs are meant those which were developed on a sound physiological and pharmacological basis, i.e., officially recognized, registered and licensed by the national regulatory authorities. My presentation is concerned with problems raised in connection with a non-official, non-orthodox remedy, which has no official recognized value, yet is used by hundreds of thousands of people. It is not really the substance itself which is interesting, but the ethical, psychological and political problems surrounding it, and we are concerned here not so much with the pitiful defense of the use of this remedy (claims of persecution, testimonials) and the simple argument of those who oppose its use, as with the fact that the very nexus of the problem concerns public and, indeed, individual rights and their relationship to official medicine.

Let us look for a moment at the case of a disputed drug, *Laetrile*, which has been promoted for about 25–30 years as a treatment for cancer. This drug has never been satisfactorily scientifically tested, nor have its safety and effectiveness been demonstrated, and its use has been prohibited by the Food and Drug Administration (FDA) yet, at least in the United States, it has become a genuine public health problem.

Over the years, proponents have claimed that Laetrile is a cure for cancer, that it is palliative, that it prevents cancer, that it is a pain killer, or that it facilitates other cancer treatments. There have been even claims that Laetrile raises the red blood cell count and thus is of value in treating sickle-cell anemia. It is said to be useful in treating parasitic disease, and to lower blood pressure in cancer victims. It is claimed that it provides relief in arthritis. But its main use is as a non-official anticancer drug. The theories about how Laetrile supposedly works against cancer (health food, vitamin) have changed over the years, according to the claims of the proponents as to what cancer is.

WHAT IS LAETRILE?

Laetrile+, amygdalin++, nitriloside, vitamin B-17, and Sarcarcinase have been used interchangeably by both proponents and opponents of Laetrile. Although

*The author is a staff member of the World Health Organization. However, the views expressed in this paper are entirely his own. The responsibility for the paper rests solely with the author.

***Present address:* Regional Office for Europe, World Health Organization, Copenhagen, Denmark.

+1-Mandelonitrile β-glucuronic acid *(Merck Index, 9th ed.* at 702) claimed to be purified amygdalin.

++D-Mandelonitrile β-D-glucosidio-6-β-D-glucoside *(Merck Index, 9th ed.* at 81).

amygdalin has been known in pharmacology for over 100 years (since 1834), the chemical compound used referred to as Laetrile was prepared in 1952 by E.T. Krebs Jr. in the United States, while working with crushed apricot pit extract which his father had prepared and studied some years earlier. Because of the variability of Laetrile formulation, obtained from varying sources of material, the FDA concluded that the term 'Laetrile' is a rather imprecise broad generic label for a group of compounds of unknown number (as has been admitted by the pro-Laetrile McNaughton Foundation from Canada in a meeting with the FDA's Ad Hoc Committee on Oncology experts in 1971 for data obtained prior to 1963). The above Committee thus declared that 'uncertain identity of the drug tested make the best results obtained questionable* (1). In the United States, Laetrile has been promoted by the 'Committee for Freedom of Choice in Cancer Therapy Inc.', the 'International Association of Cancer Victims and Friends', a selected array of individuals and a certain number of physicians (claimed to be about 1,200), and in Canada by the North End Medical Center of Montreal.

The 'natural food factor' or 'drug' has been produced under various names** in Mexico, and is being smuggled into the United States; according to press reports (2), it is, next to marijuana, 'the second biggest contraband substance'. The Mexican government gave provisional approval to manufacture the drug in 1974 (contingent upon the presentation of evidence of Laetrile effectiveness in treating cancer) to two laboratories (Cyto Pharma of Mexico) but cancelled it in 1976 because no positive results were obtained in research carried out at the Medical Center General Hospital. The decision to ban Laetrile has been appealed by Laetrile advocates, and is now in the Mexican Courts. It is also produced clandestinely in the United States; recently (1977), 112 tons of apricots were seized in Wisconsin.

A number of preliminary initial testing results on animals in which claims were made regarding the positive effects of Laetrile – Sloan-Kettering Cancer Center (of New York), Southern Research Institute (Birmingham, Alabama), Scind Laboratories (University of San Francisco, California), Pasteur Institute (Paris), Institut von Ardenne (Dresden, German Democratic Republic) and others, e.g. patient testimonials collected in the book *Laetrile Case Histories* by J.A. Richardson and P. Griffin – have all been found by the Investigation of the Commissioner of the FDA in an extensive report as methodologically wrong, incorrect, non-consistently confirmed by later investigation, insufficiently demonstrated, not supported by well-documented clinical investigation, or were preliminary work which was disclaimed by the same institutions, and never published in any scientific journal. In summary, they did not give any conclusive evidence that bitter almonds are effective in inhibiting the growth of tumors.

*'Drugs from different sources should be considered as drug products or formulations, the equivalence of which cannot be assumed on the basis of present pharmacopoeial standards', *WHO, Euro, 7406*, p. 5. Copenhagen, 1973.

**Bee-17, Aprikern, Kemdalin, Apricap, Amigdalina, containing 30–150 mg p. tablet, although the label can declare 500 mg amygdalin.

LAETRILE TOXICITY

The initial assumption has been that although Laetrile might be ineffective, it was thought not to be dangerous, although it has been surmised that the presence of the enzymes β-glucosidase, oxynitralase and glucoside amygdalin together in apricot (*Prunus armeniaca, Prunus amygdalus Batsch, Prunus persica*) pits could present the potential for combinations that would release hydrogen cyanide (hydrocyanic acid = prussic acid) in the individual consuming the extract of the pits. However, there are documented cases of poisoning, some fatal, due to consumption of apricot pits or kernels. (Laetrile is given in a dosage 200 mg/person/day.) Potential toxicity has been implicit in the statement of Laetrile proponents that amygdalin products should never be given by mouth, since hydrochloric acid in the stomach is capable of hydrolysing the drug. In a 1954 document, it explicitly stated: 'not to be taken orally' (1). It was stated that Laetrile was 40 times more toxic orally than parenterally. (Such hydrolysates, it was claimed, selectively affect only the cancer cell in vivo.) Amygdalin, a cyanogenetic glucoside can be hydrolysed by microbial β-glucosidase enzyme in the small intestine to a sugar and mandelonitrile, which by further enzymatic action releases benzaldehyde and cyanide, a potent and rapidly acting cellular respiratory poison. There is admittedly little β-glucosidase in human tissues or in purified amygdalin extracts, but the enzyme can be present in other foods, thus presumably ensuring the breakdown of amygdalin in the gastrointestinal tract (3). Lettuce, mushrooms, certain fresh fruits, green peppers, celery and sweet almonds all contain this enzyme. Thus, ingestion of any of these uncooked foods with amygdalin could produce cyanide intoxication. The cyanide radical (which is not prussic acid) can also be released from many proteins in meat, milk, eggs etc. Poisoning due to nitrilosides, or by ingestion of apricot seeds, or some tropical plants in the United States and elsewhere, has been demonstrated.* The adverse reactions attributed to Laetrile are more difficult to single out as they might be due to cytostatic or radiation treatment or to the underlying cancer itself. However, recent studies in California have listed 17 deaths among 37 cases of poisoning caused by fruit kernels containing cyanide, of which one by Laetrile. Serious adverse reactions have been reported from Georgetown University in Washington; an 11-month-old New York girl died of subacute cyanide poisoning after accidentally eating five of her father's Laetrile tablets (9). In California, a 17-year-old girl died following voluntary ingestion of the contents of several ampules of Laetrile injection (10), and an adult woman in the course of her Laetrile treatment by cyanide poisoning. Small amounts of cyanide can be degraded in the body by a thiosulfate transulferase (rhodanase), but large amounts of exogenous thiosulfate are necessary to neutralize a massive dose of cyanide. The major damage in the brain is small hemorrhages in the white matter, especially in the cerebellum, and severe degeneration of the Purkinje celis. 'Cytotoxic hypoxia produces dizziness, vomiting, hypotension, shock, stupor, coma, and if the therapy for cyanide poisoning is not prompt, progressing to irreversible respiratory failure and death' (11). Other adverse reactions reported from Laetrile include hemoglobinuria,

*Toxicity by chemically related substances, e.g. glucoside linamarin present in cassava in Africa, and other foods. See Refs. 5 and 6.

gastrointestinal hemorrhage, headache and diarrhea, allergic reactions such as dermatitis and acute episodes of fever, and paresis of the oculomotor and palpebral musculature* (12). Since the use of this 'remedy' takes place outside the official medical establishment and, in addition, as there is no system of complete monitoring of adverse reactions, it is probable that some cases of non-lethal cyanide poisoning have been overlooked, and they are, and might be in the future, more frequent than is known at present. It cannot be maintained any more *prima facie* that Laetrile is non-toxic.

Samples of Laetrile have been furthermore proven to be adulterated with dipyrone (500 mg in each tablet) or were microbiologically contaminated (bipolarly budding yeast and fungal hyphae), contaminated with methyl and isopropyl alcohols or with leakage of some ampules. Pyrogen reaction in rabbits has been noted at a dose of 100 mg/kg (13). An additional impurity of unknown toxic potential – amygdalinamide – has also been identified in the injectable formulation (14).

LAETRILE CONTROVERSY

The use of Laetrile has been opposed by practically all scientific bodies, among others: the American Cancer Society, the U.S. National Cancer Institute, the American Medical Association, the Canadian Food and Drug Directorate, and the Mexican Medical Association. Laetrile has not been recognized internationally, and has been registered only in two countries. Following the warning of the World Health Organization which describes potential dangers in the use of the drug, most countries of the world have prohibited its use or importation, and 'by definition unavailable' in any of WHO's member states throughout Western Europe.**

In the United States the Commissioner's report concludes: 'Neither Laetrile nor any other drug called by the various terms mentioned above nor any other product which might be characterized as 'nitriloside' is generally recognized by experts qualified by scientific training and experience to evaluate the safety and effectiveness of drugs to be safe and effective for any therapeutic use' (1).

The position taken by the FDA to oppose free sale and distribution of Laetrile as a worthless therapeutic or nutrient was thus both justified and understandable. It felt that it should protect the patients (and physicians) from the consequences of their own inability to obtain objective information on the drug and from those who are anxious, for profit, to mislead them. In its 70 years (Pure Food and Drug Act of 1906) history the FDA has put hundreds of such cures out of business and has gained respect and credibility in the process. Why, then, is Laetrile a public health problem? Why was the FDA challenged in court?

*In January 1979, a 3-year-old child with leukemia was reported as suffering from cyanide poisoning in Plymouth, motivating the Court to give the State the legal custody of the child. This case was appealed to the Supreme Court (Mass.) by the lawyers for the child's parents.

**In Switzerland one company does sell 'small quantities of Laetrile' 'exclusively to cancer research scientists' primarily in Western Europe (1). Although the West German response to the State Department's inquiry indicated that Laetrile is not available there, it is well known that a clinic in Hanover has been using the controversial drug for many years (8). It is claimed that amygdalin has been used also in Japan, the Philippines and elsewhere.

Among many fashionable drugs (both scientific and quack) there are some which attract a large following, particularly in the field of cancer, and which become a national issue. (See the cases of Chamlee's Cancer Specific of 1930, glyoxylic acid in 1940, NT B-15 pangamate in 1949, Hoxsey Cancer Treatment in 1950, Krebiozen 1951, later called Calcaron, Rand vaccine in 1966, and Laetrile in the 1970's (15).) All of these, except Laetrile, considered a major health fraud in the United States today, have been successfully opposed on legal and on scientific and ethical grounds, and eliminated by the FDA, a model pioneer regulatory organization. With Laetrile the FDA has been at least temporarily defeated. Seventeen States of the United States have legalized Laetrile often with huge margins in both houses*; in three, the State legislature had voted down a bill legalizing the drug interstate, and in two, the Governors vetoed Laetrile bills. One has a suit pending requiring the production rights. In Alaska, Laetrile may be prescribed by doctors, and an Oklahoma judge legalized the importation of Laetrile from Mexico under specific conditions. (The patients had to go across the border for treatment or to rely on smuggled drug.) All this happened on popular demand in an emotional polemic atmosphere and with a polarization of minds. Laetrile is considered unique among cancer remedies in that it has become as much a political issue as a medical one. The Laetrile controversy raises some serious problems which it would be interesting to examine briefly.

Certainly the advocates of Laetrile have not been able in 25 years, since Laetrile appeared as a cancer cure, to convince either the medical profession or the authorities that it is efficacious, but they have successfully maintained that even if the drug does not work, people still have the right to take it because they deserve 'freedom of choice', at least if the drug involved is not overtly toxic.

This issue goes deeper than the unscrupulous motives of the Laetrile proponents who profit** from it, and has been addressed by the FDA as follows: 'The very act of forming a government of course necessarily involves the yielding of some freedoms in order to obtain others. In passing the 1962 Amendment to the Act – the Amendment that requires that a drug be proven effective before it may be marketed – Congress indicated in its conclusions that the absolute freedom to choose an ineffective drug was properly surrendered in exchange for the freedom from the danger to each person's health and well-being from the sale and use of worthless drugs.' The FDA arguments were placed firstly on the 'protection of the citizens'. The Commissioner's report quotes:

- 'When the freedom to accept any drug for treatment and the freedom to injure oneself collides, a judgement must be made; stop signs or restrictions on turning at certain corners, restrict any freedom in driving, but at the same time, they protect any freedom from hurting myself and others in traffic' (1).
- 'For the patient ignorant of the inertness of Laetrile as an anticancer drug, there is an overriding concern that he not be denied of his individual freedom by

*Passage of State legislation does not protect from applicable civil constitutional sanctions under the Federal Food, Drug and Cosmetic Act, nor offers immunity from malpractice suits.

**A California physician who was convicted of conspiring to smuggle Laetrile charged $50 for a single injection, worth a few cents, and deposited more than $2.5 million in a single bank account between 1973 and 1976 (15).

untimely death from cancer from having relied on Laetrile to help. This is a cruel depravation of individual freedom, since the patient does not get a second chance' (1).

- 'Acceptance of the privacy of the freedom to choose medical therapies cannot be tolerated by complex modern, industrial society, and this cannot afford to let the nation's health concerns be governed by a distorted definition of that great symbol "freedom" which would return in practice anarchy to the realm of health' (1).

The FDA contends that the choice is not free: 'The patients are confronted with enormous pressure to use Laetrile instead of conventional forms of therapy'; 'the emotional trauma of a cancer diagnosis severely impairs the patients' and the familes' ability to engage in rational decision making process'; 'the choice of Laetrile therapy by persons under the severe stress associated with the discovery of cancer, and in response to misinformation presented persuasively by Laetrile proponents, cannot be regarded as choice which is free'.

While such arguments are understandable to a larger part of the medical community, they sound hollow to the public. Even more so are the FDA reasonings in refuting the possibility of limited use of Laetrile to terminal patients only. 'Such an approval would be theoretically justified only on the grounds that since such patients might be considered beyond the help of other therapies, Laetrile cannot hurt them'. Although approval of a drug for use by terminal patients is not possible under the Act, arguments were expressed: (1) there is no such thing as a 'terminal' patient; (2) allowing the use by a subgroup of cancer patients would lead to an increase in the use by patients who could be helped by legitimate therapy. The report* quotes: 'medical history is full of miracles; no one knows if, and when, any patient is going to die'.

The Commissioner concludes that restricted approval 'would lead to needless deaths and suffering among (1) patients characterized as "terminal" who could actually be helped by legitimate therapy and (2) patients clearly susceptible to the benefits of legitimate therapy, who would be misled as to Laetrile's utility [illegible] the limited approval program, or who would be able to obtain the drug through the inevitable leakage in any system set up to administer such a program.'

The third alternative – use concurrently with other therapy – has been rejected on ethical grounds; it has not been shown by any sound scientific evidence that the administration of Laetrile along with other therapy may not either make such therapy more dangerous or interfere with its effect*. Holland states, referring to the eventual testing of the drug on patients: 'One does not seek further information on why *not* to use Laetrile. If there is no good reason to do something, the best reason exists not to do it (emphasis in original). Thus, the same reasons that justify the law's ban on use of drugs not shown to be effective form an equally strong basis for the ban on that use where the use will be concurrent with other therapy.'

The FDA refuses the testing in the absence of proof that Laetrile is efficient, a logic which the proponents have failed to understand; how to prove the efficiency if

*Commissioner's Decision, pp. 71–73.

it was not tested, 'claiming' prejudice and conspiracy*. The National Council on Drugs (anti-Laetrile) has pleaded for a clinical test.

The National Cancer Institute has announced in 1978 that it will submit to the FDA an application to clinically test Laetrile in terminally ill cancer patients. The decision is being based on a recently completed NCI review of the record of patients who had taken the drug. Proponents of Laetrile on the basis of some clinical reports, a number of them favorable, have repeatedly appealed to the FDA for permission to conduct controlled tests of Laetrile's effectiveness, but it was refused because few scientists and experts have supported it. In the absence of such a test, the debate and the accusations could only have continued, as indeed they have.

The Commissioner of the FDA stated: 'We do not believe the retrospective review done by NCI to demonstrate any effectiveness of Laetrile, but there are *other reasons* (emphasis added) that we all recognize, that a controlled clinical trial might be desirable and NCI has been persuaded by them' (16).

DISCUSSION

The emotion behind the Laetrile movement includes more than a simply hysterical religious fanaticism; most people involved (and patients) believe without reservation that the chemical is beneficial (17). It is more than an issue of, what we believe, a useless remedy.

E.J. Ingelfinger (18), former Editor of the *New England Medical Journal*, wrote: 'As a cancer patient myself, I would not take Laetrile under any circumstances. If any member of my family had cancer, I would counsel them against it. If I were still in practice, I would not recommend it to my patients. Yet, perhaps, there are some situations in which rational medical science should yield and make some concessions. If any patient had what I thought was hopelessly advanced cancer, and if he asked for Laetrile, I should like to be able to give the substance to him to assuage his mental anguish, just as I would give him morphine without stint to relieve his physical suffering.' Deploring the 'tendency of national organization and leaders interested in cancer research to overwhelm the public with electric guitar-like clatter in extolling the progress of conventional cancer research' he stated that patients 'driven by desperate hope, demand the substance in numbers proportional to all the many cancers that appear to be resistant to conventional therapy, as well as to the latest chemical agents that the National Cancer Institute and its investigators are testing.' The prohibition of an agent offering hope, even if by all objective standards ineffective, would only increase demand for it. 'Under these conditions, the FDA and other controlling agencies might be most effective in eliminating this quack drug, not by legal prohibition, but by permitting its sale and use. Prohibition, however, should be replaced by accurate record-keeping, so that patients given the

*The National Cancer Institute has tested Laetrile in animals on 5 separate occasions between 1957 and 1975, without finding any evidence that Laetrile either cures or inhibits the growth of cancer cells. In 1972, three petitions signed by 43,000 people were sent to the President of the United States requesting experimental testing of Laetrile.

agent can be identified and followed' and an evaluation made after about two years (18) (a central registry of amygdalin deaths, and regular monitoring so as to insure that extensive additional scientifically based information is rapidly obtained, on the basis of which a decision as to restriction or full general release can be taken).

The discussion that followed raised the questions: Has Laetrile been successful in some cases because it is actually a placebo? Can Laetrile be ethically permitted to be universally available before it is proven to be safe and effective? Is it ethical to test a drug, when enough empirical evidence is available showing that it is useless, personal testimonials notwithstanding? Can a trial be ethical, since an honest explanation of efficacy does not supersede the imperative: clinical trials should be conducted in the belief that they will bring good, rather than merely guarantee absence of harm (19).

'The efficacy evaluation of old drugs on the market is a special problem, particularly if the legislation is changed and efficacy is suddenly required as a condition for the sale of drugs. Most of the earlier investigations on such drugs do not stand up to modern standards, while clinical experience may very well show the drugs to be efficacious or at least may have convinced the clinicians of their efficacy. It will often be most difficult to convince the clinical investigators of the importance of covering this field with more modern trials. The size of the problem may be shown by some figure from the USA. The number of new drugs in the United States for which efficacy is considered to be proven is approximately 5000, whereas the number of so-called *grandfather* drugs is unknown, but is believed to range between 200,000 and 300,000' (20).

Some traditional unorthodox remedies still enjoy popularity, and are even increasing in popularity, such as Chinese medicines, natural remedies (acceptable if given by mouth, but not as injections), etc. These substances pose sensitive issues to those drug regulatory authorities bearing a 'statutory responsibility for their control'. Recourse to the scientifically based toxicological and clinical evidence regarded as mandatory to establish the safety and efficacy of newly synthetized chemicals is not feasible. This has led many national authorities to adopt a flexible balance between cultural requirements and popular demand on the one hand, and protection of the individual from hazard and unreasonable exploitation on the other (21). Will any controlled experiment, if carried out, convince the public and the cancer patients? Has the medical profession been sold on the curability of disseminated cancer and unwilling or unable to stick with a losing situation, without abandoning the cancer patients and so failing to keep the patient's respect and trust (22), once the diagnosis has been ascertained, and when the patient loses faith in the established treatment methods? Is the end of therapeutic alliance between patient and his physician not an indictment of the profession as well as society or the quack cures? Is it ethical for the doctor to nourish the patient's mystical belief in (cancer) medication? (22). Has the public not been led exactly by the medical profession to panaceomania (23) to expect an easy, spectacular cancer cure, which is not available, while neglecting cancer-provoking substances such as tobacco? 'The government has established a connection between cigarette smoking and cancer, but it believes its responsibility in the matter is discharged by requiring the manufacturer to include a notice on the package that – cigarettes may be dangerous to human health.' Why would it not be logical to pursue the same principle with Laetrile? Why 'should not government permit its sale and require the manufacturer to state on the label that scientific research has not been able to identify any properties in Laetrile that have an anti-cancer effect? This puts the decision squarely up to the patient and the doctor, which is where it belongs' (24). The moral dimension of the problem is that danger alone is never a sufficiently persuasive argument for the public to justify the prohibition of any drug, substance or artifact (25). After all, many substances and objects in daily use are just as harmful as the substances the regulatory agencies want to prohibit (e.g., guns which are much more dangerous but are not prohibited and which cancer patients not infrequently use). T. Szasz wrote: 'Alcohol is one example of individualistic against collectivistic attitude to ethic.' Thus 'the dangerous drug should be treated more or less as alcohol is treated now.' 'Every individual is capable of injuring or killing himself. This potentiality is a fundamental expression of human freedom. Self-destructive behaviour may be regarded as sinful and penalized by means of informal sanctions. But it should not be regarded as crime (or mental disease) – justifying or warranting the use of the police powers of the state for its control. Therefore it is absurd to deprive an *adult* (emphasis added) of a drug (or of anything else) because he might use it to kill himself.' Thus this is not an area of government's intervention. Many people regard freedom of self-medication as a fundamental right, the limiting condition being the inflicting of actual harm to others. 'In the matter of health, a vast and increasingly elastic category, physicians play important roles as legitimizers and illegitimizers. This, in short, is why we regard being medicated by a doctor as drug use and self-medication (especially with certain classes of drugs) as drug abuse.' 'Our present concepts of drug abuse articulate and symbolize a fundamental policy of scientific medicine – namely, that a layman should not medicate his own body, but should place its medical care under the supervision of a duly accredited physician' (25). 'What may be less obvious is the interest of the laity: by delegating responsibility for the spiritual and medical welfare of the people to a class of authoritatively accredited specialists, these policies – and the practice they ensure – relieve individuals from assuming the burdens of responsibility for themselves' (25).

In the case of Laetrile a large number of patients want this responsibility. Is it ethical to deny it to them in a situation where the professionally offered relief is open to doubt? 'After all is said and done,' wrote Szasz (in the context of so-called drug abuse), 'the issue comes down to whether we accept or reject the ethical principle John Stuart Mill so clearly enunciated: "The only purpose (he wrote in *On Liberty*) for which power can be rightfully exercised over any member of a civilized community against his will, is to prevent harm to others. His own good, whether physical or moral, is not a sufficient warrant. He cannot rightfully be compelled to do or forbear because it will make him happier, because in the opinion of others, to do so would be wise, or even right ... In the part (of his conduct) which merely concerns himself, his independence is, of right, absolute. Over himself, over his own body and mind, the individual is sovereign."' (25)

Could the cancer patients, provided they have been properly informed (free, voluntary, informed, understanding consent, and protected against financial victimization) be deprived of the right to individual dignity and liberty to choose, even if the opinions on therapeutic value of a substance differ from that of the professional one? Should patient and family not have, at that particular point, the dominant role in making decisions particularly in a terminal illness? How much should a regulating agency, even such a good one as the FDA, regulate? Clearly regulation on drug quality and safety are indispensable on a national and international level (for our part, we would like to see the FDA strengthened). Should not the effort of the regulating agencies, in this particular case, assure the proper information of the medical profession and the public, but not go further? There is a tolerance in matters of vaccinations and in refusal of any treatment by certain religious sects. Or should they do more?

The Laetrile phenomenon is also seen as a protest against the medical establishment* and against professional medicalization. This has been played down or denied by the medical profession (and the pharmaceutical industry). However, there is an unease of the public in respect of the resource misallocation and of the absolute power which the medical profession has in matters of health in deciding what is best for the patients, including the arbitrary power of the mental health profession, psychomimetic drugs, intrusion of the bureaucratic or the legal system etc. in private life. Is there not a protest against regulatory barriers to a competitive health care system, high cost, unnecessary medicalization, examinations (of so-called defensive medicine or made simply for profit), unnecessary surgery or stay in hospitals to fill the beds? The protest against the practices of life maintenance at all costs in pain and suffering imposed by medical technology, and prevalent customs, legal or religious influences (instead of patients' or relatives' choice) might have found an expression in the Laetrile controversy, displaced as it may be. Such issues are beyond the scope of this article, but without a subconscious distrust of the medical profession, needed but not loved, a distrust certainly not devoid of some experience, this controversy about a doubtful remedy could not have reached its present proportion.

Even ethical, scientific 'modern medicines are such potent weapons that it is generally agreed that the sole responsibility for their sale, production and use can no longer be left entirely to the manufacturer and prescriber' (26); hence specific legislative provisions aimed at protecting the right of the ultimate consumer not to be exposed to unwarranted risk to health. While this last principle has unchallengeable validity, it is insufficiently applied in other areas (e.g., food additives, industrial risks) and is often rejected by the consumers in other attempts to compulsory self-protective measures as infringement of personal liberty (e.g., seat belts).

The widespread use of Laetrile is in part a consequence of the publicity given to it. Is it surprising that the public reacts, when even official new drugs are heavily promoted on television, radio, and newspapers even before the drug is known to the medical profession**. The authorities are suspected of cynicism by some segments of the population. The information compiled by the International Agency for Research on Cancer covering more than 300 substances shows that about 25 chemicals or manufacturing processes are at present generally accepted as causing

*If it is true, e.g., that 20–40 million Americans use marijuana, the protest against professional advice and regulatory agencies is difficult to disregard.

**United States pharmaceutical companies spend about $1 billion per year on 'all promotional activities' (27).

cancer in man (28). The action in respect to such substances is at best sluggish. For example, The Environmental Protection Agency announced on January 13, 1979, that it will reduce the allowable amount of pronamide, a pesticide commonly found on lettuce, which has caused cancer in laboratory mice. However, 'EPA has concluded that for all uses the economic benefit outweighs its risks'. Confronted with such statements, is it surprising that some people/cancer victims or their relatives conclude that whether to use Laetrile or not, is their right?

In January 1979, the question of Laetrile has gone to the Supreme Court. The justices have voted that the controversy is valid, and they will study the lower court rulings that have permitted the substance's use by terminally ill cancer victims. The highest court in the country will decide whether the federal government may ban Laetrile. The legal language does not know the word compassion. The justices' eventual decision may hinge on the *privacy right* of cancer victims – whether the government may limit the treatments available to persons suffering from a disease for which there is no known cure. Although putting the issue solely on a legal or scientific basis, whatever the Supreme Court decision might eventually be, it will leave many people doubting whether it will stop dispute on a matter which is considered by many as not suitable for a purely legalistic but rather a pragmatic, empiric approach. In short, the Supreme Court can eliminate a fake drug, but not the problem which is a personal, individual and philosophical one.

REFERENCES

1. Kennedy, D. (1978): *Laetrile, Commissioner's Decision, July 29, 1977*, pp. 1–73. Fr. Doc. 77-22310, Govt. Printing Office, 0-246-920.
2. Diamond, G.E.B. (1977): Cancer research – Who profits? *Harvard polit. Rev., 5*, 17.
3. Dukes, M.N.G. (1978): Remedies used in non-orthodox medicine. In: *Side Effects of Drugs – Annual 2: A worldwide yearly survey of new data and trends*, Chapter 46, pp. 383–387. Editor: M.N.G. Dukes. Excerpta Medica, Amsterdam.
4. Gunders, A.E., Abrahamov, A., Weisemberg, E. et al. (1969): Cyanide poisoning following ingestion of apricot *(Prunus armeniaca)* kernels. *J. Israel med. Ass., 176*, 536.
5. Osunstokun, B.O. (1973): Ataxic neuropathy associated with high cassava diets. In: *Monograph IDRC-010e*, pp. 127–138. International Development Research Centre, London.
6. Conn, E.C. (1973): In: *Cyanogenetic Glycosides in Toxicants Occurring Naturally in Foods*, 2nd ed., pp. 299–308. National Academy of Sciences, Washington, DC.
7. Ross, J.F. (1977): The harmful effects of Laetrile apricot kernels, and other cyanogenic fruit and vegetable materials on human beings; and the ineffectiveness of Laetrile as a therapeutic agent in patients with cancer. Statement presented to Subcommittee of Health and Scientific Research, Committee on Human Resources, U.S. Senate, 95th Congress, July 12, 1977, First session. In: *The Banning of The Drug Laetrile from Interstate Commerce by FDA*. Government Printing Office, Washington, DC.
8. Lehman, P. (1977): Laetrile: The fatal cure. In: *FDA Consumer, Vol. II, No. 8*, pp. 11–15. Report from the Georgetown University Washington. *Washington Post, July 25th*.
9. Braico, K.T., Humbert, J.R., Terplan, K.L. and Lehotay, J.M. (1979): Laetrile intoxication. *New Engl. J. Med., 300*, 238.
10. Sadoff, L., Fuchs, K. and Hollander, J. (1978): Rapid death associated with Laetrile ingestion. *J. Amer. med. Ass., 239*, 1532.

11. Lewis, J.P. (1977): Laetrile. *West Med., 125*, 55.
12. Smith, F.P., Butter, T.P., Cohan, S. and Schein, P.S. (1977): Laetrile toxicity: a report of two cases. *J. Amer. med. Ass., 238*, 1361.
13. Davignon, P.J. (1977): Letter to the Editor: Contaminated Laetrile: a health hazard. *New Engl. J. Med., 297*, 1355.
14. Kennedy, D., Whilehorn, W. and Martin, E. (1977): Toxicity of Laetril. *FDA Bull., Nov./Dec.*, 917.
15. Janssen, W.F. (1977): Cancer quackery: past and present. *FDA Consumer, 2*, 27.
16. *FDA Consumer* (1978): Cancer Institute to ask Laetrile Study. *12*, 3.
17. Dugan, W.M. (1977): Letter to the Editor: Reactions to laetrilomania. *New Engl. J. Med., 297*, 220.
18. Ingelfinger, F.J. (1977): Letter to the Editor: Laetrilomania. *New Engl. J. Med., 296*, 1167.
19. Lipsett, M.B. and Fletcher, J.C. (1977): Ethics of Laetrile clinical trials. *New Engl. J. Med., 297*, 1183.
20. Liljestrand, A. (1973): The comparative efficacy of drugs in clinical pharmacological evaluation in drug control. In: *WHO Report on a Symposium, Heidelberg, 1972. Euro 7406*, p. 53. Copenhagen.
21. WHO (1977): *Drug Information PDT/DI/77, 2, April, June*, p. 2.
22. Craddock, A.G. (1977): Letter to the Editor: Reactions to laetrilomania. *New Engl. J. Med., 297*, 220.
23. Thompson, D.K. (1977): Letter to the Editor: Reactions to laetrilomania. *New Engl. J. Med., 297*, 219.
24. N.C. (1977): The U.S. Government and Laetrile. *Newsday, 1977.* Reprinted in *Saturday Review, 10.1*, pp. 10–16.
25. Szasz, T. (1972): The ethics of addiction: an argument in favour of letting Americans take any drug they want to take. *Harper's Magazine*, pp. 74–79.
26. Dunlop, D. (1978): Good practices in the manufacture and quality control of drugs. Basle Pharma Information, 1971. In: *Health Aspects of Human Right to Developments in Biology and Medicine.* WHO, Geneva.
27. Kaplan, N. (1979): The support of continuing medical education by pharmaceutical companies. *New Engl. J. Med., 300*, 194.
28. International Agency for Research on Cancer (1978): *IARC Monograph on the Evaluation of Carcinogenic Risk of Chemicals to Man, Vol. 1–17.* Lyon, 1972.

DISCUSSION

Dukes: Mr. Chairman, not a question but a comment. May I put an analogous European case on the table? This is the case of vasolastine which is manufactured and sold in The Netherlands and also internationally. This drug was rejected by the Netherlands National Committee some years ago. It is advertised for curing myocardial infarct, gangrene, a whole series of other complaints including atherosclerosis and so on. It is injectable and only injected by doctors. It was found to contain water and the remnants of disintegrated enzymes and was rejected on lack of evidence of efficacy and on lack of a fixed constitution. But safety was not one of the grounds of rejection. The company appealed to the Queen and the appeal was referred to the Privy Council which after some years of deliberation upheld the Committee's decision. At that stage the drug was withdrawn from the market, but in Holland as in the United States, there is a considerable movement for freedom of pharmaceutic practice among patients particularly who blame present drug registration as being a conspiracy between the medical profession and the large drug industries. The Secretary of State decided to exempt this drug from the action of the Drugs Act believing that certain patients needed it and that they should be free to use it.

This matter has not yet been settled, but it looks very much as if it will be exempted from the provisions of the Drug Act. In view of the international sale of this drug with more than 30 indications, this is raising an issue very similar to that of Laetrile, although in this case, safety does not appear to be involved. I think it should be put on the table here. One more small point as regards Laetrile, the thing that has struck me in the international literature is that Laetrile imported from the States is different from Laetrile coming in from Mexico and that it is not a constant product even when brought in from one particular country. If people are to be given a quack remedy or unofficial remedies, then perhaps there should be some guarantee that they are at least of constant composition.

Payne: May I ask for clarification of your position with respect to the regulation of Laetrile? It seems to me that in citing John Stuart Mill you were hinting that you would oppose any regulation of a drug such as Laetrile that might in fact be proven fertile by human experience. We have, for example, statutes against suicide even in a nation like the United States and, therefore, I am interested in clarifying to what extent you would argue that perhaps our own Anglo-American legal tradition is misplaced or misdirected?

Velimirovic: Well, let me first comment on Dr. Dukes's statement. Probably Laetrile which has been used in a West German clinic for many years and now in some other places, in Switzerland and so on, might be somehow different, but if it is amygdalin, if it is made of apricot kernels or pits, then, it must belong to the same group, at least toxicologically. It is very difficult to accept any claim made by the proponents of Laetrile, because the substance tested is always somewhat different from the one which was tested previously.

Now, referring to my own position and this is strictly my own, if a patient has terminal cancer, give him everything he wants, whatever official medicine says. This is my position after observing a number of children with cancer. So, if it has been explained that this drug has no recognized scientific value, that it is not recommended by doctors, and that there are possible dangers, if all this has been explained and the patient still wants to take Laetrile, give him Laetrile. Many people go to Lourdes in France. At least, in those last months or years of his life, usually they are only months, give him the right to decide what he wants to do with those that remain.

The balance between benefit and risk: The dilemma of the drug legislator

BARBRO WESTERHOLM*

Apoteksbolaget AB (The National Corporation of Swedish Pharmacies), Stockholm, Sweden

Risk-taking is part of everyday life. In order to gain time we take the risk of travelling by car and by air. For pleasure we spend time sailing, skiing, and swimming – sports that all carry certain risks. From our knowledge of the size and kind of risk and the benefit which we gain, we find the benefit/risk ratio acceptable.

Administration of drugs means risk-taking, a fact known long before the birth of Christ. Homer (950 B.C.) said about drugs that many were excellent when mingled, and many fatal (*Odyssey, IV*). Galen (131–201 A.D.) warned against the dangers of badly written and obscure prescriptions. Rhazez (860–932 A.D.) advised: 'If simple remedies are effective, do not prescribe compound remedies.'

At first it was up to the individual physician to judge if the benefit of a drug treatment outweighed the risks. A number of drug catastrophes in Western countries (Table 1) led to amendments to their Drug Acts and society has now taken over part of the responsibility for the benefit/risk evaluation.

PRECAUTIONARY MEASURES

Thus, regulatory agencies have been established to ensure that drugs are adequately tested before they are marketed. Such tests include chemical-pharmaceutical,

TABLE 1. *Examples of drug catastrophes affecting drug legislation in Western countries during the last 100 years*

Drug	Adverse reaction	Year and reference
Chloroform	Sudden death	1880 (21)
Arsenic	Jaundice	1922 (22)
Sulphanilamide in diethylene glycol	Death from poisoning	1937 (23)
Organic tin (Stalinon)	Death from poisoning	1954 (24)
Thalidomide	Congenital malformations	1961 (25)
Diethylstilbestrol	Vaginal adenocarcinoma in offspring	1970 (26)

**Present address:* National Board of Health and Welfare, S10630 Stockholm, Sweden.

pharmacological-toxicological, and clinical investigations. However, one can never predict all the effects a drug may have in man from the results of animal tests because of species differences. Some adverse reactions are rare or appear late and are therefore impossible to discover during clinical trials. It would not be feasible to conduct trials of such a size and length that all such reactions could be found without running the risk of delaying the application of valuable drugs in medical practice.

In order to tackle this problem, a number of countries have established monitoring centers to which physicians are requested to report suspected adverse reactions, so that serious adverse reactions may be detected at the earliest possible moment. Furthermore, these centers forward their reports to the World Health Organization (WHO), where an international drug monitoring center was established in 1968.

On the basis of reports in the literature, from drug manufacturers, and to the drug monitoring centers, regulatory agencies continuously follow what happens to drugs on the market and take the necessary precautions when indicated. This is usually a balancing between therapeutic benefits and risks. The difficulties in such balancing are best illustrated by a number of examples reflecting how we in Sweden have looked upon various drug problems. Although my paper is based on Swedish experience, I would be surprised if other countries had not encountered the same problems.

ORAL CONTRACEPTIVES

The oral contraceptives are a good example of a group of drugs constantly subjected to evaluation and monitoring.

Drugs containing estrogens and progestogens were approved in Sweden in 1960 for the treatment of various gynecological disorders. It was well known that the drugs were used for contraceptive purposes abroad, but Sweden showed some reluctance to approve this indication since it meant the use of potent drugs in healthy women. Here the necessity of an acceptable benefit/risk ratio was more obvious than in instances where drugs were used for diseases.

In 1961 the first suspicion arose that oral contraceptives might cause thromboembolic disease (1). In the medical press this suspicion was followed by a number of others. The Swedish drug regulatory agency reported the suspicion to the medical profession and recommended restrictive use of the drugs. Physicians were also asked to report suspect cases to the authorities. Experience abroad was continuously followed, but although case reports appeared and coagulation studies were carried out, no data proving a cause-effect relationship were found.

In May 1964 the Swedish authorities had a discussion about the advisability of a more general use of oral and certain mechanical contraceptives. There was a rumor about that oral contraceptives were available on the black market and it was obvious to all present that for the individual woman it must be safer to obtain her oral contraceptive from a doctor than second-hand from a non-medical person. The result of the discussion was that drugs containing estrogens and progestogens were accepted for contraceptive use provided efficacy and safety were proven. In a special letter the medical profession was informed about the mechanism of action of oral contraceptives, efficacy, dosage, and proven and suspected adverse reactions (thromboembolism, liver damage).

During the following year thromboembolic and jaundiced cases ensuing the use of the pill were reported to the Swedish authorities (2, 3). The authorities therefore decided to issue a letter in which increased cautiousness in prescribing of the drugs was recommended. Furthermore, the medical profession was asked to report adverse reactions to oral contraceptives to the newly established Adverse Drug Reaction Committee.

A working plan was laid down in order to obtain an estimate of the risks with oral contraceptive treatment, mainly focusing on thromboembolism and jaundice.

Thromboembolism

Thromboembolism was studied by investigating to what extent women were hospitalized because of thromboembolism and their contraceptive use. Due to the limited number of patients available for study the investigation had to be extended over a long period of time and was not published until 1971 (4). The results of the investigation led to the same conclusion as British and American investigations had come to in 1967 (5), 1968 (6, 7), and 1969 (8): women using oral contraceptives run a greater risk than non-users of developing thromboembolic diseases.

Various studies were then undertaken in order to find risk patients. Thus, in an American-English-Swedish collaborative study it was shown that women belonging to blood type 0 run less risk of developing thromboembolism when on the pill or in connection with pregnancy than women with other blood types (9).

In an English-Danish-Swedish study it was shown that the risk of thromboembolism was higher with high doses of estrogen preparations than with low dose ones although it was underlined that the type of progestogen also played a role (10). In England the observation led to a very quick withdrawal of the high-dose preparations and to the introduction of oral contraceptives with low estrogen doses. In Sweden the high doses of estrogen combinations were withdrawn from the market in 1973 when it was obvious that they could be replaced by combinations with a lower estrogen content.

Jaundice

The other problem – jaundice – was solved more easily. By inquiries to the departments of infectious diseases 205 cases of jaundice in women using the pill were found during the period 1965–1969 (11). Most of the women were taken ill within 3 months of medication. The characteristic symptoms were nausea, severe pruritus, and jaundice. As a rule, the women recovered quickly following cessation of medication. Histology of the liver showed a typical picture of intrahepatic cholestasis. The clinical picture was very similar to the jaundice seen in late pregnancy. Furthermore, jaundice in pregnancy was found to be more common among these women than among controls who had been on the pill for more than 2 years without any problem (12). The conclusion drawn from the data presented as well as from similar experiences mainly from Chile (13) was that jaundice is a risk in oral contraceptive treatment. The size of the risk with the preparations used in the sixties was somewhere around 1:4000 in the Swedish population and greater in women with a history of jaundice in late pregnancy.

The view to-day is that the beneficial effects of the pill outweigh the risks. However, there are certain risk groups who should avoid oral contraceptives, namely women above the age of 35 who are heavy smokers, women with a history of thromboembolism and women with a history of jaundice or severe pruritus in late pregnancy.

LEVEL OF SUSPICION AND PRESENTATION TO THE PUBLIC

While thromboembolism was still only a suspected adverse reaction to the pill and not a proven one, it was intensively debated in the mass media, presented as a true reaction by some writers and as a false alarm by others. Such a debate is questionable since the readers become both worried and confused by the disagreement between experts. It is quite clear that the public should be informed about adverse reactions, but the question is how much evidence should be available before publication. Two examples of false alarms might exemplify what happens when: (a) a suspected reaction with very little evidence is further investigated after presentation to the public; (b) when the suspicion is further investigated before presentation to the public.

Suspicion investigated after presentation to the public

In the Autumn of 1972, McBride in Australia presented 3 possible cases of malformations after intake of tricyclic antidepressants (14). This became known to the mass media on a Friday afternoon when it was difficult to get experts' comments. The experts whom the mass media succeeded in contacting could not say much since they did not have access to the original data. During the following weekend the headlines of the Swedish newspapers and on the newspaper-stands were dominated by information about malformations following medication with tricyclic antidepressants. What harm this news caused patients on tricyclic antidepressants we have not been able to measure.

During the same weekend the Australian regulatory agency worked hard and cabled regulatory agencies around the world to give details about the 3 cases and the agency's evaluation of the matter. Investigations were started in several places and the following results were obtained. In the Australian cases the intake of drugs was not well documented. Thirty instances of mothers who had taken tricyclics in pregnancy in Australia and 300 others from other parts of the world were not accompanied by birth defects (15).

It is difficult to draw firm conclusions concerning the risks of tricyclic antidepressants in early pregnancy, but the available data show that quite a number of women have used the drugs in early pregnancy and given birth to healthy children. In Sweden pregnancy is not regarded as a contraindication to the use of tricyclic antidepressants. However, as with all other drugs, they should only be used when they are actually needed.

Suspicion investigated before presentation to the public

In the Autumn of 1970, a physician reported Down's syndrome in the children of two young mothers who had taken oral contraceptives before pregnancy. He suspected a cause-effect relationship. At the same time one hospital in Sweden reported an increased number of births with Mb Down during the preceding 8 months. The hospital had no suspicion about the cause.

For those who are not familiar with Down's syndrome or mongolism it can be mentioned that it is due to a chromosomal aberration with a trisomy of chromosome pairs 21–22 or translocation of parts of these chromosomes. The clinical signs are mental retardation of varying degree, a curious facial configuration, and a dwarfed physical state.

The two reports led to an epidemiological study of Down's syndrome in Sweden (16). All records of children with the diagnosis of Mb Down born in the years 1968, 1969, and 1970 when oral contraceptives were widely used were requested from all pediatric and gynecological departments, all boards for provisions and services to the mentally retarded, and all cytogenetic laboratories in the country. The cytogenetic laboratories contributed 24% of the cases which had not been recorded via the other channels. The total incidence (1:755) was found to be lower than in earlier Swedish investigations carried out before the use of oral contraceptives had begun. This was probably due to a reduction in the mean maternal age at childbirth.

It is well known that the risk of getting a child with Down's syndrome increases with age – a fact proven also in this epidemiological study. The incidence in mothers aged 20–24 years was found to be 1:1352 while it was 1:67 in the age group 40–44 and 1:16 above the age of 45 years. It was only in the highest age group that a significant increase had taken place. It is unlikely that oral contraceptives played a role in that group since its use of the drugs is much lower than the use in lower age groups. With this conclusion the study was presented to the authorities in the Spring of 1971.

The remarkable thing about the study was that it involved a great many people and nothing came out about it in advance. It is easy to imagine what would have happened if the suspicion had been spread and maybe regarded as truth before the study was completed.

HOW TO INVESTIGATE

It is obvious that the type of investigation to prove a cause-effect relationship, to determine incidence, and to find out who is at risk varies with the type of drug and the type of reaction.

Since resources – especially scientific ones – are scarce it is important to evaluate the level of significance for each suspected reaction before starting a project. Resources allocated to minor problems may not be available when the real problems turn up.

WHEN AND HOW TO TAKE ACTION

Especially the example of Down's syndrome raises the questions: When should regulatory measures be taken? How much proof is needed before action? It takes time to collect evidence and in the meantime the public has to be protected.

The action taken by the regulatory agency will depend on: (1) the level of suspicion, (2) the severity of the reaction, (3) the severity of the disease for which the drug is used, (4) the availability of alternative drugs, (5) the incidence of the reaction and (6) the possibility to detect who is predisposed.

With regard to Down's syndrome, sufficient data were obtained very early during the investigation to convince us that there had been no change in incidence and therefore the investigation could be completed without any undue hurry. But, if an increase in incidence had been detected at an early stage, the situation would have been much more difficult. An increase in incidence does not prove the cause behind the increase. To find the cause, interviews had to be made with the mothers of the damaged children and with control mothers with regard to exposure to various chemical agents including drugs. To have condemned the pill because of the first two suspected cases would have been wrong since the mothers might have been exposed also to other agents. If on a loose suspicion action is taken concerning the suspected agent, one might miss the real villain of the piece with a number of new victims as a result.

HOW TO TAKE ACTION

The type of action taken can be: (1) withdrawal of the drug, (2) placing on prescription, (3) relabelling, (4) information to physicians, other medical personnel and the public.

An illustration of the first type of action is the *withdrawal* of dipyrone because it caused an unacceptably high number of cases with agranulocytosis (17).

In Sweden meclozine was *put on prescription* because of suspicions about teratogenic action in humans. These suspicions could later be refuted (18, 19).

The oral contraceptives are good examples of drugs which have undergone *relabelling* several times.

Information is a difficult thing to tackle. The effect of warnings issued by the Swedish Adverse Drug Reaction Committee is illustrated by the following two examples.

In 1967 the Swedish Drug Agency issued 3 warnings against drugs containing dipyrone (17). A marked drop in the nation-wide sales of the drugs was not obtained until after the 3rd warning. All 3 warnings were published in the *Swedish Medical Journal* and sent as letters to the Swedish physicians. Only the 3rd warning appeared in the mass media. I do not favor this route of information to physicians, but it was certainly effective. Since then, the mass media publish information from the Adverse Drug Reaction Committee – usually in a balanced way.

The second example shows the difficulty of assessing which source of information is the most effective when warning physicians (Fig. 1). Sales figures for practolol decreased following the information about adverse reactions to the drug. It is

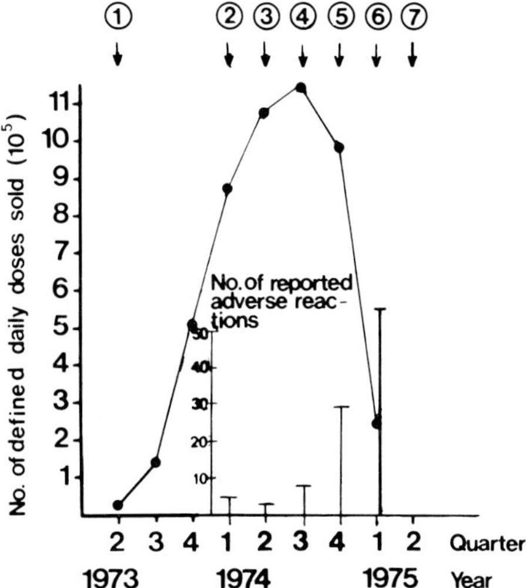

Fig. 1. Sales figures and adverse reaction reports for practolol in Sweden. 1 = NDA approval, 2 = evaluation by *Swedish Medical Journal*, 3 = adverse reactions reported in *British Medical Journal*, 4 = information from ICI to physicians, 5 = information in medical and lay press, and warning from the Department of Drugs and ICI, 6 = further reports in medical journals, 7 = withdrawal of registration.

impossible to separate the effect of the mass media information from the effect of the direct information to the physicians (20).

FINAL REMARKS

I have tried to present the efforts made in order to guarantee the public that the benefit/risk ratios of drugs are acceptable. We have to accept serious adverse reactions if the total benefits of a drug outweigh the risks. The individual patient who encounters the adverse effect, however, might find it unacceptable. We should make strong efforts to learn from occurring adverse effects who is at risk and to teach physicians to be on the alert for the unexpected because the unexpected might be related to the drug treatment.

Sir Winston Churchill has described a situation – also very true with respect to drugs. I hope we can all help to improve it. 'Men occasionally stumble over the truth, but most of them pick themselves up and hurry off as if nothing had happened.' (Sir Winston Churchill 1874–1965).

REFERENCES

1. Jordan, W.M. (1961): Pulmonary embolism. *Lancet, 2*, 1146.
2. Ask-Upmark, E. (1966): Oral contraceptives: post or propter? *Acta med. scand., 179*, 463.
3. Larsson-Cohn, U. (1965): Oral contraceptives and liver function tests. *Brit. med. J., 1*, 1414.

4. Böttiger, L.E. and Westerholm, B. (1971): Oral contraceptives and thromboembolic disease. *Acta med. scand., 190*, 455.
5. British Medical Research Council (1967): Risk of thromboembolism in women taking oral contraceptives. *Brit. med. J., 2*, 355.
6. Inman, W.H.W. and Vessey, M.P. (1968): Investigation of deaths from pulmonary, coronary and cerebral thrombosis and embolism in women of childbearing age. *Brit. med. J., 2*, 193.
7. Vessey, M.P. and Doll, R. (1968): Investigation of relation between use of oral contraceptives and thromboembolic disease. *Brit. med. J., 2*, 199.
8. Sartwell, P.E., Masi, A.T., Arthes, F.G., Greene, G.R. and Smith, H.E. (1969): Thromboembolism and oral contraceptives: An epidemiologic case-control study. *Amer. J. Epidemiol., 90*, 365.
9. Jick, H., Slone, D., Westerholm, B. et al. (1969): Venous thromboembolic disease and ABO blood type. *Lancet, 1*, 539.
10. Inman, W.H.W., Vessey, M.P., Westerholm, B. and Engelund, A. (1970): Thromboembolic disease and the steroidal content of oral contraceptives. *Brit. med. J., 2*, 203.
11. Westerholm, B. (1970): The liver and the pill. In: *Skandia International Symposia. Alcoholic Cirrhosis and Other Toxic Hepatopathias*, pp. 251–258. Nordiska Bokhandelns förlag, Stockholm.
12. Dahlén, E. and Westerholm, B. (1974): Occurrence of hepatic impairment in women jaundiced by oral contraceptives and in their mothers and sisters. *Acta med. scand., 195*, 459.
13. Orellana-Alcalde, J.M. and Dominguez, J.P. (1966): Jaundice and oral contraceptive drugs. *Lancet, 2*, 1278.
14. McBride, N.G. (1972): Limb deformities associated with iminodibenzyl hydrochloride. *Med. J. Aust., 1*, 482.
15. Morrow, A.W. (1972): Limb deformities associated with iminodibenzyl hydrochloride. *Med. J. Aust., 1*, 658.
16. Lindsjö, A. (1974): Down's syndrome in Sweden. *Acta paediat. scand., 63*, 571.
17. Böttiger, L.E. and Westerholm, B. (1973): Drug-induced blood dyscrasias in Sweden. *Brit. med. J., 3*, 339.
18. Sadusk Jr., J.F. and Palmisano, P.A. (1965): Teratogenic effect of meclizine, cyclizine and chlorcyclizine. *J. Amer. med. Ass., 194*, 987.
19. McBride, W.G. (1969): An aetiological study of drug ingestion by women who gave birth to babies with cleft palate. *Aust. N.Z. J. Obstet. Gynaec., 9*, 103.
20. Westerholm, B. (1976): Sources of information on adverse reactions and drug consumption. In: *Clinical Pharmacy and Clinical Pharmacology*, Chapter 10, pp. 153–164. Editors: Gouveia, Tognoni and Van der Kleijn. Elsevier/North Holland Biomedical Press, Amsterdam.
21. McKendrick, J.G., Coats, J. and Newman, D. (1880): Report on the action of anaesthetics. *Brit. med. J., 2*, 957.
22. Medical Research Council (1922): Toxic effects following the employment of arsenobenzol preparations. *Spec. Rep. Ser., 66*.
23. Geiling, E.M.K. and Cannon, P.R. (1938): Pathogenic effects of elixir of sulfanilamide (diethylene glycol) poisoning. *J. Amer. med. Ass., 111*, 919.
24. Wade, O.L. (1970): *Adverse Reactions to Drugs*. William Heinemann Medical Books Ltd, London.
25. Lenz, W. and Knapp, K. (1962): Die Thalidomid-Embryopathie. *Dtsch. med. Wschr., 87*, 1232.
26. Herbst, A.L. and Scully, R.E. (1970): Adenocarcinoma of the vagina in adolescence. *Cancer, 25*, 745.

DISCUSSION

Tognoni: Dr. Westerholm has correctly stressed the importance of timely release of epidemiological results and data, in order to avoid misuse of incomplete and unclear information. On the other hand, she underlined the importance of education of public opinion to a benefit/risk approach, which can best be obtained via the mass media. Do you not think that what we need first is to educate also ourselves and the authorities in dealing actively with the mass media? In many countries, under- and misreporting possibly depend on the current attitudes of the medical profession to the correct use of the mass media.

Westerholm: It is indeed very difficult to decide when to inform the public. Premature publication is always wrong, as is delayed publication. In order to get balanced information, we organize press conferences and distribute hand-outs with the facts. Usually the press handles this information in a very balanced way. It is when one single newspaper picks up news which it wants to be first to publish that the harm might occur.

Böttiger: I would like to add that we do have a positive cooperation with newspapers in Sweden. A week before this Conference, the Swedish Association for Medical Sciences held a full-day meeting for doctors and medical journalists in Sweden. We are trying to train and teach even the newspaper people and I think there have been fairly good results from that cooperation.

Shin: Are contraceptives sold without prescription in Sweden?

Westerholm: They are on prescription in Sweden. They can be prescribed by certain midwives who have had a certain training, but they are all on prescription and my opinion is that they should remain on prescription.

Ballin (M.): I have one comment regarding the fact that the harm/risk of discontinuance of a drug cannot be measured. In the United States we had at least one occasion to measure the risk. When well-meaning legislators held public hearings on birth-control pills, hundreds of thousands of women abandoned birth-control pills without having equally effective alternative methods. They, therefore, were subjected to a tremendously increased risk of unplanned and/or unwanted pregnancies with greater thromboembolic, medical, psychological, sociological and economic risks.

Herxheimer: One of the difficulties in communicating information about adverse effects to the media is that the background and context cannot be given with sufficient attention. Do you have any experience of integrating this sort of information with health education programs for the public, on TV, radio, and so on?

Westerholm: We have very recently started educational programs on the TV and they are not frequent but popular. I don't know the impact on the public in the long run yet.

Hama: Reference has been made to the use of dipyrone and many doctors did not, on the first occasion, respond to the warnings issued. What, in your opinion, were the causes for non-reaction? I am afraid that the warnings to doctors, in some cases, are not strong enough or do not have enough impact. I think that's one of the reasons why doctors did not respond to the first warnings you mentioned.

Westerholm: I think most of them did not notice the warning until it appeared in the mass media. Now I must be fair and say that the slide shows an event from 1966. The situation might have changed since then, but we have not been able to measure it since all warnings now appear in both medical and lay press.

Present limitations and future possibilities of drug surveillance in Italy

GIANNI TOGNONI[1], CRISTINA BEGHER[1], FABIO COLOMBO[1], MARIA INZALACO[1], MARIA MANCINI[1], and GIUSEPPE MASERA[2]

[1]Laboratory of Clinical Pharmacology and Lombardy Regional Center for Drug Information, Mario Negri Institute and [2]Department of Child Health, University of Milan, Milan, Italy

Italy has very little, if any, positive information to offer on how an official policy against drug-induced suffering should be established. We still have in our practice clioquinol, aminophenazone, noramidopyrine and chloramphenicol, and we have no established tradition of drug monitoring.

Our interest here is therefore to discuss two points: (1) how far the problems of Japan in the drug field are shared by other countries; (2) what lessons can be learned from recent initiatives developed in Italy with the main objective of creating a sensible and more informed public opinion in health care, and specifically in the drug field.

Before starting specific discussion I want to make the general comment that when the drug situation is like that which exists in Italy, the first step must be to try to eliminate the daily harm caused to patients and to health education by useless drugs (in one large survey they accounted for up to 80% of all prescriptions). Long and intensive education is needed to reach this goal, which is a prerequisite for giving credibility and reliability to legal and administrative measures.

THE SITUATION IN ITALY

The highly unsatisfactory drug situation in Italy, espacially with respect to criteria for drug prescription and monitoring, is evidenced by the absence of Italian investigators and health authorities in the international literature in this field. Some of the reasons and a brief description of the dimension of the problem have been the subject of recent reports (1–3). Important and quite substantial changes have been made to the legislation over the last 4 years, following pressure from inside the country (mainly development of regional drug programs), Common Market legislation requirements, and approval of new legislation for the National Health System.

The new laws and rules, however, have only made more evident the gap between what should be done and what is being done. Basically sound criteria for drug selection have been used as a cover-up in the preparation of a national formulary more oriented to the market than to health (4). Strict requirements for the approval, withdrawal and surveillance of drugs are annulled at the outset by the absence of any technical support at the central level or any policy of coordination between national and regional authorities (5, 6).

It would be repetitive to analyse the causes of the lack of interaction between the Ministry of Health, pharmaceutical industry, and the university milieu.

As the purpose of this conference is the realistic assessment of what is being or could be done to monitor and avoid drug-induced sufferings, it seemed more useful to describe the existing situation and foreseeable trends using two sets of data: (a) examples of public statements and research findings, from the recent and very recent past; (b) profile of ongoing and developing projects in the field of drug surveillance.

PRESENT LIMITATIONS

The Ministry of Health's position

Three quotations below from the official periodical *Bulletin* mailed to all doctors and pharmacists (7) give an idea of how problems related to drug-induced diseases are dealt with at the Ministry level.

Chloramphenicol
Following a vast campaign against the still widespread use of mainly fixed-dose combination products containing chloramphenicol for trivial diseases (the indications listed in the leaflets distributed to the public include: 'viral infections, measles, mumps, upper respiratory tract infections' (8)), the 1977 March issue of the *Bulletin* comments on contraindications and precautions as follows: 'already known (?) hypersensitivity to the drug'; 'drug-induced aplastic anemia can follow mainly higher and chronic dosage regimens, but is rare in Southern European populations'.

Aminophenazone-containing products
This class of products is still one of the most widely prescribed for ambulatory patients (9). Attempts to discourage its use have so far been only marginally successful, and have met with strong opposition from the industry and a carefully observed silence from the Ministry. Only after the tumorigenic risk through nitrosamine formation was underlined, was a statement released in the following terms: 'We have received information from other EEC countries that animal data show possible *undesired interactions* between aminophenazone and food components. The leaflets should therefore be amended as follows: Take these drugs one hour before or three hours after meals' (*Bulletin*, Feb. 2, 1977). As a further step aminophenazone is now being replaced by other (pyrazolone!) derivatives without the amino-group.

Oral contraceptives
The following comments are found among the guidelines given for their use (February 1977): 'Age is not a limiting factor: it should be noted moreover that use of oral contraceptive preparations can usefully postpone the menopause.' No mention whatsoever is made of the risk associated with smoking habits.

As the above quotations refer to well-documented problems and are not anecdotes, they can reliably be assumed to represent the background of reticence of the Ministry and demonstrate that little can be expected beyond wishful declarations.

Research findings

Two examples from investigations made by our group seem appropriate to illustrate the degree of awareness of drug-associated risks in clinical practice.

Psychiatric care

A survey of drug utilization of 5 psychiatric hospitals included the analysis of 2000 medical records, with a check of how they corresponded with actual practice by interviewing prescribing doctors and examining nurses' notebooks. 27% of all patients were treated chronically with neuroleptics, in most instances associated with benzodiazepines. In all, side-effects were mentioned only 24 times. The protocol did not provide for any detailed reporting of the actual rates of appearance of side-effects, though many (such as marked sedation, extrapyramidal symptoms, frank dyskinesias) were, as might be expected, revealed by the data collected in the wards.

Cardiac and cerebrovascular disorders in young women

Discharge diagnoses from Lombardy hospitals coded ICD 410–414 and 430–436 were retrieved for women aged 15–50 years for the years 1976–1977 as part of a retrospective case-control study, still in progress. Enquiry about smoking habits was documented in 20.5% of cardiac cases and in 14.8% of cerebrovascular patients; type and/or length of contraception was reported only occasionally (5.3% of reviewed cases) (10).

Comments

The 'model' situations discussed so far reveal the heart of the problem for Italy. A long tradition of denying drug-associated risks has created an unfavorable cultural background for any epidemiologically oriented surveillance. No public funds or human resources have been allocated to monitor drug effects (with the recent and very limited exception of the WHO – National Monitoring Center) (11). Technical skills are not available within the Ministry of Health, in industry or in the universities. Public opinion cannot rely on well-informed and critically balanced information when a new and/or sensitive issue is to be discussed. Reactions of denial of risk (chloramphenicol was first documented as a risk factor in 1975; see above for oral contraceptives) can therefore be expected to alternate with displays of fear (see the very recent case of clofibrate and clioquinol, for which a judicial indictment has been requested by small groups of consumers and of antivivisectionists (!) respectively). Obviously neither represents a rational basis for sound and timely judgement, or a satisfactory starting point for changing things.

FUTURE POSSIBILITIES

The systematic, progressive introduction of therapeutic hospital formularies (begun in 1973) can be considered a real qualitative innovation on the drug scene in Italy. A large number of doctors inside and outside the hospitals are adopting a more critical approach to drug selection and prescription, and this is the most promising trend on which ongoing and planned drug surveillance initiatives are based (1–3, 12, 13). The primary objective of all current efforts is to reverse the negative tradition documented above. The choice of techniques, strategies and fields of investigation is always aimed first at education, at the same time trying to confirm and strengthen existing evidence and to produce original data by research. Examples of programs activated at various levels of the health system are listed in Table 1. Before presenting briefly the specific projects, it should be emphasized that their common aim is to establish permanent and reliable networks for drug surveillance, through which to promote a better-informed public opinion.

TABLE 1. *Ongoing projects*

	Area of interest	Monitors	Methodology
Hospital	Acute cardiac cerebrovascular disease in women <50 years	M.D.'s Hospital pharmacists	Case-control
	Blood dyscrasias	M.D.'s Nurses	Prospective surveillance of hospital admissions Case-control
	Drugs used in perinatal care	M.D.'s Hospital pharmacists Nurses	Drug utilization review Prospective surveillance of in-patients
	Complications of antihypertensive therapy	M.D.'s	Prospective surveillance of hospital admissions
Ambulatory	Criteria of use of psychotropic drugs and documentation of side-effects	All health workers in 14 community mental centers	Prospective periodical survey of cases with problem-oriented records
	Drug therapy for ulcerative gastroduodenal pathology	Italian Federation of General Practitioners	Auditing of prescriptive and diagnostic patterns
General practice	Contraceptive practice	Gynecologists General practitioners Community health centers	Cohort study

Oral contraceptives (Table 2)

Two projects have been started during the last 6 months. A cohort study based largely on English experience (14) is recruiting general practitioners in all regions into a scheme designed to ensure close surveillance of data collection and an efficient chain for distribution of information. Each participating doctor receives a dossier of selected literature 3 times a year. Regional meetings are planned every 6 months, and intensive seminars for larger geographical areas will be scheduled annually, at which in addition to updated information, methodological problems will be discussed. A case-control study centered on acute cardiovascular pathology (15) now embraces 12 hospitals. The Italian Society of Hospital Pharmacists (SIFO) has assumed direct responsibility for training monitors, who under this program will also learn how to deal more generally with drug surveillance. The project has also been included in the training of doctors who participate in the program for the development of clinical pharmacology at the hospital level sponsored by the National Research Council (CNR).

Drug-induced blood dyscrasias (Table 3)

This problem has received increasing attention mainly in pediatric patients, after reports of fatalities due to chloramphenicol (8), documentation of the massive use of dangerous compounds (9), and heated debates at well-attended meetings (16). After a pilot retrospective study of cases with blood dyscrasias in all hospitals in the Lombardy Region (17), prospective collection of data has been instituted, including a case-control study on agranulocytosis and aplastic anemia as part of a large international program. The latter will include all age groups. All admissions to hospitals in the Lombardy Region (catchment area of 9,000,000 people) and the Umbria Region (catchment area of 1,000,000 people) will be monitored. The pilot phase of center recruitment, form testing and monitor training was completed by March, 1979.

CONCLUSIONS

Only in late December, 1978, after more than 10 years of debate and projects, was

TABLE 2. *Oral contraceptives*

Case-control study	5 teaching and 7 general hospitals with 17,500 beds Monitors: 5 hospital pharmacists; 7 M.D.'s Reference center: Drug Epidemiology Unit, Boston	
Cohort study	Doctors already recruited (after 4 months): 700 Points of surveillance:	
	Each point has a minimum of 5 monitors, each of whom supervises at least 5 doctors	Northern Italy: 19 Central Italy: 10 Southern Italy: 13
	Reference center: Dept. of Community Medicine, Oxford	

TABLE 3. *Blood dyscrasias in pediatric patients*

Pilot retrospective study	*Agranulocytosis* 3 cases possibly drug-related	*Drugs* (no. of cases) Cotrimoxazole (1) Cotrimoxazole + chloramphenical (1) Pyrazolone + sulfonamides (1)	*Aplastic anemia* 22 cases possibly drug-related	*Drugs* (no. of cases Chloramphenicol (8 Chloramphenicol + cotrimoxazole (1) Cotrimoxazole (3) Cotrimoxazole + pyrazolone (1) Pyrazolone (4) Pyrazolone + sulfonamide (5)
Prospective study	Controlled collection of all blood dyscrasias admitted to 100 departments of pediatrics, grouped in 7 geographical areas Case-control study of agranulocytosis and aplastic anemia admitted to the same hospitals			

the law establishing a new basis for the National Health Service approved; it is meant to be fully applied over the next few years. All matters relating to drug registration, marketing, use and surveillance have received priority, since on the one hand, much more work has been produced in this area than in any other, and on the other hand, a common legislation is being enforced for all EEC countries, pushing Italy to comply with at least the minimal requirements. The need for surveillance and information on drug risks is especially stressed. Although this official framework looks promising, the sudden conversion cannot but be regarded with some perplexity. Who is going to do the things that have been so beautifully written? The key questions appear to be:

1. *The distribution of responsibilities and duties between the central and regional authorities* The Istituto Superiore di Sanità is by no means equipped to face the tasks assigned to it by the law. On the other hand, the experience gained by doctors and hospitals during the preparation of therapeutic formularies puts the Regions in a good position to activate carefully controlled drug surveillance programs, which could be easily coordinated within general guidelines set by panels of qualified representatives balanced between the Regions and Government. The bureaucratic experience does not so far look reassuring even to an optimistic observer.

2. *The potentially positive role of Federations of doctors* has to be adequately tested after a very promising and challenging start (2) (Table 1). A rapid cultural turnover does not seem likely, as young doctors do not yet receive any specific instruction in drug evaluation and epidemiology, at least during medical training and post-doctoral courses.

3. *The pharmaceutical industry* recently went through an important phase of internal reorganization but still largely lags behind an acceptable level of awareness and research activity. The strong interactions with other European countries will

definitely facilitate the enforcement of better legislative principles. Greater and easier exchange of products to be marketed is however not equally reassuring as it could simply mean a spread of the unsatisfactory quality of drug experimentation and surveillance which (with the exception of the U.K.) is common in the EEC countries. Plans for post-marketing surveillance are just being discussed and should become effective within a few years.

4. *The role of consumer organizations* is still rather weak and confused. The multiplication of judicial indictments is hardly documented and is not followed by education campaigns. However, a more balanced view on drugs is slowly gaining ground in the mass-media. This process is favored by widely distributed publications which combine scientific documentation and popular language (18–21).

REFERENCES

1. Tognoni, G. et al. (1977): Drug utilization studies and change of therapeutic practice. In: *Epidemiological Evaluation of Drugs*, pp. 17–28. Editors: F. Colombo, S. Shapiro, D. Slone and G. Tognoni. Elsevier/North-Holland, Amsterdam.
2. Tognoni, G. (1978): A therapeutic formulary for Italian general practitioners. *Lancet, 1*, 1352.
3. Tognoni, G. et al. (1978): Drug utilization strategies within regional programs on drug control and evaluation. In: *Advances in Pharmacology and Therapeutics, Vol. 6*, pp. 101–112. Editor: P. Duchêne-Marullaz. Pergamon Press, New York.
4. De Brabant, F. (1979): *L'Industria dei Farmaci è Malata*. Edizioni del Lavoro, Rome.
5. *Gazzetta Ufficiale della Repubblica Italiana, 216*, 9/8/1977. Decreto Ministeriale, 28 luglio 1977.
6. Interregional Commission for Therapeutic Formulary (1979): Policy Statement in response to the Ministry of Health. Perugia.
7. Ministero della Sanità (1977): *Bollettino d'Informazione sui Farmaci*. Istituto Poligrafico dello Stato, Rome (See *Lancet*, 1979, *1*, 37.)
8. Masera, G. et al. (1976): Il cloramfenicolo oggi. *Prospett. Pediat., 22*, 245.
9. Franzosi, M.G. and Tognoni, G. (1979): Drug use in pediatric ambulatory practice. *Riv. ital. Pediatr., 5*, 21.
10. Balotta, F. et al. (1979): Studio preliminare di fattibilità sul rischio di patologia acuta cardiaca e cerebrovascolare in donne in età fertile che assumono contracettivi orali. In: *Consiglio Nazionale delle Ricerche. Progetto Finalizzato 'Biologia della Riproduzione'*. Rome, February 5-6-7.
11. Rossini, L. and Leone, L. (1977): Sviluppo del programma internazionale di farmacovigilanza nel nostro paese. *Rass. clin.-sci., 53*, 1.
12. Del Favero, A. (1978): Development of a regional and hospital formulary and the impact on drug utilization. *J. clin. Pharm., 3*, 75.
13. Martini, N. and Bozzini, L. (1978): The monitoring of drug use and Regional Therapeutic Hospital Formularies (RTHF). *J. clin. Pharm., 3*, 137.
14. Vessey, M. et al. (1976): A long-term follow-up study of women using different methods of contraception. An interim report. *J. biosoc. Sci., 8*, 373.

15. Slone, D., Shapiro, S. and Miettinen, O.S. (1977): Case-control surveillance of serious illnesses attributable to ambulatory drug use. In: *Epidemiological Evaluation of Drugs*, pp. 59–70. Editors: F. Colombo, S. Shapiro, D. Slone and G. Tognoni. Elsevier/North-Holland, Amsterdam.
16. Masera, G. et al. (1978): Emopatie da farmaci nell'età pediatrica. Anemie aplastiche, agranulocitosi, anemie megaloblastiche. *Min. pediat., 30*, 1463.
17. Masarone, M. and Perone, M. (1978): Emopatie da farmaci. In: *Attuali indirizzi di Prevenzione e Terapia nelle Emopatie Infantili*, pp. 41–44. A.I.E.I.P., Milan.
18. Del Favero, A. (1977): *Il Problema dei Farmaci.* Il Pensiero Scientifico, Rome.
19. Mancini, M. and Tognoni, G. (Eds.) (1978): *Farmaci e Gravidanza.* Il Pensiero Scientifico, Rome.
20. *Informazione sui Farmaci.* Bollettino del Servizio di Documentazione Scientifica delle Farmacie Comunali Riunite di Reggio Emilia.
21. Franzosi, M.G., Pisacane, A. and Tognoni, G. (1979): *Bambini e Farmaci.* Il Pensiero Scientifico, Rome.

DISCUSSION

Dukes: Dr. Tognoni mentioned a lack of technical staff in the central health administrations. Is this a quantitative or qualitative problem? Are particular disciplines lacking?

Tognoni: Both quantitative and qualitative. There are very few and they are not qualified for epidemiological surveillance. They have currently to use all their time for bureaucratic work and for nothing else.

Kimbel: Dr. Tognoni, you mentioned in your excellent paper that you have worked out a list of drugs which should be used in general practice. I believe in Italy you call this the 'prontuario'. Is it an official list or only a recommendation to the general practitioner? Is it for all patients or only for those in some public health insurance?

Tognoni: The 'prontuario' is not an official list. It was prepared by a large group of general practitioners working for 10 months, but is by no means approved. It was very fiercely attacked by the central authority because they said that any list of drugs or any comment about drugs outside the official list was confusing.

Hermann: Dr. Tognoni, the funding of programs for development of information is a problem for many countries. What do you think about adopting standard information developed on an international basis?

Tognoni: We are currently using English literature and material from all over the world. We have rules on what should be considered reliable sources, and we translate a lot. But a national policy cannot be based on translations, adaptations etc. Moreover, medical strategies and educational programs must be constructed in close contact with the cultural background of the country if they are to be effective.

Böttiger: I agree with Dr. Tognoni that hospital formularies and other such guidelines must be developed in very close cooperation with the physicians in the country where they are going to be used. You cannot throw a book at the heads of physicians: they won't use it, and they will not accept it. Hospital formularies are very valuable; we have over the last 15 years developed hospital formulary committees in all major hospitals, and they also have some kind of liaison and conferences.

Westerholm: What are you going to do about writing medical records? How are you going to improve them?

Tognoni: I have no definite answer, as you can imagine. However, some steps have been taken. The evidence collected by the retrospective surveys which I quoted in my report has been used to promote the adoption of standard forms and more rigorous procedures which could improve, at least, the 'drug' section of the medical records. Some results have already been obtained in pediatrics.

Specific attention is also being given to the teaching of good record-keeping in the clinical pharmacology training of nurses: we felt that when an atmosphere of accuracy pervades the wards, doctors will feel obliged or at least invited to take more seriously their duty to collect and record information about drugs and the events which might be related to them.

Böttiger: I think that one of the most important pieces of information in medical records is a very complete report of the drug regimen and its effect. I will remind you of the paper by Dr. Yoshimatsu from Japan which mentioned that chloramphenicol was not listed at all in the hospital records of patients treated for aplastic anemia.

Mashford: I think that the data obtained by intensive hospital monitoring are of great value but up to now it has not been sufficiently stressed that this has great educational value, not only for the people involved, but for the others. If you have some nurses asking the residents why they gave a particular drug and what they felt about the result, it has a very marked effect in upgrading the whole practice in a ward.

Tognoni: We used intensive hospital monitoring within the BCDSP as an educational tool. But it would be impossible and ineffective to use such a technique for education on any large scale. We need more flexible approaches, and we prefer to raise the interest by projects in various places and fields which involve a large variety of health workers. They will then be able to create better practices.

Non-separation of medical practice and drug dispensation

A background of drug-induced sufferings in Japan

SHINTARO ASAKURA, SADAO OGAWA, KOZO TATARA
and NOBUAKI SHIBAIKE

Department of Public Health, Osaka University Medical School, Osaka, Japan

In the Western countries it is customary for a patient to be given prescriptions by his doctors, and to take them to a pharmacist for dispensation of the drugs. In contrast, Japanese patients usually receive drugs directly from the clinic or hospitals which they visit. Thus, our system does not separate medical practice and drug dispensation. This may be difficult for physicians from Western countries to understand.

We here discuss three topics: first, the reasons why the Western system did not become established in the early modernization of Japan; second, the recent trends in the system, including the attitudes of the Japan Medical Association (JMA) and the Japan Pharmaceutical Association (JPA), the stop-and-go policies of the Ministry of Health and Welfare, and the questionable activities of the pharmaceutical industries; and third, our own views, from the standpoint of prevention of drug-induced suffering in Japan.

THE SYSTEM OF NON-SEPARATION OF MEDICAL PRACTICE AND DRUG DISPENSATION

For over a thousand years, until the Meiji Restoration in 1868, Japanese patients were treated with the method of 'KANPO-I-GAKU' (traditional Japanese Medicine), in which the doctors always administered their drugs to the patients.

In 1868 it was proclaimed by the Meiji Government that Western medicine was to be adopted. In 1874, 'I-SEI', the first fundamental law (1) concerning medical services, was instituted for the modernization of Japanese medical practice. This law, consisting of 76 Articles, declared: (1) the establishment of a health care system under the Ministry of Education, (2) the establishment of a modernized educational system, (3) a licensing system for doctors, (4) a modernized system for regulation of drugs.

In Title 41 of the 'I-SEI' (2), 'Doctors must give prescriptions, not drugs, to patients'. However, the second class doctors (KANPO-I) were permitted to give drugs directly if they wished. Thus, although in theory the Meiji Government decided to separate medical practice and drug dispensation, it is questionable whether this was really intended.

At that time, according to the survey of the Ministry of Home Affairs, there were

28,262 doctors in Japan, comprising only 5274 doctors of Western medicine and 23,015 of traditional medicine (3). As for the Western medical schools, Tokyo Medical School was opened in 1867, Osaka in 1869 and Nagasaki in 1870. However, by 1874 these Western medical institutions, except Tokyo, were closed again (4,5). In regard to the Western pharmaceutical schools, there was only one faculty, in the Tokyo Medical School, in which only 20 students studied modern pharmacology (6).

These figures reflect the discrepancy between the reality and the Government's expectation. Therefore, the Meiji Government planned to materialise the idea of 'I-SEI' first in only three prefectures (Tokyo, Osaka and Kyoto). Similarly, the second class doctors were permitted to give drugs directly to patients (7).

Of greater importance, however, were the following: (1) In 1874 the ratio of Western to traditional doctors was 1 to 5. (2) The majority of Japanese patients were accustomed over a long term to treatment by traditional medicine and, therefore, supported their traditional doctors. (3) The Meiji Government was aware of the superiority of Western medicine through the War prior to the Restoration, but for the above reasons, was not able to discard traditional medicine completely, and allowed second class doctors to continue to dispense drugs.

'YAKU-RITU', THE LAW CONCERNING REGULATION OF DRUGS

The Meiji Government enacted several laws concerning drugs (8). The licensing system for drug production was decided in 1876, the law of regulating drugs in 1880, and the Japanese Pharmacopoeia in 1886.

In the 1880's small-scale pharmaceutical industries developed in Japan. Dr. N. Nagai established the 'Dainippon Seiyaku Corporation' in 1885 and planned to supply drugs at prices cheaper than those imported. However, the volume of imported drugs increased every year. S. Shibata (9), a famous pharmacist, pointed out that the volume of imported drugs in 1890 was four times as much as in 1885.

The pharmaceutical industries in Japan intended to secure the market for themselves at the time when 'YAKU-RITU' (10) was enacted. However, it resulted in conflicts between the JMA and the JPA. JPA were against the dispensing of drugs by doctors.

At first S. Shibata was leader of the drafting committee of 'YAKU-RITU', but Dr. T. Hasegawa and other representatives of JMA soon joined. The Governmental explanation of 'YAKU-RITU' (11) was: 'Medicine and pharmacology are two independent disciplines. In Western countries the division system has been practised for the sake of developing both of these studies and medical practice. However, in Japan traditional medicine and pharmacology have been inseparable. For two thousand years the doctors' incomes depended largely on the drugs they administered. Patients also expected a doctor to dispense drugs. Thus, this system should not be abolished overnight.'

There were many conflicts between the JMA and the JPA. The main contention formed part of T. Hasegawa's statement (12, 13), April 8, 1890, at the meeting of the JPA: 'The JPA supports the new system. Should the system be enforced by law, however, patients would have to pay both prescription fees and doctors' fees, which would increase their financial burden. They would need to rely more on the governmental relief fund. I am afraid our Government cannot afford it.'

After World War II, Dr. W.H. Wandel, an advisor to the Occupation Powers, tried to persuade the JMA of the necessity of the division system. Dr. Takahashi, President of the JMA, claimed: 'If the system is carried out, an increase in total medical expenditure is inevitable'. It was surprising how closely it resembled Hasegawa's statement of many decades before.

RECENT TRENDS IN THE SYSTEM OF MEDICAL PRACTICE AND DRUG DISPENSATION

The pharmaceutical industries, which were not greatly damaged in the Second World War, regained their pre-war production levels in 1950. They continued to grow because of the increased demands of the Korean War, the establishment of National Health Insurance, and the increase in the number of medical institutions. During 1960–65, the volume of 'over the counter drugs' comprised half of all drug production (Table 1). Therefore, pharmaceutical industries made further efforts to arrange the distribution of OTC drugs to prevent cutting of prices. In 1963 the Tanabe Seiyaku Corporation adopted a policy of resale price maintenance. It was followed by the Sankyo Corporation, the Chugai Seiyaku Corporation and the Daiichi Seiyaku Corporation in 1964, and by the Fujisawa Yakuhin Kogyo Corporation and the Takeda Seiyaku Corporation in 1965. However, our pharmaceutical industries were not yet big enough to engage in international competition.

In 1967 the Japanese Government decided that a foreign investment be permitted up to 50% of all funds. Since this decision, many policies were adopted for the protection of big industries, i.e., the fundamental notification concerning recognition of drug production in 1967, the re-assessment of drug efficacy in 1973, and the adoption of a material patent system in 1974.

From the point of view of national finance, in 1975 the total expenditure on

TABLE 1. *Trend in drug production*

Year	Total*	Ethical drugs*(%)
1960	1760	933 (53%)
1961	2181	1239 (57%)
1962	2656	1471 (55%)
1963	3411	1887 (55%)
1964	4232	2382 (56%)
1965	4576	2703 (59%)
1968	6890	4883 (71%)
1971	10604	8262 (78%)
1974	16997	13819 (81%)
1977	24583	20570 (84%)

*a hundred million yen.

(Based on (1) 'Nihon No Iyakuhin-Sangyo', and (2) 'Kokumin-Eisei No Doko' (Kosei No Shihyo, 1962, 1966, 1972, 1975, 1978)) medicine amounted to 5% of the Gross National Product, and the total cost of drugs was 33% of the total medical expense cost (Table 2).

In 1973 Dr. Takemi, President of the JMA, admitted that the division system would be 'acceptable, if the consultation fee were raised'. The Ministry of Health and Welfare decided to raise the prescription fee from 100 to 500 yen, in 1974. Following this, the total number of prescriptions increased sharply and the number of dispensing pharmacists also increased (Table 3).

However, the development of the division system is affected by a number of political and economic factors and, at present, it is too early to predict its rate of growth.

IS THE DIVISION SYSTEM REALLY USEFUL FOR THE PREVENTION OF DRUG-INDUCED SUFFERINGS?

There have been many drug-induced sufferings in Japan, for example SMON and chloroquine retinopathy, which were said to be caused by excessive and long-term use of the drug (14). There is not enough evidence to determine whether the division system reduces the consumption of drugs. It is even more difficult to predict whether it will reduce drug-induced sufferings.

Is it essential for the prevention of drug-induced sufferings that the doctor and pharmacist practice separately in medical care? Is it not more important that the

TABLE 2. *Average medical expenditure and drug expenditure in health insurance payments (per patient per month)*

Year	Total*	Drug expenditure*(%)
1960	1263	303 (24%)
1963	1859	606 (33%)
1966	2766	1055 (38%)
1969	3814	1502 (39%)
1972	5587	2100 (38%)
1975	8499	2807 (33%)

*yen.
(Based on 'Shakai-Iryo Chosa' (Ministry of Health and Welfare, 1966, 1969, 1975))

TABLE 3. *Total drug expenditure at insurance pharmacies and number of prescriptions*

Year	Drug expenditure*	Number of prescriptions
1965	32.6	3744901
1967	40.8	4469072
1969	49.8	4738426
1971	64.8	4743493
1973	86.7	5142906
1975	261.5	14379875
1976	428.7	20205028

*a hundred million yen.
(Based on 'Kokumin-Eisei No Doko' (Kosei No Shihyo, 1978))

members of the medical team, including the doctor, the pharmacist and others, should re-examine their respective roles?

We should like to present an example of co-operation between a doctor and public health nurses which detected an unknown adverse reaction to clioquinol (15). In 1969, a flood occurred in N. Machi, Toyama. The Health Department of the City distributed clioquinol tablets to 310 residents, with the hope of preventing an epidemic of dysentery. They gave instructions to take five times the usual dose. One hundred and forty-seven persons took the tablets. Of these, 18 complained of gastro-intestinal disturbances and 19 of neuro-psychiatric disturbances, including euphoria, disorientation and unconsciousness. The team diagnosed these symptoms as acute intoxication of clioquinol, which was not well recognized before H.E. Kaeser's report (16).

We can learn a lesson from this case. It is of paramount importance that a team consisting of medical and other workers really endeavour to collaborate.

REFERENCES

1. *The Development of the Medical Care System in Japan,* p. 14. Ministry of Health and Welfare, 1976. (In Japanese.)
2. *The Development of the Medical Care System in Japan (The Edition of Dates)*, p. 41. Ministry of Health and Welfare, 1976. (In Japanese.)
3. *Analytical Study of the Development of the Medical Care System in Japan,* p. 45. Ministry of Health and Welfare, 1976. (In Japanese.)
4. Ikematu, S. (1932): *An Historical Study of the Non-Separation System of Medical Care and Drug Dispensation*, p. 220. Genkaido, Tokyo.
5. *The Development of the Medical Care System in Japan*, p. 76. Ministry of Health and Welfare, 1976. (In Japanese.)
6. *The Development of the Medical Care System in Japan*, p. 86. Ministry of Health and Welfare, 1976. (In Japanese.)
7. Ikematu, S. (1932): *An Historical Study of the Non-Separation System of Medical Care and Drug Dispensation*, p. 230. Genkaido, Tokyo.
8. *The Development of the Medical Care System in Japan,* p. 112. Ministry of Health and Welfare, 1976. (In Japanese.)
9. Ikematu, S. (1932): *An Historical Study of the Non-Separation System of Medical Care and Drug Dispensation*, p. 315. Genkaido, Tokyo.
10. *The Development of the Medical Care System in Japan (The Edition of Dates)*, p. 368. Ministry of Health and Welfare, 1976.
11. Ikematu, S. (1932): *An Historical Study of the Non-Separation System of Medical Care and Drug Dispensation*, p. 238. Genkaido, Tokyo.
12. Ikematu, S. (1932): *An Historical Study of the Non-Separation System of Medical Care and Drug Dispensation*, p. 245. Genkaido, Tokyo.
13. Ikematu, S. (1932): *An Historical Study of the Non-Separation of Medical Care and Drug Dispensation*, p. 251. Genkaido, Tokyo.
14. Ogawa, S. (1974): An historical study of the SMON disaster. *Yakuji, 16*, 129 (in Japanese).
15. Ogawa, S. et al. (1975): Acute intoxication of clioquinol in 33 patients. *Igaku No Ayumi, 94*, 206 (in Japanese).
16. Kaeser, H.E. (1970): Akute zerebrale Störungen nach hohen Dosen eines Oxychinolinederivates. *Dtsch. med. Wschr., 95*.

DISCUSSION

Velimirovic: Do the traditional doctors dispense so-called ethical drugs, or only traditional medicines, which I assume account for the differences between the total and the ethical drugs in the production figures in Table 1? Is this proportion covered by any insurance scheme?

Asakura: There seems to have been a misunderstanding. The 'Kampo-i' or the traditional doctors existed mainly between 1800 and 1900. There are very, very few traditional doctors now in Japan.

Velimirovic: What then is the 16% of the total amount of drug production in 1977 which is not designated as ethical?

Asakura: This refers to over-the-counter drugs, which are not ethical drugs.

Shin: The problem in separating medical practice from drug dispensing is that in our country there is a continuing conflict of interest between pharmacist and physician. For example, you can get a drug at the regular drugstore, and the pharmacist can also prescribe it, at a price that is ordinarily lower than when it is prescribed by doctors.

At medical school very few courses are offered in pharmacology, so physicians gain their knowledge about drugs by experience or perhaps from pharmaceutical representatives. Pharmacists ought to know more about drugs, but how many pharmacists pursue any continuing education? If this is the present situation, and it may not be easily improved in the near future, mere separation of medical practice from drug dispensing does not seem to be the answer.

Asakura: Regarding your first point, for a pharmacist to dispense medicine solely on the basis of the patient's account of his symptoms is very rare in Japan. This is controlled.

Herxheimer: I would like to ask, if only 3% of the dispensed drugs are dispensed by the pharmacists, what on earth do the pharmacists do for the rest of the time?

Asakura: They sell over-the-counter drugs and cosmetics, but they only handle 3% of the drugs which are dispensed according to the national health insurance system.

Shiino: I am a pharmacist. About 5 years ago, I discussed this very point with pharmacists from European countries. One of the reasons why the separation does not exist in Japan could be the difference in social position between doctors and pharmacists. It may perhaps be necessary to change the pharmacists' period of training to 6 years, like the doctors', to raise the level of the social position of the pharmacist.

Problems in monitoring systems for adverse reactions to drugs

MICHIO TSUNOO

Department of Pharmacology, Nippon Medical School, Center for Clinical Pharmacology, Tokyo, Japan

The Center for Clinical Pharmacology was affiliated with the Department of Pharmacology in April, 1966. Immediately afterwards, the monitoring system for adverse reactions to drugs was established, and the Center started monthly publication of drug information for physicians. These activities have been continued to date.

When the Center opened, the School had three affiliated hospitals: the main hospital (700 beds), and two branch hospitals (each 200 beds). Three physicians from three hospitals were placed in charge of these activities. Two of them belonged to the Department of Medicine, and one was a dermatologist.

In 1966, the first year, 71 reports were received: 59 were reported by the Department of Dermatology, followed by the Departments of Medicine (5 reports), Pediatrics (4), Ophthalmology (2) and Radiology (1).

In 1967 and 1968, 29 and 72 reports, respectively, were accepted, most of them coming from the Department of Dermatology. During these three years, there were very few serious adverse reactions except for one case of chloroquine retinitis reported by an ophthalmologist.

The reports from this Center, the Japanese Department of Welfare, and the WHO Monitoring Center will be compared over a relatively long period:

Center for Clinical Pharmacology (1969–1973) A total of 375 cases was reported by the Departments of Dermatology (289), Medicine (29), Urology (10), Otorhinolaryngology (9), Surgery (7), Ophthalmology (6), Pediatrics (5), Gerontology (4) and Obstetrics and Gynecology (4). The top 5 drugs in respect of adverse reactions were benzalkonium ointment (27), ointment of flumethasone + fradiomycin (17), sulfamethoxazole (16), chloramphenicol (13), and flumethasone cream (12).

Japanese Department of Welfare (1967–1973) The total number of cases was 1,896. The top 5 drugs were rifampicin (193), chloramphenicol (71), ethambutol (63), benzalkonium chloride (29) and bleomycin (29).

WHO (1968–1973) The total number of cases was 55,657. The top 5 drugs were ampicillin (6,213), ethinylestradiol + norethisterone acetate (3,451), sulfamethoxazole + trimethoprim (2,978), and isoniazid (2,759).

The patterns of the three reports over the long period differ from each other.

Since in a shorter period, reports might be biased, the WHO's reports will be examined:

WHO (October –December, 1975) The total was 1,115 cases. The top 5 drugs were BCG vaccine (197), sulfamethoxazole + trimethoprim (172), ampicillin (152), nitrofurantoin (124) and clindamycin (78), with BCG vaccine taking first place.

However, annual reports give a different picture:

WHO (1975) A total of 5,277 cases was reported. The top 5 drugs were ampicillin (855), sulfamethoxazole + trimethoprim (748), practolol (477), isoniazid (473) and nitrofurantoin (387). BCG vaccine (305) was sixth.

In the three years 1976–1978, the Center collected 120, 134 and 91 reports, respectively. As already mentioned, most of them were submitted by the Department of Dermatology, and a few by the Department of Medicine.

Besides adverse reactions, WHO's reports include fatal reactions, neonatal malformations, carcinogenicity and drug dependence. However, no such reports have been received by the Center over 13 years.

Analysis of the adverse reactions by the Center shows that skin disorders were the most frequent, followed by general, gastrointestinal and liver-biliary disorders. These patterns are almost similar to those of the WHO.

Finally, the problems will be discussed in relation to the three different reports during the longer period mentioned above.

The top 5 drugs of the Center included three topical preparations as well as sulfamethoxazole and chloramphenicol. The Department of Welfare's report comprised two drugs for tuberculosis, as well as chloramphenicol, benzalkonium and bleomycin, which was discovered by a Japanese. The WHO's list, however, included three chemotherapeutics, an oral contraceptive, and a psychotropic agent. These different patterns raise several questions about the monitoring systems.

First, were the monitoring systems biased, especially the first two? Does the WHO report indicate the true frequency of the usage of drugs? Is a spontaneous report better than a questionnaire? Are physicians suspicious about the confidentiality of the monitoring system, and afraid of medical suits? For the monitoring system to be valid, the cooperation of physicians is most necessary. These problems should be considered at governmental level. Experience over a decade reveals the following problems in the monitoring system of the Center:

1. The budget is fixed ad hoc.
2. The Center is located outside instead of inside the hospital.
3. The staff lacks clinicians nominated jointly with the hospital.
4. There is no direct contact with out- and in-patient clinics.
5. Clinicians are so enthusiastic to cure patients that they are not greatly concerned about adverse reactions.
6. As a result, voluntary reports are biased, and it is hard to generalize from them.
7. Is the refund system of the Government necessary?
8. In the clinical protocol, besides other clinical parameters, should adverse reactions be itemized?
9. If so, is a computer easily available to collect adverse reactions?

DICUSSION

Kimbel: I can confirm Professor Tsunoo's experience that the availability of a computer in a hospital does not ensure that information on adverse drug reactions is fed into it. The same holds true for data on drugs given to individual patients in West Germany where the hospitals are reimbursed at a flat rate per patient by Public Health insurance.

Tsunoo: I think the computer is used to calculate medical costs. However, why can we not use it to detect adverse reactions? Would that invade the clinician's privacy?

Inman: I noticed that most of the reports shown by Professor Tsunoo mentioned drugs that have been marketed for quite a long time and the patterns were very similar to those in my country. I would like to ask how sensitive he feels the system is to newly introduced drugs?

Tsunoo: In the case of new drugs, since we use the spontaneous monitoring system, it is the doctors who take the initiative. Whether the drug is already established or newly marketed does not matter. I think that both an intensive monitoring system and cooperation by the doctors are necessary.

Westerholm: I am interested to know how you reacted to the information in the WHO documents. For instance, when you saw BCG vaccine heading the list, did you query those reports or did you look at your own BCG reaction patterns?

Tsunoo: In Japan we have a large number of tuberculosis patients and we use BCG vaccines extensively. They do induce adverse reactions such as a rash or blisters on the surface of the skin and so I was not surprised by the WHO report.

Shigematsu: Dr. Tsunoo, when you received the report on the adverse reactions to BCG, did you question the source of the report?

Tsunoo: No. I just accepted the report as it stood.

Comparison of the drug affairs acts of different countries, and problems of the amendment of the Japanese Drug Affairs Act in session

KANTARO NAGANO, YUKIO ONISHI and JUNRI OZAKI

Members of the SMON Litigation Attorneys Group for Plaintiffs in the Tokyo District Court, Tokyo, Japan

As the lawyers who have been deeply committed to the court cases of the harmful side-effects of drugs, we would like to make some recommendations for the improvement of Japan's new Drug Reform Act, now being discussed in the Diet.* Our recommendations have been made with references to comparative studies of similar drug acts of other countries: The F.D.C. Act of the U.S.A., The Drug Act of the U.K. (reformed in 1968), The Law on the Reform of Drug Legislation of the F.R.G. (reformed in 1976), the Directives relating to the Drug Acts of the E.E.C. and others.

PURPOSE OF THE DRUG ACT

The history of the development of medical products has been one of increasing disaster caused by their harmful side-effects. Ever since the thalidomide catastrophe, in particular, which brought about irretrievable damage to health in a total of 10,000 innocent babies of many nations, every government has made sincere efforts to ensure the safety of all drugs.

In Japan we have experienced two large drug-induced disasters – one involving thalidomide, the other quinoform. The latter, which came to be known as the SMON catastrophe, resulted in the greater number of casualties. (Therefore, the need for guaranteeing the safety of drugs is also imperative in Japan.)

With this in mind, the newly proposed Drug Reform Act should, first of all, make clear its aim of ensuring the safety of all medical products. However, a close examination of this Act has revealed that it does not have any article which clearly states this aim. This could easily result in a lack of guiding principles in the Cabinet Orders guaranteeing the safety of medical products, since these Orders will be based on this new Drug Act.

Therefore, Japan's new Drug Reform Act should, above all, carry an article declaring that the Government will make a maximum effort to ensure the safety of drugs.** On this point, 'The Law on the Reform of Drug Legislation' of the F.R.G. (1976) is noteworthy.

*The Diet passed the Bill, with some amendments, in October, 1979.

**The new Drug Reform Act clearly states that one of the aims of the Act is to ensure the safety of drugs.

CLINICAL TRIALS OF DRUGS

As the Appendix (1) shows, other nations have regulated by laws or by guidelines the clinical trials of new drugs. In Japan, however, we regret to say that there have been no such regulations, except in the case of a very few special medical products. In this respect, the newly proposed Reform Act, along with those regulations specified in the Appendix (1), should be more closely considered.

Clinical trials should be regulated for ethical and legal purposes to safeguard the welfare of the subjects who are, after all, human beings. These trials should also be scientifically regulated to guarantee the safety and efficacy of the drugs being tested. Here, it should be remembered that improperly conducted clinical trials are not only unethical but illegal.

In regulating drugs, the principles of the Declaration of Helsinki, adopted by the World Medical Association's 29th Assembly held at Tokyo, October 1975, should be included. The regulation of preclinical trials is also essential to meet the ethical and scientific requirements.

Next, we shall make some specific recommendations regarding preclinical and clinical trials.

The new Reform Act entrusts the Minister of Welfare with the power to make legislation concerning clinical trials. Japan's former method of ensuring the safety of drugs with the Cabinet having sole jurisdiction could not have prevented the unprecedented SMON catastrophe. Therefore, we think that the basic essentials concerning drug safety should be regulated by laws and the details decided by the Cabinet.

Preclinical trials

Clinical trials must conform to generally accepted scientific principles and procedures, and must be based on accurately run preclinical trials. Therefore, the trials should meet certain standards. At least the following items should be regulated (cf. FDC Act and GLP of the U.S.A.).

1. The equipment for testing should meet the standards of legislation.
2. Government authorities should be allowed to inspect the testing equipment.
3. Tests should be performed by licensed experts. The evaluations of such tests should be reviewed by an independent committee appointed for this purpose.
4. All the important results obtained, whether favorable or unfavorable, should be submitted to competent authorities along with the protocol of clinical trials.
5. If the documents of a preclinical trial are later found to contain any false statements or to have concealed unfavorable results, permission to conduct the clinical trial or approval of the manufacture of the medical product concerned should be immediately revoked.
6. In order to ensure the observance of these two stipulations, the investigators of the trials should keep all the documents of the tests for a legally regulated period. The government should also be given the power to request submission of the documents if necessary.

Clinical trials

In order to ensure the safety and human rights of the subjects, clinical trials should at least comply with the following requirements:
1. The clinical investigators should submit to the Government a protocol which has been reviewed by the specially appointed independent committee. It should include a clear and detailed description of the purposes of the trials, the number and selection of the subjects, and the duration of the trials, along with all the documents relating to the preclinical trials.
2. Clinical trials may be permitted by the Government and only by the Government.
3. The Government may require immediate suspension of the trials or a modification of the program when serious adverse reactions occur.
4. The clinical investigators may be required to recall all the investigational drugs at the Government's request.
5. The consent of each subject should become effective only when he has had a full explanation of the purposes and procedures of the tests, a sufficient description of the attendant discomforts and possible risks involved, and, having fully understood these items, has decided by himself to participate in the testing program. As a general rule, consent should be in writing.
6. The interests of the subjects should always prevail over the interests of science or society.
7. The equipment used to investigate the trials should meet the standards regulated by the Cabinet.
8. The trials should be performed only by experts qualified by the legislation of the Cabinet.
9. When any serious adverse reactions have been detected, the clinical investigators should immediately notify the Government, the sponsor, and the other clinical investigators.
10. The clinical investigators should keep all the documents concerning the clinical trials for required periods, and the Government should be empowered to request the presentation of any documents.
11. In making the required documents for admission of new drugs, all the data of the clinical trials, whether favorable or unfavorable, should be presented. The admission will be revoked if false statements or concealed facts have been found.

ADMISSION OF NEW DRUGS

The procedure for the admission of new drugs should be conducted as scientifically as possible in order to confirm the efficacy and safety of the drugs. When there is any doubt as to the safety or efficacy of a new drug, it should not be admitted.

The new Drug Reform Act, which is more progressive than the present one, specifies the conditions under which a drug would be refused admission to the open market as a safe and reliable medical product. However, if we compare the standards of drug admission of the new Reform Act with those of the Drug Acts of various other countries, we think that the new Reform Act is still deficient on this point. Therefore, we think that the following regulations need to be added.

Efficacy

The efficacy of a new drug should be proved by 'substantial evidence'. The term 'substantial evidence' means evidence consisting of clinical investigations in evaluating the effectiveness of the drug involved, and concluding that the drug actually has the effect(s) it purports to have under the normal conditions of its prescribed use. The frequent use of a drug lacking therapeutic efficacy may cause unknown side-effects which could later prove very harmful. In order to avoid future tragedies caused by the harmful side-effects of drugs, substantial evidence showing efficacy is necessary.

Safety

When medical products have not been adequately investigated under the conditions of their prescribed uses, when the results of the investigations have proved the medical products concerned to be harmful, or when their safety has not been sufficiently proved, applications to admit these drugs should be rejected. As a rule, when any serious side-effects of a drug are suspected or when there are other safer medical products with similar clinical effectiveness, this drug should not be admitted. It is important to note here that the new Reform Act only stipulates that a drug be refused admittance if its harmful side-effects outweigh its therapeutic efficacy. This, by itself, is insufficient to guarantee the safety of drugs and could lead to dangerous consequences.

Preclinical and clinical trial documents

First of all, it should be clearly required that all documents and material obtained from preclinical and clinical trials be forwarded to the proper authorities and that both favorable and unfavorable data be included. The trial reports should be in keeping with currently recognized scientific knowledge. These regulations should be promulgated and continually adjusted to comply with new scientific discoveries pertinent to the drugs in question.

Drug labeling

Drugs can turn into dreadful poisons when they are misused because of inaccurate information. Therefore, drug labeling is an essential item in judging the efficacy and the safety of drugs (cf. Appendix, 3). In Japan, specimens of drug labels should be submitted for examination in applying for admission, as in the U.S.A. Applications should be rejected or admission revoked when drug labeling proves to be false or misleading in any way.

The contents of the drug labels should also be regulated. The following should be included as minimum essentials: the fields of application, the effectiveness, the method of application, the duration of application, the standard dosage, the contra-indications, and the side-effects of the drug.

The duration of admission

The Reform Act legislates that drugs should be reviewed when their licenses for admission expire after 6 years. However, in order to examine more closely the effects and safety of drugs on the open market, we suggest that a renewal system, practiced in some other countries, be adopted (cf. Appendix, 4).

As new information concerning the efficacy and safety of drugs is accumulated daily, it is possible that previously undetected side-effects of certain drugs turn up. Therefore, the admission of new drugs should be subject to a renewal system which accommodates possible changes in the status of drugs when their efficacy and safety are at issue (e.g., European nations adopted the 5-year renewal system). At the renewal, any new information regarding the efficacy, safety, and labeling of the drug should be examined.

The Reform Act defines the objects of revaluation of drugs as those designated by the Minister of Health and Welfare. This definition is improper, however. Rather, revaluation should be conducted on all medical products already admitted, and the standards of revaluation should be the same as those of the initial evaluation. Under the present system of renewal in Japan, drugs 'whose efficacy can be suspected' and those whose efficacy has already been substantially proved are treated equally. The justification for this is questionable.

Full exposure of information concerning drugs

All information about a drug presented at its application for admission, the renewal of its licence, and its revaluation should be open to the public.

POST-MARKETING SURVEILLANCE

Drugs experience an incomparable degree of use after being marketed and their side-effects, unknown at the date of admission, may frequently not be discovered until later. In order to protect the public from harmful side-effects of any drug, it is essential that information concerning the efficacy and safety of drugs be collected, recorded, and analyzed after marketing as a basis for proper regulation measures (cf. Appendix, 5).

Collecting information about drugs after admission

The Government should collect all necessary information about the efficacy and safety of drugs: they should order hospitals and drug manufacturers to submit clinical data, and they should examine medical publications concerning the drugs in question. The Reform Act does not clearly require that drug manufacturers collect such information nor does it oblige the Government to do so.

The danger of depending on drug manufacturers alone as information sources is obvious in the case of the SMON catastrophe, where the drug manufacturers in question continued to conceal unfavorable information concerning quinoform. Therefore, the Reform Act should clearly stipulate that the governmental authorities work independently in collecting information about drugs. Drug manufacturers, also, should be obliged to collect information about drugs from clinical trials and medical publications, and submit it to the governmental authorities. Futhermore, after the marketing of certain specified medical products, the governmental authorities should oblige the drug manufacturers to conduct clinical trials, collect information about the safety and efficacy of the drugs in question, and to report this to the authorities. These obligations should be clearly stipulated as conditions for the admission of any specified medical product.

Measures based on information about drugs – Revocation of admissions

The new Reform Act defines the conditions for revocation of admissions as follows: 'The Minister of Welfare should withdraw admission if...'

In general, the regulations of this Reform Act are insufficient in comparison with those of other nations (cf. Appendix, 6). However, the Reform Act should clearly require that the admission of a drug be revoked in any of the following cases:

1. When, for some reason, there is no substantial evidence concerning the efficacy of a drug.
2. When there is any evidence that questions the safety of a drug.
3. When any false statement is found in the documents of application.
4. When the applicant is found to have concealed unfavorable data from either the preclinical or clinical trials.

The Reform Act should clearly require that the governmental authorities have the right to order drug manufacturers to change drug labels when the essential information contained on the labels has been subject to change.

CONCLUSION

Unfortunately, in recent years medical products have caused serious impairment of health to great numbers of people – so much so that their diagnostic or therapeutic values alone are insufficient to justify their manufacture.

As declared in the Constitution of Japan, the Government is responsible for guaranteeing the human rights of all its citizens. This accepted responsibility naturally obliges the Government to protect the public from dangerous medical products and from the dangerous side-effects caused by drugs. Therefore, it is imperative that the Government regulate and strictly control the commercially motivated drug manufacturers, and fulfil its obligations to the public by realizing effective policies in securing the safety of all drugs.

With the hope that our proposals will be given serious consideration by the proper governmental authorities, we would like to conclude this report by expressing our sincere gratitude to all those who so kindly assisted and supported us in various ways. We pray that our combined efforts may bring about some hope and assistance to the many people still suffering from the harmful side-effects of drugs.

Note added in proof In June of 1979, to our great sorrow, we lost our very good journalist friend to whom we owe a tremendous debt in making this report. We wish to express here our heartfelt gratitude to the late Mr. Haruo Miyano.

APPENDIX

This material comprises excerpts from the *Pharmaceutical Affairs Law* and *Drug Regulations Reform Act Proposal* of Japan regarding the following points:
1. Regulation on Clinical Trials
2. Regulation on Admission Authorization
3. Regulation on Labeling
4. Regulation on Revaluation, Admission Authorization, and Renewals
5. Regulation on Post-Marketing Surveillance
6. Regulation on Revocation, Withdrawal, or Suspension of Admission of new drugs.

Because of limitation of space, the Drug Affairs Acts of other countries mentioned in the text could not be included in this Appendix.

1. REGULATIONS ON CLINICAL TRIALS

Pharmaceutical Affairs Law (Japan)

There is no regulation. However, for any person intending to supply such drugs designated by the Bureau of Drugs, such as anti-tuberculosis drugs, anti-cancer drugs and drugs for therapy of leprosy, for the purpose of clinical trials, it is required to submit a plan of the clinical trial with samples of the drugs to be used at least 2 weeks prior to its supply.

Drug Regulation Reform Act Proposal

Any person requesting permission to perform a clinical trial in order to obtain evidence for the application for admission of a drug shall do so according to the standards as prescribed by the Ministry or Health and Welfare Ordinance, and he must submit in advance the plan for the clinical trial to the Minister of Health and Welfare. (80–II)*

The Minister of Health and Welfare may order the person handling the drug to take such necessary measures as cancellation, change etc., sufficient to prevent the occurrence of danger to public health in any way. (80–II–3)**

2. REGULATIONS ON ADMISSION AUTHORIZATION OF NEW DRUGS

Pharmaceutical Affairs Law (Japan)

In the case where an application has been made for manufacture of drugs or quasi-drugs which are not recognized in the Japanese Pharmacopeia by any person who intends to manufacture them, the Minister or Health and Welfare shall, after investigation of the name, ingredients, quantity, dosage, efficacy, effect, etc., thereof, give approval for each item. (14–1)

The person who has obtained approval under the preceding paragraph may, in case he intends to change a part of the matter or matters approved with respect to said item, request approval in regard to such change. (14–2)

*Article 80–2
**Article 80–2, Paragraph 3

Conditions may be attached to the licenses or approvals under the provisions of this Law.

The conditions under the preceding paragraph shall be limited to those of the minimum degree necessary to prevent the occurrence of injury to health and sanitation, and shall be such as not to impose unreasonable obligation on persons who obtain the license. (79)

Drug Regulation Reform Act Proposal

In the case where an application has been made for manufacture of drugs by any person who intends to manufacture them, the Minister of Health and Welfare shall give approval for each item. (14–1)
The Minister of Health and Welfare shall investigate the name, ingredients, quantity, dosage, efficacy, effect, etc.* of the drug before granting admission. Admission shall not be granted if:
1. The drug is not recognized to have the efficacy and effect as stated in the application.
2. The drug has far more harmful effects compared to its efficacy and effect so that the drug is recognized to have no value for medical use.
3. The drug is considered inadequate as prescribed by the Ministry of Health and Welfare Ordinance. (14–2–1, 2, 3)

Any person seeking admission must submit with his application the necessary informational documents as regulated by the Ministry of Health and Welfare. (14–3)

If a change in a section of an application already authorized is necessary, that section of the change in the application may be submitted for admission. (14–4)

3. REGULATIONS ON LABELING

Pharmaceutical Affairs Law (Japan)

Drugs shall have in the attached paper or on their container or wrapper a statement on such matters as enumerated in the following respective items:
1. Precautions necessary for the use and handling thereof, such as usage and dosage;
2, 3, 4 omitted. (52)

[The clause concerning precautions necessary for the use of a drug include the warning of side-effects, contraindications and other special precautions (cf. Guideline of Ministry of Health and Welfare).]

There shall not be stated on the paper attached to drugs, container or wrapper (including the inner wrapper) thereof or on the drugs themselves, any matter which is false or likely to lead to misunderstanding of said drugs, any efficacy or effect which has not been approved under the provision of Article 14, or any usage, dosage or duration for use which is dangerous from the health and sanitation point of view. (54)

Drugs violating the provision of Articles 52 and 54 shall not be sold, supplied or stored or exhibited for the purpose of sale or supply. (55)

Drug Regulation Reform Act Proposal

Same as stated in the *Pharmaceutical Affairs Law.*

*In the new Drug Reform Act, 'the side-effects of drugs' is also listed here.
**In the new Reform Act, a clause concerning 'the duration of the application of the drugs' is added.

4. REGULATIONS ON REVALUATION, ADMISSION AUTHORIZATION, AND RENEWALS

Pharmaceutical Affairs Law (Japan)

There is no regulation by Law.

According to the guideline set by the Ministry of Health and Welfare, since 1971, revaluations of drugs have been carried out according to their categories of application or active constituents.

Drug Regulation Reform Act Proposal

Application for revaluation of new drugs shall be submitted within three months after the completion of a period of six years as from the date of the admission with those documents prescribed by the Ministry of Health and Welfare Ordinance.

Upon revaluation of the drug, the Minister of Health and Welfare shall confirm that there are no grounds for refusal (14–II).

Drugs designated by the Minister of Health and Welfare shall be revaluated by the Minister. The drug shall be revaluated in the light of scientific knowledge currently prevailing at the time when the drug is revaluated on the condition that there are no grounds for refusal. (14–III).

5. REGULATIONS ON POST-MARKETING SURVEILLANCE

Pharmaceutical Affairs Law (Japan)

There is no regulation.

The law contains no direct article regulating post-marketing surveillance of drugs. However, in the case of new drugs, the Minister may impose conditions that the applicant for the new drug shall collect the information relating to the side-effects and notify the Ministry of this information. Ordinarily, the drug manufacturer notifies the Ministry of such information relating to the side-effects according to the guidelines set by the Ministry of Health and Welfare. (cf. Guidelines of Ministry of Health and Welfare)

Drug Regulation Reform Act Proposal

Doctors or others who are dealing with drugs in their business and profession shall make an effort to cooperate with drug manufacturers in collecting the information necessary for adequate usage of the drug. (77–II)

The manufacturer who has been granted admission authorization to manufacture the new drug shall, as prescribed by the Ministry of Health and Welfare Ordinance, make further investigations concerning the usage of the drug, and shall report the results of the examinations to the Minister of Health and Welfare. (14–II–4)

6. REGULATIONS ON REVOCATION, WITHDRAWAL, OR SUSPENSION OF ADMISSION OF NEW DRUGS

Pharmaceutical Affairs Law (Japan)

There is no regulation by Law.

Such measures as suspension of marketing, renouncement of admission etc. are taken in accordance with the guidance of the Ministry of Health and Welfare.

Drug Regulation Reform Act Proposal

The Minister of Health and Welfare shall revoke an admission of a drug if he finds one of the grounds for refusal, which has subsequently developed or existed at the time of its issuance. (74–II–1)

The Minister may revoke or change a part of an admission if he finds:
1. that it is necessary to change a part of the matter admitted for preventing any danger to public health;
2. that all or part of necessary documents for the revaluation of the drug are not submitted by the manufacturer on time, or that false information is stated in the submitted documents;
3. that the admitted medical product has not been manufactured or imported for a period of over three years. (74–II–2, 3)

In the case of revocation or changing of a part of an admission the Minister may order the applicant to take such necessary measures as recalling, etc.

If a person who has received an order from the Minister of Health and Welfare does not obey such orders, or if it is urgently necessary, the Minister may cause a competent official to destroy such articles in question, withdraw them from the market, or take other necessary measures. (70)

The Minister of Health and Welfare may order the person handling a drug to take such measures as suspension of the selling or supplying of the drug and other necessary measures sufficient to prevent the occurrence of danger to public health. (69–II)

DISCUSSION

Dukes: In The Netherlands as in Japan, we have been rather slow to introduce legislation in respect of clinical trials. In fact, we have not yet introduced this, although it is in preparation. I want to emphasise that when you attempt to learn from the experience of countries which have already done this, it is very necessary to define what you are trying to do. No one wants to inhibit bona-fide research by unnecessary regulations and unnecessary bureaucracy.

In your own country, Mr. Nagano, you find there are two main problems. The first is that clinical trials may actually harm patients and the second is that they may be useless.

Now, as far as the harm is concerned in our country, we were pleasantly surprised to find very little. Both drug companies and investigators are far too cautious and perhaps far too afraid of the legal consequences to take unnecessary risks. On the other hand, the performance of entirely useless research, or pseudo-research, which is intended simply to produce publications to give the superficial impression that a drug is efficacious and safe, is an alarming problem. It is a waste of clinical capacity and space in the journals.

Our proposed solution in The Netherlands is to avoid, as far as possible, completely centralized control of clinical trials. There will be central approval of the drug before it goes to clinical trial, as in Britain and in the United States. But quite separate from this, the protocol for individual investigations can always be approved by local committees. This not only speeds things up, but also has an important educational merit. If, within any region, the physicians themselves have to form a committee to decide whether a protocol is acceptable, they will have to distinguish meaningful from meaningless research.

Kimbel: I fully agree with Dr. Dukes that too stringent regulation of clinical trials may impede progress in pharmacotherapy, provided all essential prerequisites are met, e.g. peer review or governmental approval of protocol, informed consent of patients, and full disclosure of negative results. As yet, no guidelines have been issued in the F.R.G., as provided for in the new German Drug Law which became effective on January 1, 1978. Almost all university medical faculties have, however, already established Ethical or Peer Committees to approve protocols for all research on human beings. The Federal Council of Physicians recently resolved to establish Ethical Committees within all State Councils of Physicians and proposed to the Federal Government the adoption of the WHO guidelines on clinical evaluation as the regulations required by the new German Drug Law. There is still a striking lack of clinical pharmacologists in the F.R.G. Clinical trials are relatively safe due to the constant expert supervision of patients or volunteers; the risk of a disaster is much greater after a drug is put on the market. An up-to-date drug law should therefore contain provisions for proper post-marketing surveillance of drugs. A comprehensive drug law should also ensure that complete, balanced and objective information is received by both the physician and the patient. The information for the patients (package inserts or leaflets given with the drug) should be intelligible to them and contain clear instructions on what to do when adverse effects occur, but avoid listing all possible side-effects simply for legal reasons, as this might induce the patient not to take the drug; the rate of non-compliance is alarmingly high in several countries.

Johnson: It is good to know that countries such as The Netherlands are extending controls to clinical investigations. The use of local committees would certainly be very valuable in educating their members. However, I would like to point out that review by local committees has not been successful for improvement of protocols in the United States. There have been two major studies of institutional review boards, as they are called in the U.S.A., by Bernard Barber and by Bradford Gray. In both it was noted that, while committees will intervene to alter informed consent forms, they do not monitor protocols for their scientific usefulness. There are two reasons for this failure. First, members of local committees usually lack the expertise in biostatistics, experimental design and other specialities necessary to review protocols. In contrast, physicians employed by the Food and Drug Administration normally have these skills. Secondly, members of local committees are reluctant to criticise each other. Professional criticism is not a highly-accepted behavior within the same medical fraternity. Therefore, if a country decides to rely on local review of protocols, it is important that the committees have some ‘outsiders’ as members.

Böttiger: With regard to control of clinical trials, we have in Sweden a combination of local and central approval. There are 7 local committees in the central regional hospitals of Sweden’s 7 health care regions, and there is the central approval committee within the Department of Drugs. The local committees are mainly concerned with the ethical aspects.

I would also like to point out to Mr. Nagano, who stated that the government must itself collect information, that the government cannot know where to find information, especially early suspicions of adverse reactions, if the doctors are not required to report such reactions.

Tognoni: I strongly support the approach of Dr. Dukes and Dr. Böttiger. A further comment however seems to be needed in relation to countries like Italy, Japan, Germany and others, where for a long time ahead we shall be deficient in the necessary expertise. Procedures should be envisaged for intensive monitoring of the quality of the evaluations made by various regional committees. All too commonly, at least in our country, protocols and papers are certified by 'academic authorities' which do not have any scientific acceptability, but which constitute the documentation accepted for approval and for advertising. Some measure should be devised whereby independent peer bodies include members with accredited expertise in the field of clinical trials and/or drug evaluation.

Iodochlorhydroxyquin tablets and their governmental control in the Japanese market

KIYOSHI YAMASHITA

Attorney-at-Law, Japanese Society for Hygiene, Osaka, Japan

In certain countries the use of certain drugs is regulated from the viewpoint of safety, while in others it is not. This difference in attitude may be explained as arising from the relation between (a) the pharmaceutical industry intent on producing and selling its merchandise for profit, although fully aware of the possible risks involved in its own products and (b) the nation as a whole claiming the preservation of human life and health. Therefore in countries where the nation's demand for governmental control over the drug industry is not strong enough, the government is not likely to keep strict control of regulations.

This is the case with iodochlorhydroxyquin (chinoform) and allied compounds. The use of chinoform is now subject to strict governmental regulations in advanced nations but in developing African countries (e.g. Morocco, Tanzania, Egypt, Lesotho, Malta), in the Middle East (e.g. Lebanon, Jordan), in South-East Asia (e.g. India, Malaysia, Sri Lanka), and in Latin America (e.g. Equador, Guatemala, Brazil), such regulations are limited. In Japan, formerly, no regulations whatsoever existed.

It will be seen that the relation of the two opposing factors mentioned above also applies in the case of chinoform.

THE SITUATION UP TO 1945

In the 1930s when chinoform was established as effective for the cure of amebic dysentery, it had sufficient reason to find a worldwide market.

After the end of World War I, cases of amebic dysentery increased and received attention in English and French colonies. Many cases of amebic dysentery were reported in the Mediterranean regions, Northern Africa (Egypt, Morocco, Algeria, ect.), India and South-East Asia, as well as amongst people long engaged in active service in these parts of the world. Also in the United States, especially in the State of California, many cases were found.

During World War II, this situation did not change and the market for chinoform was maintained as before.

By contrast, the Japanese market for chinoform was not consolidated until the end of World War II (1945). Some of the reasons are as follows:

(a) In about 1932, Ciba attempted to export chinoform tablets to Japan, where it expected to develop the first market for chinoform as a cure for gastroenteric disorders such as intestinal tuberculosis and catarrh. But Ciba's attempt did not materialize because the Japanese Foreign Exchange Control Order in force in, and

after, 1933 stood in the way of the importation of chinoform as an internal medicine. Other reasons were that in 1937 the Japanese Government adopted the policy of encouraging the use of home-produced drugs, and finally, that chinoform was included on the list of dangerous drugs (separanda).
(b) Outbreaks of amebic dysentery, otherwise called Manchurian, Korean, or Taiwan dysentery, were occurring with great frequency in Manchuria (now Northeastern China), Korea and Taiwan, all then colonies belonging to Japan. For the cure of this particular disease, Emetine (ipecac root) and chinoiodin (chiniofon, Yatren) were in use as a substitute for chinoform and held the market to the disadvantage of chinoform tablets.
(c) During the period from the penetration of the Japanese Army into Manchuria and Mainland China, through to the end of the Pacific War, the Japanese Ministry of Health and Welfare took the lead and produced chinoform tablets. The products were used for military purposes. At this time Ciba and other companies were under the Wartime Controlled Economy System and the formation of a market for chinoform was out of the question (the estimated output of chinoform was about 400 kg in 1939 and about 800 kg in 1941–44).

As a result of these circumstances the first step was taken to encourage SMON disorders.

As World War II intensified, chinoform was included in the war-time Japanese pharmacopeia before its safety had been established. In 1943, the Drugs, Cosmetics, and Medical Instruments Acts were passed. In the Acts chinoiodin (chiniofon, Yatren) was included among the drugs designated for consumption, and chinoform was dismissed from the 1939 list of dangerous drugs and thenceforth was not controlled.

THE SITUATION AFTER WORLD WAR II UP TO 1951

After World War II, from 1945 to 1951, there existed no market for chinoform tablets (the output of chinoform amounted to approximately 600 kg only).

Defeated in the War, Japan lost all her overseas territories and chinoform, as a cure for amebic dysentery, was to disappear from the scene (during and shortly after the War, the Japan Medical Association regarded chinoform as applicable only to amebic dysentery). At best, chinoform was employed in a small way to prevent the epidemics that were expected to break out due to the unfavorable conditions in post-war Japan (shortage of materials, lowered standards of public hygiene, and the return of more than 4 million demobilized soldiers from abroad). In fact, only 546 cases of amebic dysentery were found throughout Japan in 1950. The Korean War did not help to form the chinoform market within Japan, for the Americans demanded emetine and carbarsone rather than chinoform.

As seen from the above, for some time after the end of the Second World War there was no market for chinoform in Japan, but unfortunately during this very period another basis for SMON disorders was laid.

In 1948, with the effectuation of the Constitution of Japan, basic human rights to life and health were proclaimed. The preservation of human life and health was considered central to administrative efforts. (In the same year the WHO Charter came into effect, and the definition of health as described in the Foreword to the Charter will throw some light on the nature of the new Constitution.) With the establishment of the Constitution, the Drugs, Cosmetics and Medical Instruments Acts were revised.

But the Government acted contrary to the nature of the Acts. The safety of chinoform was not examined as it should have been.

Four reasons may be given for this: (1) The Japanese Ministry of Health and Welfare started a system, whereby any drug was given a general licence as long as it was included in the pharmacopeia, either of Japan, or of any advanced nation. (The tragedy of thalidomide is a by-product of this system). The Government was nothing other than the general agent of pharmaceutical companies for sales, production and importation. (2) The Ministry of Health and Welfare rejected the suggestion made by the Japan Medical Association that chinoform be excluded from the pharmacopeia. (3) A minor drug company, Yashima Chemicals, purchased the production facilities of chinoform from the Government. In 1951 chinoform was officially registered in the pharmacopeia. This was done by those in the Government responsible for the wartime production of chinoform. Also in 1951 the Government licensed the production of chinomin tablets, each containing about 50% of chinoform. Here chinomin was seen as a remedy for gastroenteric disorders rather than amebic dysentery. Of course, no safety check on chinoform was made. The collusion of the Government and the drug industry was only too evident. (4) What is most important, the Government gave tacit consent to the free and unlimited dosage and duration of this drug.

LARGE-SCALE PRODUCTION OF CHINOFORM, 1953–1962

By 1950 the total output of medicines for gastroenteric disorders was one-ninth of the market for internal drugs (household medicines).

In 1953 Ciba set up branch companies in Japan and launched into the Japanese market. Ciba also started large-scale production, and sales of chinoform tablets were made under a tie-up with Takeda, the biggest pharmaceutical company in Japan. At the same time, Tanabe, one of the largest drug companies in Japan, took over Yashima Chemicals to produce and sell chinoform on a large scale. (Later, Tanabe was able to recover from poor business, thanks, presumably, to the profit made from the above transaction.) In this way, chinoform first established its market in Japan. The Government gave the drug industry a free pass for the production and importation of chinoform.

Consequently, Ciba, for instance, increased its sale of Entero-Vioform as follows:

1953	38.3 kg	1958	2549.3 kg
1954	176.5	1959	3683.9
1955	341.5	1960	4518.8
1956	742.7	1961	6958
1957	1558.9	1962	8448

(In 1962, when Ciba set up its own manufacturing plant in Japan, the amount in circulation, including imported Entero-Vioform, totalled 23.4 tons.) It should be noted that chinoform was used mainly as a medicine for general gastroenteric troubles, that its dosage was not limited and that no side-effects were recognized. No attention was paid to chinoform as a dangerous drug. It would be no exaggeration to say that Japan was a hot-bed for the development of the chinoform market.

The Government was not active in regulating the production of chinoiodin and gave the pharmaceutical industry a free hand to produce and sell it. The Government also encouraged the large-scale sale of chinoform. (a) Until 1970 when the sale of chinoform was finally prohibited by the Government as many as 158 different forms of chinoform tablets were produced and consumed in Japan. (b) More than 40% of medical expenses went for medicines. The National Health Insurance, overdosage and mass consumption of drugs helped to develop the market for chinoform. The Government gave consent to an unlimited dosage for chinoform and in so doing acted in the interest of the drug industry. (c) The Drugs, Cosmetics and Medical Instruments Acts revised in 1960 prescribed chinoform tablets as digestives and widened the range of their application. (According to USP, their application was limited to amebic dysentery disorders and to use as an anti-protozoan). (d) The Government neglected to include chinoform amongst dangerous drugs.

Thus the Government, far from controlling the use of chinoform, cooperated with the drug industry to flood the market with it. Surely the Government was at fault in encouraging the mass consumption of chinoform through the National Health Insurance system established in 1955, and in neglecting to regulate its dosage.

PROHIBITION OF CHINOFORM

Eight years after the prohibition of chinoform, in 1970, the Ministry of Health and Welfare started to re-examine legal regulations on drugs from the viewpoint of their safe usage.

As is well known, Japan experienced the tragic Minamata and Itai-itai disorders caused by heavy metals such as mercury and cadmium. Governmental regulations followed to prevent them.

Thalidomide gave rise to tragedies but the responsibility was not definitely assigned.

Disasters of SMON were brought to court. It was only after litigation was brought against the Government and the drug companies concerned for the payment of compensation, and after the defendant lost the lawsuit at 4 different courts (Kanazawa, Tokyo, Fukuoka, Hiroshima) that the reformation of drug laws at last came to the fore. This, on the other hand, may be taken as a sign that the nation's efforts to preserve life and health had come to bear fruit.

CONCLUSIONS

In order to establish the safe use of drugs in general, it is necessary for nations to exchange views and combine efforts for the preservation of life and health, since drugs are used regardless of national boundaries. Also, it is urgent to repudiate 'medicinal colonialism' prevailing in countries where the use of chinoform is not strictly controlled.

It is our duty to supervise the behavior of the Government and the drug industry, from the interdisciplinary viewpoints of medical science, pharmacy, jurisprudence, economics and business administration.

ACKNOWLEDGEMENTS

Thanks are due to Prof. Yonezo Nakagawa, Tetsuo Takano, Kiyohiko Katahira and more than 20 attorneys in Kanazawa, Tokyo, Fukuoka, Osaka, Kyoto and Shizuoka, for their suggestions that were valuable for the writing of this paper.

DISCUSSION

Katahira: Already before World War II, clioquinol was used not only for amebic dysentery but also for intestinal tuberculosis. The first application of clioquinol was amebic dysentery. After World War II, the application was widened for use in gastrointestinal disorders in general, and a maximum dose was ignored. Although it had once been classified as separandum, it was removed later from the list. It seems that the Government was forced to abandon its strict policies under pressure from the industry.

Velimirovic: This interesting paper shows the difficulties of introducing laws and regulations for clinical trials and drug use even in highly developed countries. We can all learn from this story. But while mechanisms exist in developed countries to put legislation into effect once this has been decided upon, and instruments such as the EEC (European Economic Community) directives, WHO Scientific Group Guidelines for Evaluation of Drugs for use in Man, CIOMS, Council of Europe and recommendation of the Declaration of Helsinki which can easily be put to work, the situation is different in many Third World Nations, where the Government has very little control over the usage or testing of drugs.

It is a 'free for all' importation, limited only by the countries' ability to pay. The demand could be artificially created, particularly for drugs whose efficacy is not self-evident. Recently there has been an enormous outpouring of literature concerning the influence of science and technology on drug policy. But it appears that the pharmaceutical industry is interested not in supporting, but rather in weakening the position of regulatory agencies, and in maintaining the dependency of developing countries, as well as high costs (drugs sold at a much higher price than in the originating country).

Thus came the WHO initiative to promote selection of essential drugs, quality assurance and drug procurement, building up of efficient drug distribution systems and the development of local or regional production of the most commonly used essential drugs on a step-by-step basis.

For several years the WHO has expressed concern that drugs intended for export are not always subjected to the same quality-control procedures as those produced for the home market. In this case, developing countries lacking adequate laboratory facilities for drug analysis are placed at a particular disadvantage. To redress this unsatisfactory situation, WHO has sought to extend and unify schemes already operated by the health authorities of some exporting countries who issue a certificate on request to foreign importers with respect to drugs that have been subjected to statutory control. Thirty-one countries have agreed to participate through designated national authorities.

It is envisaged that the health authority of the exporting country will certify on request whether a specific product offered for export is available on the home market, and whether the manufacturer has been found, on inspection, to comply with defined standards of practice in the manufacture and quality control of the drugs. In the case of products not authorized for sale or distribution in the exporting country, the reasons will be explicitly stated and, when relevant, grounds for refusal of registration will be disclosed.

It is hoped that these arrangements will foster international understanding on inspection and control procedures, and stimulate a broader discussion of identified product defects. It is important to appreciate, however, that the scheme is concerned primarily with quality rather than the inherent safety of drugs, and that it devolves from existing national provisions relating to drug registration and pharmaceutical inspection.

In many developing countries, where drugs account for as much as 40% of the entire health-care budget, the drug supplies are not enough even to meet essential needs and the health service infrastructure required for efficient drug distribution is gravely lacking. Under these conditions it is clear that the information on the use and adverse effects of drugs after their registration, and the development of new methods to further these purposes, is inadequate. The only solution which appears to me, is for an international, non-governmental initiative to carry out an objective analysis of existing toxicological requirements, and for the WHO to organize international exchanges of data for effective post-marketing surveillance of adverse drug reactions and new drug uses.

Improvement of the law and procedures to relieve drug-induced suffering and to prevent its occurrence: Lessons from the clioquinol lawsuit and other cases in Japan

KIYOHIKO KATAHIRA[1], AKIRA SAKUMA[1], KUGAHISA TESHIMA[2] and HIDEHIRO SUGISAWA[2]

[1]Department of Clinical Pharmacology, Medical Research Institute, Tokyo Medical and Dental University, and [2]Department of Health Sociology, Faculty of Medicine, Tokyo University, Tokyo, Japan

There has been a variety of drug-induced complaints in Japan since about 1955, which has produced a great many victims (see Table 1). To solve this problem, it is necessary for the sufferers so far to be fully compensated and carefully relieved and for satisfactory countermeasures to prevent any more such tragedies to be worked out and implemented. We think that these are not separate matters. The elucidation of the mechanisms producing drug-induced complaints will at the same time indicate to us who should be responsible for promoting measures of prevention.

Taking this viewpoint and considering the lessons from the past such as the clioquinol intoxication case in Japan, we should like to make some suggestions on how the law and procedures should be revised.

CHARACTERISTICS OF AND SOCIAL FACTORS IN DRUG-INDUCED SUFFERING IN JAPAN

The studies summarized in Table 1 revealed the following three points. First, drug-induced complaints were frequent and became an object of public concern around 1955. Secondly, at the start some of the cases were 'drugstore-induced disease' caused by what are called 'over-the-counter' (OTC) drugs as symbolized by the thalidomide case; later, most of the cases were 'iatrogenic disease' due to administration and/or injections provided to patients at medical institutions. Thirdly, many victims were caused throughout Japan from the 1960's to the 1970's by the extension of drug application, increased dosages, and prolongation of administration, as symbolized by the clioquinol intoxication case.

The above-mentioned were the phenomenal characteristics of drug-induced complaints in Japan. What social factors were involved?

Kiyohiko Katahira, one of the authors, made an examination of this problem from the social scientific viewpoint and the results are embodied in Table 2. They were reported at the symposium organized by the Japan Federation of Bar Associations on February 17, 1979.

TABLE 1. *Major drug-induced sufferings in Japan (as of 1978)*

Name of drug (or event)	Year/month coming into open	Initial event	Outline (according to facts clarified)	Sufferers' action	Countermeasures
Penicillin shock	1956/5	Prof. Odaka's death from shock	108 shock deaths between 1953 and 1956		Application of shock test. Synthetic penicillin developed
Thalidomide	1961/11	Lenz's report	1,200 cases of babies (estimated) born with limb deformity etc.	Parents' Group organized. Case brought before District Courts of Nagoya, Kyoto and Tokyo in and after June, 1963	Withdrawal of drug announced in Sep. 1962, 10 months after Lenz's report was published. Out-of-court settlement in Oct. 1974. 'Ishizue' started
Ampoule-contained remedies for cold	1965/2	Sudden deaths in Chiba Pref. etc.	38 deaths between 1959 and 1965		Termination of production. New standard of combination determined
Experiment of xenalamine	1965/3	Sufferers pleaded infringement of human rights	In 1963, employees of Kowa Co. took the drug, 17 of whom were hospitalized and one died	Appeal was laid before Civil Liberties Bureau of Tokyo Legal Affairs Bureau	Recommendation by Ministry of Justice. Compensation by Company
Experiment on human subjects in Nanko Hospital	1966/3	Newspaper reports	New drug experimentally given to mental patients; about 20 persons suffered and 3 died	Bereaved families filed action against hospital	Out-of-court settlement made

Vaccinations	1970/4	Parents of affected children instituted a lawsuit	Many suffered from serious side-effects of vaccinations, mainly made by Takeda Ltd.	Case brought before Sapporo District Court	Certain conditional requirements for vaccination settled. Change of vaccine strain. Relief measures taken
Clioquinol (SMON)	1970/9	Suspension of clioquinol	Many suffered from the drug especially between 1955 and 1970, resulting in more than 10,000 patients with SMON	Sufferers' Group organized. They presented case to 23 District Courts in and after May, 1971	Sales ban. Research on cause and remedy. Out-of-court settlement made among some of parties concerned after 1977. Judicial decisions given after 1978
Coralgil	1970/11	Sales ban because drug caused hepatic disorder	More than 1,000 cases of fatty liver were seen between 1963 and 1970 (estimated)	Sufferers' Group organized. They brought case before District Courts of Niigata and Tokyo in and after Nov. 1971	Sales ban
Streptomycin	1971/9	Sufferers filed an action	Many cases of loss of hearing	Sufferers filed action in Hakodate in 1967. Another case was brought before court	Judicial decisions given in 1973 and 1978. Thorough revision of contents of package insert
Chloroquine	1971/10	Sufferers appealed directly to Minister of Health and Welfare	Cases of visual disturbance of 100-1,000 (estimated by Science and Technology Agency) or more than 1,000 (estimated by groups of sufferers)	Sufferers' Groups organized. They presented the case to District Courts of Yokohama and Tokyo etc. in and after Feb. 1973	Drug designated as a powerful drug. Precautions notified. Study group organized. Judicial decision given in 1978

Table 1 (*continued*)

Name of drug (or event)	Year/month coming into open	Initial event	Outline (according to facts clarified)	Sufferers' action	Countermeasures
Ethambutol	1971/11	Warnings by Dr. Ohtori et al.	25 cases of intoxication with drug seen even only in Osaka University Hospital between 1969 and 1971. 171 persons suffered between Feb. 1967 and Jan. 1968 (according to surveys conducted by Lederle Co. etc.)	Case brought before the Kobe District Court in Aug. 1972	Precautions revised
Vaccines	1973/6	Parents of sufferers instituted a lawsuit	1,482 persons were certified as sufferers from vaccines such as smallpox, whooping cough, diphtheria, polio and influenza etc.	Case brought before Osaka District Court also in July 1975	Improvement of vaccine, increased amount of compensation. Re-examination whether vaccination obligatory or voluntary. Vaccination Act revised and relief system legislated
Quadriceps contracture	1973/10	Many outbreaks in Yamanashi Pref.	Number of sufferers throughout Japan was said to be about 3,000 according to survey by Ministry of Health and Welfare or more than 7,300 according to survey through independent physical examination by supporting groups	Case brought before court after 1963. National Group organized in 1974	Notification by JMA. Research Committee of Ministry of Health and Welfare established

Blood-sugar level reducing drugs	1974/6	Warning by Dr. Ninomiya	500 sufferers were seen over 10 years, 50 of whom died (estimated)	Case brought before Osaka District Court in April 1973 (defendants limited only to doctors concerned)	Precautions revised. Judicial decision given in 1977
Deltoid muscle contracture	1974/12	Many outbreaks in Iwamizawa	379 patients found only in Iwamizawa and its outskirts (Asahi Shimbun)		
Combined vaccine	1975/1	Some deaths in Aichi and Gifu Prefs.	164 persons submitted notifications of suffering between Oct. 1970 and Feb. 1972	Sufferers filed action as group in and after June 1973	Suspension of vaccination
Chloramphenicol	1975/7	Parents of affected children made a complaint	Aplastic anemia was caused due to chloramphenicol	Case brought before Tokyo District Court also in Dec. 1975	Limitations placed on use including indications

From Katahira (1976)

TABLE 2. *Social factors in repeated occurrence of drug-induced complaints in Japan*

I. Factors promoting or facilitating occurrence of drug-induced complaints
1. Drug companies' attitude of pursuing their own interests, and their policies of mass-production and mass-consumption while making light of or ignoring the safety of drugs
2. Government's attitude of fawning upon (major) drug companies, and the medical and pharmaceutical administration making light of the safety of drugs
3. Easygoing attitude toward drug therapy among general medical workers, especially among doctors
4. Tendency to fawn upon the drug companies in the medical and pharmacological fields

II. Reasons why repeated occurrence of drug-induced disorders was not prevented
1. Failure to establish a scientific approach in the medical and pharmacological fields
2. Tardy response of medical workers, especially doctors, toward drug-induced disorders
3. Failure of health education of the general public
4. Lack of awareness by people of public health and human rights

The author divided these factors into two rather than one, as generally practiced, because he thought it absolutely necessary to grasp this problem dynamically in order to clarify the aggravating factors. There are many factors involved, but the primary cause seems to be the neglect by the Government and drug companies of the safety side of drugs at the time of policy making.

As Japanese, we cannot forget that, in the case of thalidomide, the number of patients redoubled because the Japanese drug companies and the Government ignored Dr. Lenz's report and continued to sell or to allow the sale of the drug for about 9 months after its publication. In addition, contrary to the rigid regulation restricting the indications for clioquinol in the United States in 1961, in Japan the indications were extended during the same period. The drug was consumed in large quantities, and resulted in many SMON patients.

Therefore, it is imperative that the responsibilities of the Government and drug companies be clearly defined.

THE PROCEDURES FOR RELIEF OF DRUG-INDUCED SUFFERING

As is clear from Table 1, the Japanese sufferers whose health and lives have been greatly damaged have made claims against the drug companies and the Government for reasonable compensation and relief through litigation or other means. But in most cases it takes a very long time before compensation is paid or relief is instituted. There remain many cases for which no compensation has been granted. For example, the thalidomide case was settled out-of-court in 1974, but that was 11 years after the case was first brought to court. Another example is the clioquinol intoxication (SMON) case, in which, although a proportion of the patients has accepted out-of-court settlement, no overall compensation or relief has yet been implemented despite an 8-year struggle since the sufferers first brought the case to court in 1971.

The reason why it takes so long is that the assailants do not readily recognize their responsibility for the damage. This is proved by the attitude of the defendants in the SMON case who repeatedly appealed to the higher court even after 5 lost cases. In the case of civil trial, the plaintiffs must adduce evidence. That is, they must prove the relationship between the drug regarded as the cause and the disturbance suffered by the victim, the degree of the damage, and the legal responsibility of the defendant. The civil suit has been the only possible procedure.

Since 1973, in the protracted course of the lawsuit, the sufferers and lawyers raised loud cries about the necessity of a system to give quick relief to the sufferers. On the other hand, the Government and the drug companies were forced to take some countermeasures, and it resulted in their beginning to study relief procedures in about 1971.

In response to the 'Report of the Study Group on Relief Systems for Sufferers from the Side-Effects of Drugs' (hereinafter called the Report), the Ministry of Health and Welfare submitted an 'Outline of the Bill of Law Concerning Relief of Drug-Induced Health Damage (tentative name) – "Proposal"' (hereinafter called the Proposal). In February, 1979, the 'Bill of the Relief Fund for Drug-Induced Sufferings' (hereinafter called the Bill), to which the findings of the Central Pharmaceutical Affairs Council was attached, was presented to the Diet. When this Bill is passed, it is planned for the Relief Fund to be established in October of 1979 and the Law to be effected in April of 1980.

The Report, the Proposal and the Bill have aroused severe criticisms from the sufferers' groups, lawyers associations and researchers. Examining these three, we feel that the relief system for which the Government is to legislate includes serious problems as mentioned below.

1. Deletion of the clause 'Health and Welfare Sevice'

The Bill states that the Fund is established for the purpose of 'providing quick relief to the patients suffering health damage due to the side-effects of drugs' by giving a medical fee benefit to the sufferers. However, what is actually provided for the 'quick relief for health damage' is 'treatment fee and medical benefit, impediment pension, allowance for bringing-up handicapped children, survivorship annuity or a lump-sum allowance for the bereaved family, and funeral expenses' – namely, only cash benefits. The clause 'Health and Welfare Service' which the Report or the Proposal once referred to has completely disappeared. Is this what is called 'quick relief for *health damage'*?

The most significant finding from the study of the SMON sufferers was their desire to restore their lost health and to make a decent life. Therefore, provision of 'quick relief for health damage' should aim at treatment and rehabilitation, a swift application of reasonable medicare, and appropriate welfare services. Of course, the object of the cash benefits should not be restricted by the government ordinance, but the level of the benefit should be raised and effected.

2. Rejection of absolute liability

Absolute liability is not adopted in the Report for the reason that it will exert great economic and social pressures upon the people and organizations concerned. Following this, the Bill has been worked out on the principle of liability arising from negligence, in which no benefit will be given 'when there is a person who is evidently responsible for compensation'. The first problem is that the relief is likely to be at a low level, should this system be made a benevolent 'system' in which the legal responsibility is separately provided. A similar characteristic was given to the relief system for vaccination cases. The second problem is that, regarding the recognition of a third person's responsibility by the Fund or the Minister of Health and Welfare, if such a third person denies the fault, the sufferer has to appeal to the court and cannot have compensation paid until the decision is made. In order to establish a truly quick and sufficient relief, absolute liability must be introduced as it is in the Indemnity Law.

3. Disqualification of sufferers before the start of the system

The provisions of the Bill are restricted to those suffering from damage after enforcement of the Law; previous suffering is to be excluded. This is a remarkable retrogression from the Report which stated that past damage was to be relieved to some extent. For whom is the relief law enacted, if the victims now suffering are ineligible? We think it only just for the existing sufferers to be eligible and, moreover, that the level of relief should not be lowered or the right to claim compensation not diminished in cases in which out-of-court settlements or juridical decisions have been made and fixed.

4. Centralization of power of judgement

In the Bill, it is provided that 'the Minister of Health and Welfare gives judgement by taking the remarks of the Central Pharmaceutical Affairs Council' into consideration when the Fund requests the case to be studied for the qualified system of application. However, when the qualification of the application system is adopted, it is very likely that a good deal of work will for long be left undone. For quick relief, the judgement of a cause-effect relationship between drug and damage should be made by the Government, and decision-making should be left to the local authority.

5. Miscellaneous points and conclusions

In addition to the above-mentioned fundamental problems, there are many points to be examined in the Bill, such as the amount of Government subsidies and the appointment of people to represent the drug companies as councillors of the Fund. As a whole, the Government seems to have no intention of thoroughly examining the mechanism by which drug-induced suffering is produced. Their intentions seem to lie only in diluting their responsibilities as well as those of the drug companies, and providing 'relief' only by a low level of cash benefits which are expected to deter people from disputes. A Bill of this kind will not only fail to bring about a real relief for sufferers, but even promote the occurrence of further drug-induced complaints. Absorbing the lessons from past drug-induced complaints such as the thalidomide or clioquinol cases, we should establish a relief system in which restoration of the situation is the central purpose. The specific responsibilities of the drug companies and the Government must also be clearly defined in the law for compensation of damages.

THE PHARMACEUTICAL AFFAIRS LAW AS A COUNTERMEASURE FOR PREVENTING DRUG-INDUCED SUFFERINGS IN THE FUTURE

Simultaneously with the establishment of the relief system for sufferers from drug-induced complaints, the Japanese Government is planning to revise the existing Pharmaceutical Affairs Law.

The present Pharmaceutical Affairs Law was enacted in 1960 by separating the former Act of 1948 from the Pharmacist Law and by modifying it. If the present Pharmaceutical Affairs Law is to be revised, this will follow its exercise for about 20 years.

In order to cope with the repeated occurrence of drug-induced complaints as shown in Table 1, the Government has taken the step of providing administrative guidance in the form of a 'Notice of the Director of Pharmaceutical Affairs Bureau', but no step to revise the Pharmaceutical Affairs Law itself. At the start, the Ministry of Health and Welfare took the stand that administrative guidance was sufficient to meet the problems, even if no revision were made in the Pharmaceutical Affairs Law. However, once the sufferers filed an action with the court, the Ministry avoided its responsibility for the reason that there is no clearly defined provision in the Pharmaceutical Affairs Law. This provoked sharp criticism as 'an action at variance to a large extent with its own former conduct' (remark made by Judge Kabe at the Tokyo SMON lawsuit, January 17, 1977).

'The Bill for Partial Revision of the Pharmaceutical Affairs Act' (hereinafter called the Bill) was presented to the Diet on March 31, 1979. It is intended to legalize approval for production of a drug, re-evaluation, monitoring, GMP and emergency work order etc., which have so far all been basically instructed by administrative guidance. This is a step forward. However, the central problem is who has the responsibility for these decisions and under what organization or system they are to be carried out.

As we have stated, we think it natural that drug companies and the Government should be responsible for the implementation of these matters. Nevertheless, there was an occasion when a clause of the original bill drafted by the Ministry was deleted at the request of industry; it spelled 'drug companies have a responsibility to offer effective as well as safe drugs to society'. Moreover, few of the provisions are expressed by the words 'the Ministry of Health and Welfare must (or should)...' whereas many of them state 'the Ministry of Health and Welfare can (or may)...', thus reducing the responsibility of the Ministry. We cannot agree that the Pharmaceutical Affairs Act should be revised in this direction. It should be made more stringent.

There are many factors to be considered. For example, the Government itself, not only the drug companies, should monitor the adverse drug reaction, and the authority of the organization of the Pharmaceutical Affairs Council should be strengthened etc. However, the fundamental issue is to alter the attitude towards the drug administration.

REVISION OF THE MEDICAL INSURANCE SYSTEM

The existing Japanese Medical Insurance System is said to be one of the factors in the Japanese overusage of drugs. This system is generally called the numerical (points) system of rating (a piece-work system) in which the total fee payment is calculated according to the kind of medical treatment or the number of times of treatment. The drugs are listed in an official price list called the ‘Price Standard for Medicines’. Because medical institutions can buy drugs at prices cheaper than those printed in the ‘Price Standard for Medicines’, the difference between cost and price claimed provides income for medical institutions. On the other hand, the numerical points for consultation, medical guidance or nursing are relatively low. We think that the existing system should be changed so that consultation, medical guidance and nursing are properly evaluated and medical institutions can be operated without depending on the consumption of drugs.

CONCLUSION

We have stated how the law and provisions for the relief and prevention of drug-induced complaints should be altered. We think the core of this problem lies in the establishment of a relief system, revision of the Pharmaceutical Affairs Law, and revision of the Medical Insurance System. They are all urgent. In the Federal Republic of Germany, Sweden and the United States, the establishment of a relief system and/or revision of the Pharmaceutical Affairs Law have already been implemented or are under examination. It is necessary for us to learn from the experiences of foreign countries and even more important to absorb the lessons of drug-induced suffering in Japan, so that we can remove the stigma ‘Japan – Kingdom of Drug-Induced Sufferings’.

SUMMARY

This paper is mainly concerned with problems of the law and procedures for the relief of suffering induced by drugs and its prevention.

Although many sufferers have been distressed for years, the issues of reasonable compensation and relief have remained unsolved. This is partly because the present Japanese law and system are full of flaws. The Japanese Government is now preparing to establish a new system for the relief of drug-induced suffering. The following points should be considered: (1) absolute liability should be introduced; (2) new relief laws should be applied to existing sufferers; (3) the aim of rehabilitating the patient to the state prior to the disorder; and (4) the clearly-defined responsibility of each drug company and the Government for compensation of the sufferers.

As for prevention of future suffering, the causes of past cases must be elucidated by interdisciplinary studies. We cannot but point out that a major factor causing so many victims is that drug companies and the Government have long neglected to give full consideration to the safety of drugs. Therefore the responsibility of each drug company and the Government for securing and controlling the safety of a drug must be clearly defined in the future Pharmaceutical Affairs Law. It is also important that the current Japanese Medical Insurance System be revised so that medical institutions operate without depending on the profit from administration of drugs.

REFERENCES

1. Katahira, K. (1976): Drug-induced sufferings and the health of people. In: *Health and Life*, pp. 76–77. Editors: Iibuchi and Nomura. Shinohara Publ. Co.

DISCUSSION

Nagano: The Federal Republic of Germany stipulates a relief fund in its legislation on pharmaceutical affairs. As far as I know, in Sweden, they have recently established a national insurance system. Is there anything problematic in the area? Are there any complaints from the victims regarding your system which has already been in effect? I would like to put these questions to Dr. Kimbel and Dr. Böttiger.

Kimbel: The new drug law provides an insurance fund for the victims of drug sufferings where neither the physicians nor the pharmaceutical company committed a criminal act willfully. This provides full protection for everybody who may be harmed by the adverse effects of drugs. The pharmaceutical industry reached an agreement with a pool of insurance companies in West Germany to cover this insurance. As with all insurances, e.g. automobile liability, there is a limitation to the amount. But this limitation is fairly generous, namely one million Deutsche Mark per patient, about equivalent to the insurance coverage of the automobile driver.

As to the second question, namely, what was done in the past for sufferers from drug-induced diseases, I may refer to the out-of-court settlement of the thalidomide victims where a large amount of funds was provided by the Grünenthal Company.

Böttiger: The situation in Sweden is very similar to that described by Dr. Kimbel for West Germany. We now have a national insurance system in operation, since I think it was on 1st July of 1978 when all the manufacturers of drugs joined together to take out a policy with the pool of insurance companies. In Sweden, there are also certain limitations. The sufferings have to be a certain degree. For instance, the working capacity of the patient must be reduced by at least 50%. The first settlements and the first payments have been made in respect of 3 or 4 patients. It is too early to tell about any problems or complications, but the system has been working smoothly so far.

Control of therapeutic drugs in Sweden

LARS ERIK BÖTTIGER

Department of Internal Medicine, Karolinska Institute and Hospital, Stockholm, Sweden

Governments and drug consumers/patients all over the world to-day take great interest in therapeutic drugs, the systems for controlling them, their availability to the public and the benefits and risks involved in using them. Governments and health authorities for obvious reasons have become more and more concerned about the safety and efficacy of drugs, and also, although to a lesser degree, of the costs of drugs. The public, at least in the industrial countries, is becoming better informed about drugs – and also more concerned about safety. One aspect of this is the marked tendency to be found, e.g., in Sweden, to turn 'back to nature' and to use 'natural' remedies (herbs, concoctions etc.), that are considered to be absolutely safe. A further step in the same direction is an overt *pharmacophobia*! Newspapers and TV programs have published so many grossly unbalanced reports of the dangers of drugs without any mention of their positive values that patients are scared to use the drugs prescribed for them and necessary for their recovery and health.

A well-developed system for governmental control of drugs – before and after marketing – is mandatory to guarantee that the public gets effective and safe drugs. The developed countries all have such systems, although the emphasis in various countries lies on different parts of the control line. Most of the developing countries, on the other hand, are in a position where they have to build new control organizations and have to look elsewhere for guidance and information on how to proceed. A valuable help in this task is a recently published international comparison of systems for controlling the use of therapeutic drugs (1).

Sweden has long traditions in the field of drug control. Already in 1913, those substances were defined that were to be regarded as drugs, and to be made available only in pharmacies ('Apotek' in Swedish), which sell drugs only. In 1934, it became compulsory to 'register' (the Swedish term for approve) a drug at the National Board of Health and Welfare before the drug could be sold – still only through pharmacies. It was stated already at that time that the safety and the efficacy of the drug should be proven. The actual wording of the law was that the authorities should investigate 'whether the composition was suitable and whether the drug had been shown to be able to prevent, cure, or alleviate disease or disease symptoms in man or animal'. In 1964 a new law, the present Drug Ordinance, was passed. In essence, it has the same meaning as the old one, although a number of definitions and regulations are much more specific.

THE DRUG ORDINANCE

The important statements in the 1964 Drug Ordinance are that a drug, in order to be registered (approved), (1) must be of *good quality*, (2) must have *proven efficacy* (the Swedish wording literally means that the drug should be 'medically suitable', which includes somewhat more than pure efficacy), and (3) *must not*, during normal use, *cause adverse reactions out of proportion to the intended effect*. Such are the bare legal specifications. It is up to the Board of Drugs to interpret the demands of the law and take the final decision whether a drug should be registered or not.

Good quality is the most simple prerequisite. It is self-evident and need not be discussed. The proven efficacy, or whether the drug is 'medically suitable', on the other hand, can be discussed at length, not to say endlessly. The official Swedish guidelines refer to 'well-presented and controlled investigations of therapeutic properties' as the basis for evaluation. It is also stated that 'no weight as evidence can be attached to undocumented claims and testimonials or to speciously reasoned assertions'. Nothing is said about the origin of the controlled clinical trials; the important factor is their quality. Thus, local trials are not a necessary part of the required documentation.

One aspect of these regulations is that *all* drugs for which efficacy can be demonstrated have to be registered, regardless of how many identical or similar preparations are already available in the country.

Another aspect is that 'proven efficacy' is not synonomous with 'medically suitable'. A narcotic drug might have proven efficacy in alleviation of pain, but if the tendency for abuse has been demonstrated to be too great, such a drug could be denied registration on the grounds that it would not be 'medically suitable'. However, this type of ruling has not been used for a long time, perhaps because all manufacturers are aware that the Swedish authorities have always been very strict and negative regarding registration of narcotics and have taken several such substances off the market (amphetamines, methylphenidate (Ritalin) and anorectic drugs).

The wording on adverse reactions is interesting in that the legislator has accepted that adverse drug reactions are a reality, and that the positive and negative effects of a drug have to be balanced against each other. The present debate in Sweden sometimes seems to indicate that one believes that therapeutic drugs entirely without negative effects can be obtained. This is – and will remain – a dream, although in Hamlet's words 'devoutly to be wished'. It is my belief that, on the contrary, we shall have to face a time with more effective and more specifically directed drugs, but with *increased* risks of adverse reactions.

It is important to realize that we have to live with adverse drug reactions – as we have learnt to live with complications in surgery – and that the patient much more often than now must be actively involved in the discussion whether a drug should be used or not. A patient with gallstones often wants to get rid of his gall-bladder – at all costs. What about the patient with rheumatoid arthritis? – does he want to get rid of his pain and stiffness, even if certain risks are involved? The answer cannot be given by the physician alone, only by the patient after an informative discussion between patient and doctor of the pro's and con's of the suggested drug.

THE REGISTRATION (APPROVAL) PROCEDURE

When a manufacturer wants a new drug registered in Sweden, he sends an application to the Department of Drugs, which is part of the National Board of Health and Welfare. The task of evaluating an application, which is performed almost entirely on the basis of written documentation submitted by the drug manufacturer, ends in a written protocol, reporting and discussing the new drug, with special emphasis on pharmaceutical, pharmacological-toxicological and pharmacotherapeutic properties.

This protocol is put before the Board of Drugs, which is a separate body unconnected with the Department of Drugs. It has 10 members, who are appointed by the crown and represent basic specialities such as pharmacy and pharmacology and such clinical specialities as internal medicine, psychiatry, infectious diseases and clinical pharmacology. The chairman is a judge from the Supreme Administrative Court.

The Board of Drugs decides whether a drug should be registered, acting upon all the documentation submitted by the manufacturer, but mainly upon the protocol produced by the Department of Drugs. The two bodies act entirely separately. The Department of Drugs undertakes a strict, matter-of-fact evaluation of the submitted documentation, stating whether it is sufficient in amount and quality. The Board of Drugs, on the other hand, has to make the final decision on whether the documentation fulfils the demands of the law.

UNREGISTERED DRUGS

Unregistered drugs may be sold only under special conditions. The main stipulation is that a physician must apply to the Department of Drugs for a *license* to be allowed to prescribe a specific amount of the drug for an individual patient. The licenses generally fall into one of the following three categories, viz. (1) drugs withdrawn from the market by the manufacturer because of uneconomically low sales; (2) drugs pending registration, when international experience may warrant limited use under strict supervision, and (3) special narcotics (e.g. amphetamines) that are forbidden and thus not registered in Sweden. The greatest restriction is applied to granting such licenses and the Department uses independent medical consultants for each case.

PROPOSED AMENDMENTS TO THE DRUG ORDINANCE

As already mentioned, in recent years the discussion of drug problems, mainly availability and safety, has been very active in Sweden. Also, the situation has been influenced by the international discussion of the so-called 'drug lag', which is taken to imply that patients are prevented from getting new and valuable drugs because the bureaucratic regulatory agencies take such a long time to process the application and to make their final decisions on approval. In 1977, the Swedish Government appointed 3 committees to study the situation and to suggest such alterations and improvements as might be indicated. The 3 committees should work with the *cost of drugs, information problems* and *the control system*, respectively.

My task was to analyze the control system, including present legislation. The work led to a number of proposals to the government, meant to improve the drug situation in Sweden.

One part dealt with the inner work of the Department of Drugs, for which I proposed a 10-point program to make the work more effective – with the main purpose of decreasing the 'processing' time of an application for registration (NDA). At the present time, it is too long – an unfortunate fact, apparent not only in Sweden but in several countries working with similar control systems, e.g. the U.S.A.

The inner organization is of little interest from an international standpoint. Suffice it to say that my program, among other things, contained suggestions for an increase in *international* cooperation in the field of drug control, for an *increased use of outside expertise*, for evaluation of new drugs – it is important to ensure that the medical specialists are in agreement with the general attitudes of the control agency – and for the use of *computer programs* to handle the complicated affair of the work-up of an application.

The suggestions regarding legislation are of more general interest. The main issue from that aspect was to introduce some possibility of denying registration on the ground that a *drug is not necessary* – there are already sufficient similar or identical drugs available on the market. In this context, it is of interest to compare Sweden with Norway which for many years has had a regulation saying that a drug should be not only 'medically justified' but also 'considered necessary'! Although the medical situation in the two countries is similar, this has resulted in a moderate but definite difference in the number of drugs available. In 1977, Sweden had 2836 different preparations registered and Norway 1933, i.e. Norway had 30% fewer drug preparations on the market. It is my definite opinion that there lies a medical risk in too many synonymous drugs – no physician can possibly be well instructed in the detailed use of 10 different beta-blocking agents! – all with small differences in pharmacokinetics and pharmacodynamics, differences which, although small, nevertheless might be a matter of life or death in an individual patient.

Other amendments to the Drug Ordinance proposed in my report were an increased possibility for the authorities to withdraw drugs from the market which can no longer be regarded as 'medically suitable' and 'registration with restrictions'. These suggestions call for a few comments.

Both stem from the fact that the Swedish legislation may be said to make it difficult for a manufacturer to get a drug through the registration process into the market, but it has turned out to be much more difficult for the authorities to reverse the process, i.e. to withdraw the registration once it has been granted. A recent ruling from the Administrative Court of Appeal has taken the position that once the Board of Drugs has decided that a drug is medically suitable, it will always remain so. This may be correct from a legal point of view, but certainly it is not true in the medical sense. We have a few drugs in Sweden that were registered 25–30 years ago. It is obvious to anybody with any knowledge of developments in the drug field that the chances are great that those drugs to-day would never have passed the Board of Drugs and been registered. The main problem is that they are ineffective or have a less suitable composition, not that they are unsafe. The quoted ruling would indicate that the Department or Board of Drugs would have to prove that the drugs are ineffective. Unfortunately, it is very difficult to prove that something does not exist!

Thus, my first suggestion was that if doubt had been cast on the efficacy of a drug, it would be up to the manufacturer to prove that the drug *still* is medically suitable.

My second suggestion – 'registration with restrictions' – would be of importance along the same lines. The most important use of such a restriction would be the use of a so-called Phase 4 procedure, i.e. a drug could be temporarily registered until the adverse reaction situation had been further clarified by more widespread and common use of the drug. Should it turn out that the fears for specific adverse reactions were unjustified, the restriction is lifted by the Board of Drugs; if they were justified, registration is immediately withdrawn. There are other possibilities to use registration with restriction, but I will not go into them now.

Taken together the 3 amendments suggested by my report would, in my opinion, give a better dynamic to the drug market – there would be some hindrance at the entrance to the market and, at the other end, at the outlet the possibilities to get drugs off the market would be greatly facilitated.

Finally, I would like briefly to discuss a few other suggestions that I consider to be of great importance, viz. more knowledge about *drug consumption*, about how drugs are used and by whom and for what. It is only with good consumption studies – conducted by and in the hands of the drug regulatory agencies – that they really can fulfil their task of providing the public with good and effective drugs without unnecessary risks of adverse reactions. And the work with *adverse drug reactions*, discussed by myself in another lecture, must be balanced against consumption studies. Let me give you two examples. Phenformin – an old drug against diabetes – has recently been taken off the Swedish market after a comparison of consumption and adverse reaction patterns had demonstrated that, although the total number of adverse reactions for phenformin and metformin was the same, there were considerably more cases of lactic acidosis and deaths after phenformin than after metformin (2). Nitrofurantoin, one of the most commonly used drugs for infections in the urinary tract, rather frequently causes pulmonary complications, that in some instances proceed to pulmonary fibrosis and death. A recent study has demonstrated that the complications from the other most commonly used drug, a sulfonamide preparation, remain at a constant level, but that the pulmonary reactions to nitrofurantoin not only have increased in number, but also and more important in relation to the amount of drug sold and used (Fig. 1). This is not the place to go into a medical discussion of this problem. I mention it only as an example of a combination of consumption and adverse reaction studies.

Finally, all measures by the controlling agencies fall short if the drugs available on the market are not used in a proper fashion by the physicians, on correct indications, in correct dosage and with the precautions and controls necessary. There is much to be done in the field of education in pharmacotherapy. There are a few academic chairs in this field, pharmacotherapy, but they are very few indeed. We need more *clinical pharmacology* – to investigate the clinical properties of the drugs we use – but we also need *much more education* in *pharmacotherapy*, how

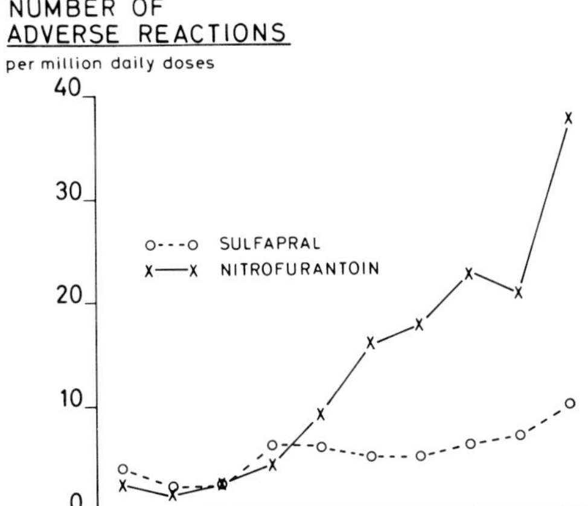

Fig. 1. Number of adverse reactions reported for Sulfapral and nitrofurantoin respectively in relation to the number of daily doses sold.

and when to use an available drug. This education to-day must have two target groups: the active generation of physicians, who never have been given a formal education in therapy with modern drugs, and medical students, who will handle the drug therapy of tomorrow!

REFERENCES

1. *Controlling the Use of Therapeutic Drugs. An International Comparison.* Editor: W.M. Wardell. American Enterprise Institute for Public Policy Research, Washington, DC, 1978.
2. Bergman, U., Boman, G. and Wiholm, B.-E. (1978): Epidemiology of adverse drug reactions to phenformin and metformin. *Brit. med. J., 2*, 464.
3. Böttiger, L.E. and Westerholm, B. (1977): Adverse drug reactions during treatment of urinary tract infections. *Europ. J. clin. Pharm., 11*, 439.

DISCUSSION

Tognoni: In order to have a more complete and realistic picture of the type of work performed by the Department of Drugs, would you please comment briefly on: (1) How many people are actually working in the Department, and what are their qualifications? (2) How many manufacturers are submitting applications for drug registration? This information would be of interest for countries (like Japan, Germany, Italy, which are represented in today's session) where many firms are present and the work required would be rather heavy, and possibly difficult because of pressure from industry and lack of appropriate manpower.

Böttiger: Well, in the Department of Drugs, there are approximately 125–130 people at the present time. There are at least 15 M.D.'s with academic training, while 4 have the status of full professor. There are also a number of trained pharmacists to help in the evaluation of the applications.

With regard to the number of companies, we have close to 10 major companies in Sweden, although only 4 or 5 of them are making serious and extensive research. Additionally, there are some 50 foreign manufacturers represented in Sweden. The number of applications, at the present time, is around 250 a year for new drug approvals.

Tognoni: I would like to add that we have already introduced rather severe regulations for clinical trials, and we are making them even more strict as from January 1st of next year.

The activities of the Federal Chamber of Physicians of West Germany in preventing drug-induced suffering

KARL H. KIMBEL

Drug Commission of the German Medical Profession, Cologne, Federal Republic of Germany

The suspicion that the occurrence of aplastic anaemia and the administration of chloramphenicol may be more than coincidental led to the chain of events which culminated in the United States in the establishment of the Adverse Reactions Registry of the American Medical Association in 1952. In the Federal Republic of Germany the adverse effects of a thorium-X-containing preparation, which was even recommended for use in children, and the abuse of appetite suppressants induced the Drug Commission of the Federal Chamber of Physicians, which was established in 1950 as a successor to the Drug Commission of the German Society for Internal Medicine dating back to 1911, to issue warnings to all physicians and to call on them in 1958 for the first time to report adverse drug reactions to the secretariat of the Drug Commission. However, it took another 2 years and a full day of discussion on drug-induced diseases at the Annual Meeting of the German Society for Internal Medicine in 1961 before the spontaneous monitoring system became operative in the Federal Republic. Understandably, when the thalidomide disaster became evident late in November 1961, it could not have contributed much to its discovery. If it were not for the serendipity and perseverance of Professor Lenz, whom we have the honour to have among us, many thousands more children in the Federal Republic would be cripples now and the catastrophe would have spread to many more countries.

From humble beginnings, the spontaneous monitoring system for adverse drug reactions in the Federal Republic of Germany grew to contribute today the second-largest number of reports to the Research Centre for International Monitoring of Adverse Reactions to Drugs of the World Health Organization (RCIMARD). Until last year the Drug Commission received some support from the Federal Government for maintaining its Monitoring System in the public's best interest. After cancellation of this support for administrative reasons, our commission is now financed exclusively by contributions from the two main professional organizations. There are especially no grants from the pharmaceutical industry; we maintain, however, close scientific relations with the Drug Safety Departments of most ethical drug companies.

Where does our information come from and how do we secure a continuous input? At present, we have about 3,500 physicians on file, who report regularly. A breakdown according to specialities is given in Table 1. General practitioners and

TABLE 1. *Reports according to disciplines (1967–1976)*

	In hospital	In private practice
General practice	—	1,574
Internal medicine	1,045	629
Paediatrics	184	141
Neurology and psychiatry	99	46
Anaesthesiology	103	—
Surgery	125	29
Dermatology	39	135
Gynaecology	34	78
Otorhinolaryngology	12	74
Urology	59	20
Orthopaedics	5	38
Ophthalmology	12	26
Radiology	17	19
Pulmonology	9	17

internists contribute the majority of reports. In spite of much better diagnostic facilities, hospitals and university clinics still lag behind. There may be two reasons for this: (1) the discussion of adverse reactions during ward rounds and at clinical and pathology conferences apparently satisfies the demand for further information and dissemination and (2) the publication of the adverse reactions and further future observations may be interfered with by early reporting. Both are obviously not valid reasons and, as far as the second is concerned, the Drug Commission refrains from publishing any data without the written consent of the reporting physicians. The same confidentiality holds true for inquiries on details of reported cases by interested physicians or regulatory authorities, except in the case of imminent hazard. Another valid reason is the lack of clinical pharmacologists in almost all regional hospitals and a great number of university clinics. The recently established subspeciality of Clinical Pharmacology requiring 2½ years training in Departments of Clinical Pharmacology or qualified clinical institutions after a basic training in experimental pharmacology may remedy this in the near future by providing assistant physicians reponsible for the monitoring of clinical departments for adverse drug reactions. We are not too keen about the services which a clinical pharmacist could render in this respect. We feel that only a well-trained physician would be able to recognize and to evaluate new and even uncommon adverse reactions. Nevertheless, a clinical pharmacist could be extremely helpful in contributing facts about changes in prescribing habits, drug usage in general and possible drug interactions. The dispensing pharmacist, on the other hand, is an invaluable source for the detection of adverse reactions to drugs sold over the counter. He is also aware of misuse patterns of non-prescription drugs and even of patients soliciting prescriptions for drugs of abuse from different physicians. He may resolve inexplicable adverse drug effects as interactions of drugs prescribed unknowingly by several physicians to the same patient. We enjoy in the Federal Republic efficient cooperation with the Drug Commission of the German Pharmacists. The army of detail men from the pharmaceutical industry (8000 in the Federal Republic of Germany) could be a powerful force in soliciting and collecting reports on adverse reactions to drugs. If well trained, they could even assist the busy practitioner to complete and forward report forms to the National Centre. But only a small number of mostly research-oriented companies assist the Drug Commission by supplying reports received on their products and advising the detail men in charge to help in securing missing information. This is in spite of the statutory obligation on all 550 member firms of the Federal Association of the Pharmaceutical Industry in the Federal Republic of Germany. This may have been the reason why the German Regulatory Authority, with the new Drug Law coming into force, insists that all drug houses report regularly on all adverse drug reactions of their products they learn from their detail men or from physicians directly. Reporting by physicians to their National Centre remains – as before – voluntary.

Participation in a spontaneous monitoring system constitutes a substantial additional burden on the busy physician. We do not feel that the occasional proposal to compensate him financially for additional examinations and for writing an elaborate report would be advisable or even helpful. It would probably attract those few who are less interested in the patient's benefit than in remuneration. We found that physicians in our country are mostly interested in the information and advice they could get on the adverse drug reaction reported. Our National Centre therefore replies to each report with a personal letter to the reporting physician. Where possible, the mechanism of the adverse effect is explained and the frequency of occurrence given. He is often advised on how to prevent or mitigate future reactions of this kind and where drug blood levels could be determined in critical situations. In the case of drug hypersensitivity reactions, lists of other drugs containing the incriminated active ingredient are supplied, so that they can be avoided even by other physicians treating the patient, this being of considerable importance in a country now with up to 120,000 registered drugs. This workload of nearly 5000 reply letters per year taxes the physicians in charge and the transcription centre of our secretariat considerably, but we feel that feeding back information of value to the practising physician is a strong motivation for him to participate. The means to motivate the physician to continue cooperating seem to be even more important than those to induce him to join the spontaneous monitoring system. His first report, after all, may well have dealt with an intriguing new drug reaction or an incident concerning him personally, so he would like to share it with other colleagues. The faithful reporting, however, of less exciting but nevertheless important adverse drug reactions is likely to tax his patience. How did we meet this problem? First of all, we reduced the paperwork to the bare minimum. The National Drug Monitoring Systems are almost all of the spontaneous type and serve to generate signals rather than to supply quantitative data. It is therefore for them more important to receive a few relevant facts in good time than to be supplied with more elaborate data at a later stage. If additional data appear to be necessary during follow-up, they may be obtained over the phone or by a visiting physician sent by the National Centre. We differ in this respect from the Drug Safety Departments of the drug companies whose predominant interest is in exculpating their suspected drugs. Secondly, report forms should be at hand at the doctor's office and in his bag for house-calls. The German Physicians' Journal (*Deutsches Ärzteblatt*), distributed free of charge to all 150,000 German physicians, contains therefore a one-page report form every other week (Fig. 1). Short forms, modelled on the

Bericht über unerwünschte Arzneimittelwirkungen (auch Verdachtsfälle)
an die Arzneimittelkommission der deutschen Ärzteschaft · Haedenkampstr. 5 · 5000 Köln 41

Bei dem Patienten (Anfangsbuchst.)	m/w	Geburts-datum:	Größe: in cm	Gewicht: in kg	Beruf bei ♀ schwanger seit:

wurde(n) am:		folgende unerwünschte Arzneimittelwirkung(en) beobachtet:	Dauer (Std., Tage)
1.			
2.			
3.			

Bis zur Nebenwirkung wurden gegeben:	Tagesdosis	p. o., i. v. usw.	von (Datum)	bis (Datum)	wegen:
1. (ausl.)					
2.					
3.					
4.					

Welche dieser Mittel wurden schon früher gegeben und wie wurden sie vertragen? Wie zuvor numerieren! Lfd. Nr. genügt.

Weitere nichtmedikamentöse Behandlung, diagnostische bzw. therapeutische Eingriffe, Bestrahlung, Schrittmacher?

Grundleiden, weitere Leiden, Stoffwechselstörungen, berufliche Exposition, Genußmittelabusus, Arzneimittelmißbrauch, Diätgewohnheiten:

Allergien und Überempfindlichkeit gegen andere Arzneimittel:

Laboratoriumsdaten: Hämatologie, Harnanalyse, klin.-chem. Untersuchungen. Wenn mögl. Befundblätter beilegen!

▼ Art d. Unters.	Datum: ▶			▼ Art d. Unters.	Datum: ▶		

Therapie und Ausgang der Nebenwirkung(en): ggf. Ort und Zeit der Obduktion, wenn mögl. Obduktionsbefund beilegen!

Name und Anschrift des Arztes: ggf. Name und Anschrift der Klinik: Meldung an Gesundh.-Behörde: ja - nein

Bericht an Hersteller: ja - nein

(Stempel) (Stempel) (Unterschrift)

Deutscher Ärzte-Verlag GmbH, 5000 Köln 40

Fig. 1

British Yellow Card, are sent twice a year to all practising physicians (Fig. 2); in the near future the official prescription pads for publicly insured patients (more than 90% of the West-German population) will be interspersed with small postcard-sized report forms, like those our British and Israeli colleagues already receive. In addition, all reply letters to reports received contain new forms. Finally, formal reports should not be the only form accepted: short free notes and telephone calls may contain just as important information.

There is no doubt that spontaneous monitoring systems provide the mainstay of information on new and unexpected drug reactions. This is already evident when considering the number of patients monitored. In 1977 there was 1 general practitioner per 2261 inhabitants in the Federal Republic of Germany. Even if a certain drug is given to only 6 in 1000 people (e.g. antidiabetic biguanides) and considering that also specialists (1 per 2192 inhabitants) may participate in drug treatment, each doctor may encounter about 10 patients thus treated in his practice. The cooperation of only 4000 physicians as in the Federal Republic of Germany would thus ensure that adverse reactions occurring in 1 in 10,000 patients could have a chance of being detected, provided the necessary examinations have been or could be done. Even a multicentre study at a number of large clinics may not be able to provide observations on 40,000 patients treated with the same drug except for frequently used substances like antibiotics or sedatives. This and the rather small amount to be spent per adverse drug reaction in a spontaneous monitoring system are sound reasons for extending and improving the existing spontaneous monitoring systems.

Spontaneous monitoring systems may be the most important, but by no means

Bei dem Pat.: (Anfangsbuchst.)	m / w	Geburts-datum:	Größe: in cm	Gewicht: in kg	Beruf:

wurden am:	folgende Arzneimittelnebenwirkungen beobachtet:	Dauer (Std., Tage)
1.		
2.		
3.		

Bis zur Nebenwirkung wurden folg. Arzneimittel gegeben:	Tagesdosis	p.o., i.v. usw.	von (Datum)	bis (Datum)	wegen:
1. (auslös.)					
2.					
3.					
4.					
5.					

Welche dieser Mittel wurden schon früher gegeben und wie wurden sie vertragen?

Weitere nichtmedikament. Behandlung, diagn. bzw. therapeut. Eingriffe, Bestrahlung?

Grundleiden:

weitere Leiden:

Allergien und Überempfindlichkeit gegen andere Arzneimittel:

Therapie und Ausgang der Nebenwirkung(en):

Fig. 2

the only or the most efficient monitors (or hypothesis generators) of new adverse drug reactions. The Drug Commission encouraged therefore as early as 1970, backed by a resolution of the Annual Meeting of the Federal Chamber of Physicians, the establishment of Intensive Monitoring Centres at several university clinics in the Federal Republic. The first pioneering work was done in Heidelberg by Professor Weber followed by Professor Kewitz in Berlin, who joined the Boston Collaborative Drug Surveillance Program, and more recently by Professor May in Bochum who succeeded in incorporating several large municipal hospitals in addition to the university clinics in his ambitious project. While in Berlin every patient in a department of internal medicine is monitored systematically for any signs and symptoms of adverse effects and his drug history is carefully taken, the other institutions depend on regular inquiries by trained physicians visiting the wards to collect all adverse reactions encountered. The problem with intensive monitoring is that it is relatively costly (it is financed by substantial grants from the Federal Ministry for Research and Technology) and yields relatively few clues about new adverse drug reactions. It supplies, however, invaluable information on the frequency and course of adverse reactions frequently observed during in-patient care.

The Drug Commission of the German Medical Profession considered therefore early other less costly means of signalizing the occurrence of new or the increase in already known significant adverse drug reactions. Some of the more severe of them can be diagnosed or at least confirmed by special examination or laboratory tests, or become evident, finally, at autopsy. We enlisted therefore the help of pathologists, haematologists and neurologists, to name just a few disciplines, to call to our attention any new or increasingly occurring symptomatology which may perhaps be drug-related. There are, e.g., only a few haematologists in the Federal Republic who are consulted to evaluate bone marrow films in aplastic anaemia cases. They could, like the former Registry on Drug-Induced Blood Dyscrasias of the American Medical Association, serve as collecting points and as a liaison between the physician taking care of the individual patient and be able to supply the drug history to the National Centre. This kind of collaboration with specialists where certain symptoms are being channelled proved to be very helpful: e.g., in following up the first cases of biguanide-induced lactacidosis, in dispelling the suspicion of a correlation between mammary carcinoma in males and spironolactone administration, and in clarifying the incidence of liver tumours in women on oral contraceptives. Unfortunately, there are no morbidity statistics broken down enough in the Federal Republic to serve as indicators for possibly drug-induced abnormalities, e.g. an increase in cerebrovascular incidents in young women on oral contraceptives. A similar situation exists with regard to drug-induced malformations, where only a fraction of all children with malformations recognizable at birth are reported. There is, however, a comprehensive study on almost 50,000 pregnancies in the process of evaluation, which is expected to yield information on the teratogenicity of many of the more frequently used drugs in the Federal Republic.

The Secretariat of the Drug Commission, in collaboration with the Computer Centre of the German Cancer Research Centre in Heidelberg, maintains a data bank with standardized data on all 20,000 reports on adverse drug reactions received since its inception in 1962. In addition, the original files are available for more detailed information. While data from spontaneous monitoring systems, for reasons well known, do not yield to general statistical evaluation, they still may be searched for some interesting parameters, such as age distribution, drug interactions, duration of drug administration etc. Nevertheless, we see the main purpose of such systems in their signal-generating function. To become aware of a new important adverse drug reaction at the earliest possible moment is one vital prerequisite to prevent drug-induced suffering, but to verify a causal relationship and to determine frequency are other indispensable obligations. A single report on a suspected relationship of an adverse event and a drug given at the time of its occurrence may be purely coincidental. If this report finds its way into a national or international data bank, to which parties other than the National Centre have access or if it is even published in the medical literature, a valuable drug's reputation may be damaged beyond repair. The data of a spontaneous monitoring system deserve therefore, in our opinion, the same protection as the evidence leading to an honest man's accusation of having committed a crime until his guilt is proven in court. We all know that this is not easily accomplished, because to confirm or dispel the suspicion, more evidence has to be sought and the physicians from whom such evidence is expected to be obtained must be fully informed about all already known facts. A grave responsibility rests with the National Centre and its advisory board, in our case the 40 active and 80 corresponding members of the Drug Commission, and the Regulatory Agency, to weigh carefully the possible threat of the suspected adverse reaction to the patient population involved against the therapeutic benefits of the drug to be restricted in its use or even withdrawn from the market. To be included in these considerations has to be another, no less important question: if the drug or drugs, which will replace the preparation withdrawn, may not pose an even greater risk, if not only by the fact that experience with this drug is rather short or the data on it not up to today's standards.

Being aware of these problems, the Drug Commission of the German Medical Profession has worked, since its inception in 1950, closely with the Regulatory Agency of the Federal Republic of Germany, the 'Bundesgesundheitsamt' (BGA). The German Physicians insisted on a comprehensive drug legislation, which was finally passed in 1976 and came into effect on January 1st, 1978. Before this was achieved, the Drug Commission delegated members to the 'Drug Safety Council' ('Beirat Arzneimittelsicherheit') which drafted in 1970 a regulation to coordinate measures and means of information in the case of suspected adverse drug reactions, the so-called 'Stufenplan'. This regulation provided for the cooperation of the Regulatory Agency, the Drug Commission, the State Health Ministries (being the executive power) and the manufacturer involved, but did not specify the necessary steps in detail to maintain the flexibility required for the optimal handling of different events. The new German Drug Law of 1976 establishes for the first time the duty of the Regulatory Agency (the 'Bundesgesundheitsamt') to collect and to evaluate centrally all risks, especially adverse reactions, interactions with other substances, contraindications, adulterations of drugs and to coordinate the measures which have to be taken according to this law. Paragraph 63 of this law provides that the Minister for Youth, Family and Health issues by means of a common administrative regulation, with the consent of the Federal Council ('Bundesrat'), a Procedural Plan ('Stufen-Plan') to fulfil the duties imposed in Paragraph 62 of the law (cited above in part). Paragraph 62 obliges the Regulatory Agency to cooperate in its duties with the World Health Organization, the Regulatory Agencies of other countries, the German State Health Authorities and the Drug Commissions of the Professional Chambers (Physicians, Veterinarians, Dentists, Pharmacists) and other institutions, whose duties comprise the collection of drug risks.

The second draft of the Procedural Plan has been submitted to all parties concerned; they took the opportunity to propose changes and modifications. The Plan establishes the Drug Commissions in their past voluntary and private role to collect and evaluate all reports on adverse drug reactions received from the members of their profession. They have to submit their findings to the Regulatory Agency at certain intervals. They are also given the task of advising the members of the profession on proper drug usage. The chairmen of the Drug Commissions are invited with the Health Officials of the States to regular Routine Sessions at the Agency to discuss matters pending. Actual drug-safety problems are dealt with in ad-hoc Sessions, where manufacturers' representatives and experts join the participants in the Routine Sessions. The procedure has already been used in connection with the withdrawal of clofibrate.

The Drug Commission has suggested the establishment of an Advisory Committee to coordinate all measures to evaluate and establish a causal relationship of adverse drug reactions to facilitate the decisions of the Regulatory Agency. The Committee has already been appointed and convened to draft a general policy plan.

DISCUSSION

Takano: You told us that clinical pharmacology has a training period of 2½ years. In the Federal Republic of Germany, do you have the ordinary pharmacists' training course before that?

Kimbel: This is a training course for physicians for 2½ years in pharmacology, experimental pharmacology, and clinical pharmacology in a clinic. There is no established training for clinical pharmacists in the Federal Republic of Germany, but we do have several excellent Institutes of Pharmacology in Frankfurt and several other places where trained pharmacists can receive an additional training in pharmacology, so that they can serve as hospital pharmacists, for instance in the capacity of a clinical pharmacist.

Nagano: Could you please explain what 'Stufenplan' is?

Kimbel: The former 'Stufenplan' provided for 3 steps (as the word 'Stufen' in German means), so that if there was some evidence, but unconfirmed, of a drug risk, the Drug Committee of the Germany Chamber of Physicians had to sit together with representatives from the Federal Institute of Health and the manufacturers to discuss further measures to investigate the causal relationship and the frequency of the drug.

Step 2 was if there was a confirmation of evidence or strong evidence that there was a relation between the drug and the adverse effect. In this case, a warning to the physicians had to be issued in the 'German Physicians Journal' and steps taken to restrict indications or the duration of administration. For instance, as the clioquinol cases became known in the Federal Republic of Germany, the German Drug Commission at once got together with the manufacturers involved and representatives of the Federal Institute of Health to limit the duration of administration of clioquinol to no more than 2 weeks and in most cases to 1 week.

Step 3 involves a restrictive action that means the withdrawal of the drug or a severe limitation of the indications.

The new Drug Law provides for new procedures in Articles 62 and 63. According to a draft of the New Regulations, the Government, i.e. the Federal Institute of Health, calls for an ad-hoc meeting in Berlin. This happened for instance 2 months ago when the clofibrate study of WHO became known.

In addition to the ad-hoc meetings at the Federal Institute of Health, there are regular quarterly meetings on current problems where items such as increasing abuse of drugs, labelling changes or lack of information to physicians are discussed.

After such an ad-hoc or routine conference in Berlin, the Federal Institute of Health announces that a decision will be taken within a certain period of time. For instance, a meeting took place on clofibrate on March 19th, and on April 18th a decision was published by the Federal Health Office on further steps to be taken. So, the new 'Stufenplan' is different from the current one in that the Federal Institute of Health has now taken the initiative to act first while in the past this was a cooperative effort between the Federal Institute of Health, the Committee on Drug Safety and the manufacturers.

Sugisawa: In 1979, according to the Japanese newspapers, a second thalidomide tragedy could arise in West Germany. There were 950 cases of malformations due to a hormone preparation which was produced by the Schering Company. A similar drug has been sold in Japan under the name of 'Onogynon' by the Japan Schering Company. Are you aware of these incidents?

Kimbel: I assume you refer to the suspected relation between hormonal pregnancy tests and malformations in babies born to women thus tested. The Drug Commission of the Federal Chamber of Physicians warned the German Medical Profession in 1973 of a possible teratogenic effect of hormones given in early pregnancy and repeated the warning with regard to hormonal pregnancy tests last year. The Federal Institute of Health of the Federal Republic of Germany convened recently a meeting of experts from all over the world to discuss the evidence presented in the recent literature. It came to the conclusion that conclusive proof of a causal relationship was still lacking but that there is no longer a place for hormonal pregnancy tests. The question whether progestogens should still be used in threatened abortion remains to be extensively discussed.

Dukes: I would like to support what Dr. Kimbel has said. If sex hormones given in pregnancy do injure the fetus, they probably do so by disrupting implantation (by stimulating the uterine wall) rather than by specifically injuring the fetus. This would explain the very diffuse pattern of malformations reported – a situation which is quite different from that of thalidomide.

A further point here is that the need for hormone administration in pregnancy is dubious. Hormonal pregnancy tests have been superseded by in-vitro tests and pregnancy maintenance with progestogens is very probably not effective. The slightest suspicion of harm therefore justifies the abandonment of such methods.

Tognoni: There is a wide use of hormones for maintaining pregnancy in Italy and we have advised about the lack of data on efficacy. But doctors do not trust our warnings too much and so we were forced to run a double-blind clinical trial which has just been completed. The results will be presented in July at an international meeting but they are completely negative.

SESSION III: LEGAL AND SOCIAL ASPECTS OF DRUG-INDUCED SUFFERINGS

Outline of the SMON litigation proceedings in the Tokyo District Court

KENGO OHASHI

SMON Litigation Attorneys Group for Plaintiffs in the Tokyo District Court, Tokyo, Japan

The full details of the litigation proceedings in the Tokyo SMON case will not be considered; rather general principles will be assessed with a view to future action for the early relief of victims.

In Japan, SMON litigation proceedings are taking place in 23 district courts and 4 higher courts with 4,720 plaintiffs (actual patients, 4166). The Tokyo District Court handles over half the cases (2,525 plaintiffs of whom 2,302 are patients). These figures apply as of March 6th, 1979. In July, 1977 when the first proceedings were completed, there were 2,000 plaintiffs. However, the number increased, and the number of plaintiffs in the Tokyo District Court was especially large compared with other district courts. The specific characteristics of the litigation proceedings in the Tokyo District Court are thus illustrative.

Firstly cases were presented relatively early in 1971 so that the actual proceedings began earlier, compared with litigation in other district courts.

Secondly the court is an independent body but is part of the state organization. Therefore, the proceedings in Tokyo, the state capital, influence other district courts.

Thirdly the plaintiffs' group of lawyers presented a comprehensive case incorporating all individual cases. In other district courts, the plaintiffs lived within the domestic area of the court, while in the Tokyo litigation the plaintiffs were from all over the country. Therefore, the proceedings had a nationwide impact.

Finally the plaintiffs and lawyers were divided into three groups, and if a consensus was not achieved, differences arose among them.

PROGRESS OF THE TOKYO SMON LITIGATION PROCEEDINGS

General progress

There were basically three stages. Firstly proof of a causal relationship between clioquinol and SMON was required; this process began on January 2nd, 1974, and ended on January 2nd, 1975. Nine witnesses were examined 24 times. The second aspect concerned liability; from January 20th, 1975, to April 14th, 1976, 15 witnesses were examined. The third stage examined witnesses to prove damage and lasted from April 26th until May 18th, 1976, when witnesses were examined three times; of the 27 witnesses, 4 were foreigners.

The court proceedings from individual points of view

To gain relief for such great numbers of plaintiffs, it was necessary to conduct and complete the proceedings as rapidly as possible. In this regard the method of individual recognition is important. That is to say, a precondition for optimal compensation was that the plaintiff should be established as a SMON patient or otherwise and damages clarified. The extent of damage took into account medical, social and domestic aspects and the settlements adjusted accordingly.

The fundamental aspect is of course the medical, and expert judgements were required. Therefore, statements from plaintiffs and defendants in the initial stages were contradictary or hostile. The lawyers for the defence requested all medical records and the lawyers for the plaintiffs stated that such approaches would only prolong the proceedings.

As a method for individual recognition the second group of lawyers requested examination by a team of expert witnesses, to assess the presence and degree of SMON disease in individual patients. A medical report from the family doctor was initially used and when this was insufficient, other reports or certificates were employed.

The first group accepted the same method for assessing the presence of SMON disease but was at first against the procedure on its degree. However, they later agreed in toto. The third group disagreed on the grounds that rejection (cut-off) would ensue and because the final result would take a very long time. They insisted that individual recognition should be made by the court by individual interview and written medical records etc. The court accepted the request of the first and second groups and exercised its authority over group three.

The team of expert witnesses consisted of 15 members selected from the Research Commission for SMON. The examination by experts comprised written reports and supplemental interviews.

On May 12th, 1976, judgement was given and on September 25th, 1976, was rendered for 154 victims. These were the first proceedings. There were further settlements for 1,653 victims on March 5th, 1979, and among these final judgement now applies to 1,430 victims. At present there are no unrecognized victims. (Throughout the country, 16 district courts have now examined a total of 2,418 victims for recognition, the number of the reported cases being 1,876.)

The degree of damage is classified as follows: first degree (minor cases) 18%; second degree (medium extent) 48%; third degree (severe cases) 34%. These figures apply to litigation in the Tokyo District Court while nationally the values are 19%, 46% and 35% respectively. The SMON Research Commission conducted their own study on 1,527 victims according to these data and found: first degree 38%; second degree 41% and severe cases 22%. Relatively speaking, the value of 34% for the severe cases is larger as a result of the court.

For individual recognition, examination is conducted on respective plaintiffs. In the first rulings all 154 plaintiffs were examined but for the remaining more than 2,000 victims, it is considered impractical to conduct similar assessments. It is quite reasonable that a small number of plaintiffs can represent the others and testify to the actual distress of their social and family life in the presence of a judge. In this respect there is agreement among the three groups.

The settlement and court ruling

One of the major characteristics of the result of the Tokyo SMON litigation proceedings was that for similar kinds of cases, both a ruling and settlement were obtained while in others court rulings were made. Two kinds of approaches are thus apparent in the Tokyo SMON litigation proceedings. (In Kanazawa, Fukuoka and Hiroshima District Courts, the court rulings were rendered, but no settlements were obtained.)

The settlements were supervised by the court, which provided a kind of settlement plan acceptable to both parties: this has great significance.

The settlement had the following characteristics: normally defendants present the amount of financial payment as stated in the text and incorporated in the protocol; in the present cases, however, the causal relationship between clioquinol and SMON and also the liability of the Government and pharmaceutical companies were both incorporated in the protocol. The plaintiffs requested, as a precondition for settlement, admission and apology from the Government and pharmaceutical companies. The court accepted the request and the court stated their opinions with respect to the settlement processes. The high relief for settlement was disclosed beforehand. Thus, those involved in the case knew that the final ruling would not, in substance, be totally different from the one the court had presented beforehand. In calculating the level of compensation for the extent of the disease, age and whether the victim fully supported the family, whether housewives had children were all considered. Once settlement was concluded, the victims knew or were able to predict the amounts of compensation money to be awarded.

Such approaches also applied to litigations in other district courts besides that in Tokyo, including Okayama, Kochi and Osaka District Courts.

Cases in which nursing expenses and permanent expenses were not incorporated in the ruling were challenged. The result of the Tokyo District Court spread or were applied to other district courts in Japan and played a fundamental role in giving overall relief for the victims.

Tanabe Pharmaceutical Company has not yet agreed to the settlement approach.* However, the state has agreed to pay to the victims one-third of the compensation on the basis of the separate settlement. As of March 5th this year there are 2,302 patients, of whom 46% (1,055 patients) have already obtained settlement. In detail, 473 patients obtained a complete settlement and 582 patients obtained a separate settlement. In this connection it may be said that throughout the country 532 victims have obtained a complete settlement and 650 victims a separate settlement; 1,182 victims in all have received approximately 17.5 billion yen. However, even now there are many victims who have not obtained compensation. An early complete settlement is expected and it is hoped that the victims will accept settlement according to the approach outlined.

*About 1 month after KICADIS, this company was compelled to agree to the settlement.

17 items on the so-called permanent policies

HIROSHI KANEDA, FUMIO SUZUKI and TSUTOMU KIGASAWA

Tokyo 2nd Group of Plaintiffs for SMON Litigation, Tokyo, Japan

PROGRESS

The first civil action for SMON victims was brought in May 1971, before the Tokyo District Court, and was concluded in September 1976, after five years of trials. The judge then endeavoured to effect settlement and made public the opinions of the court in January and in April 1977. The proposals for settlement were accepted by most of the plaintiffs and defendants, the state, the Ciba-Geigy Japan and Takeda Chemical Industries and the first settlement was effected before the court in October 1977.

The court expressed the opinion that the plaintiffs and defendants should together discuss the so-called permanent policies, that is, the rehabilitation of the SMON patients, research on medical treatment, expenses incurred by the patients, the costs of hospitals and equipment for the patients, and other facilities.

For this purpose the plaintiffs submitted a report of basic demands, summarized in 17 items, to the court in July 1977. The demands were reviewed by a meeting of delegates of the plaintiffs and defendants and lawyers under the auspices of the court. Subsequently, since similar settlements were effected at the Okayama, Kochi and Osaka District Courts, the delegates and lawyers took part in this Tokyo meeting. Fourteen such meetings have so far been held. In the beginning the plaintiffs explained the severe consequences to their daily lives, and detailed their concrete demands. The delegate of the State then proposed some of the permanent policies which the State might be able to realize immediately.

THE CONTENT OF DEMANDS

The first and second items illustrate the basic principles behind the demands. The plaintiffs make a strong plea for the prevention of further drug induced sufferings.
1. The defendants should make it clear that there is the causal relationship between the administration of clioquinol and the occurrence of SMON disease and also that they had a responsibility for this occurrence. The defendants should apologize to the plaintiffs and take part in the discussion to atone for the offence.
2. The defendants should deeply reflect on the occurrence of SMON, and then take measures for the prevention of future drug induced sufferings. In regard to the

amendment of the Pharmaceutical Affairs Act, the state should take steps to revise the Act fundamentally, taking the plaintiffs' opinions into consideration.
3. The defendants should at once start to establish a top-level organization to study methods for the medical treatment of the SMON patients. The remedies which the organization develops should be made available to patients throughout the country. (In spite of several years of study in Japan, effective remedies have not yet been developed. The patients' first hope is for alleviation of their pain and a cure for complications caused by their physical inconvenience.)
4. For the future remedy of SMON patients, the defendants should bear the whole expense of the doctors with whom the patients consult.
5. Hospitals should be designated for the treatment of SMON patients in accordance with the need in each prefecture, and rooms and beds should also be specially reserved. Arrangements for entering hospitals should be simplified.
6. The expenses for going to or staying in hospital, such as transportation fee or taxi charge, should be paid to each patient according to his or her demand. A simple procedure for payment should be devised.
7. The expense for staying at the hot spring sanatorium for rehabilitation and transportation charges should be paid according to the patient's demand. A simple procedure for payment should also be devised.
8. A system should be devised for a group of doctors, including neurologists, to conduct periodical examinations of the physical therapy for bedridden patients at home, and home-help should be provided. The state should bear the expenses of sending doctors and home-helps.
9. The defendants should pay for heating systems or equipment which the patients require in their homes and the upkeep. The defendants should also pay other expenses to improve the living surroundings. A simple procedure for payment should also be established.
10. A system should be formulated for the patients to receive periodically acupuncture, and moxocausis and massage every month, without cost.
11. The defendants should meet the cost of drugs such as a herb medicine which cannot be obtained from the health insurance. A simple procedure for payment should also be established.
12. The defendants should, on presentation of the receipts, pay for the equipment necessary for the patients in their daily life. A simple procedure for payment should also be devised.
13. The defendants must provide a telephone in every patient's home and pay its monthly expense.
14. The defendants should provide a 'SMON Note' or 'Certificate' for each patient so that they can immediately be identified as a SMON victim, and operate a system for patients to obtain the above-mentioned privileges by presenting this document.
15. All the above-mentioned benefits must be adjusted if there is a rise in prices.
16. In case the agreed measures should not be enforced, another meeting should be held for discussion. In this case, machinery for adjustment should be established.
17. Since it may take a long time for all the decisions to be made, the defendants should prepare an office for the plaintiffs' use and pay for its equipment and maintenance.

SUMMARY OF BUDGET

1. The costs of the remedial measures and medical services are as follows:
a. The cost of construction of two new wards for the clinical study of SMON is estimated at *1,590 million yen.*
b. The yearly expenditure of the SMON Reseach Committee is estimated at *200 million yen.* The committee will lay emphasis on a joint study with oriental medicine with the aim of relieving palsy, pain and strain.
2. The cost of 2,400 sickbeds to be installed for nervous diseases such as SMON is estimated at *1,104 million yen.*
3. The future expenses are estimated as follows:
a. A Government subsidy for the cost of patients under the health insurance of *300 million yen.*
b. A subsidy for the cost of hospital admissions of *220 million yen.*
c. A subsidy for the cost of nursing of *730 million yen.*
The annual total expense is thus estimated at *1,250 million yen.*
4. A subsidy for taxi fares necessary for going to or entering hospital of *594 million yen.*
5. It is planned that 30 tickets for using the hot spring sanatorium will be given to each patient every year. The estimated cost is *1,500 million yen.*
6. The subsidy for patients to purchase two sorts of herb medicine is *840 million yen.*
7. The subsidy for patients to purchase necessary equipment is *100 million yen.*
8. The cost of periodical examination by doctors and helpers of serious patients at home is *420 million yen.*
9. The cost of heating systems and the improvement of living surroundings is *2,200 million yen* yearly.
10. A subsidy for each patient to have a telephone; the total cost of installation is *900 million yen* and of maintenance is estimated at *600 million yen* yearly.
11. The expense for the plaintiffs' office, with necessary equipment and maintenance, which includes rent, clerical expenses, wages etc. is *53 million yen* yearly.

PATIENTS' ACTUAL CONDITIONS

1. As for the physical damage, most patients have abnormal sensory disturbances such as paralysis, pain and stiffness, forcing their daily lives to be inactive. A national survey indicates that 19% of the patients cannot walk at all and 33% need a crutch or a walking aid.

14% of the patients have become blind or have serious optic disturbances and another 64% are losing their eyesight. 60% have developed complications in the stomach, intestines, heart, liver or kidneys, and have to be periodically examined by a doctor. Especially serious cases who cannot walk and are bedridden have become too weak to have meals ten years after falling ill, and about 200 of them died last year. Most had been nursed in their homes, and their families were worn out with the long nursing.

For several years after falling ill, all the patients had changed their hospitals in the search for an effective remedy and some had paid about two or three million yen in one year. During this period, many patients lost their employment and had a hard life. It is estimated that 61% of patients are undergoing hardship and 21% are in dismal poverty.

2. At present, all but 2 or 3% of the patients have returned home and only visit the hospital or clinic for acupuncture, moxocausis or massage.

The reason for leaving hospital is that the physicians had no positive measures for remedy to offer and the patients could not bear the heavy cost. But the patients at home always suffer complications caused by lack of physical movement. Periodical examinations are necessary to diagnose complications in the early stages. Acupuncture, moxocausis and massage are absolutely necessary for alleviation of pain and prevention of complications. Most patients now rely on the above two methods, but they have difficulty in meeting the expensive doctor's fee or taxi fare, and are forced to reduce the number of hospital visits.

The patients desire rehabilitation treatment for at least one month a year, but cannot afford it. Only few patients can go to a sanatorium. In case they need to enter hospital, it is very difficult to secure immediate admission to a good hospital. National hospitals have a few beds for SMON patients but these may be very far from their homes, and the beds may be already occupied by other patients. Since in public hospitals a bed charge and the cost of nursing are borne by the patients, only few can stay in hospital.

The state is planning to increase the number of beds for SMON patients and to change national tuberculosis sanatoria into SMON sanatoria. However, as long as they fail to develop effective remedies, to redistribute the national hospitals and solve the problem of charges, it cannot be said that the SMON problem has been settled.

3. As already stated, 61% of the patients are in severe economic circumstances, and patients who have lost their positions by falling ill cannot get their jobs back, so the future still offers them nothing.

The improvement of home equipment to make their lives easier is still unfulfilled. What the patients first of all ask for is the completion of heating systems, the possibility to revive acquaintanceships by telephone conversation and the supply of aid devices.

The families of patients are suffering a heavy economic load, have got tired by the long period of nursing and have forfeited their health. If this condition is not changed, any happiness in the family will be lost and all the SMON patients will fall into a critical situation.

It is urgently necessary for basic permanent policies to be established.

INSTITUTION OF POLICIES RESULTING FROM THE DISCUSSIONS

As mentioned above, 14 discussion meetings have already been held and the Ministry of Health and Welfare has started to put into effect the policies decided at the discussion in November 1978.

1. A counter to promote the policies for SMON patients was prepared in every

prefectural office throughout the country.
2. Arrangements were made for patients to enter the national hospitals and national sanatoria. The former provide the beds for short periods of treatment and the latter for long periods.
3. Two wards will be constructed in 1979 for the purpose of clinical studies and for developing remedial measures.
4. In respect of SMON patients, health insurance will be applied to the acupuncture, moxocausis and massage treatment.
5. Loans for living expenses are mandatory for SMON patients who find it hard to make a living.
6. More than two kinds of walking aids or other equipment are given to the SMON patients if necessary.

THE OPINION OF PATIENTS

It is considered that these policies are not actually put into effect very satisfactorily. As a result, there is quite a big difference between the plaintiffs and the defendants about the permanent policy for the relief of the SMON patients.

The state has made a budget for the policies in 1979, but it is less than one fifth of the amount needed for the demands made by the patients.

The defendants have already lost their cases at eight district courts throughout the country. The plaintiffs decided to accept settlements for the purpose of promptly relieving the serious cases. It is urgently required for the defendants to show their good faith by the establishment of permanent policies and providing the budget for their realization.

DISCUSSION

Payne: Have the plaintiffs requested the defendant drug companies to bear the duty of carrying out research on the alleviation of the victims' sufferings?

Kaneda: Takeda and Ciba-Geigy have committed themselves to cooperate over permanent policies, but Tanabe has not agreed to this. The Tokyo District Court ordered us to consult among plaintiffs and defendants to propose permanent policies and the court is providing us with the utmost assistance.

The prolonged litigation for drug induced suffering and provisional disposition

KATSUYA TAKAHARA

SMON Litigation Attorneys Group for Plaintiffs in the Okayama District Court, Okayama, Japan

Many litigations in Japan have tended to extend over long periods. This trend is most apparent in litigations concerned with public pollution and hazards, and drug induced suffering. For example, major pollution related litigations, such as the Minamata litigation in Niigata and Kumamoto prefectures, the Itai-Itai disease litigation (a disease of extreme pain and bone deformation caused by the industrial waste containing cadmium and other heavy metals), and the Yokkaichi asthma litigation (asthma caused by fumes from the Yokkaichi industrial complex), have taken from 3 years and 3 months to 4 years and 10 months between the initial filing of the suit to the court decision. The thalidomide litigation, the first drug pollution related litigation in Japan, took 11 years from the initial filing to the settlement in October 1974.

The reasons for such prolonged litigations are that the defendant corporations as well as the state persisted in the claims that there were no causal relationships and that foreknowledge was impossible; the result was that the court room ended up in scientific debate. Another reason is that too many plaintiffs are involved and proof of individual damage takes a very long time. In May of 1971 the first SMON litigation was initiated in the Tokyo District Court and similar suits have been filed in 23 other district courts; but all have taken a very long period of time.

It seems to be usual that the time from the outbreak of the disease to the initial filing of the suit takes a long time, during which the victims have their livelihood threatened by unemployment, divorce etc. These victims must think of ways in which to get necessary medical and living costs and many sell property and fall into debt. The prolonged litigation only adds to the suffering and hardship of the victims. The necessity of avoiding prolonged actions is obvious and efforts must be made to secure the necessary, immediate medical and social aid for victims while the suit is still in progress.

The plaintiffs' lawyers in the Okayama SMON suit used the provisional disposition system to partly eliminate some problems and provide certain immediate social and medical expenses.

The following considers the importance and our experience of the provisional disposition system. Under the Japanese code of civil procedure the following systems exist:

1. System of provisional settlement.
2. System of provisional disposition concerning disputed subject matter.
3. Provisional agreement to temporarily settle matters.

The first two measures freeze the property of the other party. Provisional

TABLE 1. *Provisional disposition by district courts courts (As of April 15, 1979)*

Name of District Court	Date of application	Number of applicant	Date of decision delivered	Admission	Withdrawal	Rejected	Reservation	Amount admitted (per plaintiff) (¥ 10,000)	Period	Examination completed
	May 12, 1978	23	May 19, 1978	23				10,15 or 20 per month	for 6 months	yes
Tokyo	May 16, 1978	123			123					
(1st Group)	May 29, 1978	45						45		
	Aug. 30, 1978	63	Dec. 22, 1978	30	33			10,15 or 20 per month	for 6 months	yes
	Jan. 18, 1979	26			26					
	April 5, 1979	10			10					
Tokyo	Mar. 28, 1978	115	May 19, 1978	115				10,15 or 20 per month	for 6 months	yes
(2 nd Group)	May 2, 1978	56	Dec. 22, 1978	55	1			10,15 or 20 per month	for 6 months	yes
	Nov. 30, 1978	29	Dec. 22, 1978	13	16			10,15 or 20 per month	for 6 months	yes
	Dec. 6, 1978	25	Jan. 31, 1979	6	19			10,15 or 20 per month	for 6 months	yes
	Dec. 6, 1978	26	Jan. 31, 1979	24		2		10,15 or 20 per month	for 6 months	yes
Tokyo	Apr. 5, 1978	36	May 19, 1978	28	8			10,15 or 20 per month	for 6 months	yes
(3rd Group)	May 1, 1978	80	May 19, 1978	41				10,15 or 20 per month	for 6 months	yes
			Dec. 22, 1978	34	2		3	10,15 or 20 per month	for 6 months	yes
	Nov. 14, 1978	40	Dec. 22, 1978	34				10,15 or 20 per month	for 6 months	yes
			Mar. 30, 1979	5				10,15 or 20 per month	for 6 months	
			Apr. 9, 1979			1				
Yokohama	May 1, 1978	1	Jun. 1, 1978	1				Yen 250 as provisional payment 15 per month	for 6 months	no
	Dec. 15, 1978	1	Dec. 27, 1978	1				15 per month	for 6 months	no

Osaka	July 3, 1978	10	Aug. 18, 1978	8				10 or 20 per month	for 6 months	no (incl. bereaved family)
			Sept. 22, 1978	1	1			10 or 20 per month	for 6 months	no
	Aug. 10, 1978	111	Oct. 23, 1978	77		34		5,10 or 20 per month	for 6 months	no (incl. bereaved family)
Kyoto	July 14, 1978	11	Sept. 21, 1978	11				4,7,9,10,12,13,14 16,20 or 22 per month	for 6 months	yes
	Nov. 28, 1978	17	Dec. 25, 1978	15		2		3,5,6,7,8,9,13,14 or 18 per month	for 6 months	no
Shizuoka	June 30, 1978	48	Oct. 11, 1978	20				15 or 20 per month	for 6 months	yes
			Jan. 16, 1979	13				10 or 15 per month	for 6 months	yes
			Mar. 8, 1979	6			9	10 or 15 per month	for 6 months	yes
Sapporo	Oct. 4, 1978	15	Dec. 11, 1978	15				7,12 or 20 per month	for 6 months	yes – 13, no – 2
Kanazawa	Oct. 19, 1978	49	Dec. 26, 1978	37			12	5,7,10,15 or 20 per month	for 6 months	no

settlement ensures the right to claim for money, and it prohibits the transfer and mortgaging of property by the other party. In the system of provisional disposition of disputed subject matter, the disposal of specific articles is prohibited. The provisional agreement to temporarily settle matters on the other hand aims to remove the anxiety arising from continuing and prolonged dispute and is an interim measure that will go on up to the conclusion of the suit.

For example, if a person is seriously injured in an automobile accident, he may file a suit for a compensation of damage or if a worker is unreasonably laid off, he may file a suit for wrongful dismissal. The provisional disposition system orders the other party to make provisional socio-medical payments to protect the livelihoods of the victims while the suit is in progress.

To obtain such court orders the claimant must prove the right to such security and the necessity of these measures. After the request is made in the court on principle, there will be an examination that will not go through all proceedings. It is the sole discretion of the judge to decide whether or not other parties should be examined. Furthermore, when the claim is admitted, the court may order the claimant to deposit a certain amount of money to act as an alternative for presumptive proof or to cover possible damages that the other party may incur while the process is put into effect.

Now we are most concerned with the provisional disposition system related to a temporary settlement. In the Okayama Prefecture alone the large outbreak of SMON disease from 1965 has produced over 1,000 patients to date. In December 1973 we initiated suits against Japan Ciba-Geigy, Takeda Chemical Company, Tanabe Pharmaceutical Company and the state. Immediately thereafter, many victims came forward demanding litigation and at present there are 144 plaintiffs, with 72 to 80 more in preparation.

In March of 1978 lawyers requested provisional disposition from the Okayama District Court to gain immediate living and medical expenses of the victims for the reasons:

The greatest controversy in the SMON litigation was and remains the causal relationship between SMON and clioquinol. The SMON Research Commission, later reorganized into the SMON group of Special Disease Research Committee of the Ministry of Health and Welfare, reported in 1972, in 1975 and repeatedly in 1977 that there can be no doubt that a causal relationship does exist between the two. Of the defendants, Japan Ciba-Geigy and Takeda Chemical Company and the state agreed in January 1977 and in April of the same year to accept Judge Kabe's tentative clauses of settlement. As a result, in October 1977 in the Tokyo District Court we were able to see the realization of this settlement.

Unfortunately, however, the victims who were covered by this settlement were only those that had used clioquinol manufactured and sold by Japan Ciba-Geigy and Takeda Chemical Company. The victims that had been using the Tanabe clioquinol or who had been simultaneously using Tanabe clioquinol as well as Ciba-Geigy and/or Takeda clioquinol were not covered by the settlement. This was because Tanabe Pharmaceutical Company had persistently insisted on the virus hypothesis which states a virus cause of SMON disease and had repeatedly refused to accept Judge Kabe's settlement plan. In the Okayama Prefecture, in spite of the expert opinions on clioquinol and SMON, the settlement was applied in only 20 out of the 55 plaintiffs. For the remaining 35 settlement could not be realized. That is to say that 10 years after the outbreak of the SMON disease, the same victims, bearing the same hardships and sufferings, were divided into two groups according to the pharmaceutical company that produced the clioquinol that they took.

As mentioned, the prolonged litigation was already adding much pressure to the hardship of the victims. At this point in time we anticipated that a long time would be necessary for decisions to be reached in this suit in the Okayama District Court. The plaintiffs' lawyers thus decided to apply for provisional disposition. However, other obstacles had to be overcome first for the request to be admitted.

Provisional disposition by its very nature entails the pre-judgement period. Therefore, the request was for an order to give pre-payment of a part of the final compensation. However, in cases of public pollution of drug induced suffering, provisional disposition had only been given in very special cases. In addition, the Okayama District Court was still in the middle of the controversy with the Tanabe Pharmaceutical Company as to whether SMON was actually related to clioquinol. Therefore, it was thought it would take extreme courage on the part of the judge to order provisional disposition. The timing of the request was thus carefully chosen, being made on the day following the victory of the SMON litigation in the Kanazawa District Court.

This request was admitted by the Judge of the Okayama District Court on March 27th. The Court ordered the Tanabe Pharmaceutical Company to pay a total of yen 61 millions, from a maximum of yen 4.2 millions to a minimum of yen 800,000, an average of yen 1,967,742 per victim. The court decided that examination of the Tanabe Pharmaceutical Company was unnecessary and that the claimant did not have guaranty money on deposit. The lawyers group then visited the Tanabe Pharmaceutical Company's main office in Osaka and made attachment to bank accounts and assets in the president's office. By doing so, all the payment ordered was obtained. The Okayama District Court decision is notable from three points of view:

Firstly, the decision has opened the way for the relief of the victims while the litigation is still underway. As the litigation tends to be prolonged, this is extremely significant. Secondly, this decision has become a model and has been followed by other district courts so contributing to the relief of the victims throughout Japan. As described in Table 1, during the 6 months following this decision in the Okayama District Court, a maximum of yen 20–22 million and a minimum of yen 3–10 million per plaintiff every month were given out in the Tokyo, Yokohama, Osaka, Kyoto, Shizuoka, Sapporo, Kanazawa District Courts. It is expected that similar decisions will be taken in other district courts. Thirdly, disciplinary actions against the Tanabe Pharmaceutical Company were obtained.

However, complete satisfaction has not been achieved, since it took 4 years and 3 months after the initial filing of the suit. The central problems of the day to day life of the victims are far from being solved. As mentioned above, the causal relationships between SMON and clioquinol has been the center of controversy. The SMON Research Commission already in March 1977 reported that there can be no doubt that the causality exists. If this decision had been reached earlier, relief for the victims could have been provided earlier. Provisional disposition is not the only solution and it is urgently necessary to establish a permanent relief system for the victims of drug induced sufferings.

Finally, it is a great pleasure to report that on August 4, 1978, plaintiffs' lawyers were given provisional attachment of immovables against Tanabe Pharmaceutical Company.

Foreseeability in lawsuits for drug-induced injuries

JUNICHI MATSUNAMI

Attorney, Toyama, Japan

Drug-induced injuries in Japan up to 1945 largely resulted from impure medicines. Mass production has resulted in pollution problems from the manufacturing processes and the inevitable mass consumption of the products has caused drug-induced injuries and food poisoning of sorts. Examples include the many injuries induced by thalidomide, Coralgil, chinoform (clioquinol), chloroquine etc.

Fierce protests from the injured made the Japanese Government undertake, with poor grace, legislation for the relief of drug-induced suffering. However, since relief measures were inapplicable for victims under civil liability towards individuals, lawsuits against the drug companies and/or the Government were required. Current judicial precedents, constructed around liability for negligence rather than contract point out that the sufferers should prove negligence in suits against the pharmaceutical companies and/or the Government, until a new preventative law against drug-induced injuries is instituted and based on entirely different concepts of liability without fault. However, such proof, essentially as regards foreseeability of drug injury, would be very difficult for the plaintiffs. To reduce such difficulties for the victims, it has been argued that once a drug-induced injury has occurred, it should be assumed that the pharmaceutical companies producing the drug and the Government permitting to manufacture have committed negligence. There have been several recent decisions, creating precedents, that have accepted this concept. However, such decisions cannot be presumed since contrary concepts and precedents have also been applied.

On the premise that assailants are obliged to pay great attention, two approaches have been used regarding judgements and theories concerning public hazards and drug-induced injuries: one considers the level at which prediction is possible, while the other concerns the scope and application of predictions.

The former approach is based on the following characteristics of the substance in question: (1) hazard to man probable; (2) occurrence of an actual hazard in man; (3) hazard unreasonable in proportion to the therapeutic benefit; (4) hazard similar to a predicted disease; (5) hazard and disease similar; (6) hazard and disease share common features; (7) hazard almost identical with disease; and (8) hazard itself produces disease.

Companies causing public hazard and drug-induced injuries have so asserted themselves that the recognition of the hazard itself, namely (8), is the only prerequisite for predicting hazard. However, this claim is so trivial, because prediction should be based on avoiding strategies towards materials likely, or known, to be hazardous.

By precedent, some recognition on level (1) has been sufficient to predict the hazard and doctrines supported these conclusions. Therefore, in lawsuits concerning drug-induced injuries, as well as public hazards, against pharmaceutical companies and the Government who had exclusive information and knowledge on the substance, we argued that surveys on the nature and the extent of the toxicity should have been carried out and the results made public. If levels (1) and (2) were known, the hazard should have been considered predictable and negligence was present if action had not been taken.

Medicine is a special case in that if a drug was recognized as being on level (3), it should not be used without further advanced surveys; it could even be said that full responsibility should be taken for all hazardous results regardless of its use. In the actual SMON lawsuit, considering the slow evolution in the courts, the five steps of arguments were adopted and proof was based on recognitions of (1) to (5) including the hazard-disease association (neurotoxicity).

There is another approach. When the plaintiffs brought lawsuits for SMON at Tokyo, Fukuoka, Kanazawa, Hiroshima and other places in 1971–1973, only the literature concerning neurotoxicity reported by Hangartner (1965) in animals and by Berggren and Hansson (1966) in man was known. Although the report of Gholz and Arons (1964) was later submitted to the court, it seemed hopeless to go back further to older ones.

Since SMON had already occurred in the late 1950s, it was necessary to find reports on the neurotoxicity of chinoform (clioquinol) published up to about 1955 to win suits for all patients in every era. This was the most difficult problem when the SMON lawsuit started. At that time it was known that the Aachen district court in the Federal Republic of Germany had closed a criminal action for injury induced by thalidomide against the Grünental Company and this gave hope for our eventual success. The decision regarding the prediction of thalidomide teratogenicity stated that if a compound or its derivatives comes under suspicion of teratogenicity, possible injury should be suspected or likely.

In this respect chinoform (clioquinol) is a halogenated oxychinoline derivative and possesses a chinoline nucleus. Thus, if chinoline, oxychinoline and their derivatives were neurotoxic, chinoform (clioquinol) might be expected to be neurotoxic given the known structure-activity relationships. We then attempted to survey the literature on neurotoxic derivatives. This type of work is readily and rapidly done by pharmaceutical companies or Government but it wasted much time and labor for non-experts in this field. The reports were eventually found and used in the SMON lawsuit: chinoline (Biach et al., 1881; Heinz, 1890; Stockman, 1894; Foster, 1894; Santesson, 1895, etc.), oxychinoline (Carlottenburg, 1906, 1907; Macht, 1928; Takase, 1937; Crescitelli, 1950, etc.), aminochinolines (Wiselogle, 1941; Schmid et al., 1959, etc.), chinine and its derivatives.

These reports demonstrated various neural disturbances, including paralysis, convulsions, psychomotor seizure, nystagmus and visual disorder. In addition, they more than adequately suggested that chinoform (clioquinol) with the same chinoline nucleus was likely to induce similar neural disturbances. In 1973 documentation was submitted to the court insisting that: 'Since chinoform (clioquinol) is a derivative of chinoline and it was well known that the chinoline core has harmful effects on the central nervous system, blood and liver, it was reasonable to suspect that chinoform might have similar hazardous actions.'

In this connection, a visual disorder caused by chinine was first reported by Graefe in 1857. Jess, in 1913, gave details of an optic toxicity of chinoline as a part of chinine. Furthermore, Schanz et al. also reported optochin and eucupine as possibly causing optical injuries. At a meeting of natural scientists and physicians, held in Bad Nauheim, Germany, in 1920, Jess gave a lecture entitled 'Dangerousness of chemotherapy for eye, especially on a component of chinine and its derivatives able to induce severe injuries of optic organs', and judged the toxic effect on retina to be due to chinoline. In the next year he stated: 'Analysing which component of chinine is essential for the visual disorder, it can be concluded that chinoline has particularly hazardous toxicity' and 'the optical toxicity of chinine and its derivatives is evidently due to chinoline'; and he thus issued a broad warning that chinoline-containing drugs could provoke optical injuries.

This warning was given about 40 years before Hobbs et al. reported that chloroquine caused a visual disorder. In a lecture to the General Meeting of the Ophthalmologist Association of Rhein-Westfalen in Essen in 1960, the hazards of chinoline-containing drugs on the retina were stressed. When Berggren and Hansson reported in 1966 that an infant taking chinoform (clioquinol) had symptoms of optic atrophy, it did not surprise those who knew that chloroquine contains a chinoline nucleus; the *Lancet* pertinently stated: 'These observations are not surprising, since irreversible retinopathy is well known after long-continued administration of chloroquine and 4-aminochinolines' (*March 30*, 1968, p. 679). It might therefore have been assumed that the results of Jess associating optical injury with chinoform (clioquinol) had been taken into consideration.

The progress of the SMON lawsuit promoted the understanding of the possible toxicity of drug analogs and the concept of structure-activity relationships; the literature on chinoline derivatives has now spread to other plaintiffs outside this area.

Pharmaceutical companies argue that only slight structural modifications change activities. Since such a complete loss of previous activity after partial structural change might not always occur, the structure-function argument still applies until it can be verified that the activity in question is completely lost after partial structural alteration.

The presumption that structural analogs have similar functions has been argued by plaintiffs; the toxicity of chinoform as a chinoline derivative has gradually been adopted by the courts.

Initially the Kanazawa District Court gave a decision but no judgment on this problem. In the second decision by the Tokyo District Court the toxicity of chinoline derivatives was considered to be reference material for that of chinoform. In the third decision by the Fukuoka District Court the toxicity of the particular drug as a chinoline derivative was assessed on the basis of the clinical observations on the toxicity of chinoform (clioquinol) as reported by Gravitz and others; this decision affirmed the assumption of the toxicity of analogous compounds as follows: 'If any nerve disturbances due to chinoline and its derivatives were predictable and correlated with SMON, it must be judged that SMON itself was predictable'. 'It had been already reported that oxychinoline derivatives and chinoline as their structural core caused neural disturbances in animals, before developmental studies on chinoform (clioquinol) as an internally administered drug were carried out.' 'We could not neglect reports concerning other structurally analogous compounds. There were also reports on neurotoxic effects of 4-aminochinolines and 8-aminochinolines'. Finally, 'Accordingly, no-one could say that the development of neural disturbances was not predictable, assuming a relationship between SMON and chinoline and its derivatives.'

Finally, in the fourth instance by the Hiroshima District Court prediction of the toxicity in question was completely affirmed as follows: 'Considering both the chemical structure and process of chinoform (clioquinol), originating from chinine, then from chinoline to oxychinoline, and finally through halogenation, a severe toxicity could be suspected. In addition, it was not so difficult to know these matters from the basic pharmaceutical and pharmacological literature and related reports, and from specialized advanced publications in therapeutics and pharmacology'.

A fruitful product of lawsuits for public hazards has been the recognition of a cause-and-effect relationship using epidemiological methods. In the case of SMON suits the prediction of injuries from empirical notions that structural analogs resemble functions has also been established as a precedent.

In conclusion, I sincerely hope that these concepts will be used extensively in future lawsuits concerning drug-induced injuries.

ACKNOWLEDGEMENTS

I am indebted to Prof. A. Igata, Medical School of Kagoshima University, Prof. H. Kumaoka, Faculty of Pharmaceutics of Mukogawa Women's University, Prof. Y. Gomi, Faculty of Pharmaceutical Sciences of Kanazawa University, Prof. T. Kameyama, Cancer Research Institute of Kanazawa University and Prof. Y. Sawai, Kansai University, for their helpful advice.

REFERENCES

1. Decision of the Fukuoka District Court, 5 October, 1977. *Hanrei Jiho, 866*, 27.
2. Decision of the Fukuoka District Court, 14 November, 1978. *Hanrei Jiho, 910*, 42.
3. Decision of the Tokyo District Court, 3 August, 1978. *Hanrei Jiho, 899*, 61.
4. Decision of the Kumamoto District Court, 20 March, 1973. *Hanrei Jiho, 696*, 17.
5. Sawai, Y. (1973): On the dirty drainage from a factory. *Horitsu Jiho, 2,* 10.
6. Matsunami, J. (1977): In: *SMON Drug Induced Suffering*, pp. 205–210. Editor: T. Kameyama. Otsuki Publ. Co., Inc.
7. Hangartner, P. (1965): Troubles nerveux observés chez le chien après absorption d'Entéro-Vioforme Ciba. *Schweiz. Arch. Tierheilk., 107,* 43.
8. Berggren, L. and Hansson, O. (1966): Treating acrodermatis enteropathica. *Lancet, 1*, 52.
9. Gholz, L.M. and Arons, W.L. (1964): Prophylaxis and treatment of amebiasis and shigellosis with iodochlorhydroxyquinoline. *Amer. J. trop. Med. Hyg., 13,* 396.
10. Fujiki, H. (1971): Decision of the thalidomide clinical trial in West Germany. II. *Jurist, 494*, 101.
11. Jess, A. (1921): Die Gefahren der Chemotherapie für das Auge, insb. über eine das Sehorgan schwer schädigende Komponente des Chinins und seiner Derivate. *Von Graefes Arch. Ophthal., 104*, 48.

12. Hobbs, H.E., Sorsby, A. and Freedman, A. (1959): Retinopathy following chloroquine therapy. *Lancet, 2*, 478.
13. Jess, A. (1965): Augenschäden nach Langzeitbehandlung mit Chlorochin. *Fortschr. Med., 83*, 547.
14. Annotations (1968): *Lancet, 2*, 679.
15. Kaeser, H.E. and Wüthrich, R. (1970): Zur Frage der Neurotoxizität der Oxychinoline. *Dtsch. med. Wschr., 95*, 1685.
16. Oakley, P. (1973): The neurotoxicity of the halogenated hydroxyquinolines. *J. Amer. med. Ass., 225*, 395.

DISCUSSION

Hansson: I thank the speakers in this session for their very interesting papers, especially the foreign guests at this Conference. The information given is very important to our understanding of the situation for SMON victims in Japan.

I also have to say that it is very sad to hear that you have to fight in this way for the rights of the victims. I am convinced that I speak on behalf of all the foreign guests of the KICADIS conference when I wish you success in your struggle and a total victory for all SMON patients in the very near future.

Relief of SMON victims in Sweden

OLLE HANSSON

Department of Pediatrics, University of Gothenburg, East Hospital, Gothenburg, Sweden

At present, there are about 22 patients in Sweden known to have been damaged by clioquinol or other oxyquinoline compounds and another 10 to 12 cases are being investigated. The majority of these cases came to light after information on the Japanese situation had been given to the Swedish public, especially after a TV program on SMON and other drug catastrophies. After the TV program, I received about 400 letters from people in Sweden who believe that their problems are caused by oxyquinoline. Most of these, of course, I have been able to convince that there must be some other cause.

Until recently, the attitude of Ciba-Geigy to giving financial compensation to Swedish victims has been quite negative. They have shown no interest whatsoever. However, we have been waiting for the court decision here in Japan, and when we got a translation of the crucial parts of the Tokyo District Court decision a few months ago, one of the lawyers in Sweden who assists the patients, Mr. Sjöström, announced in the newspaper his intention to sue the drug companies and also the Swedish state.

In Sweden, if you sue the state, the Attorney-General will be the defendant in court. A few weeks ago the Attorney-General took an important initiative by arranging a meeting between the drug industry and representatives of the Swedish patients. At this meeting an agreement was reached to start negotiations for a settlement out of court to be supervised by the Attorney-General. If we cannot reach an agreement, the Attorney-General will propose a compromise. If this is impossible, the drug companies and the Swedish state will be sued.* At the moment in Sweden there are two lawyers representing the patients. One is Mr. Sjöström who unfortunately could not come to this meeting and the other is Mr. Michael Tuveson. For the negotiations in Sweden I think that the experience in Japan will be very important. First of all, the causal relationship between the neurological damages and clioquinol has been proven in the Japanese courts; secondly, the negligence of the drug companies has been proven; and thirdly, the Japanese courts have found not only the companies but also the Japanese state guilty. So, in Sweden we see no reason to spend a lot of time, perhaps many years, starting a court trial. Instead, we shall use the evidence given in the Japanese courts in the Swedish situation and we are very fortunate in having this complete translation of the Tokyo District Court. Therefore, I am very optimistic about the Swedish situation.

*In February, 1980, the negotiations failed and 40 patients have sued the drug companies and the Swedish state.

I think that the drug companies will have to realize that if they are not reasonable they will be put under great pressure from the public and their reputation and credibility will be damaged. If necessary, we are of course prepared to sue both the Swedish state and the drug companies.

My role in the negotiations is to be an independent advisor for those patients who have contacted me. The negotiations will probably start at the beginning of next Autumn. We shall have full control of the course of these negotiations and we shall not allow any prolongations.

DISCUSSION

Takahara: You said that there are 22 patients who are suffering from the adverse effects of clioquinol and other oxyquinoline componds. What do you mean by other oxyquinoline compounds besides clioquinol?

Hansson: Well, there are different types of oxyquinoline depending on which halogens are in the molecule. The most frequently used is clioquinol or chinoform, but you also have broxyquinoline which is very similar. This has two bromine atoms whereas in clioquinol you have chloride and one iodine. In fact, I think there is no substantial difference between them from the clinical point of view. Chemically they are different, so I used the term 'oxyquinoline drugs' to indicate that there is not just one type. From the chemical point of view there are 3 or 4 different compounds.

Ohashi: In Japan, it is difficult for the long period patients to obtain confirmation from the doctor that their disease is caused by oxyquinoline. In Sweden you said that there are patients who only took these drugs once or twice during the past decade. Is it easy to obtain proof from the doctor that the patient took this drug over such a long period of time or so far back in the history?

Hansson: Well, it is of course a problem that a lot of these drugs taken by many people many years ago were not prescribed by doctors nor were they given in hospitals. This means that there are no medical notes from hospitals etc. to supply to a court as proof that the patients were in fact taking these drugs. In Sweden the situation is the following: After information about the side-effects of these drugs had been given in the newspapers and on TV, patients wrote letters to me. Some of them already in their first letter very completely described their symptoms and signs, when they appeared and what their situation was after that. Sometimes I have had correspondence and asked them several questions. Also many of them have been to hospitals for investigations into their neurological damage. But in the hospital notes there is no mention of these drugs because at that time we didn't know about the connection between the drugs and their disease.

The history given by these patients is so beautifully described by them in their own words that I'm convinced that it is impossible to fake a patient's history to a doctor who is well informed about how this disorder appears. So, in my opinion, you should use the spontaneous information from patients in the same way as documents from hospitals. If the patients can give a description of their symptoms and signs which fulfils the medical criteria, then there is no reason whatsoever to doubt that they are telling the truth. I can see no difficulty in convincing a court in Sweden if necessary that these letters from the patients themselves have the same values as a brief observation by a doctor in notes from a hospital.

Lannek: I would like to add a few words to the discussion about clioquinols and broxyquinoline. I have studied the adverse effect of quinolines in dogs for several years at the Royal Veterinary College in Stockholm. In my material of 110 dogs, the intoxication was caused by clioquinols in about 95% and in 5% by broxyquinolines. In the beginning I found that the dogs which were intoxicated by the latter had received a smaller dose per kg body-weight than the former. The material was too small for statistical evaluation. In further experiments on dogs I found no difference between the preparations.

Neurological complications following Kontrast-U injections: damaged persons versus Swedish drug company 1974–1979

MICHAEL TUVESON

Erik Tuvesons Advokatbyrå, Trelleborg, Sweden

There is a special X-ray method of examination of the lumbar part of the spine called myelography. This method consists of he following: (1) intravenous injection of a blood-pressure-increasing substance, (2) spinal anesthesia, (3) subarachnoid injection of a contrast medium, and (4) X-ray pictures which are taken of the lumbar part of the spine.

The contrast medium principally used in Swedish hospitals in 1972 was a medium called Kontrast-U, manufactured by the 'Leo' drug company in Helsingborg, Sweden. The contrast medium was a solution containing 0.2 g methiodal sodium per ml. The methiodal sodium consisted of about 50% iodine and had been used in Europe for about 40 years. It was exported from the 'Leo' drug company to many different countries and was also manufactured by a drug company in Germany. About 15,000–20,000 persons were examined by this myelographic method in Sweden each year, principally to investigate pain in the lumbar region.

Since Kontrast-U could not be used for examinations in the upper part of the spine because of its neurotoxic effects, gas was usually used as contrast medium, e.g. oxygen. An X-ray examination with contrast medium produced better X-ray pictures than examinations without contrast medium. On the X-ray pictures the doctors could see the contrast filling the space like a white string, the surrounding space being grey or black. If the white string had any protuberances, it could be a sign of lumbar disease, e.g. disc protrusion. Now and then an article was published concerning the side-effects of this method. It was known that disc protrusions could cause neurological complications. The first Swedish article on neurological complications after myelography with Kontrast-U 20% was published in 1959. The authors could give no definite explanation for the complications. In 1961 animal experiments were published with reports on paralysis after Kontrast-U myelography. In 1961 and later in the 1960's other articles appeared concerning sensitivity disturbances in the hypogastrium and in the legs after Kontrast-U myelography. Two persons were myelographed in my home town in 1972 and two persons in the neighboring city during the same month in 1972. The myelographic examinations were immediately followed by a cauda equina syndrome which involves paresis of the bladder and disturbed rectal function, disturbances of potency and numbness in the perianal region and down the back of the legs. The reason for the examinations was lumbar pain. The X-ray pictures of the damaged persons did not show much and they were mainly negative. The lumbar pain declined in general, but the cauda equina syndrome remained, except in one case where it later slowly declined. The damaged persons could not control their urinary function or evacuation. They suffered from disturbances of potency and felt numbness in their hips. At first the damaged persons believed that the reason for the complications was the treatment at the hospital. Because of that they informed the hospital directors about the complications and asked for compensation. The hospital directors performed investigations and reported on the complications to the State Medical Board's committee for drug-induced suffering. From that we conclude that in the 4 original cases the doctors considered that the complications were to be regarded as side-effects of Kontrast-U myelography and Kontrast-U was reported as a suspected drug. The committee started an investigation and the matter was also reported to the State Medical Board's committee with responsibility for medical attendants. The responsibility committee also started an investigation and its work was finished in 1974. According to their findings the treatments had been normal and the doctors bore no responsibility for the complications. According to the drug committee the cause of the complications could not be assessed because of lack of information. The 4 persons then contacted our law-office and asked for our advice. Our work with the cases now started. According to two formal reports from two Swedish professors dated 1973 and addressed to the drug committee it was improbable that the anesthetic agent had caused the complications and it was more likely that the circumstances surrounding the production of the contrast medium had something to do with it. Because of these remarks we contacted the manufacturer of the contrast medium. The drug company had already withdrawn the batches in question in the autumn of 1972. A meeting was arranged at a coffee-house in the neighboring city between the damaged persons and a director of the drug company. The director did not make any statements and there were no results of the meeting. When the director left the coffee-house he did not even pay for his own coffee. The damaged persons were upset about the fact that the drug company could not even pay them a cup of coffee.

After this we concluded that there would be no results in the negotiations between us and the drug company. Time went quickly by – the drug company did not say no and they did not say yes. They told us several times that more investigations were necessary. We could not wait for years and years. The damaged persons were about 50 or 60 years old and we decided to start legal proceedings against the drug company. There was a complication, though. You could not just state that there was a connection between the contrast medium and the neurological complications. You also had to provide evidence. If the connection was proved, what about the responsibility of the drug company? Was negligence on the part of the drug company necessary for responsibility or not? What kind of negligence could be of interest? I read a lot of books concerning product liability and came to the conclusion that the following points were of interest: (1) product information, (2) control of the drug, (3) condition of production, and (4) whether there was a disproportion between the side-effect and the desired effect of the drug.

Where to begin? The pharmaceutical documents of the State Medical Board were secret. I could not get them without the permission of the drug company. I started with the problem of the connection between Kontrast-U and the complications. In one of the professors' reports to the drug committee, I could read the name of an article in a German medical publication. I wrote to the nearest university library and asked for the article. They sent me a copy of it. At the end of the article I found references to other articles. I wrote to the library again and asked for the references. In those references I found other references. I asked for these and after a few months I had a great many articles from Sweden, Norway, Denmark, Germany, France, England and the U.S.A. on my desk. Now I had to think of the translation of these foreign articles to which we referred as evidence concerning myelography with methiodal sodium. The court required that these should be translated into Swedish. The cost for those translations upon inquiry to an authorized translation bureau appeared to be very high (about a year's salary of a public servant) and I was told that it would take about one year to do this work. It was not clear who would pay for it. We solved the problem by a happy coincidence. I met a person who had the necessary knowledge and who accepted to do the job for a reasonable charge. She worked very efficiently and the translations were ready in about 6 months.

In some of the articles I found animal experiments described and very interesting things about the risk of neurological complications in connection with Kontrast-U myelography. According to several experts the anesthetic agents had nothing to do with the cauda equina syndromes. I concluded that the contrast medium was the main factor in the matter. The result of my work was that the contrast medium must be the cause of the complications. Before 1963 contrast media could be sold without registration by the State Medical Board. In 1963, however, registration must be made. The drug company sent a registration application to the State Medical Board which then asked for information concerning the pharmacological and toxic effects of the medium. After that the drug company sent a list of references to the State Medical Board. I got the list of references and the application documents from the drug company. The fact that the registration acts are secret has been a big problem. We did not receive all the material from the State Medical Board: e.g. Leo's complete correspondence with the Board concerning the withdrawal of Kontrast-U in the autumn of 1974. According the Swedish law reports on drugs which have been submitted by drug companies to the Board must not be made public except where the authorities find that it is in the public interest. According to the authorities' interpretation, individual interest (claims because of side-effects of a drug) can never coincide with public interest. Therefore we could not obtain any other reports than those which Leo allowed us to have. In the Swedish laws there is a statement that a court can order that a secret report must be made public if it can be of importance in a trial. This possibility naturally puts active pressure on the drug company to have the reports made public. It is important to get out these reports on cases of side-effects *before* suing a drug company. You will not have to go to trial against a drug company just to get the reports.

A big problem was to get experts to help us. The connection between the medical staff and the drug industry was very hard to break. I contacted Professor Shapiro, Connecticut, U.S.A., who had written one of the publications to which we had referred as evidence. I received his address through the Swedish Embassy in Washington. After that, Professor Shapiro had offered us his help and to come to Sweden to attend the public hearings. This had been made known to the public through the newspapers and the situation became easier for us. It was now easier to have some experts to help us.

It would be convenient if the medical authorities were obliged to help lawyers by referring them to experts who could give aid in cases of side-effects of drugs.

Among the references on Kontrast-U sent to the State Medical Board you could not find the animal experiments in 1961 which had been published and you could not find several other publications. In the product information you could not find warnings against cauda equina syndromes. In several of the articles which the drug company before or after registration never sent to the State Medical Board, I found remarks, among other things, of cauda equina syndromes in connection with myelographies. I now thought that I had evidence for a connection between the contrast medium and the complications and that I had evidence for negligence concerning the product information. The time had come to open legal proceedings. The proceedings were opened in February, 1976. In our legal documents we also maintained that the drug company was responsible for the complications, even if negligence could not be proved. We have no law in Sweden about strict liability for manufacturers. Swedish law cases on drugs do not exist. The primary principle in Swedish law is that negligence is necessary for liability.

After opening the legal proceedings many people in Sweden and other countries contacted us. They informed us about their cauda equina syndromes which appeared after contrast myelographies and wanted our legal assistance.

According to the court decision the oral proceedings were to be finished in March 1979, which they were. The court's decision has not yet been published.

DISCUSSION

Kojima: In these drug-induced litigations, as has already been mentioned, the experts' assistance in proving the case is very hard to obtain. You mentioned that you had to ask an expert from abroad to come to Sweden. I would like to ask two questions related to this. Firstly, do you have an expert witness system in Sweden that is related to the court? We don't have this in Japan yet. Secondly, in preparation for litigation you need experts who will give advice. Is it possible to have these people act as expert witnesses during the trial?

Tuveson: Regarding the first question, whether we have an expert witness system in Sweden which is related to the court, my answer is no. But the court can ask an expert to come to the trial or to give advice to the court, to be of aid to the court, and maybe to make a statement or whatever the court asks for.

In this way, the expert is almost a kind of expert judge since of course the judges listen to him, and I suppose that the judges do what the expert will advise them to do. In this contrast medium trial, for example, we had a Swedish professor whom the court asked to be the court's aide, and he put a tremendous amount of work into this trial. According to this professor, there was a causal relationship between Kontrast-U and the cauda equina syndrome. If now the court makes a decision that there is a causal relationship, maybe you could say that this professor has been an extra judge in the trial.

On your next question, if there is a kind of system with advisory experts which can be used in the trial, the answer is 'yes', because in the proceedings if I as attorney want advice from an expert, I will ask him to help me, and then during the public hearing he can be called by me as an expert witness. But if I lose the case, I have to pay the expenses myself.

Kojima: When this person comes forward as an expert witness in court, in Japan as a qualification he must give his opinion in a very sincere way. If, however, this same witness acted as an advisor to one of the parties, would this not be an obstacle under Swedish law?

Tuveson: The answer to your question is that it is no problem in Swedish law to have an advisor to one party because he of course knows that the other party also has private advisors, and they have to perform their work in a strictly objective way.

'Drug reform' legislation in the United States

ANITA JOHNSON

Consumer Affairs Section, Box 386, Washington, DC, U.S.A.

Public interest in prescription drugs is very high in the United States. The daily press features numerous articles on drugs. Some of these articles stress the good news about drugs – drugs under development, benefits that up-and-coming drugs are expected by the manufacturers to offer. Womens' magazines tend to prefer these good-news articles. Other articles focus on the bad news about drugs – reporting previously unknown side-effects of drugs, disappointments in therapies, high prices, etc. Bad-news articles tend to appear in major dailies but are uncommon in other newspapers and in periodicals.

The drug laws are administered by the U.S. Food and Drug Administration, which has a high public visibility. The Food and Drug Administration (FDA) has been under attack by a number of consumer organizations as being too optimistic about the value of drugs, and too slow to realize their potential for harm. The same agency has also been under attack by drug manufacturers for what they view as its excessive caution in approving drugs and excessive concern about side-effects. Recently, the FDA has also been under attack from this angle by groups that favor so-called natural medicines such as Laetrile.

With so many people having critical things to say about the FDA in recent years, it is not surprising that 'drug reform' legislation is now being considered by the Congress. This legislation has been actively pursued in both houses of the legislature and is now in similar form in both houses. While passage of this legislation is not certain, the fact that committees have been working on it for 2 years and the fact that it has the imprimatur of Senator Edward Kennedy make passage of some drug legislation in the current session of Congress a strong possibility.

I shall describe the most interesting parts of the bills under consideration and try to point out where there are strong controversies on their merits.

The drug laws in the United States require the drug manufacturer to prove the safety and effectiveness of his product prior to marketing. The drug manufacturer normally generates scientific proof of these elements himself, but he may also rely on data in the published literature about his product or similar ones. The data are submitted to the FDA which prepares evaluations on the data and approves the drug if its evidence of benefits and risks is sufficient and if the benefits of the drug outweigh the risks. The FDA evaluates the data, but does not generate it. A drug may be removed from the market if the FDA re-evaluates its worth later, but formal, and frequently protracted, procedures are necessary. By law, decisions about drugs are made at the FDA, which employs 275 new drug evaluators – mostly physicians and Ph.D's. As an informal matter, the FDA frequently calls in academics and other experts to discuss decisions in advisory committee meetings before decisions are finalized, but the decisions are made by civil servants, not outside experts. In order to *test* new drugs in humans, the law requires the manufacturer to secure approval from the FDA based on animal, chemical and other information.

One of the unique features of the U.S. drug law is a requirement that drugs be proven effective with 'adequate and well-controlled investigations, including clinical investigations, by experts qualified by scientific training and experience to evaluate the effectiveness of the drug involved...' (21 U.S.C. 355). The requirement that effectiveness be proven by well-controlled studies is a truly startling change in drug evaluation that was introduced into law together with several other measures in 1962 as a result of public horror at the thalidomide experience. Until that time, drugs were adjudged as to safety, but in general, what information about their effectiveness that was available came from testimonials and uncontrolled investigations. The best example of the fallacy of this approach to drug therapy is the case of diethylstilbestrol (DES). This drug was thought by many medical practitioners to prevent spontaneous abortion and was prescribed for millions of pregnant women. When controlled studies were conducted, DES was shown to be ineffective for that purpose. Nevertheless, DES has caused hundreds of cases of cancer in the female offspring of women so exposed, and is associated with other reproductive tract abnormalities as well.

The requirement of well-controlled trials now in the law is an important consumer protection tool. Nevertheless, after 18 years on the books, it is still unaccepted by many interested parties. The American Medical Association (AMA), the main professional association for doctors in the U.S., has called for its repeal. One would expect doctors to be appreciative of well-studied therapies, but the AMA has opposed the effectiveness requirements on the basis that the effectiveness of drugs need not undergo scientific study because their effectiveness can be adequately judged in clinical practice. Doctors in the U.S. are not, as a rule, trained in scientific procedures and the evaluation of scientific materials; the great emphasis of formal training is on clinical experience through observation in hospitals.

The drug manufacturers have also viewed the well-controlled trial requirement with disdain, although their opposition is more subtly directed at the FDA for its administrative decisions on what studies are 'well controlled'. The drug manufacturers have made a great deal of effort to convince the public that important drugs are available outside the U.S. and are being held back by the FDA because of the well-controlled evidence of effectiveness requirements. One example widely used by drug manufacturers has been the beta-blocker drugs, which the FDA has been cautious in approving for sale. Although propranolol is now approved for use in heart pain in the United States, the FDA refused approval for years because the manufacturers failed to conduct well-controlled studies. Doubts about the effectiveness of propranolol for this use remain. Several other drugs were kept off the market because of fears of their cancer-causing potential, including practolol, a drug sold in Europe but now known to be associated with serious eye damage and other damage.

The drug bills permit the 'conditional' marketing of drugs which lack controlled evidence of effectiveness if the drugs are intended for fatal or severely debilitating diseases that lack adequate therapy and if the FDA determines that there is anecdotal information from experts and animal evidence indicating their usefulness.

This 'conditional' approval continues for 3 years, or is renewed, and the manufacturer is supposed to conduct well-controlled studies in the interim. This provision is strongly opposed by manufacturers and the AMA, consistent with their view that well-controlled investigations are not essential. Consumer groups oppose this provision, saying that these conditionally approved drugs would be promoted and distributed just like fully tested drugs, before any valid assessment of their worth could be made. They also point out that patients will risk the side-effects of these drugs without understanding that the evidence supporting the benefit is soft.

DATA DISCLOSURE

A key goal of consumer groups for this legislation has been public disclosure of the scientific data upon which drug approval is based. At the present time, summaries of these data are released by the FDA, but the data themselves are not released on the theory that they are 'trade secrets'. The manufacturers oppose disclosure, arguing that these data will provide competitors with windfall information that might be used to secure approval for an identical drug from the FDA or give research leads for similar drugs. On the other hand, consumer groups argue that these data are necessary to evaluate whether or not the summaries – submitted by the manufacturers or constructed by FDA personnel from manufacturers summaries – are accurate. They say that whatever information may be gleaned by competitors is already gleaned in the summaries released by FDA (if the summaries are accurate).

In recent years, Congressional committees have spotlighted instances of misrepresentation of test data by the manufacturers. For example, there was testimony that the G.D. Searle company submitted rat studies to the FDA which, it said, showed that metronidazole, Flagyl (used for trichomonas vaginitis infections), did not cause cancer. Pursuant to a finding that metronidazole causes decreased white blood cell counts in humans, this drug was re-tested by independent scientists who found that it did, indeed, cause cancer in mice. An FDA investigator re-examined the earlier, Searle, data and discovered that, contrary to Searle's allegations, rats fed metronidazole exhibited higher rates of cancer. The FDA requires many drugs to have long-term animal studies, for cancer and other chronic effects such as cataracts, prior to approval. There has also been testimony that test laboratories hired by drug manufacturers are involved in falsification of animal studies, including the reporting of studies that were never conducted at all. One laboratory, according to investigators, has been involved in several hundred such studies. In a recent spot-check of ongoing human drug investigations, the FDA found that 10% entailed serious violations which compromised the value of the study or the patients' safety. FDA Commissioner Donald Kennedy has stated that drug company data is 'sloppy much of the time and frequently even corrupt'.

Consumer groups point out that an open data policy would provide strong incentive to produce good-quality data because the data would be open to scrutiny by everybody. They say that as long as drug tests are performed by the very party who stands to benefit the most by a finding of 'safe' and 'effective', open data will be necessary to provide adequate incentive for careful and honest practices. This view is shared by the FDA, which has consistently supported the disclosure provisions of the bill.

The FDA points out that open data will permit it to explain its regulatory decisions to the public. Now, the agency is in the untenable position of having to justify its decisions without being able to show the scientific evidence upon which the decisions are made. When drug companies claim publicly that the FDA is stifling new drugs, the FDA cannot rebut the claims.

Last, drug innovation and competition by innovation will be enhanced by data disclosure. As pointed out by the 1977 U.S. Department of Health, Education and Welfare's Report on New Drug Regulation, wasteful and expensive duplication of tests already performed by another company would be ended as will needless exposure of human subjects to drugs already deemed hazardous in earlier tests. Free exchange of scientific knowledge to the medical profession and others would fertilize drug ideas. The Report pointed out that drug companies with significant new inventions can take adequate steps to protect their interests by securing patents.

EXPORTS

Under current U.S. law, American companies may generally export only those drugs which are approved for sale in the United States. A drug must be approved for some indication in the U.S. before it can be exported (labels may differ overseas, however). The drug legislation now in Congress, with the support of the FDA, increases export of products unapproved for use in the U.S. It permits export of drugs not approved for any purpose in the U.S., unless the FDA decides that the drug is 'contrary to the public health'. Under the bill, the burden is on the FDA to stop export and to undertake formal hearing procedures if it wishes to do so. Consumer groups believe that although the FDA would have the power to stop export of some unapproved drugs, it would not, as a practical matter, undertake to do so because of the expensive procedures involved, because there are no interest groups in the U.S. to encourage the FDA to do so, and because it is unlikely that the FDA will have the information to prove that the drug is hazardous. They believe that the most common situation is that the drug will be new, and little information will be available about it either way.

The drug manufacturers argue that it is paternalistic for the U.S. government to make decisions for other countries. The FDA notes that all exported drugs would have to meet U.S. standards of purity and potency, and have to receive permission of the foreign government.

LABELING

The bill requires all prescription drugs to carry a label written for patients that describes the purposes for which the drug was approved, side-effects, instructions for use, warnings, etc. Traditionally, labels for prescription drugs have been prepared only for physician use. Sponsors of the bill note evidence that physicians are not always thoroughly familiar with the contents of the FDA-required physician labels and do not always take the time to acquaint their patients with the contents. An example of this situation cited by consumer groups is the progestogen drugs, such as Provera and Delalutin, prescribed over half a million times in 1975 for pregnancy-related conditions, long after the pregnancy-related conditions were removed from the approved indications on the physician label. Proponents of the so-called patient package inserts say the labels will educate consumers on what questions to ask their doctors about drug therapy, and permit them to take an active role in choice of therapy.

Manufacturers and the AMA oppose patient labels as an unwarranted intrusion into the doctor-patient relationship.

PRICE AND PROMOTION

The bill seeks to encourage competitive pricing of drugs by posting of prescription drug prices in pharmacies, and permitting the FDA to develop a 'formulary' of generic drugs, a list of equivalents in terms of manufacturing quality to brand name drugs or a list of non-equivalents.

New strictures on promotion of drugs are proposed. Following Congressional testimony about elaborate gifts to medical students and doctors from drug companies, the bill prohibits gifts over $5 in value. It prohibits unsolicited free samples of drugs. It restricts surveys of pharmacies. Drug companies have in the past procured pharmacists' records to locate which doctors are prescribing their products and which are not, with the aim of directing salesmen to certain doctors.

CRIMINAL LIABILITY

Under current law, corporate executives may incur criminal liability for adulterated drugs if they bear a responsible relationship in the corporation to the particular violation. This liability may attach without proof of intent or negligence, although the FDA states that it has not punished executives absent repeated violations. This provision has long been a source of great dismay to corporate officials, who believe they should not be prosecuted unless the government can prove their direct personal role in the violation. The new bill states that corporate executives may be prosecuted upon proof of their personal negligence. Consumer groups point out that negligence may be very difficult to prove since corporate executives will argue that they cannot be negligent if they delegated responsibility to a well-qualified subordinate, and followed practices which were common in the industry. Consumer groups also point out that, although not exercised often, criminal liability without proof of scienter impresses upon executives the importance of giving top priority within the company to compliance with drug laws.

POST-MARKET CONDITIONS

At the present time, the FDA has only the authority to prove or disapprove a drug.

Once a drug is approved, any doctor may prescribe it for any purpose under any conditions. One bill gives the FDA the authority to limit use of drugs to hospital use, to use only with written informed consent of the patient, etc. One case for limited distribution is the drug chloramphenicol (chloromycetin), the drug of choice for certain typhoid infections which is widely prescribed for minor infections and even colds. Chloramphenicol causes sometimes fatal blood disorders, and limitation to hospital use would cut back its distribution to the appropriate population of typhoid victims.

Thus, the bill is a mixed bag of provisions and embodies no consistent regulatory philosophy. Some provisions address consumer criticisms that drugs are underregulated and some provisions address manufacturers' criticisms that drugs are overregulated.

DISCUSSION

Payne: With respect to testing of pharmaceutical products for FDA approval, what position would consumer groups take as to the assumption of full responsibility for such testing to be taken by a Federal executive agency, such as the FDA?

Johnson: Consumer groups think it's essential in the long run to get the testing out of the control of the drug companies. However, there is very little chance of that getting through the Congress at the present time. Senator Gaylord Nelson from Wisconsin has introduced a bill where the government would act as a broker for drug tests, the government would not conduct the tests but the government would take the money from the drug companies, find out from the drug companies what the intention of the test is and then make arrangements for a respected academic or some independent hospital to do the testing. There really is only a handful of people who understand how serious the problem of low-quality data is and only a handful of people that support this.

Payne: Well, if there was a choice then between the government acting as a broker, and the government actually taking over the responsibility for the testing, which side do you think the consumer group would prefer?

Johnson: That would be a wonderful luxury for consumer groups to choose between those two. I don't foresee that we will have that luxury at least in the next decade. I don't know.

Herxheimer: Could you say something about the sorts of consumer groups in the U.S. that consider drug issues, and whom they represent?

Johnson: I'm really not prepared to answer this question, I will try off the top of my hat. There are actually not very many consumer organizations which are equipped to work on medical matters. It is very difficult. In the United States many consumer groups are employing lawyers, but it's very hard for lawyers to work on these issues without having scientists, scientific colleagues with them. So the number of consumer groups who work on drug matters and on medical therapy matters is relatively small. The most prominent group is the Ralph Nader group, the health research group. It's a very tiny group – I think the budget runs between 90,000 and 100,000 dollars a year; they employ 4 or 5 professionals, but over the years they have worked on a number of different issues like unnecessary surgeries, hysterectomy for sterilization, and unnecessary dangerous use of drugs such as tetracycline for minor infections.

Herxheimer: Do they represent anybody?

Johnson: They represent their contributors, and the same thing is true of the consumers union which has done advocacy in the medical area, and the environmental defense fund which has about 45,000 contributors. But these are voluntary contributors and usually they are very low budget organizations. Most of them operate only with a great deal of volunteer time from experts. An expert at university may be worried about a problem and call up an advocacy group and say 'Let me send you some publications on this subject. I'll help you with the vocabulary.' Many, many hours of that kind are donated by experts to consumer groups. But in general I would say consumer groups are very tiny and very undernourished in the United States.

Disclosure of hazards in international drug promotion*

MILTON SILVERMAN and MIA LYDECKER

Health Policy Program, School of Medicine, University of California, San Francisco, CA, U.S.A.

With practically no exceptions, any drug powerful enough to relieve symptoms or control a disease can also cause injury or tissue damage – and, in some cases, even death.

The size of the problem is difficult if not impossible to describe with precision. In the United States, it has been estimated that from 3 to 5% of all hospital admissions to medical services are caused by drug-induced reactions. Among patients admitted to the medical services for any reason, somewhere between 10 and 30% will acquire an adverse reaction. For patients who suffer such reactions, the hospital stay will on the average be doubled. The number of deaths attributed to adverse drug reactions in the United States has been estimated to be at least 30,000 a year and perhaps as many as 130,000 annually. The financial cost of these drug-induced reactions for hospital board-and-room expenses alone has been put at approximately $4 to $5 billion per year (1). Some experts have estimated that roughly 80% of these drug-caused disasters are predictable and most of these are preventable (2).

It has long been assumed that physicians, in whatever country they practice, are fully aware of the hazards inherent in the drugs they prescribe or administer. It has likewise been assumed that reputable drug manufacturers will honestly disclose not only the proved values of their products but also the dangers. Such assumptions can no longer be accepted.

Since at least 1973, when Dunne and his co-workers in London revealed the remarkable discrepancies in the labeling of chloramphenicol in some 20 industrialized and Third World nations (3), the labeling and promotional practices of drug firms have been seriously questioned. Some of these questions have been raised by physicians, pharmacologists, and pharmacists. Some have been raised by the parents, children, wives, or husbands of the victims.

In our effort to examine this situation more fully, a comparison was made of the promotion of 28 important prescription drugs in the form of 40 different products marketed in both the United States and 11 Latin American countries by 23 multinational drug companies. The basis for the comparison was *Physicians' Desk Reference (PDR)* (4), distributed each year to essentially all practicing physicians in the United States. It was selected not because the statements it contains are necessarily valid or free from controversy, but because those statements have been approved by an official governmental agency, the industry can live profitably if not

*Based on research supported in part by grants from the Janss Foundation, Los Angeles, and the Ford Foundation, New York.

enthusiastically with them, and the book is widely used by physicians.

The somewhat comparable volumes studied in Latin America (5–8) may mention the same product marketed by the same company, but the statements are not approved by any government agency. The companies say what they wish to say, and they leave out what they do not want to tell physicians.

The differences were striking. In the United States, the companies were restricted in their claims of efficacy to those which they could support by substantial scientific evidence and not merely by glowing testimonials. Similarly, under the law, they were required to list all necessary warnings, contraindications, and potential adverse reactions. In the Latin American countries, with few exceptions, the companies grossly exaggerated the claims for their products, and the warnings were minimized, glossed over, or totally omitted. A few examples may be cited.

In the case of Parke-Davis' Chloromycetin or chloramphenicol, physicians were advised to prescribe this potent antibiotic only for such life-threatening diseases as typhoid fever, Hemophilus influenzal meningitis, and other infections for which no safer drug was available. Physicians were warned of the risk of serious or fatal aplastic anemia and urged not to use chloramphenicol for trivial infections.

In marked contrast, chloramphenicol was recommended to Latin American physicians for the treatment of such scarcely life-threatening conditions as tonsillitis, pharyngitis, bronchitis, urinary tract infections, ulcerative colitis, staphylococcus and streptococcus infections, yaws, and gonorrhea. Appropriate warnings were given to physicians in Mexico but not to those in Guatemala, Costa Rica, and the other Central American countries.

Ciba-Geigy's Butazolidine or phenylbutazone and an 'alka' product combining the drug with an antacid were described in the United States as products that are not to be considered as simple analgesics or administered without caution. They have limited applications, usually for severe forms of specified arthritic conditions. They may cause stomach or duodenal ulcer, sometimes with perforation, and a serious or fatal blood dyscrasia. They are contraindicated in children and in senile patients. Especially in the elderly, treatment should be limited to brief periods.

But in Latin America, these products were described as useful not only in serious forms of arthritis but in a wide variety of conditions described vaguely as marked by fever, pain, and inflammation. The 'alka' form was recommended as 'especially indicated for patients with sensitive stomachs and prolonged treatments, as well as in infancy, adolescence, and advanced age'. In some countries, no contraindications, warnings, or adverse reactions were mentioned.

Four oral contraceptives were included in the study. In the United States, the only approved use was for the prevention of pregnancy (except for a high-dosage form approved for the control of endometriosis and hypermenorrhea). Physicians were warned of the risk of serious and potentially fatal thromboembolic changes.

In Latin America, one product – Norinyl, marketed by Syntex in Mexico – was described in essentially the same terms as it was in the United States. But Searle's Ovulen, Wyeth's Ovral or Anfertil, and Parke-Davis' Norlestrin or Prolestrin were recommended not only for contraception but also for the control of premenstrual tension, dysmenorrhea, the problems of the menopause, and a host of other conditions. Warnings were presented in some of the Latin American countries but not in others.

These findings have been extended now to Spain and other countries. Our colleagues have pointed out to us the striking discrepancies between the drug descriptions published for use in the United Kingdom and those concerning the same products published for use in some of the developing countries in Africa (9).

It should be stressed that these discrepancies do not involve only the promotion and labeling practices of the multinational companies. The promotion by many local companies is also marked by what independent drug experts would view as an exaggeration of claims and a covering up of hazards.

In defense of their practices, the multinational companies – American, French, Swiss, and West German – presented a number of explanations.

Physicians in Latin America, they said, were already aware of the hazards and needed no further warnings. This argument may be counted on to infuriate drug experts and medical educators, who have witnessed all too many examples of irrational and dangerous prescribing.

It is the drug detailer or sales representative, some companies said, who explains the hazards to physicians. But, in Latin America as in the United States – and probably most other countries – it is commonly noted that you don't expect a salesman to 'knock' his own product.

What we're doing, some company spokesmen claimed, is only accepted business tradition. Thus, as a Latin American drug promotion expert explained it, if your competitor claims 5 indications for his product, you must claim at least 6. And if he discloses 3 adverse reactions, you are unwise if you disclose more than 2.

The discrepancies in drug promotion, some company officials have said, are merely honest differences in opinion. For example, a spokesman may say, 'We have in our files a wealth of convincing evidence to show that our product is as safe and effective as we claim. But, unfortunately, the evidence is not convincing to the United States Food and Drug Administration. What we have, therefore, is a dispute between honest scientists'.

Such an argument might be more palatable if the company said one thing in the United States, where it is under the constant scrutiny of the FDA, and another thing throughout the world where perhaps the laws are less formidable. But it was apparent that there were differences within Latin America, with the company saying one thing in Mexico, something different in Honduras and Nicaragua, something still different in Ecuador and Colombia, and something else again in Brazil.

Finally, the companies said, whatever else you think, we are not breaking any laws. In some countries, this defense is sound; the companies were not breaking any drug promotion laws or regulations because there were no such laws. But in other countries, company assertions of innocence were apparently untrue; the drug promotion was in violation of laws clearly requiring full disclosure of hazards.

The first findings from this survey were published in May of 1976 (10) and presented simultaneously to a committee of the United States Congress (11). So far as we are aware, however, there is nothing that the Congress can do to control the promotional activities of an American firm marketing its product in a foreign country. Presumably the same situation exists in Switzerland, France, West Germany, Great Britain, and other industrialized nations. Accordingly, other steps must be investigated.

One such step was taken late in 1976, when the Pharmaceutical Manufacturers

Association of the United States introduced a resolution before the council of the International Federation of Pharmaceutical Manufacturers Associations (IFPMA), calling for prescription drug labeling to be consistent with 'the body of scientific and medical evidence pertaining to that product'. Moreover, 'particular care should be taken that essential information as to medical products' safety, contraindications and side effects is appropriately communicated.' The resolution was adopted by unanimous vote.

The IFPMA action was merely a recommendation, and not binding on its members. Nevertheless, it is now apparent that – at least in some of the Latin American countries – some of the multinational companies are altering their labeling and promotion. Claims are being limited and hazards disclosed. Some manufacturers are saying to Latin American physicians essentially the same thing they are saying to physicians in the United States (12).

But the future remains unclear. Even in Latin America full disclosure of dangers is far from universal. Many physicians remain uninformed, or misinformed – deliberately or otherwise. Their patients remain at risk and many suffer needlessly. Throughout the Third World, the problem is still present and serious.

There are drug industry leaders who have long claimed that the industry can be counted on to police itself. The record of the drug industry, or any other major industry, to police itself and control its socially irresponsible members does not seem to offer grounds for much confidence. Although some distinguished economists insist that irresponsible companies – those that market unsafe or ineffective products, or make unsupported claims – will soon lose the confidence of their customers and be punished competitively in the market place, this does not seem to happen very often in the drug business. Or, at least, it has not happened often during the last half century. Companies that have been publicly charged with making unsubstantiated or even fraudulent claims, with marketing unsafe or ineffective products – and sometimes that have been required to take those products off the market – remain in business. They remain viable. They remain profitable.

Other steps need to be considered. Certainly each country, industrialized or developing, should enact appropriate laws and regulations covering drug labeling and promotion. These laws and regulations must not merely be put on the books. They must be enforced – and enforced vigorously – and offenders must be dealt with.

Those countries which purchase substantial quantities of drugs for their own social security or health programs should consider not only the quality and price of the products but also the quality of the promotion and labeling.

The World Health Organization or some other international body should be encouraged in attempts to set up standardized drug labeling as based on the consensus of the world's medical and scientific community, to serve at least as guidelines.

And those companies which have already exhibited their social responsibility by telling the truth, the whole truth, and nothing but the truth should be applauded and supported.

In each drug company, we are deeply convinced, there are decent, honorable people who want their own firm to adopt this approach. They deserve our encouragement.

REFERENCES

1. Silverman, M. and Lee, P.R. (1974): *Pills, Profits, and Politics*, pp. 261–266. University of California Press, Berkeley, CA.
2. Melmon, K.L. (1971): Preventable drug reactions – causes and cures. *New Engl. J. Med., 284*, 1361.
3. Dunne, M., Herxheimer, A., Newman, M. and Ridley, H. (1973): Indications and warnings about chloramphenicol. *Lancet, 2*, 781.
4. *Physicians' Desk Reference* (1973 et seq.): Medical Economics, Oradell, NJ.
5. *Diccionario de Especialidades Farmacéuticas, Edición Mexicana* (1973 et seq.): Editors: E. Rosenstein, A. Martín del Campo and I. Landero. Ediciones PLM, Mexico City.
6. *Diccionario de Especialidades Farmacéuticas, Edición C.A.D.* (1973 et seq.): Editors: E. Rosenstein and A. Martín del Campo. Ediciones PLM, Mexico City.
7. *Diccionario de Especialidades Farmacéuticas, Edición E. Co.* (1973 et seq.): Editors: E. Rosenstein and A. Martín del Campo. PLM International, Bogotá, Colombia.
8. *Index Terapéutico Moderno* (1973 et seq.): Editor: P.B. de Carvalho Fontes. Serviços de Publicações Especializadas, Sao Paulo, Brazil.
9. Medawar, C. (1979): *Social Audit – Insult or Injury?*, Chapter 9. Social Audit Ltd., London.
10. Silverman, M. (1976): *The Drugging of the Americas*. University of California Press, Berkeley, CA.
11. Silverman, M. (1976): In: *Hearings Before the Subcommittee on Monopoly of the Select Committee on Small Business, United States Senate: Competitive Problems in the Drug Industry*, Part 32, pp. 15360–15391.
12. *Diccionario de Especialidades Farmacéuticas, Edición C.A.D.* (1978). Ediciones PLM, Mexico City.

DISCUSSION

Shin: Dr. Silverman has pointed out some very important points, particularly differential sales practices depending on the countries where certain drugs are sold. I believe that the solution to this question is fundamentally a moral or ethical problem rather than a scientific, technical or legal problem. For example, pollution as well as drug-induced suffering has slowly deteriorated our body knowingly or unknowingly until we are sure of apparent wicked effects.

Therefore, the question about what we all have to think of right now seems to be not simply a technical detail of how to effectively control such and such problems, including drug-induced suffering, but how to correct the state of the human mind which easily tends to become wicked by external influences, such as business interest or other immediate results.

Silverman: I agree with you completely, Dr. Shin. And, Mr. Chairman, may I add at this point one recommendation we are not making is that Japan or any other country should import the Food and Drug Administration. The problems that each of you are facing in your individual countries are your problems. You must find your own solutions with whatever help we can give, but you must find your own.

Inman: I entirely agree with Dr. Silverman's proposal that there should be no variation in ethical standards in different countries, but I would like to hear his views about the emphasis that should be placed in different countries on certain types of warning. For example, we would insist on warnings about the risk of thrombosis in women using oral contraception, but I could see no reason why such a warning should be given to women in India, where there is no such risk. When the FDA coughs other national agencies may catch a cold. The same advice may not always be appropriate in all countries.

Silverman: Well, I know we've been told that FDA is supposedly really the WHO of pharmaceuticals, which is absolutely nonsense. The FDA is a national organization and a national organization that does not have universal popularity in the United States, but it has served I think as an umpire in attempting to solve problems of the United States.

Now, whether the UK or Japan or Indonesia or any other country should follow FDA policies is something which, of course, must be determined by those individual countries themselves.

With regard to the other problem you mentioned about how much warning you give women in India about oral contraceptives, obviously the Indian Government or the Indian medical profession must decide that. We have been fascinated by the position that has been maintained, and is still being maintained, I understand, regarding chloramphenicol in many parts of the world. In the big city areas of Latin America, the general feeling among knowledgeable physicians is essentially the same as yours and mine. It should not be for the care of the common cold or sore throat. But in the jungles, in the back areas, there is a different problem, and apparently this has occurred most acutely in portions of the People's Republic of China where chloramphenicol is a marvelous antibiotic. It has a broad spectrum of activity. It works against many different infections. It is highly effective and quickly effective when taken by mouth. You don't have to inject it. It is relatively inexpensive. It has a good shelf life, but it does produce aplastic anemia.

Now apparently some countries have reached, after due consideration, the decision that they will take a calculated risk. They will risk the death of maybe a few dozen or a few hundred young people from aplastic anemia to save perhaps 50,000 lives from typhoid. Well, that's their decision, and I am delighted that each country is looking at this in its own way.

Hansson: I cannot follow Dr. Inman. Why shouldn't women in India get the same information of drugs as women in the United Kingdom? It's a question of how to give the information. I realize that it's much more difficult to give adequate information to the women and the populations in the underdeveloped countries than in developed countries. I think it is a rather dangerous attitude to have different policies for people in the developing countries.

Silverman: May I disagree with my friend Dr. Hansson. I think the important issue here is the full honesty of the drug company. How much information should it give or should it withhold from physicians in a particular area? What the physician does with this is another matter, a very important one, not the one that concerns us today.

The legal settlement of thalidomide cases in Japan*

YOICHIRO YAMAKAWA

Attorney, Tokyo, Japan

How did the thalidomide tragedy happen in Japan, and how efficiently or inefficiently did the machinery of justice work for its legal solution? In this paper I shall describe the events seen from my position as a counsel for the plaintiffs. In doing so, I hope to draw some lessons for similar cases which should not, but might, happen in the future:

HOW DID THE TRAGEDY HAPPEN?

Thalidomide drugs were originally developed by Chemie Gruenenthal Co. of West Germany and exported to other countries. In Japan they were sold for use as sleeping pills or sedatives from October 1957 by 15 drug companies which obtained permission to sell from the Ministry of Health and Welfare. Among them was Dainippon Company, Ltd. which produced and sold thalidomide under a technical assistance contract with Chemie Gruenenthal.** The Dainippon Company was responsible for more than 95% of the total sales in Japan.

On November 18, 1961, Dr. Widukind Lenz of West Germany (currently professor at the University of Munster) issued a warning that there was a danger that the thalidomide drugs might cause serious limb malformations to the embryo in the pregnant mother. This warning was quickly reported to the authorities of several countries, and considered by them to be very serious. The Land Government of Northrhine-Westphalia banned the sales of the drugs on the 27th of the same month, and the West German, English, Swedish, Swiss, Dutch and Finnish Governments promptly followed in December 1961.

Unfortunately, however, the reaction of both the drug companies and the Government of Japan was very slow. They did not take Dr. Lenz's warning seriously, but rather maintained the starting position that unless a causal relationship between the intake of thalidomide and the malformations were scientifically proved, neither the Government nor the companies would have to stop selling it. Though Dainippon sent a staff member to West Germany in January 1962 for fact finding, he did not even interview Dr. Lenz and came back with a

*Reproduced from *Equality and Freedom: International and Comparative Jurisprudence, Vol. III*, Oceana Publications, Inc., Dobbs Ferry, New York, pp. 965–969, 1977. With permission.

**Dainippon first learned from an article written by the staff of Chemie Gruenenthal how to produce thalidomide. Later, a patent dispute occurred between the two, which was finally solved by this technical assistance conctract.

superficial, one-sided report that there was no causal relationship between the intake of thalidomide and the malformations. The Japanese Government did not take any action. Thus sales of the drug continued, while the casualties increased.* It was only after a newspaper report about the thalidomide babies in May 1962 that Dainippon curtailed shipment. The withdrawal of the drugs from the market was further delayed until September 13, 1962.

We do not have any accurate information about the damage, because until the very recent settlement of the tort actions against the Government and Dainippon, both of these consistently denied any causal relation between the drugs and the malformations and accordingly made no formal or scientific survey of the damage. One study conducted by a Professor in 1963 estimated that 936 babies were born with limb malformations. However, this report has been criticized because of many methodological flaws, and its accuracy is doubted. With this single exception, there are no scientific data about how many damaged babies were born and how many of them survived.

INTO THE COURT

The babies and their families suffered multiple pain and difficulties: physical, psychological, emotional and economic. In addition, they had to suffer the prejudice and contempt of their neighbors, who believed that the malformations were caused by hereditary defects of the parents. The parents of the babies brought their case to the civil rights division of the Justice Department and the public prosecutor's office. But these official agencies did not press the investigation, and found no cause for action. Nor did the Government and the company take any steps. The victims were left alone to struggle for themselves.

In 1963, the first tort action was brought against Dainippon in Nagoya and the second case against both the Government and Dainippon followed in Kyoto in 1964. In 1965, 24 families brought a similar action against the same defendants in Tokyo. Several other suits followed. The total number of families who joined the litigation was 63. The cases in Kyoto and Tokyo were taken up by lawyers who were members of the Japanese Civil Liberties Union, who volunteered to carry out the difficult, non-paying work. Attorneys in the Tokyo case took the initiative in coordinating all the counsels involved in the cases and played the leading role in the court procedure. It was agreed between the parties that all the evidence and the transcripts of testimonies concerning the causation and negligence would be later used in the other district court. The Tokyo case was a kind of *de facto* class action in a country which does not have the class action system.

The main issues, common in all the cases, were (1) whether there was a causal relation between the intake of the thalidomide drugs and the malformations, and (2) whether there was any negligence in Dainippon's selling of the drugs and in the Government's granting of permission to do so. Thus, the foreseeability of the danger, in other words, the level of medical knowledge about the danger available to

*One expert estimated that the long delay before the curtailment of sales caused about 50% increase in the number of malformed babies.

the defendants when the drugs were first sold, was argued. As Japanese law has neither the product liability theory nor the strict liability theory, it was the weak plaintiff's burden to prove negligence on the side of defendants who were armed with powerful staffs and financial support.

The defendants fiercely denied both the issues, contending that upon all the knowledge available to them at that time, it was absolutely beyond their imagination to think that a drug which was safe for adults might be dangerous to embryos.

It took about 6 years for the Three Judges Panel of the District Court of Tokyo to finish the pretrial proceedings. During this period the court clarified the issues and the parties exchanged the elaborate briefs and presented the evidence. Most of the evidence was taken from Japanese, German, English, Swedish and American medical journals. It took a great deal of energy, time and money for plaintiff's counsels to collect it from the university libraries and to have it translated into Japanese.

Professor Lenz who visited Japan in 1965 was particularly helpful in providing the results of his long study of the thalidomide tragedy. Many conscientious Japanese scholars also provided their expert knowledge.

Finally on February 14, 1971, the trial began after the long preparation. The plaintiff's star witnesses were Professor Lenz who gave the testimony about the causation and Professor John B. Tiersch of the University of Washington who testified about the standard of the scientific knowledge concerning the side-effects of drugs upon the embryo, and the animal experiments he had conducted for the pharmaceutical companies to check the effects of drugs on the embryo. The testimonies of both professors were very strong. By December of 1973, 27 witnesses from both sides had given their testimonies and the trial was going advantageously for the plaintiffs.

TO THE SETTLEMENT

It was on December 14, 1973, close to the final stage of the long trial, that the defendants jointly declared that they would not continue to contest the case and that they wished for sincere negotiation to work out sufficient compensation for the welfare of the children, who were already between 10 to 13 years old.

The plaintiffs agreed on the understanding that the declaration meant the defendant's admission of both causation and negligence. In the first session with many TV cameras present, the president of Dainippon and a high official of the Ministry of Health and Welfare openly admitted the causation and their negligence to the children and their parents.

Thus the negotiation started. It was a long and intricate process, covering monetary compensation, various welfare measures for the children to be taken by the Government, and the establishment of a welfare foundation. Finally, on October 13, 1974, after 10 months' long negotiation, both parties reached the agreement. The essence of the agreement is as follows:

1. The Government and Dainippon admit that the thalidomide drugs caused the malformations and that they were negligent in not conducting a sufficient safety test before putting the drugs on the market and in not immediately withdrawing the

drugs from the market when they learned about Dr. Lenz's warning.
2. They apologize for their contesting the causation and negligence for more than 10 years and not making any remedies available to the damaged children.
3. They promise to make their best efforts to insure the safety of drugs and prevent a drug accident in the future.
4a. The defendants will jointly pay to each plaintiff family compensation in the amounts of 40, 33 and 28 million yen (133,000, 100,000 and 93,000 dollars, respectively) plus attorney's fees and all the costs, according to the degree of the damage.
4b. The plaintiffs have the option to receive 15 million yen ($ 50,000) in the form of an annual instalment for 60 years, which would be calculated to offset inflation.
5. The defendants will pay the same amount of money to all the non-litigating thalidomide families.
6. In addition, the defendants will contribute 500 million yen ($ 1.7 million) to the foundation which will be established to take care of the problems concerning the welfare of all the thalidomide children.
7. The Government promises to take special welfare measures for the thalidomide families in the field medical care, everyday care, education, job training and other relevant fields.

The settlement was quite satisfactory for the plaintiffs and considerably higher than the standards of compensation in ordinary tort cases in Japan. It was also unique in that:
1. the Government admitted legal liability and paid a substantial amount of money without even a district court decision (this is very rare in Japan when the Government is the defendant);
2. the compensation in the form of annual instalments to be adjusted for inflation was first adopted in Japan in this case.* It would be most suitable for the needs of young victims;
3. the defendants promised to pay the same amount of money to all the non-litigating families. The litigation played the role of *de facto* class action;
4. both the Government and the company promised to do their best to insure the safety of drugs.

THE EXPECTED ROLE OF THE LAW

What the law can do to cope with the undesirable results caused by new developments of science and technique is divided into two categories. One is to secure the safety of the products or techniques. This will be attained by tightening the regulations and procedures to screen the safety of the goods. The other is to establish a speedy and reasonable system to provide sufficient remedies once the damage has occurred.

Finally, I want to draw attention to the following points concerning the second category.

*The Swedish settlement in 1969 included the same scheme.

A. Speedy remedies

Litigation was the last and only resort for the thalidomide families. I still have frankly to admit that the machinery of justice moved very slowly for the tragic families.* There were a few reasons for this delay. Japan does not have the law of strict liability, which places a heavy burden on the usually weaker party, the plaintiff. Also, the origin of the case lay in West Germany, which made it difficult to obtain the evidence. Finally, the case involved complicated scientific issues, to which all the parties and the court were not well trained. All these conditions worked against the speedy and reasonable solution of the case. Therefore new legal machinery to lighten the burden of the plaintiff and trained lawyers is very much needed.

B. Importance of international cooperation

We received much help and useful information from many scholars and lawyers, both domestic and foreign. Without them, it would have been almost impossible for us to win the satisfactory settlement. As science and technology have deloped, they have become more and more international. Therefore, international cooperation is very important and desirable.

DISCUSSION

Johnson: The individual lawsuit is very important for compensation of individual victims of dangerous products, but the importance of these lawsuits goes beyond the compensation of the individual plaintiffs. These lawsuits have a major role in preventing injury in the future.

The lawyer in a single lawsuit acts as a detective, digging hard into facts for months and years, facts that no one else had any interest in digging out, facts that the government has not revealed, or the manufacturers have brought to light.

Once these facts are brought out by a single lawyer in a single case, frequently other product victims in the future can frequently use them to get compensation for themselves. But further than that, these facts can be used to push the government into acting, to push the government into restricting dangerous products or warning future consumers of the dangers.

It is very imporant for us to remember that product safety is not only a government function. It is also a matter for private lawyers, private lawsuits and private plaintiffs.

I am more familiar with the United States than with Japan, but in the United States time and time again it is the private lawsuits which have pushed the government to regulate on behalf of the people and forced the companies to withdraw products or to provide individual warnings. Otherwise both the government and the manufacturers would have sunk into sleep.

You may be interested to know that in the United States many large manufacturers' are now advocating a cutback in private lawsuits. They want new laws to make it more difficult for injured consumers to win in the law courts, and their argument is: We do not need private lawsuits for product safety. Our government agencies can do the job all by themselves.

This is completely false, as I am sure your own experience and what we have heard today make clear.

*The settlement of the thalidomide cases in Sweden was made in October, 1969. The West German settlement was made in April 1970 and the English settlement followed in July 1973. Mr. Ralph Nader campaigned for the plaintiffs in the English settlement.

In summary, the private action for personal injury benefits not only the individual plaintiffs but the safety of the country as a whole.

Matsunami: Mr. Yamakawa, I would like to ask about the preparatory procedures. If the whole material is to be submitted beforehand, it will lead to a prolongation of the whole proceedings. Moreover, the preparatory procedures are not open to the public.

In the case of thalidomide and the case of Tokyo SMON Litigation (First Group), we had such preparatory procedures, and I would like to know your impressions. What were the drawbacks or merits?

Yamakawa: I think this is a very difficult question to answer. In the thalidomide case, the plaintiffs filed the suit just before the termination of the statutory limitation. At that stage, there was no evidence on the part of the plaintiff to prove negligence on the part of the pharmaceutical companies and the government.

Therefore, the plaintiffs needed such a preparatory procedure. However, except in this kind of special situation, a preparatory period only prolongs the whole proceedings. This is my impression.

For the initial two to three years I think such loss of time due to preparation was unavoidable. Later in the trial I think we spent too much time in pre-trial procedures.

During the latter part of the preparatory procedures we had to collect very detailed evidence of a medical kind. However, I felt the discussion of the medical aspects could have been taken up at the open trial.

Tuveson: What do you think can be done against drug companies' efforts to prolong drug cases?

Yamakawa: This is a very difficult question, but, as I stated in my report, one thing is that the plaintiff should have the backing of legal principles such as product liability or strict liability. I understand that these are already adopted in the American courts, and the Japanese courts should follow suit.

Other than that, as a practicing attorney I really do not know how to shorten the long process of litigation.

The streptomycin lawsuit in Japan

KOZABURO YOSHIKAWA

Streptomycin Lawsuit Attorneys Group for a Plaintiff, Tokyo, Japan

OUTLINE OF THE TRIAL

Plaintiff: Tomi Aoyama
Defendants: Sankyo Co., Ltd., Kaken Kagaku Co., Ltd., Kodama Co., Ltd., Meiji Confectionary Co. and the state. (At the very beginning the physicians were also defendants. The court settlement was achieved almost at the end of the stage with the physicians and they were no longer the defendants. The settlement amounted to 20 million yen in the Tokyo District Court.)
Date of case presented: August, 1971.
Date of ruling delivered: September 25, 1978.
Damage suffered by the plaintiff: Total deafness, buzzing in the ears, trigeminal neuralgia, headache, arthralgia of both arms and legs, muscular pain, difficulty of equilibration, autonomic ataxia (imbalance) and stiffened shoulder, etc.
Content of the ruling: Plaintiff won against 3 pharmaceutical companies (Sankyo, Kaken and Kodama). The text clause stated that 8,779,060 yen are to be paid by each. The Meiji Confectionary Company and the state cases were dismissed because the streptomycin produced by Meiji was not used. The amount acknowledged was very low because 20 million yen had been settled by the physicians.
Method of approving: The investigation comprised examination of the witnesses through our consulting physician, Dr. Hayashi, by both the plaintiff and the defendants. All the other evidence was documentary, most medical literature. (I believe that this is one of the unique points about this case.)

CHARACTERISTICS OF STREPTOMYCIN

Streptomycin was widely used in Japan between 1958 and 1969 as specific treatment for tuberculosis. There are 3 types of streptomycin – streptomycin sulfate, dihydro-streptomycin and combined streptomycin which combines the two other forms. Each has different side-effects.

The present case involved the combined streptomycin and dihydro-streptomycin which cause irreparable auditory impairment. In about 1970 the production of these two drugs was banned and today only streptomycin sulfate is used.

Since the start of streptomycin manufacture, it was well known that side-effects included auditory nerve disturbances and impaired equilibrium. As mentioned, there was no controversy as to the efficacy of streptomycin in the treatment of tuberculosis and equally there was no controversy concerning the side-effects. Therefore, the issues in this case are somewhat different from those of the thalidomide and SMON litigations.

The major point at issue concerns the obligation of avoiding the consequences. There was no comprehensive survey or statistics on the incidence of auditory damage. According to the investigation carried out by the husband of the plaintiff, it is estimated that there are about 30,000 victims with such a side-effect. Under the present circumstances relief measures have not been applied.

Lawsuits for damages by victims of streptomycin exist throughout Japan. There are, to my knowledge, about 10 cases pending, and these mostly pursue negligence on the part of physicians. There is no other lawsuit in which the state and/or pharmaceutical company are also defendants. It is remarkable that we won against the pharmaceutical companies.

REVIEW OF THE RULING OF THIS CASE

From May 26, 1965, to October 27, 1966, the plaintiff received combined streptomycin, PAS and hydrazide in the treatment for tuberculosis in Omori Hospital. During this period, three 'kools' of streptomycin were administered (one 'kool' equals 50 units and one unit contains 1.0 g streptomycin). During this period there were no overt symptoms that could be regarded as side-effects.

Since then, the plaintiff from December 3, 1966, to March 4, 1971, was treated by Dr. Hayashi as an out-patient; the streptomycin was given from October 1, 1967, continuously until August 28, 1968. The first 'kool' was 51 units and the second 16 units.

During this period, facial rash, facial neuralgia, cheek swelling and other symptoms occurred. Near the end of treatment on August 7, 1969, the patient complained of the subjective symptom of hearing difficulties. However, the treatment was continued until August 28 of the same year.

Responsibility, duties and liabilities of the pharmaceutical company

(1) Violation of duty to carry out follow-up research and investigation.
(2) Violation of duty to warn physicians and public about side-effects.
These two points were taken up in court and the ruling accepted the violation of the duty to warn about the side-effects and the claim was accepted. Regarding the follow-up research etc., the ruling avoided judgement on whether there is a legal obligation. Since drug manufacturers handle large volumes of drugs, they have abundant resources to investigate side-effects, and at the same time they are in a position to collate the research of medical, pharmaceutical or pharmacological departments, various research organizations, medical institutions and organizations. In addition, since they generate profits from their products, manufacturers must attempt to ensure the safety of their drugs, even those given approval by the Ministry of Health and Welfare. In that sense, the ruling largely recognizes the duties of the follow-up investigation.

In this case, there had already been investigations of side-effects so that the symptoms of the plaintiffs could not have been prevented. That was the ruling and the plaintiffs' assertions were dismissed.

Concerning item (2), the ruling accepts that, according to the Drug Affairs Law, it is the drug manufacturers' duty to fully inform physicians of precautions and side-effects, as stated in Article 52 of the Drug Affairs Law, stipulating that drugs must have inserts, stating: usage, dosage, and necessary precautions in use and handling. The defendant pharmaceutical company claimed that there was a description of side-effects in the package insert. However, there was no description or statement concerning numbness of the lips, formication and auditory malfunction.

Related to this ruling, impaired VIII cranial nerve function was described but numbness of the lips, formication, or auditory malfunction were not given in 1968 when this case actually occurred. Since then some changes have been made and the other side-effects given. The ruling stated that the side-effects, compared with those affecting the VIII cranial nerve, were not severe. However, we cannot ignore the other damage. Therefore, the additional side-effects of streptomycin should have been clearly stated and cautions stipulated in accordance with the aims and objectives of Article 52 of the Drug Affairs Law.

As to causal relationships, it was confirmed that if the defendants stated or described the previously mentioned side-effects in the package insert, and physicians had examined renal function, etc. and checked for side-effects with audiometers etc., streptomycin could have been stopped or reduced and the consequences avoided. The ruling thus recognized the duty of the pharmaceutical companies and causal relationships. The users of streptomycin are physicians who lie between the defendant and the plaintiff. Nevertheless the prevention of side-effects lies with the pharmaceutical companies.

Liability of the state

(1) Violation of obligation to prevent side-effects and provide relief measures concerning streptomycin manufacture (Article No. 14 of the Drug Affairs Law of the Minister of Health and Welfare).
(2) Violation of the duty to instruct physicians concerning treatment of tuberculosis by the Minister of Health and Welfare.
(3) Violation by the defendants of the duty to apply appropriate treatment for plaintiffs. Duty of the state in terms of the Tuberculosis Prevention Law.

Items (1) and (2) above are similar in drug-induced-suffering litigation. Item (3) demands that the state is liable as the promotor according to the Tuberculosis Prevention Law. As to preventing side-effects, the state from the time of the written manufacturing license requires the description of side-effects, usage and precautions on the package insert. Furthermore, by notifying prefectural governors the state demands the treatment of tuberculosis, requiring physicians to carry out regular examination by audiometer etc. In this way the state applies preventive measures. The plaintiff's assertion that the state is neglecting the preventive measures is thus not justified according to court ruling. Although the assertion is dismissed, the ruling may however acknowledge the obligation of the state to take preventive measures.

In item (2) against the state, the plaintiff asserted that the state had the duty to indicate or instruct physicians in their obligation to install and use audiometers; the ruling stated (according to Item II of Article 24 of the Medical Practitioners Law) that the instruction to physicians is limited to cases where there are marked risks to the human body, public health etc.

Auditory disturbances as side-effects of streptomycin did not occur in all cases and loss of hearing was even more rare. Therefore, the risks cannot be said to be very great. Further, since the guidelines for tuberculosis treatment demand regular auditory examination there is no need to further instruct the physician in Item II of Article 24 of the Medical Practitioners Law.

With regard to item (3), the Tuberculosis Prevention Law cannot be interpreted as designating the state as actually giving medical care and, therefore, the plaintiff's assertion was dismissed.

This is the outline of the litigation.

DISCUSSION

Ohashi: Regarding the appeal in the case of streptomycin, the pharmaceutical companies appealed to the High Court. In this regard, was there any appeal filed from our side to the High Court?

Yoshikawa: No, we didn't make that kind of appeal.

Ohashi: What is the background to that?

Yoshikawa: It largely reflects the economic burden on the plaintiff, and as was reported earlier, the ruling of the first instance concerning the defeat of the state was based on the fact that the state was proceeding adequately.

Ohashi: I believe that the issue you raised was that the package insert did not appropriately describe the side-effects. Isn't there any obligation or duty then on the part of the state to provide appropriate and accurate package inserts?

Shimojima: The production and the manufacture of streptomycin in this case were carried out by 3 or 4 pharmaceutical companies. I don't think the pharmaceutical companies are specified in the medical character, etc., but how did you determine which product the physicians used?

You also said that the streptomycin produced by the Meiji Confectionery Company was not used and that for this reason the company was dismissed from the case. Are you satisfied with that decision by the court?

Yoshikawa: This is a question of specifying the product. Physicians specified which product they used produced by which company, and before filing the suit the plaintiff was told by the physician that the Meiji Confectionery Company product was used. However, during the stages of the lawsuit it was pointed out by the physician that the Meiji product was not used, and according to confirmation by the court it was established that the Meiji product was indeed not used. Physicians established which product was used by the plaintiff. Also wholesalers provided some information.

The litigations for contracture of muscle by administration of intramuscular injections, and for aplastic anemia induced by chloramphenicol

HARUKO SHIMOJIMA

Attorney, Tokyo, Japan

I. Induced muscle contracture is a condition following intramuscular injection wherein the muscle tissue becomes scarred and the fibrosis progresses in such a way as to damage elasticity and impair function. Symptomatically, in the case of the shoulder or deltoid muscle, the victim's control over his arm is limited: if he attempts to grasp his shoulder with his hand, his elbow cannot be made to lie flat against his chest; it stands out from it. In the case of the gluteus, a victim attempting to squat with both knees together will find that they swing apart of their own accord. Where the femoral quadriceps is involved the victim cannot sit up properly and in extreme cases his legs are awkwardly stiff when walking.

Litigation over such cases was initiated in four district courts including that of Kyoto. I have been involved in cases in the Yamanashi Prefecture, where of the 300 known victims 235 were plaintiffs. All were traceable to a single pediatrician who had administered intramuscular injections to every victim. In Japan as a whole, the Ministry of Health and Welfare in 1975 conducted an inadequate survey which reported a total of 3,669 victims. If, however, we add to this the number of victims who display no functional disorders but who show other after-effects, the total comes to 9,696. Finally, an interim report in 1976 made by the Japan Voluntary Physicians' Examination Group listed 7300 patients.

Most reports about the problem tend to focus on orthopedics. Up to 1959 there were 12 reported cases involving the femoral quadriceps, 8 of which were caused by intramuscular injections. In 1963 there occurred a mass breakout of 30 cases, and up to 1965 the cumulative total came to 106 reported cases.

In other countries there have been relatively fewer cases. In 1961 J.V. Todd of Britain warned that intramuscular injection may be the cause of certain functional disorders, ruling out the possibility of congenital causes, as did two other reports. In correspondence with a Japanese physician in 1964, D.R. Gunn reiterated the warning, cautioning against repeated injections of this type. T.G. Lloyd-Roberts re-examined the cases allegedly due to congenital defects and discovered that there had been a reaction in the femoral quadriceps to such injections when the patients were infants.

The large number of cases seen in Japan is due largely to the fact that doctors have too easily given injections to infants not in need of hospitalization. Looking further into the cause of this faith in the efficacy of injections, we may surmise that it arises from postwar living conditions, where food, clothing, shelter and medical services were scanty or absent; it was a time when people died merely from common colds. It was also a time when penicillin injections apparently worked miracles in cures, and inoculations worked miracles in disease prevention. At that time newspapers were the principal and almost the only medium of public information, and they tended to be full of advertisements for injectable drugs. With the development after 1949 of painlessly injectable vitamins, the pharmaceutical industry tirelessly popularized the use of injections by laymen quite capable of taking vitamins this way. The advertisements stressed only the painlessness and immediate results, and were directed not at physicians but the general public.

To cite a few examples, an advertisement in March 1949 by Shionogi Pharmaceuticals said of its Para-S injectable vitamin that it was 'almost painless, no discernible discomfort. Ladies and children can easily handle this'. Another, from Sankyo Pharmaceutical, sang the praises of its Vitamin B1 'Painless Injection'. This was, moreover, a 'premium' ad campaign, wherein anyone with three boxtops got a lottery chance (first prize was 500,000 yen).

The Health and Welfare Ministry took a laissez-faire attitude toward the drug industry and medical profession, and injections by laymen became extremely popular up to the late 1950's, when the National Health Insurance System came into existence and many of the popular drugs became prescription-only items. Nevertheless, hospitals and clinics connected with the health insurance scheme continued administering injections. It was around this time that the drug industry advertisements began to center around physicians instead of laymen. A typical advertisement in 1956 advised readers to 'go to your family doctor and ask for an Omnacillin shot. Your high fever will subside immediately'.

In 1976 the Japan Pediatricians' Commission on Muscle Contracture announced guidelines concerning the practice. The first was that 'injections should not be administered solely upon the parents' request'. This statement would be difficult to understand without knowledge of the background factors that had led parents to have such blind faith in the efficacy of injections.

In the Yamanashi prefecture case, many children received injections of Sulpyrin and antibiotics in suspension. In animal experiments, muscle contracture was seen after the first such injection.

Looking more closely at two of the Yamanashi cases, each involved dysfunctions of the quadriceps in both legs. One was a girl born in July 1968. Over the period from October 1968 to May 1971, she suffered from acute bronchitis, acute colitis, and acute pharyngitis; she had received a total of 165 injections. The other victim was a boy born in July 1969. Up to April 1973 he received 144 injections and suffered from colitis, gastritis (pharyngitis), and bronchitis, all acute, and from tonsillitis.

In Japan three circumstances contributed to the large-scale outbreak: the attitude of the pharmaceutical industry, pursuing profit at the expense of medical ethics and propriety; the laissez-faire attitude of the government regulatory authorities; and the carelessness of the medical profession in uncritically accepting these injection practices.

It was established that intramuscular injections were the proximate cause of all of these conditions. The prevalence of these cases in Japan recalls that of the SMON malady. But as the animal experiments proved, the problem is not necessarily limited to Japan, and there have in fact been such occurrences in other countries, though in smaller numbers.

Lessons can be drawn from Japan's experience in this connection, and a simple series of tests has been devised to help determine whether a child's development may have been adversely affected by intramuscular injections. Here are two:

1. The child lies flat on its stomach, face down, legs extended and together. Placing one hand on its hips, use the other hand to raise the foot up and back, bending the leg at the knee. Femoral rectus muscular abnormalities are present if the hips rise up simultaneously and the foot cannot touch the hip.
2. The child lies on its back, legs extended and together. Have it pull its foot back towards the hip while still touching the floor, the leg bending at the knee. If the calf cannot be made to touch the back of the thigh, it is evidence of femoral vastus muscular abnormality.

In some cases both of these tests may show abnormalities.

II. Another medical problem of legal interest is that related to the drug chloramphenicol, hereinafter abbreviated 'CP'. It is well known to be a cause of aplastic anemia. In the United States, where the drug was developed, the law requires that the following warning be placed on the drug. In paraphrase:

> 'Serious and even fatal blood dyscrasis (aplastic anemia, hypoplastic anemia, thrombocytopenia, granulocytopenia) are known to occur after the administration of chloramphenicol. ....It must not be used in the treatment of trivial infections such as colds, influenza, or infections of the throat; or as a prophylactic agent to prevent bacterial infections.'

To this was added in 1968 the following, also paraphrased:

> 'To facilitate appropriate studies and observation during therapy, it is desirable that patients be hospitalized.'

Nevertheless, in Japan in 1968, CP was used to treat a very wide variety of complaints, some 37 types. Examples include infant diarrhea, measles, and pre- and post-surgical prevention of infections. By 1973 the total domestic production amounted to 181.1 tons. Although in 1968 the Health and Welfare Ministry required some mention of aplastic anemia on its labeling, it was inadequate and CP continued to be used extensively without any requirement for accompanying blood tests. At last in December 1975 its use was limited to five diseases, including typhoid, and blood tests, and cautious prescription of CP came to be required.

Despite all this, the government and the pharmaceutical industry insistently denied the existence of any causal relationship. The authorities maintained that the warning was only a normal cautionary measure and that there was no direct proof of a link between CP and serious fatal disorders; the warnings were directed at ensuring the proper administration of antibiotics in general, including CP. For their part the pharmaceutical companies excused themselves by stating that they were only following the government's 'Gyōsei-shidō', that is, administrative advice; they too said that there was no causal relationship involved.

Sankyo Pharmaceutical was one of the defendants. It maintained a business connection with Parke Davis of the U.S., the original developer of CP. Sankyo continues to insist that although it has been aware of the restrictions on the use of the drug in that country, it does not recognize their necessity in view of the quite small number of cases of drug-induced aplastic anemia in Japan.

Another defendant, Kowa Pharmaceutical, concluded that the U.S. restrictions on the use of CP were purely political and not the result of medical research.

On the part of both private and public investigators the denial of the link between CP and aplastic anemia was based on the absence of an experimental dose-response relationship and of any demonstrance in animal experiments. It is true that these tests would indicate such a relationship if it existed, but the converse is not true. Human diseases or disorders do not always appear in animals.

The government in particular said it was unable to obtain persuasive results in epidemiological tests. But these 'tests' took the form of questionnaires sent to doctors, and it appears that therapeutic drugs prescribed for this problem were decided not on the basis of patients' clinical charts but only on individual recollections over the preceding six months or so. If the government had wished to deny or disprove a theory generally accepted world-wide, it might at least have done more precise research. Some investigators say that since 1964 the CP-anemia relationship has been seen in females in Japan.

If its thesis is true, i.e., that there is no causal link, this would be major medical news of international importance. In 1974 in France a doctor carelessly administered CP to a child who subsequently died. The doctor was fined. He would have been glad to know that he was not at fault by the Japanese government's standards.

The problem has long since been solved in other advanced countries. But in Japan the government and the pharmaceutical industry still condone the administration and production of large quantities of CP, and this has resulted in unnecessary deaths. Even if the compound were to be more strictly regulated in Japan, it could still be exported to other countries where regulations are less strict, or used domestically in animal feed. An international system for exchange of information is essential to prevent aplastic anemia from abuse of CP.

III. Finally, some remarks are in order about litigation over retinopathy in premature infants. This condition arises from unnecessary administration of oxygen to such babies; in extreme cases it can cause blindness. In Europe and the U.S., care is taken to administer only the minimum of oxygen necessary; by 1957 the condition in its epidemic form had been eliminated with only a normal statistical rate of incidence remaining. In Japan, however, such routine administration continues. Between 1965 and 1973, blindness was reported on an epidemic scale. Physicians have still not admitted their negligence and have even maintained that such blindness was an unavoidable consequence of the measures necessary to save the lives of premature infants. We believe, on the contrary, that doctors in general remain completely ignorant about the toxicity of oxygen to those so young. If it were administered only when necessary there is ample reason to believe that the survival rate would be unaffected. There is no reason to lag 5–15 years behind the advanced western countries in matters of this kind.

IV. In this review of three types of drug litigation in which I was involved, the common factor appears to have been extreme delay in, or even lack of, exchange of information among the victims. We can only hope that the death or suffering of more than 10,000 children arising from these causes and questionable medical practices will not be repeated abroad. Ideally there should be international pressure on the Japanese authorities, the pharmaceutical industry and the negligent physicians to advance themselves to the best world standards.

The Coralgil trial in Japan and its future problems

SHUHJI NAKAMURA and MASATOSHI KAWAMURA

Niigata Coralgil Trial Attorneys Group, Niigata, Japan

OUTLINE OF CORALGIL INTOXICATION

Prolonged use of Coralgil, a coronary dilator, produces abnormal accumulations of fat (phospholipid) as well as Coralgil in blood cells and liver. The cells are eventually destroyed, leading to systemic disorders.

Main symptoms include loss of weight, loss of appetite and systematic fatigue. Swelling of the liver and spleen and, in serious cases, liver cirrhosis and death have been reported. There have been no national surveys and accurate statistics are lacking. It is estimated that there are at least 50,000 victims, of whom 250 have died. The extent of the damage is comparable with that of SMON disease.

SIDE-EFFECTS OF CORALGIL

Coralgil is a new synthetic drug comprising diethylaminoethanol and hexestrol, and is sometimes termed DH. In 1952 the Italian Magionni Company developed the drug. Initially, the drug was reported to be effective as a coronary dilator. However, in 1961 the drug began to be used as a cholesterol-lowering drug. In 1963 the drug was introduced into Japan and sold. Soon after hematologists recognized a new disease called 'foam cell syndrome'. In 1969 a new hepatic disease was described called 'phospholipid fatty liver'. In November, 1970, animal experiments demonstrated that these two new diseases were due to Coralgil intake.

Soon after the adverse effects were disclosed, Japanese pharmaceutical companies stopped the sales of the drug. In December of the same year the sale of the drug was totally banned. It is said that since the importation of the drug into Japan until the time of the total ban, 8,720 kg of DH was sold, representing 349 million tablets (25 mg/tablet).

PROGRESS OF THE TRIAL IN NIIGATA AND TOKYO

In November, 1971, 7 victims filed a suit in the Niigata Prefecture demanding compensation for the damage caused against Torii Pharmaceutical Company and the Government who permitted the importation and the manufacture (the first trial). At present the first stage of the fourth trial is in progress. There are 22 families and 32 plaintiffs in the litigation demanding 661 million yen compensation. In Tokyo there are 3 families and 9 plaintiffs filing a suit against the same two defendants. In the Niigata District Court in 1972 the first oral proceedings were held and by June of this year the proceedings for the first filing will be concluded. During the proceedings 12 medical doctors and another 6 witnesses from the Ministry of Health and Welfare and the company appeared.

The following statements concern efforts by the plaintiffs to prove the case, to clarify the problems encountered and to assess the future progress.

Firstly, during development of DH no safety tests were conducted. As mentioned, DH comprises two molecules, of which hexestrol is a compound with strong estrogenic activity. The hypothesis that by combining diethylaminoethanol with an estrogenic compound, an effective coronary dilator would result, allowed the Magionni Company to successfully develop DH. No chronic toxicity tests were carried out during development, however.

Just before DH was released in Japan, triparanol-induced injuries occurred in the United States. This is also a cholesterol-lowering drug and its structure is very similar to that of Coralgil. Had these injuries been properly noted, the present tragic disaster of the Coralgil-induced damage could have been avoided.

The plaintiffs have stressed the following: before selling DH in Japan, the Government and pharmaceutical companies failed to carry out chronic toxicity studies in animals. According to the 1963 edition of 'Guidelines for Manufacture of Drugs' published by the Pharmaceutical and Supply Division of the Ministry of Health and Welfare, the approval of new drugs for prolonged use demands chronic toxicity tests. DH is stated to be a coronary dilator suitable for prolonged use in a pamphlet published by the company. Notwithstanding, the company did not conduct any chronic toxicity tests on the grounds that DH had been used in Italy for over 10 years and was considered safe.

The application to the Government for the approval of importation and manufacture carried an inaccurate clinical report. The Ministry of Health and Welfare did not conduct substantial reviews when granting permission. Therefore, the whole process was singularly inept; one of the plaintiff's witnesses admitted as much. In evaluating drug efficacy, no double-blind examination report was contained in the clinical material.

Regarding the pharmaceutical company's negligence, an important fact is that, in 1965, the manufacturer conducted secret chronic animal toxicity tests and although confirming the side-effects of DH, the data were not released and the drug was sold for 5 years thereafter. The secret tests were conducted because, shortly after the introduction of the drug into Japan, there was a report from a physician that liver disorders develop after DH therapy. They confirmed the side-effects of weight loss and an increased transaminase.

If the pharmaceutical company had taken precautions at this stage, then the tragic results could have been avoided. Thus the pharmaceutical company cannot deny their negligence in the light of these secret experiments.

The trial has also revealed that the state drug administration, especially the system concerned with safety, is incomplete and imperfect.

In December, 1962, a Drug Examination Committee conducted a safety test on DH to approve importation and manufacture. However, at this examination no clinical doctor was present and members of the Committee only examined the documents submitted by the company. According to the testimony of the Government witness who was in charge of the DH examination, no state funds were allocated for investigations of the drug; obviously the review was inadequate.

For the trial Italy was visited to allow examinations there. The defendants insisted that there was no negligence because in Italy the drug had been used for over 10 years prior to its introduction into Japan. This was the reason why it was considered unnecessary to perform chronic toxicity tests in animals. Although the drug was indeed used in Italy for over 10 years, can it be said that no side-effects occurred or rather that perhaps they were not seen or even reported?

Last summer a witness made contact with a professor who enabled us to visit the Magionni Company in Italy. The visit, last January, lasted 10 days and, with the cooperation of Milan University, the Magionni Company and several hospitals were visited.

The presence of DH side-effects or damage in Italy was not clarified. However, the method of use of DH in Italy was quite different to that in Japan. The pamphlet of instructions for DH states that there should be an occasional non-dosing period and it also states that a standard dosage is 75 to 100 mg per day, with a maximum of 150 mg. However, in the instructions it is also stated that this standard dosage is perfectly adequate. The pamphlet published by Torii Pharmaceutical Company does not mention a non-dosing period and gives a standard dose as 150 mg. The average weight of a Japanese is smaller than that of an Italian so that Japanese taking the same amount of tablets receives considerably more on a weight basis. Thus, the whole Coralgil intoxication in Japan reflects negligence on the part of the pharmaceutical company.

The defendants did not contend the causal relationship of Coralgil intoxication. However, the defendants insisted that individual symptoms of Coralgil intoxication were due to other diseases. To support these views, suitable parts from the medical histories of the victims were cited. These attitudes produced endless discussions of medical affairs throughout the trial.

The defendants clearly tried to prolong the whole proceedings. Therefore, although the plaintiffs thought the medical reports from doctors and the statements of the victims were adequate evidence, detailed reports from medical doctors were obtained and the doctors appeared in court to testify on the disease processes, prognoses and other symptoms of DH intoxication.

Finally, I would like to present my impressions as an attorney in this trial. Most of the victims of Coralgil were in their forties and fifties. Of course, they did have chronic cardiac disease with hypertension, etc. However, these diseases caused no major troubles in their daily lives. They took DH to alleviate these diseases, instead of which it deprived them of their lives and good health. The victims stood up and sued the pharmaceutical company and the Government to obtain fair compensation to eradicate this kind of drug-induced suffering. Seven years after the initial filing of the suit, a conclusion is being reached. In the meantime neither the Government nor the pharmaceutical company has paid any compensation. Victims have had to bear the cost of 10 million yen for the trial which has been supported by contributions from labor unions, consumer groups within Niigata Prefecture and political parties. Without the cooperation of these citizens, sincere medical doctors and personnel, the whole proceedings and fruitful results would not have come to pass.

The trial of drug-induced suffering is usually very difficult and complex, and prolonging the proceedings worsens the process. It is necessary to strengthen drug safety administration to prevent such suffering, but to compensate for actual disasters, court trials are the only way to bring early relief to the victims. I believe that systematic collaboration between attorneys and scholars, both nationally and internationally, is essential.

DISCUSSION

Johnson: Was Coralgil marketed in the United States, and, if so, what was the brand name of the drug?

Nakamura: Coralgil was not marketed in the United States. When we went to Italy we heard from the director of the Magionni Company, that the United States has very strict safety standards.

Hama: With regard to the reason why Coralgil was not marketed in the United States, I would like to put forward my personal views, as I also have conducted some research into the Coralgil disaster.

In addition to the strictness of the FDA in approving the marketing of a new drug, the close similarity between Coralgil and triparanol (MER-29) seems to be another important reason why the drug was not marketed in the United States. They are very similar in many respects. Firstly, the structure of both drugs comprises a diethylaminoethyl moiety and a synthetic estrogen. Second, they were both reported to have a hypocholesterolemic capacity. Third, the mechanism of hypocholesterolemic action was determined as being due to the inhibition of reduction of desmosterol to cholesterol. Fourth, there was a similarity in their toxicity including hepatotoxicity and the accumulation of myeloid figures in the cytoplasm of many tissues observed on electron microscopy.

In the United States, there has been much enthusiasm about the development of hypocholesterolemic drugs to prevent atherosclerosis. Many manufacturers synthetized and tested many hypocholesterolemic compounds structurally similar to triparanol. However, they failed to introduce them into clinical practice, because most of them induced the accumulation of desmosterol and were found to be too toxic. Coralgil was also tested and was considered to be one of this class of hypocholesterolemic agents.

After triparanol had been banned due to its serious adverse reactions, it was generally believed in the United States that all compounds structurally similar to triparanol were possibly too toxic for clinical use, so that manufacturers lost interest in developing this class of compounds as hypocholesterolemic drugs.

If we Japanese had learned the lesson of the triparanol case in the United States, the toxic potential of Coralgil would probably have been suspected in Japan before it was marketed.

In the United Kingdom, I have learned that Coralgil was introduced under the name of 'Cardane' by a manufacturer who carried out animal experiments indicating the definite estrogenic potency of the drug in a dose almost equivalent in the clinical dose level. The drug, however, does not seem to have ever been on the market in the United Kingdom.

I asked the Committee on Safety of Medicines (CSM) for the manufacturer's name. Dr. Greenberg, one of the members of the CSM, replied that she did not know the drug or the manufacturer's name, that the drug might never have been on the market in the United Kingdom, or if so, withdrawn as soon as it appeared. Anyway, it is very unlikely that 'Cardane' was ever marketed in the United Kingdom after animal experiments had been carried out. If this is true, it will be another important fact for the discussion on the expectability of Coralgil toxicity in Japan.

At the present time, however, we do not know what the actual name of the pharmaceutical company is who dealt with Cardane in the United Kindom. I feel that, in these respects, international cooperation is called for.

Yasuhira: In 1970, Coralgil damage occurred and its sale was totally prohibited. I would like to know the whole process of the banning of the total sales. Is it because there was causal relationship between the drug and this intoxication? I would like to know the actual results of the whole proceedings.

Nakamura: Yes, this point was taken up in Osaka University and animal experiments were conducted utilizing Coralgil. At present in the trial, the defendants, the state and the pharmaceutical company have admitted the existence of a causal relationship between the two. However, what is the problem? During the development of Coralgil, they state that they did not have enough material to foresee any side-effects at that stage, and also the actual symptoms of Coralgil are rather different. This is an internal disorder and it's different from the symptoms seen in SMON and thalidomide. Since the diseases in victims in their forties and fifties will be in the senile form, it is very difficult to actually prove that those diseases are due to Coralgil. The defendants have stated that those diseases are all due to diseases other than Coralgil intoxication. Therefore, the whole proceedings have been prolonged. With respect to product liability, this is negligence without fault, which under Japanese law is not acknowledged. Unless negligence is confirmed, no liability will be put on the defendants.

Johnson: In the United States, the state is not liable for drug injuries or failure to remove drugs from the market in a timely way. I wonder, as a matter of policy, whether it is a good idea to sue the Japanese state. Some of your cases do proceed against the state as well as against the manufacturer.

There are really two reasons why I have reservations about making the state the defendant. One is that it's questionable whether the taxpayer would pay for injuries which ultimately were preventable entirely by the manufacturer.

Secondly, it puts the state in a defensive position, allying the state with the manufacturer at the very time when you want the ministries to be helping the plaintiff as much as possible. I think that those are the reasons why the courts in the United States have refused to impose liability on the U.S. Food and Drug Administration in these cases. In the United States liability is only against the manufacturer.

Shimojima: I myself have some doubts about taking the state as the defendant. However, when we requested the Ministry of Health and Welfare for research material and documents, they never answered our requests. For example, in the Pharmaceutical Commission, which is the body that allows or disallows the marketing of some drugs, procedure-wise and practice-wise they have taken the stand of protecting confidentiality etc. and they are very reluctant to give us information that is 10 or 20 years old. They never give us the proceedings of their meetings or any of their documents. Therefore, they never give us any information that will be favorable to our side, and even in the court they say that they cannot immediately give a response to our request for information.

Ohashi: In Japan, concerning the occurrence of these drug-induced sufferings, the medical policy of the Japanese Government is greatly involved with these events. For example, in the case of SMON you can typically observe that its mass occurrence in Japan was due to the administering of large or excess doses of clioquinol for general diarrhea, whereas in the United States this was only limited to specific types of amebic dysentery. In the United States, there was a period when the administration of clioquinol had to be stopped. But in Japan there was no indication concerning the period when the administration of clioquinol could not be continued.

Concerning the injection of Coralgil and chloramphenicol, the same thing can be said in Japan. Therefore, we believe that government policy lags behind that of other countries and must be pursued by bringing up cases against the state.

Payne: Just getting back to Miss Johnson's question, I have a little bit of unease in this respect, and I wished perhaps there had been a more general description of the legal structure in Japan prior to developing the specific presentations of Japanese lawyers. I think what's lacking here certainly is an overall legal structure in which to place the problem.

So I would appreciate one or more of the Japanese lawyers here setting forth a more complete answer to Miss Johnson's question. It seems to me that part of the problem, as Mr. Ohashi said, was that in the Japanese Constitution, first of all, there is a specific article setting forth the responsibility of the state for the welfare of the Japanese citizens.

But apart from that, I think maybe some Japanese attorney or professor here could comment on the fact that in Japan there is not the problem of sovereign immunity that we have in the United States, so that direct actions against the state are much easier in Japan than in the United States where we have to worry about statutory exemptions, or for the case law interpreting those statutory provisions.

Quite apart from that, without trying to provide an answer to the second question which is the wisdom, as an attorney, of suing the state, thus driving the state into an alliance with the defending companies, I think the action of the Japanese attorneys is much more understandable generally from the fact that in Japan, the executive agencies are always in a continuing program of consultation and exchange of views with the industries they regulate, much more so than in the United States.

So the state would not be driven into an alliance against its will with the industries because it is already in alliance with these industries. I would very much appreciate one of the Japanese attorneys here detailing the kinds of cooperation and consultation that go on between the Health and Welfare Ministry and the drug companies.

Johnson: We have that problem, too, in the United States, by the way. Attorney Shimojima's comments about making the government dependent in order to obtain necessary documents is a very good one. In the United States, we have the Freedom of Information Act which permits plaintiffs, any party, to get a great deal of documentation from the government agencies, but in addition government documents are obtainable by subpoena from non-parties to a lawsuit. Is that true in Japan? Can you take discovery from non-parties?

Judicial administration in multi-district mass litigation

TAKESHI KOJIMA

Faculty of Law, Chuo University, Tokyo, Japan

I myself am not directly involved in the SMON lawsuit, but I believe that the skill of judicial administration plays an important role in this kind of multi-district mass litigation and the impact of the administration is extremely large. I am carrying out research from the academic point of view on complicated multi-district mass litigation, and I would like to report my views to you.

I would like to divide my presentation into 3 parts: (1) the concept of the universalization of justice, (2) the coordination of multi-district litigation, and (3) the selection between settlement and court rulings or decisions.

CONCEPT OF UNIVERSALIZATION OF JUSTICE

Article 32 of the Constitution guarantees the right of trial or justice to its citizens. Guarantee of access to justice is provided in the Constitution so as to universalize the protection of rights. Unless justice is easily accessible to ordinary citizens, rights guaranteed in substantive laws will only be an empty promise and effective feedback of danger through presentation of negative information to the court will become difficult. But in reality, the path to justice is very hard with many obstacles standing in the way. If we are to rely only on litigation, it is difficult to relieve the victims of damage when the damage is still slight or to inhibit the aggravation of damage. For universalization of access to legal justice, what can be called a comprehensive system of justice must be conceived by skilful combination of various legal relief measures so that the different needs of the various parties and cases can be met. At the same time, various new measures to facilitate access to justice such as class litigation and collective litigation must be introduced.

SIMPLIFICATION AND COORDINATION OF MULTI-DISTRICT MASS LITIGATION

As can be observed in the SMON case, product liability litigation now usually takes the form of multi-district mass litigations with numerous cases presented to local district courts scattered throughout Japan, reflecting the mass production and mass sales of the products in modern society. These types of litigation, in which the evidence in the hands of the victims is often sparse, make each individual trial an unbearably heavy burden on the victims.

In litigations over drug-induced suffering, the central issues are common. If the generic evidence from some cases can be applied to others so as to avoid repetition, the burden of examination on the part of the courts will be lessened, while at the same time the energies of the parties will be greatly saved. Furthermore, if the common issues are centrally determined, differences in the judgements due to disparity in ability to proceed with litigation can be avoided, contributing to securing just decisions as well as preventing inequality or unfairness amongst parties.

One possible device for attaining this goal is the concept of model litigation by selecting one or more test cases. If the results of a pioneer suit can be applied to other litigations efficient examination of mass litigation can be carried out.

We believe that there are various ways of implementing model litigation. There are two situations: one in which mass litigation is concentrated in one court and the other where it is handled by a number of courts in remote districts. In the first, a priority in the examination schedule should be given to the selected model suit, and from this point, all cases can be consolidated according to Article 132 of the Code of Civil Procedure. Thus, the result of examination of evidence in model litigation can be used as a common basis for all suits that are consolidated. If multi-district litigation is handled by numerous courts in various parts of Japan, except for cases where discretional transfer based on the Article 31 of the Code of Civil Procedure is possible, the results of the examination cannot be applied to other relevant suits through consolidation. In these cases, the record of the model litigation can be presented as documentary evidence. In the latter situation, the model suit can function most effectively if based on prior agreement. However, even without prior agreements, it can greatly contribute to the efficiency of a relief system or systems.

Even when examinations on common issues such as negligence or the causal relationship are completed, individual issues such as the causal relationship relevant to each plaintiff remain important. Standards for the approval of such causal relationships and indemnity are clearly set out in the model suit. It is rational for the court to make use of testimony by experts such as physicians. Since divergences of opinion concerning diagnostic methods etc. are likely to occur, a number of expert witnesses are desirable. In such cases special consideration should be paid in disqualifying expert witnesses to prevent the situation in which none is left.

According to the judgement by the Tokyo Upper Court of May 19, 1978, concerning one of the 14 appointed expert witnesses, the court approved the challenge by one of the defendants. The defendant was unable to trust him because he had provided expert opinions privately to the plaintiffs outside of court.

However, it is reasonable in such cases to consider the balance between experts inclined towards the plaintiffs, those inclined towards the defendants, and neutral experts, in deciding whom to exclude. Such experts do not provide the final judgement, that is the prerogative of the judges.

The aim of the challenge system is not the unconditional pursuit of absolute impartiality but to provide the possibility of exchanging the experts for better alternatives.

SELECTION BETWEEN SETTLEMENT AND COURT RULINGS

In such complicated litigations, the decision between a settlement and a court ruling is a difficult matter because there are many people involved. It is very difficult to make prompt and wise decisions because there are often differences of opinion amongst the parties. We can normally expect greater and more effective action or ripple effects when legal rulings are obtained. But in cases which rest only on a weak foundation, an unfavorable decision may be detrimental to the plaintiffs' interests. If the judge recommends a settlement of quasi-arbitration type on the basis of legally established facts, we can expect ripple effects or action in line with the court ruling. Furthermore, since appeals to higher courts, thus delaying relief, will not be made after settlements, their merits are high. However, in rulings, if the court has proceeded rapidly, giving priority to the model case, and if, in the first instance, the judgement was accompanied by a provisional enforcement, early relief can be fruitfully achieved.

Concerning provisional enforcement, there are many cases in which the total sum of the claim was accepted, and there is probably no impediment to approval of provisional enforcement of the total sum claimed. There are other means of securing early relief. One such is rather drastic, namely the provisional disposition order for pre-payment of an indemnity. Some such provisional disposition orders have been made. One noteworthy ruling was made by Yokohama District Court on 28th of November, 1979, when a monthly payment of 150,000 yen for living expenses and a lump sum payment of 2.5 million yen for reimbursement of loans and moving house were approved at a relatively early stage on basis of the diagnostic chart and the certificate of drug administration, even before the examination of expert witnesses. Since for victims of drug diseases the medical treatment may not yet be developed, the mere payment of an ordinary level of indemnity will not provide sufficient relief for the victims. This raises the necessity of a system of relief which surpasses existing legal principles. In such cases, aside from legislative reform and administrative measures, settlements offer the most effective approach at present.

In the end, whether to seek a court ruling or a settlement must be made for each case individually, and we cannot conclude that court rulings are invariably better. What is important is to respect the desire of the parties involved, and not to force the opinions of experts or lawyers. If the party is to go to law, there must be a reasonable possibility of a favorable outcome, otherwise the party must be persuaded to accept a settlement.

THE FUTURE

I would like now to look towards the future. Administration of multi-district litigation is still at the threshold. The task of advancing the unexplored frontier and of establishing appropriate practice in this field depends on the capability and insight of lawyers. Furthermore, the cooperation in a common objective between judges and attorneys of both the plaintiffs and defendants is extremely important. If a bond of confidence allowing cooperation over procedural matters in spite of heated discussion on the merits of cases, I am sure that we can eventually establish good practices in judicial administration. We now greatly need lawyers with high ideals, with a philosophy backed by new ideas and concepts, so that social justice may be guaranteed for all citizens.

DISCUSSION

Matsunami: At the very end, Professor Kojima emphasized the importance of cooperation between those concerned. I agree with this approach but there are some difficult points. I speak as a person actually involved in litigations. You talked about some of the defects of multi-district litigations. Apart from what you have mentioned, another drawback is that lawyers for the plaintiffs can only gain experience of a single case in one district court, but lawyers for the defendants can appear in cases in all the district courts throughout Japan. Therefore, lawyers for the plaintiffs are at a disadvantage compared with those for the defendants. There are some merits, of course; in my experience, data from interrogation of the best witnesses are often actually used in other courts.

Good as well as bad rulings are provided by different district courts. Such rulings do influence each other, and there are also opportunities for public opinion and experts to criticize. Therefore, later rulings may be an improvement on earlier ones. However, if you select a pioneer litigation, such opportunity for improvement will be lost.

In any litigation, there is the problem of whether you can obtain the best counsel in that particular court. In the Tokyo SMON case, there are three groups of lawyers for the plaintiffs, and I do not think that we have provided for the utmost cooperation between them.

In addition, the appointment of the judges is sometimes questionable. I wonder whether they are always the most capable judges for the particular type of litigation, and there is always the fear that there may be changes. If appeals are made, there is the question of whether the court of appeal is reliable.

Kojima: Thank you very much for your very detailed analysis. I agree with many of the points that you raised. Mass litigation, such as in SMON and other cases, is extremely complicated, however, and even if drug-induced sufferings are reduced by future measures, there will still be many mass litigations resulting from traffic accidents and nuclear accidents. Under such circumstances, you have to create a judicial procedure to meet the needs of the citizens.

There are three possible approaches. One is by individual lawsuit, and another by integrated or unified lawsuits. Model litigation comes somewhere between the two. Unless the involved parties can cooperate with each other, there will be a heavy burden on the courts. Then, the Diet will try to introduce a legislative measure to concentrate the litigations into one jurisdiction.

Of the three possibilities, I believe that model litigation, which would make unnecessary any rigid legislative measure for concentration, is the best.

SMON and a doctor's responsibility

HIROKUNI BEPPU

Department of Neurology, Tokyo Metropolitan Fuchu Hospital, Tokyo, Japan

What have doctors learned from the SMON disaster, with its more than 10,000 victims throughout Japan? Is it possible for doctors, who encountered SMON, to prevent a repetition of such drug induced suffering?

These questions, and my own personal regret at having prescribed clioquinol, are the main motives for this survey.

MATERIAL AND METHODS

The subjects for this survey were randomly selected from general practitioners around Fuchu-city, in the west part of Tokyo, and from doctors at the Tokyo Metropolitan Fuchu Hospital and its affiliated hospitals.

We sent each of them a questionnaire concerning current knowledge of clioquinol intoxication, opinions on adverse drug reactions, and views on individual actions regarding SMON. To compare differences of opinion we also sent the questionnaire to the doctors of the group boycotting Tanabe's products, who may be regarded as the most sensitive to drug induced suffering. (Tanabe is a pharmaceutical company that denies its responsibility for SMON.)

The questionnaires were sent to 174 doctors and 104 returned them (60%). The classification of these 104 doctors according to clinical speciality was: 46 physicians, 11 surgeons, 15 neurologists, 3 neurosurgeons and 29 others, 40% being general practitioners and the remainder hospital doctors.

Sixty percent of all the replying doctors had examined or treated SMON patients. To the question if they had prescribed clioquinol, 56% gave affirmative answers. Ten doctors had personal experience of prescribing clioquinol to SMON patients, and those who had produced SMON patients accounted for 4% of the total.

ACQUAINTANCE WITH REPORTS ON THE TOXICITY OF CLIOQUINOL

Seven papers were selected to assess the acquaintance with adverse reactions to clioquinol.

1 . (a) Grawitz' report: a paper recommending 0.5 g of Vioform 3 times daily for 30 days to treat amebiasis. In the course of treatment however, the author observed one case of transverse myelitis (1).

(b) Barros' report: a report of two additional cases of myelitis in the course of clioquinol therapy. Barros clearly indicated the neurotoxicity of clioquinol, and warned against Grawitz' recommendation (2).

2. David's warning: a proposal to limit the administration period of clioquinol and to prohibit its use in non-amebic diarrhea, to avoid the adverse reaction to clioquinol (3).
3. Gholz and Arons' report: a paper on the long-term prophylactic use of clioquinol, in which 20 out of 4000 cases showed an abnormal gait during the course of therapy (4).
4. Hangartner's and Schantz' reports: both reports described convulsive seizures, coma or anxiety states in cats and dogs after Enterovioform or Mexaform. After realising these adverse reactions, the CIBA Pharmaceutical Company sent a circular to veterinarians advising them to stop using the drugs for veterinary treatment (5, 6).
5 . Berggren and Hansson's report: a paper on optic atrophy which developed during the treatment of acrodermatitis enteropathica with clioquinol.

All these papers were used as documentary evidence by the Tokyo District Court in the SMON suit. Figure 1 shows the awareness of the doctors of these papers. The dotted area represents those who knew the papers. Seventy-seven percent knew none of them (7).

POSSIBLE AVOIDANCE OF THE SMON DISASTER

If these papers had been known at that time, would general doctors' prescriptions of clioquinol have been different? Was it possible to have avoided the SMON disaster if this information had been relayed efficiently?

Figure 2 shows the possible changes in the doctors' attitude towards prescribing clioquinol had they been aware of the papers. The graph at the top left represents

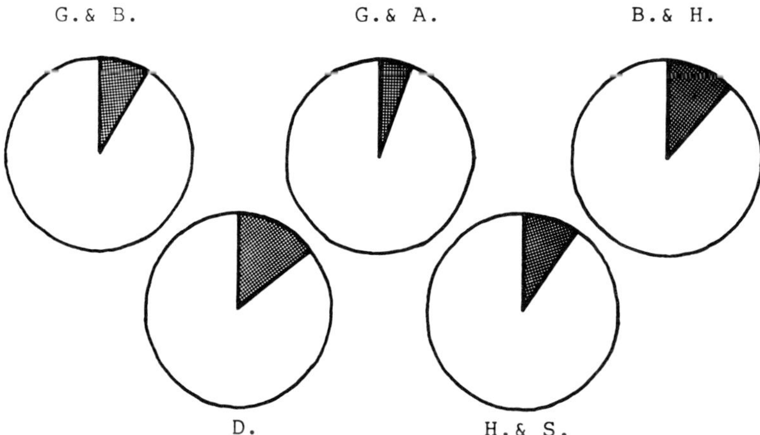

Fig. 1. Acquaintance of doctors with papers on adverse reactions of clioquinol. For explanation, see text.

the papers of Grawitz and Barros. Thirty-three percent of doctors answered, 'Clioquinol would have been changed to other drugs', and 38% answered, 'Would have been more careful about the prescription of clioquinol'. The doctors who answered 'Would have been no change even if his paper was known' comprised only 3%.

The graph at the top center is for David's warning, and the top right is for Gholz and Arons. The bottom left is for Hangartner and Schantz, and the bottom center is

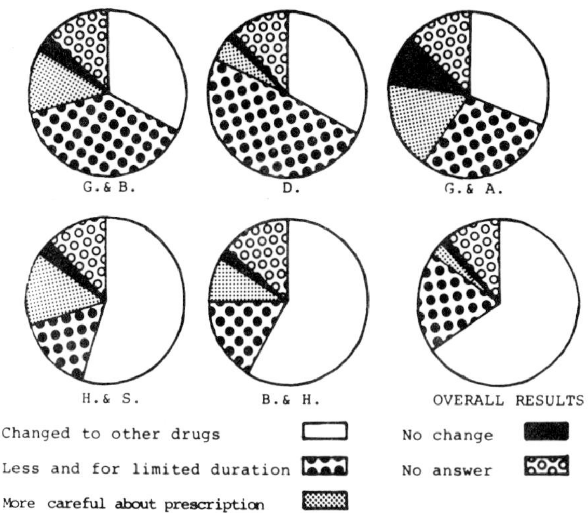

Fig. 2. Had doctors been aware of papers on adverse reactions, would their prescription of clioquinol have been different? For further explanation, see text.

for Berggren and Hansson. The bottom right shows the overall results of these graphs. If they had known all these papers, 65% would have changed the prescription of clioquinol to other drugs, and 19% would have prescribed less and limited the administration period.

This is of course speculation, but it is possible to draw conclusions with respect to the prevention of another SMON disaster.

REASONS FOR THE MASS OUTBREAK OF SMON IN JAPAN

In response to questions about the reasons for the mass outbreak of SMON in Japan, 66% suggested lack of general sensitivity to adverse drug reactions by doctors in Japan. The lack of communication about drug information was mentioned by 60%, and defects in a medical system in which the prescription of drugs is the biggest source of revenue, by 34%.

In addition, 'too close contact between drug makers and medical world' and 'too much advertising by drug companies' were mentioned by 31% and 26% of doctors respectively.

Only one doctor chose infectious factors as a cause of SMON. From these results SMON seems to be generally recognized as a clioquinol induced disease, in spite of the vast propaganda against the SMON-clioquinol theory by the pharmaceutical companies.

DOCTORS' RESPONSIBILITY

How do doctors feel about their responsibility for SMON? Figure 3 shows that some responsibility was felt by 87% of doctors, and 30% felt seriously responsible for SMON. The recognition of such responsibility depends on personal experiences with SMON. Among the doctors who had never treated SMON patients, 10% denied doctors' responsibility. On the other hand, of doctors who had treated SMON, 92% admitted some responsibility, while only 2% denied responsibility. And more especially, of those who had prescribed clioquinol to SMON patients, 56% admitted serious reponsibility and none denied it.

As to why doctors are responsible for SMON, 'Deficiency in gathering information' and 'Careless prescription without doubting its effectiveness' were mentioned, but the most common answer was 'No matter what reasons there were, the doctor is responsible for his prescription'.

Twenty-one percent of doctors pointed out the role of doctors in supporting today's medical system of excessive drug usage. In other words, doctors are responsible both as individuals and as members of the medical profession.

The five doctors who denied the doctors' responsibility attributed it to a communication problem in the system or to the government, and they felt that individual doctors could not change this.

What should doctors do when reflecting upon the SMON disaster? Answers are

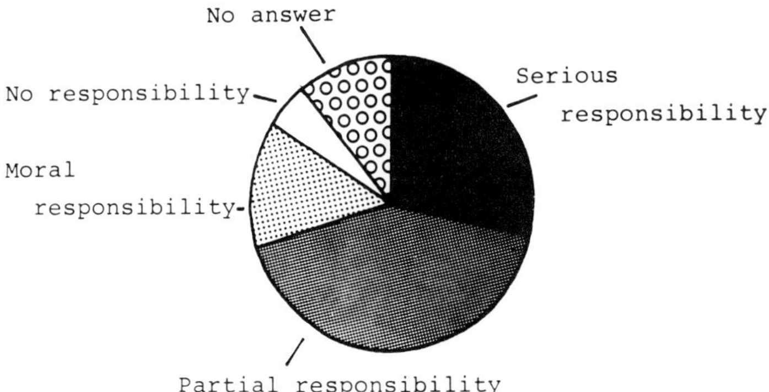

Fig. 3. What doctors felt about responsibility for SMON.

shown in Figure 4. 'Revision of the system to prevent drug induced suffering', was the reply of 77% of doctors. The second most common answer from 51% was to reform the medical system to reduce excessive drug use. These two answers stress the prevention of further drug induced suffering. Answers 3, 4, 5 and 7 concern the direct relief of SMON victims. However, 3 and 4 are easy to say but extremely difficult to execute. Most doctors who knew enough about SMON did not select these answers, but instead 5 or 7 were often selected. 'Severing the overly close connection with drug companies' was also often mentioned by both general practitioners and hospital doctors.

THE PROBLEMS IN GETTING DRUG INFORMATION

To the question whether they receive enough drug information, 59% answered 'Not enough' or 'Almost none'.

A lack of authoritative publications for relaying reliable information and an absolute shortage of information was the feeling of 75%. The main sources of drug information are shown in Figure 5. The largest source is the literature or advertising material from pharmaceutical companies, though doubtful in reliability. The second largest source is personal communication between colleagues, which is sometimes convenient and effective but sometimes irregular and not always reliable. The third source is the medical associations and their publications. Today's medical associations, however, are subdivided into so many special fields that comprehensive and practical information cannot be expected. Information from government sources is at present inadequate.

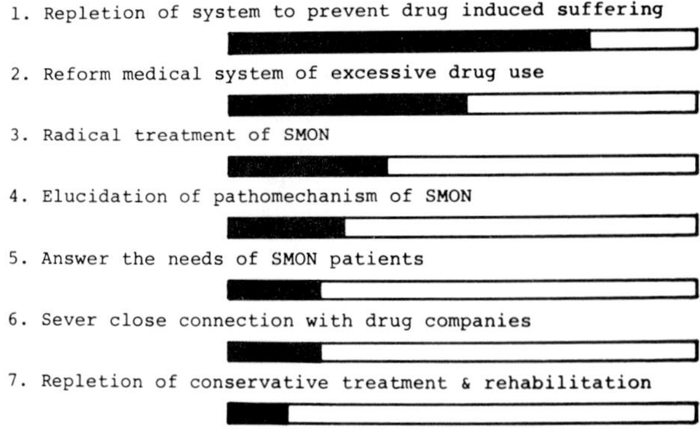

Fig. 4. What should we do when reflecting upon the SMON disaster?

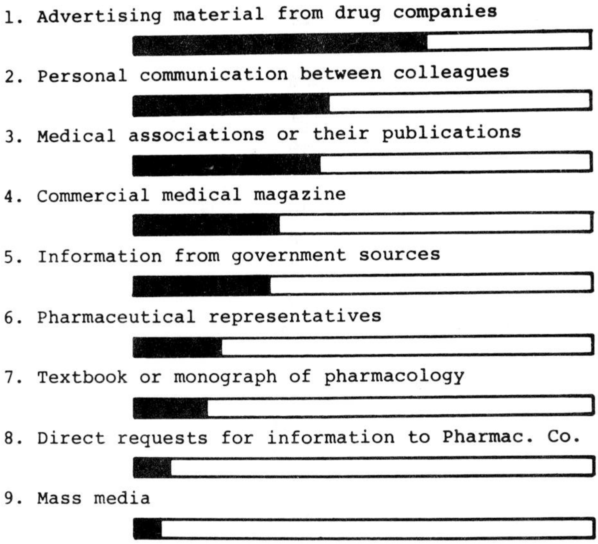

1. Advertising material from drug companies
2. Personal communication between colleagues
3. Medical associations or their publications
4. Commercial medical magazine
5. Information from government sources
6. Pharmaceutical representatives
7. Textbook or monograph of pharmacology
8. Direct requests for information to Pharmac. Co.
9. Mass media

Fig. 5. Main sources of drug information.

CONCLUSION

SMON is well known by most doctors in Japan, and there are very few who doubt the causal relationship between clioquinol and SMON. Many doctors feel seriously responsible for SMON. Most of them, however, are not aware of papers on the toxicity of clioquinol published prior to the ban in 1970. If they had been aware of these papers, most of them thought they would have stopped or modified prescription of clioquinol.

The lack of doctors' sensitivity concerning adverse drug reactions in Japan and the communication problem of drug information are regarded as the most probable reasons for the mass outbreak of SMON. Most doctors are not satisfied with the drug information they presently receive.

The most common sources of drug information are advertising material from drug companies, personal communication between colleagues and the medical associations. Information from government sources is not effectively distributed.

From these summaries, there remains obviously a risk of repeating the SMON disaster. Drug induced suffering is not avoidable simply by the effort or knowledge of individual doctors. Integrative reforms in the communication system for drug information are necessary for future prevention.

REFERENCES

1. Grawitz, B. (1935): *Sem. med., 42,* 525.
2. Barros, E. (1935): *Sem. med., 42,* 907.

3. David, N.A. (1945): *J. Amer. med. Ass., 129*, 572.
4. Gholz, L.M. and Arons, W.L. (1964): Prophylaxis and treatment of amebiasis and shigellosis with iodochlorhydroxyquinoline. *Amer. J. trop. Med. Hyg., 13*, 396.
5. Hangartner, P. (1965): Troubles nerveux observés chez le chien après absorption d'Entéro-Vioforme Ciba. *Schweiz. Arch. Tierheilk., 107,* 43.
6. Schantz, B. and Wikstrom, B. (1965): *Sven. vet. T., 17*, 106.
7. Berggren, L. and Hansson, O. (1966): Treating acrodermatitis enteropathica. *Lancet, 1*, 52.

DISCUSSION

Dukes: Mr. Chairman, I have a comment and a question. My comment stems from Dr. Beppu's remark that had the physicians been aware of these publications, they might have behaved otherwise. I would like to say something about the possibility of a physician being aware of papers such as those he cites.

For three years we have been working with the production of the Side Effects of Drugs Annual, which is supposed to be an encyclopedic international review of adverse reactions and which has facilities available which the average physician does not have.

Let me quote some figures to you. We have analyzed material from about 2,000 journals all over the world. About 60,000 reports on adverse reactions appear yearly. Of those 60,000, about two-thirds are misleading in that they are promotional and produced largely at the instigation of drug companies as promotional material and entirely misleading as to the adverse reaction information.

About 20,000 are left for screening by medical people. The ultimate screening results in about 4,000 which do contribute to new knowledge about adverse reactions, quantitatively or qualitatively, 4,000 new publications a year which ultimately get into the Annual, and of those 4,000 many contain allegations and pointers which are at least as serious as those pointing to SMON in the various periods during the 1960s.

Of those 4,000, only a tiny fraction appears in Japanese, and indeed about a third appears in languages other than English – a tremendous and formidable problem. Obviously one cannot reasonably expect the physician to process this information himself, while he is going to rely on the transmission of this information into the advertising material on which he so greatly depends, or on government channels of information which must be highly selective.

Now my question: Does Dr. Beppu believe that Japanese physicians really know what they are prescribing? Do they have sufficient knowledge of chemistry and pharmacology to understand which drug they are giving? If so, they are exceptional because the information I have seen from other countries presents a very unfavorable picture of the physician's knowledge of the drugs he has given. He does not know commonly when giving a drug under a trade name what the constitution of that drug is, and particularly when giving a combination he does not know what the constitution of that combination is.

What does Dr. Beppu think about the Japanese physician's knowledge of the drugs he has given, as to their characteristics, more particularly their identity?

Beppu: Thank you very much for your valuable information, your figures are extremely significant. As you say, physicians must know what kind of drugs they are prescribing. Personally I do not think that I have adequate knowledge. I think Japanese doctors are lacking in that respect also.

As for the SMON disaster, changes have occurred and some improvements have been made, largely due to our daily efforts, but we just cannot leave this to individual doctors' efforts and present knowledge. We must regard the problem in a larger perspective. There is too much information at present. How to select the right information is the biggest problem for physicians.

For the average doctor in his normal practice, and in order to avoid any disasters, this is something that we must work towards in the future.

Kurahashi: In the Okayama Prefecture we have seen a large number of SMON outbreaks, and I have conducted a survey on 144 of the plaintiffs. We examined the administration history of these plaintiffs. There were very few cases in which the general practitioners prescribed the drugs to the patients. A large number of the plaintiffs received the drugs from large hospitals, and all these hospitals hold very authoritative positions in our society.

As for the period of administration, it varied from 50 days to 100 days for 27 cases. The largest was 200 days of administration.

The administration situation of clioquinol in Japan is characterized by the fact that many of the patients had taken clioquinol by prescription from the doctors.

As Dr. Hansson mentioned in his data, a large number of patients had been continuing their prescription over a long period of time. I do not feel, therefore, that this is very characteristic of Japan. A large dosage over a long period of time seems to be characteristic. I am not a clinical physician, and I really do not know the reason why it had been continued over such a long period of time and in such large doses.

Do you, Dr. Beppu, have any explanations or comments on this fact?

Beppu: My personal opinion concerning the SMON disaster is that we were told that clioquinol was a very safe drug and this is one of the reasons for the long period of administration. At that time, there was much debate about the use of antibiotics, so if it was made as a safe drug, many doctors felt it was better to use these drugs rather than antibiotics.

As for the prolonged use of these drugs, we can say that the doctors are too busy with too many patients. Therefore, they were not in a position to reconsider, or they were pressurized into long periods of administration. When one gives long prescriptions, there must be a period, a checking point, between the prescriptions.

The actual condition of drug induced sufferers, especially those with SMON, and the restoration to their original state. Based on the results of a nation-wide survey of SMON

TOSHIO HIGASHIDA

Department of Public Health, Kansai Medical University, Osaka, Japan

Whole families have been suffering from the pains and physical disturbances of SMON for a number of years. This report is concerned with some of the characteristics of Japanese drug induced suffering and measures for their prevention. It is based on a nation-wide survey and also on a study in Osaka of the actual condition and medical care of SMON patients.

A nation-wide survey of the actual situation of SMON patients was conducted in 1977 in 24 prefectures, about half of the total number of prefectures in Japan. 1,812 patients responded, 531 male, 1,281 female. 9% were under 39 years old, 44% 40–60 years old, and 47% over 60 years old. 10% were hospitalized and 90% nonhospitalized.

The actual symptoms were as follows (Fig. 1). Almost all of them had difficulty in walking; 7% were bedridden and 50% needed crutches or a walking stick.

90% had sensory disturbances, which were mainly in the lower half of the body and limbs: pain, strangulation and paralysis. 13% suffered from blindness and serious optic disorders. Over 50% needed various kinds of help in their daily lives. 60% suffered from various complications.

In addition to the physical pains they also suffered emotionally. They felt that their diseases were unlikely to be cured and encountered difficulties in their daily lives. 15% of the patients felt desperate and some of them even attempted to commit suicide.

The actual state of medical care for SMON patients is very inadequate. SMON patients need diverse, sufficient medical care and assistance.

The nation-wide survey revealed that one-fourth of all non-hospitalized patients desired to be admitted to specialized institutions. They also requested some kind of therapy, such as acupuncture or needle electrode, massage, hot spring therapy or medical rehabilitation. Bedridden patients asked for personal nursing and help.

50% of the patients are in need of special help in daily life. However, only a few actually receive such help or nursing and in most of the cases the burden is borne by family members.

Most of the families with SMON patients are exhausted. The members of some have fallen ill and are unable to work, decreasing the income. Sometimes divorce or family separation occurs, and some children may be obliged to forego marriage or

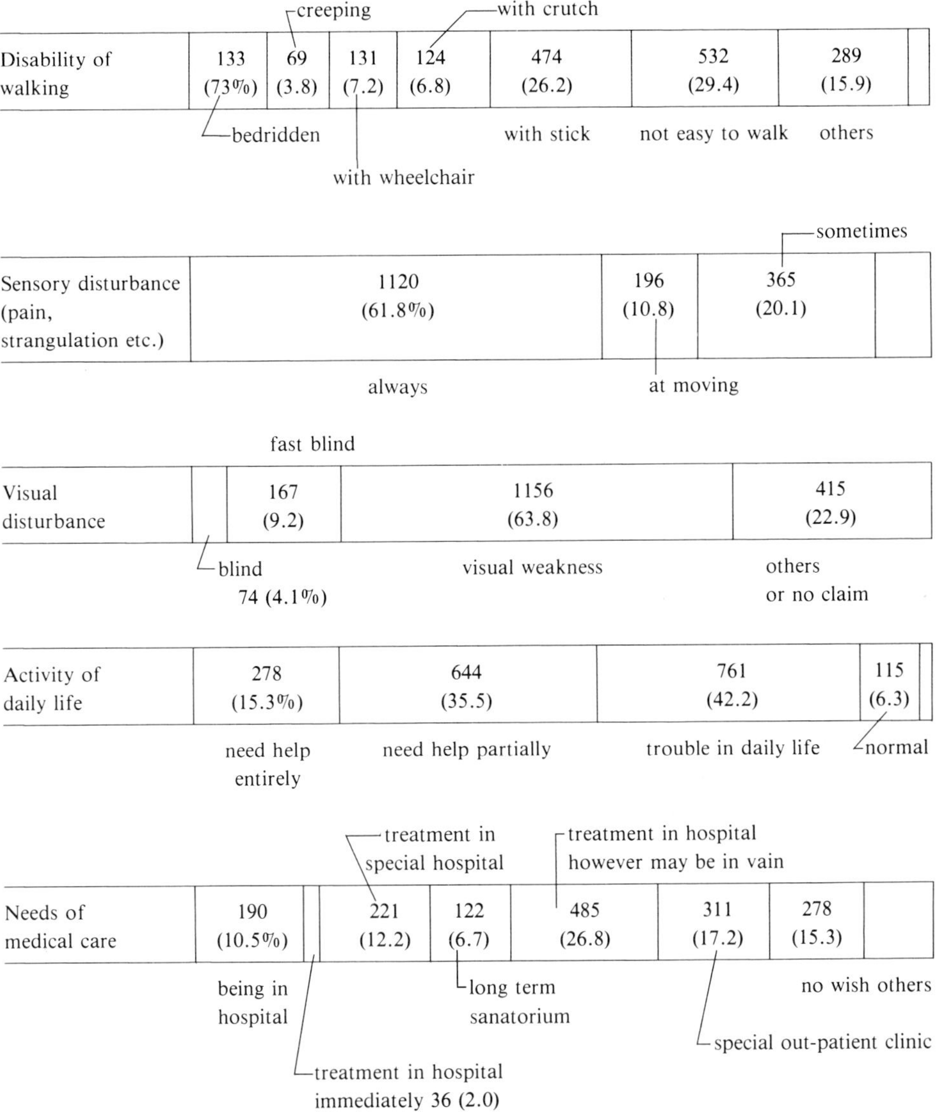

Fig. 1. Actual situation of SMON patients and need of medical care (1812 persons in 24 prefectures, 1977).

entrance into a school of higher grade. Therefore, the dispatch of home helpers and nurses is one of the most urgent requirements. Financial assistance is also called for.

With respect to the hospitalized patients, medical care and nursing are so inadequate, that one-third of them want to be transferred to more suitable conditions.

However, the patients need substantial amounts to meet hospital charges and fees for helpers, acupuncture therapy, massage and transportation to medical institutes (Table 1).

TABLE 1. *Needs of medical services (patients at home)*

No. of persons surveyed	1622	100.0
Admission to special hospital or sanatorium	379	23.4
Family doctor in neighborhood	266	16.4
Medical attention in a special hospital	477	29.4
Rehabilitation center for out-patients	295	18.2
Home visits by physical therapist	169	10.4
Therapy for pain	362	22.3
Electrotherapy	257	15.8
Acupuncture therapy	257	15.8
Massage	634	39.1
Hot spring therapy	512	31.6

(answers overlapping)

They are in a difficult economic situation and suffer from poverty. 60% of the patients have difficulties in their daily lives and about 50% are so poor that they need financial assistance and loans; some of them are in debt, etc. For these reasons SMON patients in a lawsuit are obliged to choose a 'settlement approach' with the defendants.

The housing situation is also serious. 20% of the patients live in houses which are unsuitable for their disability and 32% need repair work to their houses. Also heating facilities and telephones are necessary.

A follow-up study in Osaka has shown an increase in the number of patients with a deterioration of the disease and, recently, an increase in the death rate.

As regards compensation and medical care for the SMON victims the legal judgements by the courts confirmed the guilt of the defendants, the government and the pharmaceutical companies, and their obligation for compensation of the victims.

However, the defendants lodged appeals to the higher court and tried to take a 'settlement approach'. To tell the truth, the current legal standard or structure in Japan is deficient in relation to compensation for 'health victims' and in respect of the human rights of the people by the government. The essential demand of 'health victims' is the restoration of their original physical stituation, and the guarantee of sufficient medical care, rehabilitation, and security of livelihood.

SMON victims themselves are not at fault. Their state is due entirely to the wrongful acts of the government and pharmaceutical companies. Essentially, the government has legal obligations to restore the human rights of the victims, as stipulated by the Constitution of Japan.

To provide sufficient medical care and assistance to victims throughout the country, appropriate governmental action should be taken, based on the principles of complete sharing the burden by the guilty parties. Also local governments should take immediate action to relieve these victims. From this point of view the party of SMON victims had demanded the enactment of a special law.

The government should now conduct a nation-wide survey to determine exactly the needs of SMON victims and the present state of the clioquinol episode, including the discovery of latent victims.

At present a bill for 'an Act for a Fund for the Relief of Drug Induced Sufferers' is being considered. However, this draft of 'an Act for a Fund' aims only to reduce the financial burden of the guilty party. It may lead to 'the relief of guilty pharmaceutical companies', but not to the genuine relief of their victims and it is doubtful if it will help to prevent the further occurrence of drug induced sufferings.

The characteristics and prevention of drug-induced suffering in Japan

TOSHIO HIGASHIDA

Department of Public Health, Kansai Medical University, Osaka, Japan

The SMON episode illustrates the recent lack of concern about serious pollution in Japan. In a period of high economic growth, industry has pursued a policy of 'mass production and mass consumption' with governmental co-operation, often to the neglect of safety for the consumers. The drug industry has been no exception. In addition, we have in Japan unique channels for the sale and distribution of drugs, and the pharmaceutical administration lacks scientific procedures for approval of the manufacture and sale of drugs.

The Government has tended to accept the applications of pharmaceutical companies without conducting any scientific investigations of the toxicity of drugs. This has eventually led to serious episodes of drug-induced suffering, of which SMON is one. On the other hand, the FDA of the U.S.A. not only drew attention to the limited efficacy of clioquinol but also restricted its use because of its toxicity. The governmental administrations of Japan and the U.S.A. thus took opposite standpoints. The second important point is the machinery for the sale and distribution of drugs. 'Vigorous commercial advertisement creates the demand for goods and leads to mass consumption.' This includes drugs. A survey was conducted by questionnaires to 71 physicians who had administered clioquinol, asking about their reasons and motives (Tables 1 and 2). They answered that they used clioquinol mainly on the basis of statements or advice from agents of the pharmaceutical companies and they totally believed in the safety and effectiveness of clioquinol for many kinds of intestinal disturbances.

In addition, the influence of commercial advertisements for drugs in medical journals should not be overlooked. The advertisements for clioquinol appeared in

TABLE 1. *Reasons for of the use of clioquinol*

No. of doctors surveyed	71	100.0
1. Believing it a 'safe and effective drug'	45	63.3
2. Being informed that 'it has no side-effects'	31	43.7
3. Being informed that 'it causes no resistant bacteria'	8	11.3
4. Being informed that 'it is hardly absorbed in the intestines'	6	8.5
5. Being informed that 'the dosage may be increased according to symptoms'	7	9.9
6. Being informed that 'any side-effect is temporary, so the prescription need not be discontinued'	1	1.4
7. Other	5	7.2

TABLE 2. *Advertisements for clioquinol appearing in the 'Japan Medical Journal' (weekly)*

Vol. no.	Date of issue	Name of drug
1884	1960 6. 4	Entero-Vioform (Ciba)
1899	9.17	Entero-Vioform (Ciba)
1938	1961 6.17	Entero-Vioform (Ciba)
1941	7. 8	Emaform (Tanabe)
1946	8.12	Emaform (Tanabe)
1947	8.19	Entero-Vioform (Ciba)
1951	9.16	Entero-Vioform (Ciba)
1993	1962 7. 7	Emavorm (Tanabe)
1999	8.18	Mexaform (Ciba)
2000	8.25	Emaform (Tanabe)
2037	1963 5.11	Mexaform (Ciba)
2039	5.25	Emaform (Tanabe)
2043	6.22	Emaform (Tanabe)
2084	1964 4. 4	Mexaform forte A (Ciba)
2087	4.25	Mexaform forte A (Ciba)
2090	5.16	Entero-Vioform (Ciba)
2093	6. 6	Entero-Vioform (Ciba)
2099	7.18	Entero-Vioform (Ciba)
2100	7.25	Mexaform forte A (Ciba)
2101	8. 1	Mexaform forte A (Ciba)
2103	8.15	Mexaform forte A (Ciba)
2104	8.22	Mexaform forte A (Ciba)
2106	9. 5	Mexaform forte A (Ciba)
2147	1965 6.19	Mexaform forte (Ciba)
2251	1966 6.18	Mexaform forte (Ciba)
2212	9.17	Mexaform (Ciba)
2251	1967 6.17	Mexaform forte (Ciba)
2266	9.30	Mexaform forte (Ciba)
2273	11.18	Mexaform forte (Ciba)
2288	1968 3. 2	Mexaform forte (Ciba)
2305	6.29	Mexaform forte (Ciba)
2318	9.28	Mexaform forte (Ciba)
2359	1969 7.12	Mexaform forte (Ciba)
2365	8.23	Mexaform forte (Ciba)
2394	1970 3.14	Mexaform forte (Ciba)
2400	6. 6	Mexaform forte (Ciba)

the *Japan Medical Journal,* which enjoyed the highest circulation in Japan from 1960 to 1970, especially during the summer (Table 2). Also *Acta Pediatrica Japonica*, the journal of the Japanese Pediatric Society, published the same kind of advertisement every month of the spring and summer of 1964–1966, stating that clioquinol was safe even for children. The appearance of these advertisements for clioquinol coincided with remarkable increases in SMON patients.

The protection of the user should be the first duty of the pharmaceutical administration. The serious situation of the SMON patients was partly induced by the lack of medical care and social assistance, but mainly due to the negligent attitude of the

Government. It is most essential that the Government concerned should realize their responsibility to protect the human rights and health of SMON victims as stipulated by 'The Constitution of Japan', and to guarantee medical care and social assistance of the highest possible level.

The physicians should act independently of the pharmaceutical companies and respond to the trust of the patients.

Finally, I would like to cite the concluding remarks of the judgment of the Fukuoka Court: 'First, the plaintiffs are reasonably demanding the restoration of their bodies to their original healthy state. Secondly, they are making a highly moral request for the eradication of drug induced-sufferings. The timely complete relief of these patients and the eradication of drug-induced sufferings in general are, indeed, two sides of the same coin. Now, we are requested to solve these urgent national problems.'

Nature of the damage affecting SMON patients: required relief measures and systems

KYOICHI SONODA and NOBUKO IIJIMA

Department of Health Sociology, School of Health Sciences, Faculty of Medicine, University of Tokyo, Tokyo, Japan

The aim of this report is to present an appropriate means of providing compensation and relief for SMON patients and their families. For this purpose, the report mainly deals with the status of the physical, mental, economic and social damage affecting them so as to identify the structure and correlation of these factors based on the findings of a field survey conducted over the past 9 years by the health sociology task force of the SMON Research Commission.

PROGRESS OF STUDY AND SAMPLES SELECTED FOR SURVEY

A series of surveys was conducted on a total of 392 SMON patients and their families (see Table 1) in Ibara City, Okayama Prefecture (in 1970 and 1973), Toda, Warabi, and Kawaguchi Cities, Saitama (in 1970 and 1974), Tokushima (in 1972), Aichi (in 1974), Kagoshima (in 1976) and Niigata (in 1977). Of these patients, 317 were actually interviewed by the staff members of this Research Commission as the rest had moved to other areas, had died or were away from home at the time of interview, or refused to respond to the questionnaire. Incidentally, the surveys conducted in Okayama and Saitama Prefectures in 1973 and 1974, respectively, were designed to re-examine the status of the same patients interviewed previously.

Another survey was carried out in 1978 by mailing questionnaires to 299 patients who had been interviewed before, and replies were obtained from 254. Of the total respondents in the 6 prefectures covered by the survey, those in Aichi were originally selected from Group A (rehabilitated patients) and Group B (those with particularly serious damage), while the patients in the other prefectures were picked out from the list of all victims in selected areas which had been prepared by the epidemiological task force of the SMON Research Commission and the members of the Clinical Subcommittee. For the purpose of examining the status of all patients, therefore, it is necessary to eliminate the two groups in Aichi Prefecture and analyze the replies from the remaining 203 respondents.

The data obtained from these 203 patients and the results of a nationwide survey by the epidemiological task force were examined to find out the extent of their attributive biases. However, no significant difference was observed between the two surveys in respect of such comparable data as the percentage distribution of respondents by sex and age bracket or the results of analyzing their replies as to whether they suffer from impairment of the sensory organs, ambulant ability, or eyesight (see Tables 2–6).

TABLE 1. *Numbers of patients surveyed and replies analyzed*

	Interview				Mail		
	Patients selected for survey	Patients actually inter-viewed	Patients resurveyed: Patients selected	Patients resurveyed: Patients inter-viewed	No. of ques-tion-naires mailed	No. of res-pon-dents	Total no. of replies analy-zed
Tokushima (Tokushima City)	99	78			78	65	65
Okayama (Ibara City)	91	78	78	68	68	55	55
Saitama (Toda, Warabi, and Kawaguchi cities)	30	29	29	21	21	19	19
Aichi Group A (rehabili-tated patients)	52	45			45	41	
Aichi Group B (patients with serious damage)	12	12			12	10	
Kagoshima (all areas)	40	36			36	28	28
Niigata (Niigata City and neighboring muni-cipalities)	68	39			39	36	36
Total	392	317			299	254	203

TABLE 2. *Classified total by sex*

Male	60	29.6%
Female	143	70.4
Total	203	100.0

FINDINGS

Nature of the damage affecting SMON patients and their families

The nature of the damage affecting SMON patients and their families can be summarized as follows. SMON patients and their families are primarily affected by the physical impairment which the patients suffer due to the contraction of this disease. The contraction of this disease brings about a heavier economic burden on

TABLE 3. *Grouping by age bracket*

0– 9	0	-
10–19	0	-
20–29	1	0.5%
30–39	18	8.9
40–49	45	22.2
50–59	43	21.2
60–69	57	28.1
70–79	35	17.2
80 and over	4	2.0
Total	203	100.1

TABLE 4. *Patients' replies on numbness*

Always numb	167	82.3%
Sometimes numb	19	9.4
Unaffected	10	4.9
No response	7	3.4
Total	203	100.0

TABLE 5. *Patients' replies on their ability to walk*

Cannot walk at all	14	6.9%
Can walk if helped by attendants	6	3.0
Can walk by themselves by using sticks or other aids	36	17.7
Can manage to walk by themselves	85	41.9
Can walk nearly as well as before contracting the disease	39	19.2
Not affected by the disease as far as their ability to walk is concerned	20	9.9
Other	1	0.5
No response	2	1.0
Total	203	100.1

TABLE 6. *Patients' replies on their sight (multiple answers) (total no. of respondents: 203)*

Completely lost eyesight	4	2.0%
Lost eyesight nearly completely	10	4.9
Affected by declining visual power	122	60.1
Affected by narrowed visual fields	30	14.8
Eyesight not affected	40	19.7
Others	12	5.9
No response	14	6.9
Total	232	114.3

the patients' families because of increased medical and living expenses. In addition, such physical injury impairs the patients' working ability and subsequently forces them to leave their jobs or suffer a decrease in earnings. It also affects their ability to lead a normal daily life bringing about changes in roles assigned to each of their family members and, when the patients' condition reaches an advanced stage, the

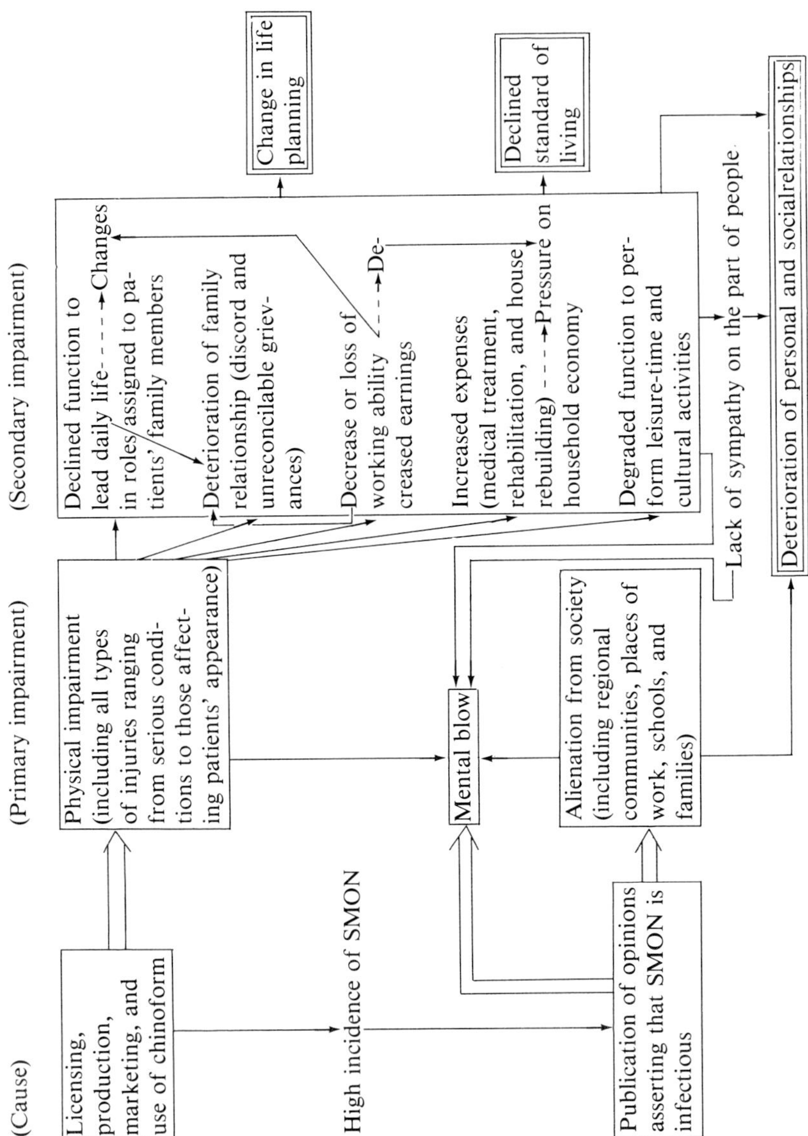

Fig. 1. Structure of damage affecting SMON patients and their families. From Iijima (5).

other family members' work load increases substantially since they have to take care of the patients. These unfavorable conditions are likely to worsen the relationship among family members, often leading to more severe discord and unreconcilable grievances among them. Besides these mental blows, the patients and their families become alienated from the community, in many instances because of the opinion maintained by some that this disease is infectious.

Figure 1 is a diagram giving an outline of the damage inflicted on SMON patients and their families.

Summary of survey results

This section deals with the physical conditions and livelihood of SMON patients and their families based on the results of a survey conducted in 1978 by mailing questionnaires to selected victims.

Physical impairment and medical care

In response to whether they were affected by numbness, more than 90% (91.7%) of the patients said that they suffered from some sort of paresthesia (see Table 4). As to their ambulant ability, only 9.9% replied that they could walk as freely as before SMON attacked them (see Table 5). Also those who said that their eyesight was not affected by the disease accounted for only 19.7% (see Table 6). As is apparent from these examples, most of the SMON victims surveyed were still suffering from a variety of physical injuries more than 10 years after the onset of the disease.

According to the survey findings on the medical care which SMON patients are currently receiving (see Table 7), more than half (52.2%) of the respondents, including those treated for some other diseases, said that they went to hospital regularly as outpatients. In addition, some 5% each replied that they were hospitalized, that they had doctors visit them, and that other members of their families went to medical institutions to get medicines only. Those replying that they saw doctors only when they felt particularly ill accounted for 18.2%, while only 11.3% said that they seldom received medical treatment. Moreover, a substantially high percentage of the respondents, or 1 out of every 4 to 6, said that they were being treated with acupuncture, moxa, or massage and were taking herbal medicines (see Table 8).

All these treatments and drugs served to increase the patients' medical expenses,

TABLE 7. *Patients' replies as to medical treatment*

Are hospitalized	14	6.9%
Have doctors visit them at regular intervals	8	3.9
Receive medical treatment at a hospital as outpatients	106	52.2
Take medicine fetched by other members of their families	9	4.4
See doctors only when particularly ill	37	18.2
Seldom see doctors	23	11.3
Others	2	1.0
No response	10	4.9
Total	209	102.8

Note: Multiple answers were allowed, but the percentages were calculated by using 203 as denominator.

TABLE 8. *Medical expenses (multiple answers)*

Doctors' fees and hospital bills	35	17.2%
Travelling expenses (for outpatients only)	43	21.2
Charges for acupuncture, moxa, or massage	46	22.7
Hospital charges not covered by health insurance	3	1.5
Attendants' fees	9	4.4
Proprietary and herbal medicines	54	25.6
Others	21	10.3
Patients who suffer no medical expense	6	3.0
No response	74	36.5
Total	291	142.4

Note: Percentages were calculated by using 203 as denominator.

TABLE 9. *Grouping of patients by bracket of total monthly medical expenses*

None	7	3.4%
Below ¥1,000	2	1.0
¥1,000–¥5,000 (exc.)	36	17.7
¥5,000–¥10,000	21	10.3
¥10,000–¥20,000	21	10.3
¥20,000–¥50,000	21	10.3
¥50,000–¥100,000	10	4.9
¥100,000–¥200,000	3	1.5
No response	82	40.4
Total	203	99.8

TABLE 10. *Patients' replies as to whether they have jobs that bring about an income*

	Total		Male patients only	
Have jobs	71	35.0%	35	58.3%
Are jobless	127	62.6	23	38.3
No response	5	2.5	2	3.3
Total	203	100.1	60	99.9

including doctors' fees and hospital bills, outpatients' travelling expenses, charges for acupuncture, moxa, or massage, hospital charges not covered by health insurance, attendants' fees, and proprietary and herbal medicines. This is clearly reflected in the fact that the patients spending ¥1,000 to ¥50,000 a month accounted for a large percentage, indicating that these expenses still remained at a substantially high level (see Table 9).

Occupational problems and financial loss

This section deals with the patients' financial loss incurred by the contraction of SMON. With regard to occupational problems arising from their reduced work capacity, 71 respondents or 35% said that they had jobs with an income, while 127 or 62.6% replied that they were jobless. An analysis of replies from the male patients only revealed that those who 'have jobs' accounted for 58.3% compared with 38.3% represented by the 'jobless' (see Table 10). As to why they were out of

TABLE 11. *Reasons for not working*

1. Physical impairment due to SMON	59	46.5%
2. Old age	28	22.0
3. No imminent need to work because other members of their families have jobs	21	16.5
4. Others	3	2.4
5. Combination of 1 and 2 above	9	7.1
6. Combination of 2 and 3 above	1	0.8
7. No response	6	4.7
Total	127	100.0

TABLE 12. *Annual income of patients by sex and age bracket (earnings of other family members excluded)*

Income \ Age group	20–29	30–39	40–49	50–59	60–69	70–79	80 and over	Total
Below ¥500,000			(2)	(3)	3(1)	1(1)		4(7)
¥500,000– ¥1 million		(1)	1(2)	2(4)	2		1	6(7)
¥1– ¥2 million	1	2(4)	2(2)	1(3)	(2)	(1)		6(12)
¥2– ¥3 million		2	2(1)	2(1)	(2)			6(4)
¥3– ¥4 million		1	4(1)	1				6(1)
¥4– ¥5 million			3	1(1)				4(1)
¥5 million and over			2					2
Subtotal	1	5(5)	14(8)	7(12)	5(5)	1(2)	1	34(32)
Unsure			(1)	(3)				(4)
No response		1			1(3)	1		3(3)
Total	1	6(5)	14(9)	7(15)	6(8)	2(2)	1	37(39)

Note: Figures in parentheses represent female patients. This table does not include the 23 male and 104 female patients who replied that they do not have any job.

TABLE 13. *Patients' replies as to their share in housekeeping*

	Total		Female patients only	
Play leading role in housekeeping	49	24.1%	46	22.2%
Take over part in housework	53	26.1	47	32.9
Take little or no charge of housework	65	32.0	36	25.2
No response	36	17.7	14	9.8

work, nearly half or 46.5% of the 'jobless' mentioned their physical impairment due to SMON as a reason (see Table 11). Asked whether they experienced any difficulty, felt pain, or worried about their physical condition due to SMON during workings hours or commuting, 50 (or 70.4%) of the 71 respondents who 'have jobs' replied in the affirmative.

When decreases in their own annual earned income and that of their families as a whole are taken into account (see Table 12), it can be readily understood how strongly they hoped for the implementation of adequate measures to guarantee their livelihood through pensions and other benefits.

Adverse effects of SMON on patients' home life and their family relationships
Physical impairment resulting from the contraction of SMON affects the patients' ability to lead a normal daily life, subsequently changing the role assigned to each of their family members. Asked how much housekeeping they took over, 50.2% of the patients said that they played the leading role in housework or that they took partial charge of this family task. When responses from the female respondents only were picked out for analysis, this percentage was as high as 65.1 (see Table 13). However, 85.3% of them complained of physical impairment affecting their ability to carry out housework freely. As a matter of course, the SMON patients' or their families' demand for the services of home helps arises from their current status as noted above.

Where the contraction of SMON has further reduced the patients' ability to lead a normal daily life, the other members of their families suffer from an increased work load because they have to take care of the patients. Questionnaires mailed to the selected patients in the 1978 survey offered 4 alternative answers to a question regarding meals, changing of clothes, bathing, excretion, and indoor ambulation: the first answer was that the patients 'need no help at all', the second that they 'can somehow manage' for themselves, the third that they 'need some help', and the fourth that they have to 'rely entirely on the help of others'. Although the respondents' answers varied somewhat with their behavior or situation, about 5% of them had to be completely taken care of, and around 10% needed some help (see Table 14). It is likely that this will develop into a more serious problem in the future when the patients grow still older.

As is apparent from the above observations, the physical impairment of SMON patients is likely to worsen their family relationships, resulting in severer discord and unreconcilable grievances among them. Meanwhile, the patients who replied that their occupation had been unfavorably affected by their disease, and those contending that their plans for old age had been disarranged accounted for more than 20% each. In addition, some 10 to 20% of the respondents said that their education, marriage, family relationship, business, planned construction of new houses or rebuilding of old ones, or the use of leisure time had been affected by their disease (see Table 15). Those replying that their family relationships were not very favorable also exceeded the 10% level (see Table 16).

TABLE 14. *Patients' replies as to how much they can take care of themselves*

	Meals		Changing clothes		Bathing		Excretion		Indoor ambulation	
		%		%		%		%		%
Need no help at all	100	49.3	89	43.8	90	44.3	95	46.8	91	44.8
Can somehow manage for themselves	62	30.5	74	36.5	68	33.5	76	37.4	70	34.5
Need some help	25	12.3	22	10.8	19	9.4	13	6.4	19	9.4
Need complete help	4	2.0	6	3.0	15	7.4	8	3.9	11	5.4
No response	12	5.9	12	5.9	11	5.4	11	5.4	12	5.9
Total	203	100.0	203	100.0	203	100.0	203	99.9	203	100.0

TABLE 15. *Patients' replies as to disarrangement of their life plan (multiple answers)*

Education	33	37.4%
Marriage	22	10.8
Family affairs	36	17.7
Business	33	37.4
Occupation	48	23.6
Housing	34	16.7
Preparations for old age	47	23.2
Plans for leisure	28	13.8
Others	8	3.9
Not particularly affected	41	20.2
No response	31	15.3
Total	361	220.0

TABLE 16. *Family relationship*

Have no trouble	88	43.3%
Enjoy fairly good family relationship in general	67	33.0
Not on good terms with other family members	24	11.8
Others	10	4.9
No response	14	6.9
Total	203	99.9

REQUIRED RELIEF MEASURES AND SYSTEMS

The foregoing sections have mainly discussed the losses sustained by SMON patients and their families as well as the circumstances they are in based on the findings of the 1978 survey. In view of this status of the SMON victims, this report gives a summary of the measures and systems which appear to be necessary to guarantee their future livelihood.

Effective therapeutics, provision of institutions, financial aid

As is apparent from paresthesia and declined ambulant ability, the physical impairment and pains that SMON patients suffer still remain unalleviated. To solve this problem, it is essential that a continuous study should be conducted to establish effective therapeutics for the disease, while providing special medical institutions and personnel on a nationwide scale for affected residents in each region. At the same time, efforts must be made to provide adequate financial aid and other measures to increase the availability of acupuncture, moxa treatment, and massage since these remedies are much in demand with many patients. Another important financial aid is to give increased benefits for indirect medical expenses such as outpatients' travelling expenses (including taxi fares) and attendants' fees.

Aids to employment, working conditions

As for the economic problems of SMON patients, emphasis should be placed on measures to offer them jobs, better working and commuting conditions, or aids to facilitate their self-employment or pay jobs that can be carried out at home. Since many of the patients are growing too old to find employment easily, it is also essential that pensions and other aids should be extended to them to guarantee their livelihood on a continuous basis.

Home helps, visiting nurses

The social and mental sufferings of SMON patients include those involved in their family relationships, which are mainly attributable to their declined ability to take part in housekeeping. This poses a particularly serious problem for female patients as well as those who live alone or who are aged and have only their elderly wives or husbands to turn to for help. In addition, seriously affected patients who need help in their daily life impose a still heavier burden on their families. For this reason, it is essential that efforts should be made to provide the services of home helps and visiting nurses.

This disease has brought about various other adverse effects on the victims and their families, including changes in the course of life they have mapped out and the loss of what makes their life worth living and pleasant. Moreover, these patients suffer from a lack of understanding on the part of those around them as well as alienation from the community due to the opinion that the disease is infectious. It can be asserted that adequate relief measures are needed to extend sufficient aid to these patients and to fully compensate them for this mental suffering and damage.

CONCLUSION – APPROPRIATE RELIEF MEASURES

An examination of the existing relief measures has revealed that except for the general social welfare and security systems, only a very few measures have so far been provided for SMON patients and their families to solve the various impediments, difficulties, and problems confronting them. These measures mainly consist of public aid covering the portion of direct medical expenses which is to be borne by patients themselves and a system established in 1978 to finance part of the charges for acupuncture, moxa treatment, and massage. These measures are apparently inadequate in view of the physical condition of SMON patients as well as the current status of their family relationships and livelihood.

It should be noted that currently these patients and their families mostly take recourse to lawsuits for damages as a means of solving their impediments and other problems. Since the existing systems provide little financial relief, it is likely that those who do not participate in such litigation may not even get relief in the form of an indemnity.

The number of patients now in action against the parties apparently responsible for their disease reaches some 4,500, which is substantially less than half of the victims (11,007 persons) listed by the SMON Research Commission. Since the total number of SMON patients in Japan, including latent sufferers, is estimated at 20,000, those who are left unrelieved are expected to reach a significantly large percentage.

Furthermore, such legal action is far from being satisfactory as a means of providing sufficient relief to guarantee the future livelihood of the patients and their families, because it is designed primarily to identify the parties responsible for the damage and to claim an indemnity from them. It must be emphasized that many problems related to the relief of SMON victims still remain unsolved or rather unattended and that this problem can never be solved by temporary compensation alone such as indemnities obtained through lawsuits or contracted sums awarded the victims in amicable settlement of the dispute between the parties involved.

Consequently, legislative and administrative relief measures are needed to permanently guarantee the future livelihood of the patients and their families as well as to provide specific services to help them in their daily lives. It can be asserted that the Diet and the Administration are required to work out such measures.

REFERENCES

1. Miyasaka, T. and Sonoda, K. (1975): Sociological aspects of SMON. *Jap. J. med. Sci. Biol., 28.*
2. Iijima, N. (1976): Life of Canadian Indians and the influence of mercury poisoning on it. In: *Proceedings, International Congress on the Human Environment, Kyoto, 1975.* Asahi Evening News, Tokyo.
3. Sonoda, K. (1978): SMON and other socially induced diseases in Japan. *Soc. Sci. Med., 12/6A.*
4. Iijima, N. (1979): *Pollution Japan – Historical Chronology.* Asahi Evening News, Tokyo.
5. Iijima, N. (1974): *Survey Report by Health Sociology Task Force, SMON Research Commission,* p. 28.

DISCUSSION

Kaneda: I earlier spoke about the permanent policies and I have calculated the compensation level. Other speakers have presented their calculations as regards compensation. With regard to the so-called permanent policies, what percentage of the budget should be borne by the government and what percentage should be borne by the manufacturers? I would like to hear your views on this.

Sonoda: This is very difficult to answer in specific terms. However, in this context the government is one of the parties involved in the whole litigation. Therefore, when considering compensation, one aspect is compensating for certain liabilities; another aspect is how to socially assist the future daily lives of the victims. Which aspect should be stressed is the problem. In the case of the SMON litigation, I think the government is the actual party involved in the whole case, so it should compensate for the liability. I think this should be stressed.

Kojima: You mentioned about 20,000 potential victims. How did you arrive at this figure, and what is the reason for this kind of calculation? How did you identify the potential victims and what methodology did you use in order to calculate this figure?

Sonoda: For the estimation of the potential victims, we can think in terms of various methods. I arrived at a figure of 20,000 victims. Within the Ministry of Health and Welfare, there is a division handling epidemiological factors, and their staff arrived at this figure after much examination and research. Also, about 2 years ago we asked Professor Igata of Kagoshima University, and he fully cooperated with us in our efforts. Within Kagoshima Prefecture the professor conducted the calculation of the potential victims. He contacted all the health centers or medical associations within Kagoshima Prefecture and tried to obtain all necessary information. Professor Igata and other professors at Kagoshima University, medical neurologists, also conducted a study and arrived at a figure that was double the number of potential victims originally expected.

Kagoshima Prefecture is just one prefecture in Japan and Kagoshima University just one state university which conducted this kind of research, and with the cooperation of the medical association and all the health centers, we arrived at this figure. Within the limited area of one prefecture it was relatively easy to gain this kind of cooperation, but I hope the same kind of research will also be made in other prefectures in the future.

Tuveson: We have heard about the experiences in different countries concerning drug-induced sufferings, and the information we had will be used in the international struggle against drug-induced suffering where there are disproportions between the efficacy of drugs and their adverse reactions.

The problems of the litigations are many, and the information we can get from this Conference will surely be a contribution to solving them. I would like to thank the speakers for their excellent contributions.

The logic of the SMON settlement and some prospects for the relief of the victims

AKIYOSHI SATAKE

National News Division, Asahi-Shimbun, Tokyo, Japan

As long as medicines and drugs have harmful aspects and faults are made in society, the drug-induced suffering will continue. However, mass outbreaks of disasters such as that of SMON must be prevented, social measures must relieve the victims. It is extremely significant that people from most professions are present at this Conference and are searching for new and better systems to prevent and/or treat drug-induced suffering. All of us present must reflect on our respective roles in this area.

In Japan the disasters of SMON and thalidomide have been experienced. Victims have suffered great pain while society has been insensitive to the extent of only adding to the suffering. A just society must understand the pain of each of its members, and the press has a primary responsibility to transmit this information. The SMON and thalidomide disasters in Japan reveal an insensitivity and lack of proper communication between the press and population at large.

Early relief to victims is essential. Victims suffer pain all the time, and for the elderly victims relief must be rapid, although it must be recognized that at best it can only provide temporary consolation and cannot re-establish previous conditions before the suffering. It is thus all the more frustrating that the Tanabe Pharmaceutical Company denies any responsibility and, at the same time, talks about relief.

The relief of the victims entails solving the problem and the application of relief. Drug litigation, especially the SMON litigation, must rapidly realize early relief for the victims, and create a system for automatic prevention for the future.

The endless courtroom debates comprised conflict between the defendants and plaintiffs and prolonged scientific debate. For the victims this is cruel time-wasting and final relief is never guaranteed.

In the SMON litigation, however, a logical and realistic measure of relief was achieved, by a 'settlement', supported by the press. This was of course based on the premise that the settlement was one in which the state and the pharmaceutical companies admitted their reponsibility and provided rational compensation. The settlement was also judged to adhere to the principle of early relief and out-of-court settlements.

It was of course vital that clioquinol was recognized as the cause of SMON, so that the endless scientific debate over causal relationships between clioquinol and SMON could be avoided. If, by circumstantial argument, a scientific relationship could be explained, the theory of probability regarding causal relationship could be applied.

Secondly, any person manufacturing or selling substances considered as inducing damage – though not specified strictly as legal negligence – is responsible for compensation. The SMON settlement is thus made under the product liability theory. This was the first case in which negligence without fault was applied to a settlement. This new concept in this country goes beyond existing laws of negligence and permitted both early relief and a basis for future litigation.

Of course, the law admits legal negligence and defendants have appealed to the higher courts on all the court rulings. However, the settlement by not defining legal responsibility has taken the position of negligence without fault and by so doing does not admit defendants' rebuttal. Negligence without fault does not yet apply in this country, and debate continues. This does not mean that there was no negligence on the manufacturers' part, but it emphasizes that, regardless of negligence, anyone propagating the damage should be responsible, a line of thought inherent in the settlement clauses.

Victory in the court clarifies defendants' legal responsibility but does not provide adequate relief under the existing law. There is no reason why we must be bound by the framework of existing laws which must be extended to provide relief. This is the only way to achieve viable laws for the future.

There is no doubt that the state and its administration were responsible in the SMON disaster. Existing drug laws lack clauses concerning the prevention of drug-induced damage and the legal responsibilities are ill-defined. Even the Tokyo District Court mentioned that the responsibility prior to 1967 cannot be applied by precedence. The settlement goes beyond the defective existing law and casts administrative responsibility in a new light. The Tokyo District Court settlement is extremely significant in that for the early relief of the victims it went beyond the existing law.

If at present relief cannot be provided, the law must be amended. The SMON settlement was a happy example in which the law was extended.

The Ministry of Health and Welfare have drafted a bill, to come into effect in April, 1980, for relief of victims of drug-induced diseases. This is one of the results of SMON litigation. The bill is formulated within the framework of the existing law, and may not assist future cases and obviate loopholes in the existing law. On one hand, the Tokyo District Court settlement presents a future legal principle, while the Ministry of Health and Welfare bill for the relief of victims of drug-induced sufferings must fail sooner or later.

The settlement plan of the Tokyo District Court is surely most significant. The dedicated people involved with this settlement epitomized the sense of mission required for this type of settlement. A most wise and dedicated judge allowed precedences to be created.

The press too have contributed to this settlement, in that the victims and the public were thoroughly informed so that society has accepted and supported the settlement. Public opinion has also helped to overcome various bureaucratic problems hampering the endeavors.

Any corporation that damages the livelihood of the citizens must recognize that its own viability will be threatened by society itself. Society must be wary of all these corporations. The basic human respect that has arisen from the experiences of Minamata disease, Itai-itai disease, the thalidomide and SMON disasters, will prevent corporations repeating similar tragedies.

Although the SMON settlement created precedents, many complex problems remain. Firstly, the Tanabe Pharmaceutical Company has avoided their responsibility and many of the victims have been omitted from the settlement. Secondly, since all the defendants appealed before the decision was made, the path for future settlements is closed to remaining victims. The Tanabe Pharmaceutical Company has refuted the Tokyo District Court settlement plan on the basis of the virus theory, which has already been dismissed both scientifically and socially. The stance of Tanabe will become increasingly difficult when society will object to its very existence.

It is merely expedient for Tanabe to persist with the virus theory, for by indulging in extensive scientific debate they hope to avoid responsibility.

The Tanabe corporation must be persuaded to argue realistically. The company must be able and made, if necessary, to compensate the victims.

The Ministry of Health and Welfare is able to supervise the activities and can no longer let Tanabe's position remain. Recently, Tanabe Pharmaceutical Company asked the Ministry of Health and Welfare to act as a representative in the settlement; this is inadequate. If Tanabe Pharmaceutical Company sincerely desires settlement, they must apologize and adhere to the Tokyo District Court settlement plan. However, Tanabe Pharmaceutical Company and the Ministry of Health and Welfare do not refer to responsibility. This is extreme pride on the part of both the Ministry and the Company.

There is also the problem of the victims who continue in the court over legal responsibility. Because of their efforts victories in Tokyo, Kanazawa, Fukuoka and Hiroshima have been seen. In cases without certification of dose, but classed as SMON patients compensation should be given. It is unfortunate that such rulings cannot be directly related to relief, since the defendants keep appealing to the higher courts.

If someone is drowned in the river, do we discuss who is responsible? The most important thing is: How should we extend a helping hand before precious time has already passed? Theory for the relief of victims is already complete. The four victorious court rulings in Tokyo, Kanazawa, Fukuoka and Hiroshima, illustrate how society has become sensitive to such problems; society wants early relief to be given to the victims. For the SMON litigations on trial victory is ensured but it must not proceed with conflict. If all appeal to the higher court, then the court rulings are meaningless for time passes and suffering continues.

For cases still under litigation, the Tokyo District Court settlement plan should be accepted and efforts should focus on the expansion of the medical facilities and the centers for recovery. Such a change must apply pressure on Tanabe Pharmaceutical Company to bring a change in their attitudes.

DISCUSSION

Silverman: It is very important that victory is not simply the conclusion of the litigation and settlement in the SMON affair in Japan. One battle does not win a war. Other countries are concerned, and there will be other drug disasters; what has been done here can serve as a guide for others to prepare for future, almost inevitable, catastrophes. Mr. Satake's paper is open for questions.

Matsunami: This is not a question but an expression of a personal opinion. I agree that settlement is one method of solution, but I cannot agree that settlement is the best method of relief. A drowning person can be saved by a helping hand, but provisional settlements provide sums of money for the victims. The problems and issues are clear, but the biggest problem is that litigation is too prolonged. I agree with Dr. Kojima's method for future litigation.

Satake: My comments are specifically concerned with SMON litigation and are not general principles. SMON litigation has lasted for over 5 years.

Teshima: When you mentioned the role of the press, wherein does the responsibility for the delay of relief of the victims lie? The state and the pharmaceutical companies were the ones responsible for the delay of relief. So to achieve early relief, I think we should not recommend settlements to the plaintiffs, rather we should aim to make the defendants admit responsibility.

Satake: The role of the press in the delay of relief is largely due to the defendants. Courtroom litigation demands that the press make judgments as early as possible, although the rights and wrongs cannot be judged fully. In complex issues, the press cannot genuinely examine or indeed judge.

Chairman: Today, the discussion focussed on four aspects: court litigation and rulings; the relief based on these; the prevention of a repetition of such disasters; the role of the press in promoting public awareness.

To date there have been four decisions and court rulings. The legal rulings only solved certain points at issue. The fact that the points were solved has shifted awareness from a minority to a majority. Such shifts in views promote preventive measures.

Sometimes the illusion is formed that when the rulings are made the problem is solved, but it is not so. Objective court criteria, once fully understood, will permit development of preventive measures. Collaborative efforts will contribute to the establishment of ethical standards between industry and the medical profession.

SMON: PANEL DISCUSSION

Etiology of SMON.
An early study and its development

TADAO TSUBAKI

*Department of Neurology, Brain Research Institute,
Niigata University, Niigata, Japan*

A peculiar syndrome which usually involves the spinal cord and the peripheral and optic nerves has recently been recognized in Japan. The first patient was described in 1955 and subsequently the number of patients increased until 1970 when their estimated number totalled about 10,000. Epidemics of this syndrome have been noticed in several cities in Japan. In 1963 I started a study of this syndrome in Kushiro city, which is one of the areas where it is most prevalent.

CLINICAL FINDINGS

The frequency of the neurological signs and symptoms of this syndrome was surveyed in Kushiro city. Sensory disturbances were the most common feature, being observed in all cases, followed by muscle weakness (95%), abnormal knee jerk (81%), abnormal jerk (68%), loss of abdominal reflex (60%), visual impairment (51%), bladder disturbance (35%), pathological reflexes (25%), speech disturbances (14%) and nystagmus (11%).

These sensory disturbances were typically seen in the lower half of the body, with an upper level not higher than D_{10} in the majority of cases. The lower extremities were most markedly affected, especially in their distal parts. Sensory disturbances rarely involved the upper extremities.

The signs and symptoms were bilateral. The patellar tendon reflex was hyperactive in 54% and hypoactive or absent in 5%, whereas the achilles reflex was hyperactive in 19% and hypoactive or absent in 38%. Consequently, hyperactive patellar reflexes associated with hypoactive achilles reflexes were seen in some cases.

It is generally agreed that in most cases abdominal symptoms – abdominal pain, diarrhea etc. – precede the neurological symptoms. However, clinical analyses of cases revealed two kinds of abdominal symptoms. They are (1) a gastrointestinal disorder that was observed in the early stage of the illness, and lasted for months or years and (2) a prodromal abdominal symptom complex preceding the neurological symptoms. Diarrhea was the most common symptom in the former group (145 cases), followed by abdominal pain (74 cases). In the latter group, abdominal pain was most common (20 cases), whereas diarrhea was very rarely seen (1 case). In this series 47 cases had no abdominal symptoms in the early stages, but in 36 cases chinoform (5-chloro-7-iodo-8-hydroxyquinoline) had been administered for prophylactic purposes after abdominal surgery.

Females were the more commonly affected, the ratio of males to females being approximately 1 to 2. Most patients were relatively old, over 40 years of age.

LABORATORY FINDINGS

The cerebrospinal fluid was essentially normal. Electromyography showed reduced interference potential and motor conduction velocity was also reduced in about a half of the cases. Electroencephalography showed some abnormalities, these being related to the severity of the neurological findings.

PATHOLOGICAL FEATURES

Symmetrical demyelination and axonal degeneration of the spinal cord posterior columns and pyramidal tracts were seen. The changes were more marked in the distal than in the proximal parts of the tracts. Axonal degeneration was more prominent than demyelination.

The same changes were seen in the peripheral nerves. In the posterior root ganglia of the spinal cord, degeneration of the ganglion cells and proliferation of the capsule cells were seen.

The same changes occurred in the optic nerves. In the retina, degeneration and disappearance of ganglion cells were seen in the ganglion cell layer.

In severe cases, nerve cells of the inferior olivary nucleus had degenerated and gliosis had occurred.

Throughout the involved nervous system, there was hardly any inflammatory reaction.

DIFFERENTIAL DIAGNOSIS

Many diseases involve spinal cord and peripheral nerves. There are some important diseases that should be differentiated from SMON: Guillain-Barré syndrome, vitamin deficiency neuropathy, carcinomatous neuropathy, diabetic neuropathy, porphyria, amyloid neuropathy, adult celiac neuropathy and demyelinating diseases. After differentiating these diseases, I am convinced SMON is a new clinical and pathological entity.

NAMES PROPOSED

Various names have been proposed for this disease. Tsubaki, Toyokura and Tsukagoshi (1) named it subacute myelo-optico-neuropathy (subsequently abbreviated to SMON) in 1965 and this name has been most widely used in Japan. It has become the accepted name since 1967 when the Ministry of Health and Welfare of Japan organized the SMON Research Commission.

ETIOLOGY

Initially a viral infection was suspected as the cause of SMON. Several viruses were reported to have been isolated from faeces, cerebrospinal fluid and other specimens. However, such findings have not been confirmed by other investigations. Etiological factors other than viruses were also considered. These included especially metabolic and deficiency or toxic disorders, but no such causes were detected until 1970 when the chinoform theory appeared.

CHINOFORM THEORY OF THE ETIOLOGY OF SMON

It had long been noted that the tongue was colored green in some SMON patients. In 1970, Takasu, Igata and Toyokura (2) paid special attention to this. In the same year, Igata, Hasebe and Tsuji (3) found two SMON patients excreting greenish urine. Yoshioka and Tamura (4) reported that this green pigment in the urine was the iron chelate of chinoform. Tsubaki, Honma and Hoshi (5) surveyed the relationship between SMON patients and chinoform administration and claimed that SMON was caused by the medication.

One hundred and seventy one SMON patients were surveyed and 166 cases (97%) had a history of chinoform administration just before complaining of the neurological symptoms.

Moreover, many important results were obtained by epidemiological studies.

1. The monthly occurrence of SMON patients and the amount of chinoform used in a hospital were correlated.
2. The annual occurrence of SMON patients and the amount of chinoform sold by a major company in Japan were also correlated.
3. The sales of chinoform in a company in 1967 in each prefecture and the annual incidence of SMON patients in 1967 and 1968 were also correlated.
4. Table 1 shows the relation between the frequency of SMON and the amount of chinoform given to patients in two hospitals (H and S). In both hospitals, no SMON patients appeared if chinoform was not given to patients with gastro-intestinal diseases. In patients given a daily dose of about 1 g chinoform for less than 13 days, very few and then only questionable cases of SMON appeared. In

TABLE 1. *Relation of frequency of occurrence of SMON to amount of chinoform given to the patients in two hospitals (H and S)*

	GI diseases not given Ch.F.		Given Ch.F.					
			H			S		
	H	S	13d>	14d<	Total	13d>	14d<	Total
SMON	0	0	1	17	18	0	19	19
SMON?	0	0	0	11	11	0	6	6
Minimal signs of SMON	0	6	3	12	15	2	9	11
No neurological signs noted	708	760	149	70	219	173	68	241
Total	708	766	153	110	263	175	102	277

patients given a similar dose of chinoform for more than 14 days, many cases of SMON occurred.

5. In the non-SMON patient group in Hospital S, chinoform had usually been given for relatively short periods of time, whereas in the SMON patient group it had been prescribed for relatively long periods.
6. The correlation of age distribution of the patients given chinoform was examined. In the older age group, there were many patients who were given chinoform for more than 14 days, and also many cases of SMON. This could explain why SMON was more prevalent in older age groups.
7. Comparisons of the incidence of SMON in groups of patients receiving or not receiving chinoform were made by Yoshitake et al., Kuratsune et al., Aoki et al. and Tsubaki et al. and all showed significant differences (Table 2).
8. The number of SMON patients diagnosed each month by neurologists of the SMON Research Committee in 1970 is shown in Figure 1. After presentation of the chinoform hypothesis of Tsubaki and the ban on the sale of chinoform by the Department of Health and Welfare, Japan, the number of new SMON patients decreased significantly. After 1971, none, or only a very few were found in Japan.

DEVELOPMENT OF THE CHINOFORM HYPOTHESIS

After we proposed the chinoform hypothesis, quite a few reports supported it, but a very few still claimed a viral origin.

Animal experiments on induced chinoform intoxication have also been carried out by a number of investigators. Tateishi and his associates (6) demonstrated pathological changes of SMON in dogs given high doses of chinoform. We have obtained similar results in dogs. The pathological features are essentially the same as those found in SMON patients.

In March 1972, the Japanese SMON Research concluded that SMON was mostly caused by medication with chinoform.

TABLE 2. *Incidence of SMON in the groups of patients with or without chinoform administration*

Authors	Chinoform administration	SMON (%)	Non-SMON	Remarks
Yoshitake et al., 1970	Yes	34 (43.6)	44	Post-surgery
	No	0 (0.0)	77	$p<0.001$
Kuratsune et al., 1971	Yes	5 (4.3)	110	Enteric disorders
	No	0 (0.0)	217	$p<0.005$
Aoki et al., 1971	Yes	17 (3.2)	515	Enteric disorders
	No	4 (0.1)	3,782	$p<0.001$
Tsubaki et al., 1971	Yes	29 (11.0)	234	Enteric disorders
	No	0 (0.0)	708	$p<0.001$

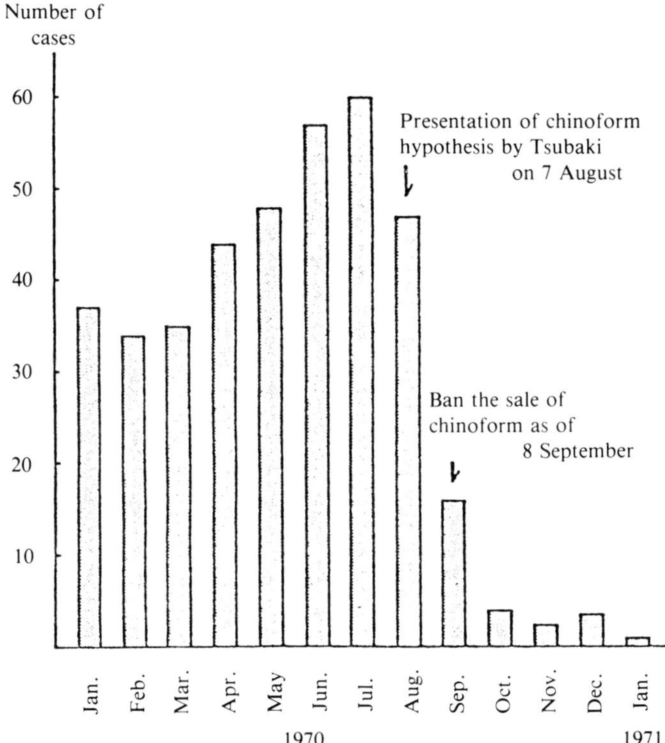

Fig. 1. Number of SMON patients newly diagnosed each month by the neurologists of the SMON Research Commission in 1970 and 1971.

COMMENT AND CONCLUSION

An early study of SMON from clinical, pathological and etiological viewpoints has been described. In particular, the long path to reach the chinofrom theory has been reviewed. Soon after we proposed the chinoform hypothesis, we noticed several reports about adverse effects of chinoform and related compounds from Sweden and a few other foreign countries. Why was chinoform poisoning as the cause of SMON not noticed in Japan for a long time? I believe that the following two points are important.

1. Chinoform was very widely used in Japan, being considered as a non-toxic and hardly absorbable drug.
2. All of the abdominal signs and symptoms were considered as a part of SMON, and it was overlooked that many of the abdominal symptoms and signs were only the reason for the use of chinoform.

I hope that the experience of the tragic SMON epidemics in Japan will prevent similar accidents in the future.

REFERENCES

1. Tsubaki, T., Toyokura, Y. and Tsukagoshi, H. (1965): Subacute myelo-optico-neuropathy following abdominal symptoms. A clinical and pathological study. *Jap. J. Med.*, 4, 181.
2. Takasu, T., Igata, A. and Toyokura, Y. (1970): On the green tongue observed in SMON patients. *Igaku no Ayumi, 72*, 539 (in Japanese).
3. Igata, A., Hasebe, S. and Tsuji, T. (1970): On the green pigment found in SMON patients. Two cases excreting greenish urine. *Japan J. Med., 2427*, 25 (in Japanese).
4. Yoshioka, M. and Tamura, Z. (1970): On the nature of the green pigment found in SMON patients. *Igaku no Ayumi, 74,* 320 (in Japanese).
5. Tsubaki, T., Honma, Y. and Hoshi, M. (1971): Neurological syndrome associated with clioquinol. *Lancet, 1*, 696.
6. Tateishi, J., Kuroda, S., Saito, A. et al. (1971): Myelo-optic neuropathy induced by clioquinol in animals. *Lancet, 2*, 1263.

Oxyquinoline intoxication outside Japan, its recognition and the scope of the problem

OLLE HANSSON

Department of Pediatrics, East Hospital, Gothenburg, Sweden

OUTSIDE JAPAN, 1934–1970

In 1934, Ciba introduced clioquinol* for oral use as Entero-Vioform. As early as 1935, 2 cases with severe neurological symptoms and signs were reported in Argentina (1, 2). The disturbances were identical to those later described as the subacute myelo-optico-neuropathy (SMON) syndrome.

One author (2) reported that when he informed the pharmaceutical company about the suspected adverse effects, '... it thanked him for the information, stating that it would advise physicians not to use the drug in excess of doses indicated in the brochure' (3).

Between 1935 and 1970, when Professor Tadao Tsubaki in Japan discovered that SMON was caused by clioquinol, the potential risks of irreversible neurological damage were already documented in the medical literature as well as in the internal files of Ciba (4, 5).

In 1962, it was reported to Ciba that several dogs treated with Entero-Vioform for diarrhea by their owners had had acute epileptic seizures, and had died (6). Ciba failed to mention that it had made similar observations in animal experiments 23 years before, in 1939! In 1965, in some countries Ciba added a warning to the package leaflet: 'Note: this formulation is not suitable for the treatment of animals.'

In 1966, the first cases of optic atrophy caused by oxyquinoline were reported in the literature (7) and directly to Ciba (8, 9). These reports were followed by several others in the literature and directly to Ciba, clearly indicating the potential dangers of these drugs.

With the first reference in 1875 (10), extensive studies showed the toxicity of therapeutic agents of the quinoline group. The non-toxicity of 8-hydroxyquinoline was emphasized by the manufacturers, but Heubner and Siegel (11) in 1926 found that toxicity varies very much with the species.

Concerning the fate of 8-hydroxyquinoline in the organism, Rost (12) had already believed in 1899 that it was excreted in the urine combined with sulfuric acid, and Brahm (13) in the same year reported that it was bound to glucuronic acid. Grabbe (14) in 1928 found that it was rapidly absorbed from the intestinal tract and that in the middle third of the small intestine most of the drug was combined with acids.

* clioquinol = chinoform = 5-chlorine-7-iodine-8-hydroxyquinoline; oxyquinoline(s) = halogenated 8-hydroxyquinoline(s).

In 1932, Palm (15) showed that 5,7-diiodo-8-hydroxyquinoline was easily absorbed from the intestinal tract in rabbits and excreted mainly with the urine in the form of conjugated sulfuric and glucuronic acid. This study was confirmed by Haskins and Luttermoser in 1953 (16).

The reports of animal experiments proving that oxyquinolines are absorbed from the intestinal tract into the body did not provoke the drug companies to investigate whether this also happened in humans. They simply denied it. However, in 1963 (17) and in 1968 (18) the absorption of oxyquinolines was reported in humans.

OUTSIDE JAPAN, AFTER 1970

After the Japanese ban on oxyquinolines in 1970 SMON disappeared in that country, while new cases damaged by these drugs are continuously reported from other countries around the world. Suspected cases are known from more than 25 countries.

However, the consequence of the absence of information, the distortion of information and the frank lies on the part of the drug companies about oxyquinolines is that not only the public but also doctors and medical authorities are ignorant of the dangers. The experience in Sweden clearly indicates that the number of known oxyquinoline victims is correlated to the available information. Ever since correct information was given, especially after a TV-program in 1977, several cases with hitherto unexplained neurological damage caused by oxyquinoline were recognized.

In 1978, 16 Swedish cases* were published (19) (Table 1). Today I know of 22 cases where a causal relationship between oxyquinoline medication and the neurological symptoms and signs is highly probable. In another 15 cases oxyquinoline cannot be excluded as the causal factor.

The majority of these cases suffer from myelopathy and/or peripheral neuropathy of varying severity. In this group women above the age of 40 predominate. A few cases have optic atrophy without other abnormalities. In 2 cases with the complete SMON syndrome, the invalidity is comparable with the most severely damaged Japanese SMON patients.

CONCLUSION

The legal statements by the courts in Japan only confirm scientific facts known for many years. For example, in the Tokyo District Court ruling of August 3, 1978 it is concluded that: (1) the cause of SMON is clioquinol; (2) none of the proofs given have substantiated that the disease is due to a virus or any substance other than clioquinol; (3) the high incidence of SMON in Japan is explained by the fact that drugs containing clioquinol were used by large numbers of people in large doses over long periods.

Hopefully the great number of SMON victims in Japan has no counterpart in any other country. However, considering the widespread and uncontrolled use of

*In February, 1980, 40 cases were discovered in Sweden.

TABLE 1. *Swedish patients with neurological disturbances after treatment with oxyquinolines*

No./Sex	Age (yr) at onset	Oxyquinoline treatment Indication	Duration	Neurological disturbance(s)
1. ♀	49	salmonellosis	26 days	M/N
2. ♀	57	diarrhea	10 days	M/N
3. ♀	57	prevention	3 weeks	O, M/N
4. ♀	44	diarrhea	4 weeks	M/N
5. ♀	46	colitis ulcerosa	several years	M/N
6. ♂	65	diarrhea	several years	O, M/N
7. ♀	56	prevention	4 weeks	M/N
8. ♀	53	prevention	36 days	M/N
9. ♀	70	chronic diarrhea + prevention	several years	M/N
10. ♂	2	diarrhea	3 months	M/N (reversible)
11. ♀	47	colitis	3 years	O
12. ♂	12	diarrhea	27 days	O, M/N (reversible)
13. ♂	24	diarrhea	2 months	M/N (reversible)
14. ♂	2	acrodermatitis enteropathica	1½ year	O
15. ♂	18	acrodermatitis enteropathica	several years	loss of color sense
16. ♀	55	colitis ulcerosa	1 day	retrograde amnesia

M/N = myelopathy and/or peripheral neuropathy; O = optic atrophy.

oxyquinoline during more than 40 years around the world and the persistent denials of the severe adverse effects made by the drug manufacturers, it is unfortunately more than probable that a vast number of children, women and men have been – and are just now – injured by oxyquinoline outside Japan.

Ciba-Geigy and many other companies are still selling Entero-Vioform and hundreds of other brands for 'intestinal disorders' and without giving warnings. Thus, the scope of the oxyquinoline problem is tremendous. I fully agree with a statement made by Professor Reisaku Kono (20) that oxyquinoline '... is a dangerous and useless drug which has a potential to cause a second SMON incidence in any part of the world. I believe that the continuation of its production and sale is a kind of crime to mankind'.

REFERENCES

1. Grawitz, P.B. (1935): *Sem. med., 1*, 525.
2. Barros, E. (1935): *Sem. med., 1*, 907.
3. Katahira, K. (1978): *J. Amer. med. Ass., 239*, 2757.
4. *Ciba Information, No. 3*. Adverse Drug Reaction Centre, January, 1970.
5. Internal document, Ciba-Geigy, May, 1976.
6. Hangartner, P. (1965): *Schweiz. Arch. Tierheilk., 107*, 43.
7. Berggren, L. and Hansson, O. (1966): *Lancet, 1*, 52.
8. Hann, L. (1966): Letter to Ciba, January 25, 1966.

9. Muntz, W. McL. (1966): Letter to Ciba, June 9, 1966.
10. McKendrick, J.G. and Dewar, J. (1875): *Proc. roy. Soc. (Lond.), 23*, 290.
11. Heubner, W. and Siegel, R (1926): *Klin, Wschr., 5,* 1709.
12. Rost, E. (1899): *Arb. kaiserl. Gesundh., 15*, 288.
13. Brahm, C. (1899): *Z. physiol. Chem., 28*, 439.
14. Grabbe, C. (1928): *Arch. exp. Path. Pharmakol., 137*, 96.
15. Palm, A. (1932): *Arch. exp. Path. Pharmakol., 166*, 176.
16. Haskins, W.T. and Luttermoser, G.W. (1953): *J. Pharmacol. exp. Ther., 109*, 201.
17. Hansson, O. (1963): *Acta derm.-venereol., 43*, 465.
18. Berggren, L. and Hansson, O. (1968): *Clin. Pharmacol. Ther., 9,* 67.
19. Hansson, O. (1978): *Läkartidningen, 75*, 3064.
20. Kono, R. (1976): Personal communication.

Follow-up aspects of the first reported case of optic atrophy caused by clioquinol

LENNART BERGGREN

Department of Ophthalmology, University Hospital, Uppsala, Sweden

In the light of our present knowledge of clioquinol toxicity I would like to give some views on the first reported case of optic atrophy.

A boy born in 1961 and suffering from acrodermatitis enteropathica since he was 6 months old was treated with clioquinol and other hydroxyquinolines. This had been current therapy since 1953 when it was empirically discovered that hydroxyquinolines improved the prognosis for the disease (1). After 14 months of treatment the boy developed an optic atrophy in both eyes. The case investigation did not reveal any disease possibly connected with optic atrophy. Furthermore, acrodermatitis enteropathica itself does not give rise to optic atrophy and no hereditary cause of the atrophy was found in the family. The fact that chemically related compounds, the aminoquinolines, might cause ocular toxicity led to a suspicion of an adverse drug effect. A report by Berggren and Hansson was published early in 1966 (2). Our findings were confirmed 3 weeks later by Etheridge et al. (3). The Swedish Adverse Drug Reaction Committee concluded in 1966 that a relationship between hydroxyquinolines and optic atrophy was suspected. If hydroxyquinolines cause optic atrophy, then this means that they must be absorbed from the intestinal tract. Attempts to obtain information on the pharmacology of hydroxyquinolines from the drug industries met with several difficulties. Disregarding that absorption was described in 1932 (4), toxicity was demonstrated in 1944 (5) and animal excretion determined in 1953 (6) the general opinion in the sixties was that since the compounds were insoluble in water they could only be absorbed in minimal quantities or not at all. By mere chance a veterinary article by Schantz and Wikström (7) came to our notice. They showed that treatment of dogs with clioquinol could lead to convulsions, ataxia and even death.

This combination of circumstances stimulated us to evaluate the absorption of hydroxyquinolines in man. The spectrophotometric method used was a further development of the method used by Haskins and Luttermoser (8). It is based on the principle that hydroxyquinolines when combined with ferric ions form green compounds. Minimal amounts of hydroxyquinolines in free form but considerable amounts of the glucuronide were found in the urine after 10 hours (Table 1). It is well known that the body deals with foreign substances by conjugating with glucuronic acid. The absorption study was published in 1968 (9). Our reports led to comments from the Editors of several medical journals in 1968–1972 (10–12) warning against an indiscriminate use of clioquinol and related compounds. The animal toxicity of clioquinol established in 1965 by Schantz and Wikström (7) as well as by Hangartner (13) led in 1968 to the surprising addition to the information

TABLE 1. *Excretion in the urine of different hydroxyquinolines after a single oral test dose*

8-Hydroxyquinolines	Dose (g)	Test subjects (N)	% Urine excretion after 10 hours Mean	Variation
Diiodo	0.30	6	4.6	2–7
Dibromo	0.25	6	10.2	1–28
Chloroiodo	0.25	6	12.6	6–21
Dichloromethyl	0.20	6	34.9	30–46
Chloroiodo	0.25	3	10.2	5–14
Chloroiodo	0.25	P.J.	13.1	
Chloroiodo	0.25	M.W.	23.5	

From Berggren and Hansson (9).

on clioquinol – 'For human use only'. Clioquinol was then sold without restriction in Sweden. The usual procedure is otherwise that established animal toxicity disqualifies a drug from human use. Clioquinol was sold on prescription on the Swedish market from 1972 to 1975 when it was withdrawn. In 1974 it was discovered that acrodermatitis enteropathica is caused by zinc deficiency, and the disease is now treated with orally administered zinc (14, 15).

The boy in our case report is now 18 years old. Since 1974 he has been treated with zinc tablets. His visual acuity is reduced to the counting of fingers at a distance of 1–2 meters. He can only read with the help of magnifying systems and even then with difficulty. He tries very hard to conceal his visual handicap and is not willing to use any conspicuous visual aid system.

What conclusions can be drawn in retrospect? It was previously common belief that clioquinol and other hydroxyquinolines were not absorbed and they were thus considered to be safe drugs. The discovery in 1968 that considerable quantities were absorbed did not lead to any change in the recommendations. It is hard to believe that relevant absorption documentation was not known earlier for a drug that had been on the market for several decades. The fact that minimal amounts of free drug but considerable amounts of the glucuronide was excreted is not a pharmacological singularity. The information that no or minimal absorption occurred was deceptive and very likely contributed to an indiscriminate use. It would probably have been better if there had been no information at all. Today it would be impossible to introduce on the market a drug with such inadequate pharmacological documentation and with such a high risk-benefit ratio such as clioquinol.

Had the data on clioquinol absorption and toxicity been better known, the cause of SMON might have been detected earlier. In our study in 1968 (9) we used a green ferric clioquinol compound to determine the amount excreted. In 1970 the observation that the green urine from patients treated with clioquinol was caused by ferric clioquinol led to the discovery of the cause of SMON (16).

The authorities should have been more disturbed by the fact that a drug which was freely sold for human use was at the same time not permitted for veterinary purposes.

Treatment of acrodermatitis enteropathica with clioquinol and other hydroxyquinolines led to 13 cases of optic atrophy (17) before it was discovered in 1974 that the disease was caused by zinc deficiency. Knowledge of the properties of clioquinol, however, could have revealed the cause of the disease much earlier. It could have been suspected that the noted favorable effects of clioquinol on the symptoms had to do with its being absorbed from the intestinal tract. Furthermore, it was known that hydroxyquinoline compounds readily form chelates with metal ions and methods of determining the presence of zinc had been published in 1964 and 1969 (18, 19). Treatment with clioquinol turned out to be two-edged. Zinc-clioquinol chelates were absorbed from the intestinal tract, and zinc had a favorable effect on acrodermatitis enteropathica while clioquinol proved to have toxic effects on the optic nerve.

The slow progress in establishing the relationship between SMON and clioquinol is instructive. It points out how difficult it is to gather facts, to put results together and to make the right conclusions as quickly as possible. Even if the situation generally is better today and legislation more rigorous and effective, the difficulties still exist (20). The increasing number of new drugs and with that an increasing potential risk of adverse drug effects put great demands on a control system. A non-commercial drug monitoring center is a necessity but can only operate effectively with a very broad international support. At present 23 countries participate in the WHO Collaborating Centre For International Drug Monitoring located in Uppsala, Sweden.

REFERENCES

1. Dillaha, C.J., Lorinez, A.L. and Aavik, O.R. (1953): Acrodermatitis enteropathica: review of the literature and report of a case successfully treated with diiodoquin. *J. Amer. med. Ass., 152*, 509.
2. Berggren, L. and Hansson, O. (1966): Treating acrodermatitis enteropathica. *Lancet, 1*, 52.
3. Etheridge, J.E. and Stewart, G.T. (1966): Treating acrodermatitis enteropathica. *Lancet, 1*, 261.
4. Palm, A. (1932): Untersuchungen in der Chinolinreihe. *Arch. exp. Path. Pharmakol., 166*, 176.
5. David, N.A., Phatak, N.M. and Zener, F.B. (1944): Iodochlorhydroxyquinoline and diiodohydroxyquinoline: animal toxicity and absorption in man. *Amer. J. trop. Med., 24*, 29.
6. Haskins, W.T. and Luttermoser, G.W. (1953): Urinary excretion of Vioform and Diiodoquin in rabbits. *J. Pharmacol. exp. Ther., 109*, 201.
7. Schantz, B. and Wikström, B. (1965): Suspected poisoning with oxyquinoline preparations in dogs. *Svensk. vet. Tidn., 17*, 106.
8. Haskins, W.T. and Luttermoser, G.W. (1951): Spectrophotometric determination of 8-quinolol and some of its halogenated derivatives. *Analyt. Chem., 23*, 456.
9. Berggren, L. and Hansson, O. (1968): Absorption of intestinal antiseptics derived from 8-hydroxyquinolines. *Clin. Pharmacol. Ther., 9*, 67.
10. Editorial (1968): Clioquinol and other halogenated hydroxyquinolines. *Lancet, 1*, 679.
11. Editorial (1971): Clioquinol and neurological disease. *Brit. med. J., 2*, 291.
12. Editorial (1972): Entero-Vioform for preventing travellers' diarrhea. *J. Amer. med. Ass., 220*, 273.
13. Hangartner, P. (1965): Troubles nerveux observés chez le chien après absorption d'Entéro-Vioforme Ciba. *Schweiz. Arch. Tierheilk., 107*, 43.

14. Moynahan, E.J. (1974): Acrodermatitis enteropathica. A lethal inherited human zinc deficiency disorder. *Lancet, 2*, 399.
15. Michaelsson, G. (1974): Zinc therapy in acrodermatitis enteropathica. *Acta Derm.-venereol. (Stockh.), 54*, 377.
16. Yoshioka, M. and Tamura, Z. (1970): On the nature of the green pigment found in SMON patients. *Igaku no Ayumi, 74*, 320.
17. Committee on Drugs (1974): Blindness and neuropathy from diiodohydroxyquin-like drugs. *Pediatrics, 54*, 378.
18. Carter, D.A. and Ohnesorge, W.E. (1964): Spectrofluorometric study of (2-methyl-8-quinolato)-zinc chelates in absolute alcohol. *Analyt. Chem., 36*, 327.
19. Smith, G.L., Jenkins, R.A. and Gough, J.F. (1969): A fluorescent method for the detection and localization of zinc in human granulocytes. *J. Histochem. Cytochem., 17*, 749.
20. Westerholm, B. (1978): The relationship between potential hazards and legislative action. Paper presented at: FIP Congress, Cannes, 1978.

Clioquinol and SMON in The Netherlands: some lessons in retrospect

M.N.G. DUKES

Department of Pharmacotherapy, Central Inspectorate for Drugs, Leidschendam, The Netherlands

Japan is a country of 113 million people; the number of suspected cases of subacute myelo-optico-neuropathy (SMON) there has been estimated at more than 10,000. The Netherlands, by contrast, has a population of only 14 million people; the number of verified cases of SMON there can be counted on the fingers of one hand, the number of suspected cases on the fingers of two. In spite of these disparities the experience of Holland can, I would suggest, add some useful annotations to the impressive account of clioquinol-induced SMON with which Japan provides us. Firstly, of course, there is the important fact that well-documented cases of SMON did occur in The Netherlands at all, a small country which in some quarters is regarded as notable – or, if you wish, notorious – for its very low consumption of drugs as compared with the rest of Europe. Secondly, the story raises some interesting points as to the minimum of medical evidence which a government agency reasonably needs in order to take action against a widely known drug. Finally, the experience in Holland confronts us with the question of the physician's responsibility for severe side-effects at a time when knowledge on these effects is not readily available.

It was early in 1970 that two verbal descriptions of ophthalmic disorders possibly attributable to clioquinol reached the Netherlands Health Authorities. Looking back on those reports, as they were submitted, one can hardly be surprised that they were simply filed with the great mass of other data reaching the Adverse Reactions Monitoring Centre, which at that time had existed on a very small scale for some 3 years. The standard reference works at that time made little reference to adverse reactions from clioquinol; vomiting, diarrhoea, rash and occasional staining of the nails and hair were listed in the books, alongside a transient increase in protein-bound iodine. Had the Adverse Reactions Monitoring Centre at that time had the facilities for very thorough literature study, however, more might have come to light; Berggren and Hansson had reported their first 2 cases of optic atrophy in 1966 and 1968, in both instances in well-known journals; Gholz and Arons had as early as 1964 found transient derangements of gait in 20 of 4000 patients treated over a long period with the drug. On the other hand, in 1970 not a single report from Japan had yet reached the Western literature, and Hangartner's pioneering veterinary publication was to be found only in a Swiss veterinary journal, unlikely to be accessible in medical circles in Holland. Evidence there was, thus, but difficulties of language and the inadequate adverse reactions documentation of a decade ago rendered it inaccessible. Had all that evidence been more rapidly to hand in 1970, later misery might have been saved.

During the next 2 years, the situation changed rapidly. In 1971, 7 publications on SMON appeared from Japan, 6 of them in the Western literature, four of them indeed in the *Lancet*. And almost at that same moment, physicians at centres in The Netherlands found themselves confronted with 4 classic cases of SMON. It was the Dutch internist Pannekoek, who, gifted with a phenomenal memory, a wide circle of national and international contacts and an associative mind, marshalled at great speed the totality of evidence against the halogenated hydroxyquinolines and ensured that it was published. As an immediate result, 3 products disappeared from the market; Entero-Vioform survived only as a prescription drug with a miniscule field of use. We may be gifted with better data banks at the present day, but in such situations as these it will perhaps always be the brilliant physician who first assembles the truth from a medley of confusing and incomplete data.

Let me describe briefly those first 4 published cases. In all of them, the product had been over-used by the standards then pertaining. One was a woman of 75 who had been suffering for some 2 years from diarrhoea and for a year from paraesthesia in the legs and difficulty in walking; there was a neurological disorder originally diagnosed as subacute combined degeneration of the cord and optic atrophy. This woman had been taking up to 1.5 g of clioquinol daily for her diarrhoea for 2 years. Most authors at that time, as I would remind you, recommended only half that dose, i.e. 750 mg/day, given for 10 days, and perhaps later for another 10.

The second patient, a woman of 37, developed a pyramidal syndrome, a mild peripheral neuropathy, and changes in the optic disc; this woman too had been taking 1.5 g clioquinol daily, but for 5 years for chronic diarrhoea; when the drug was withdrawn the condition was stabilized.

The third patient was a physician aged 69 who had undergone an anastomosis of the small intestine and had treated the resultant diarrhoea successively with Mexaform, chlorquinaldol and finally clioquinol, using the latter in variable doses of up to 3 g daily, i.e. 4 times the dose recommended at that time in the textbooks. He had been taking the drug for 15 weeks when he developed paraesthesiae in both feet and deep sensory loss. Since the cause of the complication was unsuspected, treatment with clioquinol continued. By the 9th month there was severe sensory loss and pain in the legs, and the urine appeared greenish. During the second year the patient walked with difficulty, there was sensory loss in the fingers, cramping of the hands and evidence of optic neuritis. The drug clioquinol was now suspected as the cause and it was withdrawn; there was some slight improvement in the optic condition by the time the patient died some months later from other causes.

The most striking of these first 4 cases from Holland, and the most tragic one, relates to an 18-month-old girl, referred by a general practitioner to the paediatrician because of difficulty in walking and apparent impairment of vision. Because of diarrhoea, the infant had at various times been given clioquinol, Mexaform, or both. In all she had received some 129 clioquinol. The patient was found to be completely blind.

These 4 cases, then, were the ones which put a virtual end to the career of the halogenated hydroxyquinolines in Holland. A remarkable medico-legal point is, however, raised by a fifth case, which was one of those which only later came into the public eye.

Litigation against physicians is not a prominent feature of the Netherlands scene, and perhaps this is a good thing; it solves nothing as a rule and can, if practiced regularly, derange physician-patient relationships. However, any patient can lodge a complaint against his physician with the Central Medical Disciplinary Council if he feels that he has been wrongly treated, and this may lead to the physician's being struck from the register, or suspended for a certain period. One would hardly have expected this to occur with respect to SMON, for a proportion of the victims had engaged, at least in part, in self-treatment with the drug. One disciplinary case did however arise. It involved a small boy who was treated from November 1970 until August 1971 with 1 g clioquinol daily. For a small child, of course, this was gross overdosage. By the end of the period of treatment the child, by then some 3 years old, had developed a severe and permanent deterioration of vision. The parents of the boy duly lodged a complaint against the general practitioner and – rather to the astonishment and indignation of many people in The Netherlands – the case was dismissed. The Central Medical Disciplinary Council was, it is true, of the opinion that the physician would have done well to consult a specialist when the child's diarrhoea proved so persistent, but it took into account the fact that the drug had appeared to be effective, and that it had developed a reputation for use in diarrhoea over a period of 40 years. The use of an excessive dose was not even recognized as such.

What, then, were the grounds on which the parents based their case? As you will recall, the child was treated with clioquinol from November till August. In the few months preceding the start of this course of treatment, there had been two references in the weekly *Netherlands Medical Journal* to the fact that Entero-Vioform could have a severely detrimental effect on vision. During the course of treatment, in April 1971, a warning had also appeared in the *Netherlands Drugs Bulletin*, a 4-page fortnightly journal sent free of charge by the Ministry of Health to all practitioners in the hope that they will read it. Well, the Disciplinary Council proved to be of the opinion that a physician could not be reproached for having failed to perceive any of this information, let alone read the foreign journals. The Council's decision, handed down in 1973, was confirmed on appeal in 1975.

One must doubt, in view of the storm of criticism which followed this decision by the Disciplinary Council, whether such a judgement will ever be given again. Whatever the responsibility of the pharmaceutical company selling or promoting a drug may be for the injury which that drug causes, no-one can seriously doubt that the practising physician has a responsibility to inform himself as to the risks and the limitations of the drugs which he employs, and to realize that our knowledge of those risks and limitations may change from year to year and from month to month. It perhaps does not matter very much if a physician fails to keep abreast of the literature as regards the newest in apparatus, diagnosis and surgical techniques, but drugs present an exceptional case, in which even the average general practitioner surely has a duty to keep abreast of knowledge in transition, and to be aware of even dubious risks. He can be helped, perhaps even spoon-fed with free bulletins and government circulars, but there is a certain minimum of effort which he must deliver himself.

There is a saying that it is easy to be wise in retrospect, and if one judges these events by the standards which generally pertained when they occurred, one can indeed argue whether the Netherlands authorities failed in their duty when they set aside the first two reports of SMON in 1970, or even whether this physician failed in his duty to the patient in 1971 except as regards the use of excessive doses. By the standards of 1979, however, standards which have emerged from the experience of SMON, of practolol, and of a dozen lesser drama's, one can well speak of failure. If these things occur again, we shall have only ourselves to blame.

REFERENCES

1. Pannekoek, J.H. (1972): Neurotoxische verschijnselen na clioquinol (Enterovioform). *Ned. T. Geneesk., 116*, 1611.
2. Bron, H.L.N.M., Korten, J.J., Pinckers, A.J.L.G., and Majoor, C.L.H. (1972): Subacute myelo-optico-neuropathie na het gebruik van grote hoeveelheden joodchloorhydroxychinoline (Enterovioform). *Ned. T. Geneesk., 116*, 1615.
3. Drukker, J. and Lindenburg, P.A.W. (1972): Beiderzijdse opticusatrofie bij een kind van anderhalf jaar die wellicht een gevolg is van toediening van joodchloorhydroxychinoline (Enterovioform). *Ned. T. Geneesk., 116*, 1618.
4. Van Beeck, J.A. and Scholten, J.B. (1972): Polyneuropathie na langdurig gebruik van clioquinol (Enterovioform). *Ned. T. Geneesk., 116*, 1621.
5. Anon. (1975): Uitspraak Centraal Medisch Tuchtcollege. *Med. Contact, 30*, 561.
6. Wennen-van der Meij, C.A.M. (1975): Het zal je kind maar wezen. *Med. Contact, 30*, 662.
7. Anon. (1975): Geneeskundige Hoofdinspectie overleg met K.N.M.G. na uitspraak Centraal Medisch Tuchtcollege. *Med. Contact, 30*, 662.

An international survey on the recent reports concerning intoxication with halogenated oxyquinoline derivatives and the regulations against their use*

KIYOHIKO KATAHIRA[1], KUGAHISA TESHIMA[2], HIDEHIRO SUGISAWA[2], SHIGEKI KUZUHARA[3] and REISAKU KONO[4]

[1]*Medical Research Institute, Tokyo Medical and Dental University,* [2]*Department of Health Sociology, University of Tokyo,* [3]*Institute of Clinical Medicine, University of Tsukuba, and* [4]*Central Virus Diagnostic Laboratory, National Institute of Health, Tokyo, Japan*

Halogenated oxyquinoline derivatives (HOQ)**, one of the popular intestinal antiseptics widely used for prophylactic purpose or treatment of gastro-enteritis, amebiasis, travellers' diarrhea etc., were suspended from the Japanese market in September of 1970 because of their close association with a new neurological disease called SMON (subacute myelo-optic neuropathy) (1). The action taken by the Japanese Government produced a dramatic fall in new cases of SMON and the outbreaks of the disease which occurred every year in the 1960s did not recur after 1971 (2). Many other studies of the SMON Research Commission have supported the neurotoxicity of HOQ. Nevertheless, HOQ are still being used in many other countries because SMON is considered rare. This paper surveys the cases of intoxication with HOQ (neurological disturbances) appearing after 1970, and the extent of the regulations against the use of HOQ in this country.

METHODS

Literature review

We reviewed reports on intoxication of HOQ in man (including suspected cases) in articles using the terms 'iodochlorhydroxyquin' in *Index Medicus* and 'clioquinol' in *Pharmacology and Toxicology* and in *Adverse Reactions Titles* of Excerpta Medica between January 1970 and December 1978. The weekly literature citation service by Ascatopics was also scanned using 13 key words including 'oxyquinoline', 'SMON', 'neuropathy', etc. Other literature obtained through the SMON Research Commission etc. was also included.

*This work was supported by a special grant from the Ministry of Health and Welfare of Japan.
**iodochlorhydroxyquinoline, broxyquinoline, halquinol, diiodohydroxyquinoline, chlorquinaldol.

TABLE 1. *Number of reported cases of intoxication with HOQ outside Japan*

Country	Number of cases published after 1970	Number of cases reported in the mail survey	Number of reported cases (Ciba-Geigy Ltd.)	
			1962-71[1]	1935-75[2]
U.S.A.	5* (1)[3]	4		27
Canada	1	2		1
U.K.	9 (6)	0	8	9
France	10 (3)	ca. 12	1	10
Switzerland	6 (1)		13	16
F.R. Germany	5 (3)	ca. 19	22	30
Austria	2**	0		3
Sweden	14	5	3	6
Denmark	4	9		4
Norway	0	5		3
Netherlands	7	ca. 4	9	8
Belgium	2		2	2
Poland	1			1
Spain	1	0		1
Italy	1		1	3
Finland				1
Israel	2 (2)	0		2
Lebanon	1			
Iran	1			
India	9	0****	6	11
Indonesia	3 (3)			1
Singapore	1 (1)			1
Australia	9***	0(1974,8-'75,2)	12	30
New Zealand	0	0		2
Curacao				1
Colombia				1
Brazil				2
Argentina				3
Total	94 (17)	ca. 60	77	179

[1]Documentary evidence of S.M.O.N. Lawsuit Kanazawa District Court. Hei-187.
[2]Documentary evidence of S.M.O.N. Lawsuit Kanazawa District Court. Hei-321.
[3]Numbers in parentheses are suspected cases, cases which are difficult to be determined as HOQ intoxication for lack of sufficient description or because the articles have not been obtained yet.
*Besides, Prof. Tsubaki reported a 51-year-old woman. (Tsubaki, T. Personal communication)
**Besides, Prof. Wewalka reported a 36-year-old man. (Igata, A. Personal communication)
***29 cases including these were reported at Honolulu Symposium in Jan. 1976.
****'No reports of controlled study' was the reply.

Inquiry by mail

Questionnaires to health authorities on reports of adverse effects of HOQ and regulations against their use were sent out twice. Addresses of these authorities were obtained through the courtesy of the National Institute of Hygienic Sciences of Japan, foreign embassies in Japan and Dr. Hiroshi Nakajima of WHO. The questionnaire was first sent out to 99 countries between August 20 and November 20, 1976 and from 41 countries we received replies between August 27, 1976 and July 21, 1977.

The second questionnaire was sent to 40 countries on December 30, 1978 asking them about their national situation relating to the above matters since their first reply. One country having answered to the first questionnaire that 'HOQ were not imported for use' was excluded. Answers came from 27 countries between January 16 and June 11, 1979. The report from Denmark, already received in October 1978, stating that 'HOQ were withdrawn' was also included.

RESULTS

Number and contents of the reports on HOQ intoxication

The literature survey showed that, outside Japan, 114 cases (29 in Australia) diagnosed as either SMON (including suspected cases) or HOQ intoxication were reported in 55 articles during the period January 1970 to September 1978. These cases were reported by 21 countries, Australia reporting the largest number. In the mail inquiry about 60 cases were reported by 8 countries including West Germany, France, etc. Some did not give exact records so that a few reported before 1970 may have been erroneously included. We present these figures in Table 1, in which the statistics of Ciba-Geigy Ltd. are also included for reference. The total number of reported cases was 207 from 28 countries, that is, 179 cases from 26 countries reported from 1935 through 1975 and 28 cases after 1976.

S.K., a neurologist, studied the reported cases based on clinical records of signs and symptoms described and diagnosed 74 (from 42 articles) to be either SMON or HOQ intoxication. These were classified into three groups: subacute or chronic intoxication in adults and children, and acute intoxication (Table 2a,b,c). 53 adults with diarrhea, colitis or the like, developed subacute or chronic neurological symptoms after administration of HOQ, 14 children with diarrhea or acrodermatitis enteropathica developed neurological symptoms after ingestion of HOQ (Diodoquin in most cases) and 7 cases developed acute intoxication.

In the cases of subacute or chronic intoxication, it is notable that sensory disturbances were found in 42 of 53 adult cases and that visual disturbances were the only neurological signs in 10 of 14 children. Three cardinal signs and symptoms of sensory, motor and visual disturbances in SMON were found in 13 patients. As to acute intoxication, symptoms of the central nervous system such as confusion, amnesia, etc. were described.

The doses of HOQ given to subacute or chronic cases in children before the onset of neurological symptoms, were large. 13 of 28 adults whose drug intake was clearly

TABLE 2a. *Subacute or chronic cases of intoxication with HOQ in adults (over 16 years old) outside Japan (1, 2, 3) (only cases reported in articles after 1970)*

Country	Report date	Reporter (first author, if joint work)	Sex	Age at onset (yr)	Symptoms for administration[1]	Brand name of HOQ[2]	Doses of HOQ before onset[3] (g)	Neurological symptoms
U.K.	1971.10	McEwen[1]	M	42	intrinsic allergy	CQ	ca. 26.2	S
	1971.10	McEwen[1]	F	23	intrinsic allergy	CQ	ca. 202.5	S
	71.12	Spillane[2]	F	20	vomiting, diarrhea	Entosan	5.5	SM
France	72. 8	Cambier[3]	F	66	chronic constipation	M	18	SO
	73. 4	Grenier[4]	F	75	abdominal pain etc.	M, CQ	84	SM
	73	Castaigne[5]	F	55	ulcerative colitis	EV	40 ~ 60	MO
	73.10	Latterre[6]	M	24	delusion	M, Intestopan	ca. 100	SMO
	74.11	Gendre[7]	M	59	diarrhea	M	15.6	SM
	74.12	Vitale[8]	F	56	constipation	EV	2800	MO
	76. 3	Froissart[9]	F	77	abdominal pain	M	27.6	SM
Switzerland	70. 8	Kaeser[10]	F	63	irritable colon	EV	more than 2000	SMO
	70. 8	Kaeser[10]	F	52	ulcerative colitis	EV, M	ca. 3000	SM
F.R. Germany	73	Boergen[11]	F	51	chronic diarrhea	EV	more than 1500	O
Austria	74. 3	Heilig[12]	M	80	cancer of the rectum	M, RP	ca. 750	SMO
	75. 6	Mamoli[13]	F	72	rectal cancer	RP	65	SMO
Sweden	71. 9	Osterman[14]	M	24	diarrhea	EV	45	SMO
	78. 9	Hansson[15]	F	49	salmonella	EV	6.75	SM
		Hansson[15]	F	57	diarrhea	EV	[about 10 days]	SM
		Hansson[15]	F	57	prophylactic	EV	[about 3 weeks]	SMO
		Hansson[15]	F	44	diarrhea		[about 4 weeks]	SM
		Hansson[15]	F	46	ulcerative colitis		[several years]	SM
		Hansson[15]	M	about 65	diarrhea		[several years]	SMO

TABLE 2a. *Continued*

Country	Report date	Reporter (first author, if joint work)	Sex	Age at onset (yr)	Symptoms for administration[1]	Brand name of HOQ[2]	Doses of HOQ before onset[3] (g)	Neurological symptoms
		Hansson[15]	F	56	prophylactic		[4 weeks]	SM
		Hansson[15]	F	53	prophylactic		[36 days]	SM
	1978. 9	Hansson[15]	F	70	chronic diarrhea + prophylactic	EV	[several years]	SM
		Hansson[15]	F	47	colitis		[3 years]	O
		Hansson[15]	M	18	acro. e.	CQD	[several years]	O
Denmark	72. 7	Jensen[16]	F	70	diarrhea	Joklokinol	17	SMO
	72. 7	Kjaersgaard[17]	F	41	irritable colon	EV	more than 1500	SMO
	74. 1	Dahl[18]	M	19	acro. e.	CQ	ca. 47.2	S
Netherlands	72. 9	van Beeck[19]	M	70	diarrhea	EV, M, Siosteran		SO
	72. 9	Bron[20]	F	74	diarrhea	EV, M	more than 500	SMO
	72. 9	Bron[20]	F	35	abdominal symptoms	EV	1095	SM
	72.12	Yamamoto[21]	F	27		CQ	1752	OM
Belgium	71.11	Danis[22]	M	78	colitis, enteritis	M	21 ~ 42	SO
	76	Otte[23]	M	46	abdominal symptoms	CQ		SMO
Iran	78. 9	Derakhshan[25]	M	51	colitis	EV	[8 years]	O
Italy	77.9	Fabiani[24]	F	28	Crohn's disease	CQ	2000	SMO
India	73. 9	Wadia[26]	M	21	dysentery etc.	EV		SM
	73. 9	Wadia[26]	M	42	colitis, dysentery	EV, M		SM
	73. 9	Wadia[26]	F	53	colitis	M, Enteroquinol		SM
	77. 3	Wadia[27]	F	60	constipation	M	21.6	SM
		Wadia[27]	F	60	abdominal disturbance	M	ca. 235	MO
		Wadia[27]	M	55			[80]	MO
		Wadia[27]	F	40			[45]	M
		Wadia[27]	F	65			[420]	M

TABLE 2a. *Continued*

Country	Report date	Reporter (first author, if joint work)	Sex	Age at onset (yr)	Symptoms for administration[1]	Brand name of HOQ[2]	Doses of HOQ before onset[3] (g)	Neurological symptoms
Australia	1972. 1	Selby[28]	M		abdominal symptoms	EV		SM
		Selby[28]	F		abdominal symptoms	EV		SMO
		Selby[28]	F	57	abdominal symptoms	EV	total doses	SM
		Selby[28]	F	~	abdominal symptoms	EV	18 637.5	SM
		Selby[28]	F	67	abdominal symptoms	EV		SM
		Selby[28]	F		abdominal symptoms	EV		SM
	73. 9	Reich[29]	F	18	ulcerative colitis	EV	540 ~ 1080	O

[1]Name of disease for which HOQ were used.
acro. e. = acrodermatitis enteropathica
[2]CQ = Clioquinol (Brand name undescribed), EV = Entero-Vioform, M = Mexaform, RP = Reasec-Plus, CQD = Chlorquinaldol, DQ = Diodoquin, BQ = Broxyquinoline
[3]Blank columns are due to impossibility of measuring doses for intermittent administration etc. [ ] = total dose or administration period
[4]S = sensory disturbances, M = motor disturbances, O = optic disturbances

TABLE 2b. *Subacute or chronic cases of intoxication with HOQ in children (under 15 years old) outside Japan (only cases reported in articles after 1970)*

Country	Report date	Reporter (first author, if joint work)	Sex	Age at onset (yr)	Symptoms for administration	Brand name of HOQ	Doses of HOQ before onset (g)	Neurological symptoms
U.S.A.	1973. 9	Pittman[30]	M	3.5	diarrhea	DQ	109.2	O
	74. 5	Behrens[31]	F	5⅓	diarrhea	DQ	227.5	O
		Behrens[31]	M	4.5	loose stools	DQ	more than 1000	O
	74. 7	Fleisher[32]	M	2¼	nonspecific diarrhea	DQ	762 ~ 871	O
Canada	77. 2	Carr[33]	M	4	acro. e.	EV		O
Sweden	78. 9	Hansson[15]	M	2	diarrhea		[3 months]	SM (transient)
F.R. Germany	73	Reich[34]	F	10 ~ 14	acro. e.	DQ, M-S	ca. 6000	O
Netherlands	71	van Balen[35]		1.5	Hirschsprung's disease	EV		O
	72. 9	Drukker[36]	F	1.5	diarrhea	EV, M-P	12	O
	72.12	Yamamoto[21]	F	11		CQ	33.6	SM
Poland	74.11	Papuzinski[37]		4	acro. e.	EV, Entosan		MO
Lebanon	73. 7	Idriss[38]	M	3	acro. e.	DQ	more than 500	O
Spain	74	Garcia-Perez[39]	F	2	acro. e.	CQ	280	O
India	77. 3	Wadia[27]	F	9	abdominal pain diarrhea	M	21	M

TABLE 2c. *Acute cases of intoxication with HOQ outside Japan (only cases reported in articles after 1970)*

Country	Report date	Reporter (first author, if joint work)	Sex	Age at onset (yr)	Symptoms for administration	Brand name of HOQ	Doses of HOQ before onset (g)	Neurological symptoms
Switzerland	1970. 2	Kaeser[40]	M	24	diarrhea	EV	7.5	amnesia etc.
	70. 8	Kaeser[10]	F	56		EV	3	amnesia etc.
	70. 8	Kaeser[10]	F	22		M	1.5	amnesia etc.
Sweden	78. 9	Hansson[15]	F	55	ulcerative colitis	BQ	1	amnesia
Denmark	71.11	Kjaersgaard[41]	F	21	acute gastroenteritis	EV	4	amnesia etc.
Australia*	73.12	Ferrier[42]	F	43	for preventive use	CQ	1.5	amnesia etc.
	73.12	Ferrier[42]	M	32	abdominal pain, nausea	CQ	4	disorientation etc.

*A mass outbreak that accompanied abdominal symptoms or headache etc. was reported to have occurred after 10-day-planned administration of broxyquinoline, 3 g daily, in an institute for retarded children in Australia 1965. (T.I. Robertson, Epidemiological issues in reported drug-induced illnesses–S.M.O.N. and other examples, p. 283, McMaster Univ. Library Press, 1978)

cf. In Japan an accidental outbreak of acute Emaform intoxication happened at Nyuzen-cho, Toyama Prefecture, in August 1969 when Emaform tablets were distributed free of charge for prevention after a flood. At that time 12 tablets (3 g of HOQ) were given due to wrong direction and caused 33 persons among 147 who took the tablets to develop psycho-neurological symptoms (indistinctness, disturbance of consciousness, paresthesia of hands and feet) or abdominal symptoms (nausea, vomiting, abdominal pain etc.). Average dose of 19 persons who could remember the doses was 2 g. (Sadao Ogawa et al., *Igaku-no-Ayumi,* 1975, *94*, 206) known took more than 100 g. However, 2 of them developed the disease after having taken 10 g or less. In the case of acute intoxication, doses were clearly lower, ranging from 1.0 to 7.5 g. Therefore, it seems that outside Japan sensitive individuals may also develop intoxication with HOQ even with relatively small doses.

Regulations against the use of HOQ

The results of the first inquiry are shown in Table 3. Twenty-seven of 41 countries answered that the government, companies or other agencies concerned had taken some measures (including warning) to regulate the use of HOQ. Ten other countries answered that no measures had been taken, but 4 of them were considering regulations in the future. Of the other countries, 3 (Madagascar, Guatemala, Israel)

TABLE 3. *Regulations against HOQ outside Japan (internal use only; made up as of 1976–77)*

Regulation and country (date, contents)	
Suspension of sales (4)	
U.S.A.	(Ciba-Geigy Ltd. withdrew Entero-Vioform in 1972)
Taiwan	(The use of compounds was banned from Jan. 1972, but samples are still allowed to be on market)
Norway	(The Board of Drugs decided to withdraw all preparations from the market since Jan. 1974)
Sweden	(Ciba-Geigy withdrew the register of Entero-Vioform in May 1975)
Only prescription (11)	
New Zealand	(Since 1970; direction was given not to exceed 7 g in total in May 1972)
Denmark	(Since Feb. 1972; the amendment was made according to the reports on S.M.O.N.)
Netherlands	(Since Jul. 1972; 'the risks of the drugs have also been made known to physicians through direct government circulars and publications in the Drugs Bulletin')
Bulgaria	(Since Feb. 1973; on the grounds of reports from WHO and international medical literature)
Malaysia	(Since Apr. 1976; controlled under Poisons Ordinance)
Austria	(Since Oct. 1976; to be prescribed not more than five times during a six-month period)
France	(Since 1972; controlled under table C of 'substances vénéneuses', and limitation of dose and duration etc.)
Australia	(Except Victoria State)
Canada	(Regulation was taken recently)
Iraq	(The Committee for the Selection of Drugs recommended that the physicians and the public must be warned of the possible hazards of the indiscriminate use of these drugs)
Portugal	('The sale of them is subject to the presentation of medical prescription.')

TABLE 3. *Continued*

Limitation on dose and duration etc. (7)	
Ireland	(From 1971; duration within 2 weeks)
F.R. Germany	(From Aug. 1972; the Federal Health Office and the German Physicians' Drugs Committee published recommendation to be used within 750 mg daily ×7 days. 'It is expected these drugs be subject to compulsory prescription before long')
D.R. Germany	(2 preparations among 3 were limited to 750 mg ×7 days and importation of the other was stopped after Jan. 1976)
U.K.*	(Since May 1973; 'manufacturers have agreed that self-medication should be limited to courses of not more than 7.5 g separated by intervals of at least 4 weeks')
Rumania	(Since Apr. 1974; the Drug and Drug Monitoring Commission decided to modify the box leaflets to prescribe within 750 mg ×28 days)
Hungary	(The National Institute of Pharmacy has limited the continuous administration to one month at the most for safety's sake)
Czechoslovakia	('Only the general dosage scheme for these drugs has been early adopted appropriately')
Warning on adverse effect, etc. (3)	
Thailand	(The manufacturer must warn users as 'This drug may cause neurological symptoms of leg and eye')
South Africa	(Steps have been taken locally to propose to firms involved that a caution be included on the label of these drugs, etc.)
Italy	(The Committee for Proprietary Medicinal Products of the C.E.C. has underlined the risk for the use of these drugs in Nov. 1976, etc.)
Others (2)	
El Salvador	The drugs are used except for the persons having sensitiveness to iodine or of thyroidism)
Cyprus	('Their use is limited')
Nothing, but comment was described (4)	
Afghanistan	('The Ministry of Public Health will take action......when reliable reports ......are received......')
Spain	(Regulation 'is possible')
Lesotho	('The government will send out a warning to all practitioners......and encourage them to follow their patients on these drugs and report any adverse effects they can observe')
Jordan	(Not prohibited, but 'the subject is undergoing studies by the Health Authorities')
Nothing (6)	
India, Democratic Yemen, Monaco, Malta, Zambia, Ecuador	

*After this survey, the use of clioquinol was limited only on prescription in the U.K. in 1977.

did not answer this question, and one (Nauru) answered that HOQ were 'not imported for use'.

The results of the second inquiry are shown in Table 4. Comparing them with the replies in the preceding survey, it is clear that no country has loosened regulations, and that, on the contrary, more stringent controls have been introduced in 20 countries. In particular it is noticeable that Entero-Vioform was withdrawn in New

TABLE 4. *Regulations against HOQ (internal use) outside Japan (according to replies from 28 countries between Oct. 1978 and March 1979. New regulations are in italics)*

Regulations and country (date, contents)	
Suspension of sales (7)	
1. U.S.A.	(Ciba-Geigy Ltd. withdrew Entero-Vioform in 1972)
2. Norway	(The Board of Drugs decided to withdraw all preparations from the market after Jan. 1974)
3. Sweden	(Ciba-Geigy withdrew the registration of Entero-Vioform in May 1975)
4. *New Zealand*	*(The company withdrew Entero-Vioform in 1978)*
5. Taiwan	(The use of combined preparation was banned after Jan. 1972; *simples are subject to prescription)*
6. *India*	*(The use of combined preparation was banned. Simples are subject to prescription)*
7. *Denmark*	*(The Danish Board on Adverse Reactions to Drugs decided to withdraw derivatives of oxyquinoline as from May 1978)*
Only prescription (15)	
1. Bulgaria	(After Feb. 1973)
2. Malaysia	(After Apr. 1976)
3. Canada	
4. Iraq	('But in actual fact, the sales have not gone down significantly, despite the legislation of the Drug Establishment made several years ago')
5. Portugal	*(Some literature or leaflets were improved)*
6. Australia	*(Available on prescription only in all states)*
7. *Ireland*	*(Between 1976 and 1977)*
8. *F.R. Germany*	*(A new case of intoxication was reported)*
9. *D.R. Germany*	*('Only 1 halquinol containing preparation is available by prescription. Two drugs with phanquinone and halquinol/phanquinone existing in a very minute supply are distributed by special application only. But the complete withdrawal of both is planned')*
10. *Italy*	*(A new case (or cases) of intoxication was reported: in print)*
11. *Monaco*	
12. *Lesotho*	('...but they are actually available freely through pharmacies and patients normally request them without consulting their physicians')
13. *Israel*	*('Because of other preferable available drugs for the same indication, the use of quinolines has declined')*
14. *Afghanistan*	*(Avicenna Pharmaceutical Institute has decided to stop the importation of chloro-iodo-hydroxyquin but di-iodohydroxyquin is still imported)*
15. *Hungary*	*(For the use of Mexaform, Mexase)*

TABLE 4. *Continued*

Warning, limitation on dose, etc. (4)	
1. Cyprus	(The Drug Council intends to revoke the marketing licences of all preparations containing clioquinol and its derivatives')
2. *Democratic Yemen*	*('The Therapeutic Committee has recommended its supply only on prescription')*
3. Thailand	*('They have been classified as dangerous drugs)*
4. South Africa	*('Sold through pharmacies only under personal supervision of the responsible pharmacist')*
Others (2)	
1. El Salvador	(The Ministry of Public Health and Social Assistance plans to work out the countermeasures to be taken)
2. Zambia	('Available through pharmacies. Demand very limited')

Zealand, and combined preparations were banned in India as they were in Taiwan. The replies from East Germany and Cyprus also attracted our attention.

These surveys show that the number of countries where HOQ is banned or rigidly regulated has increased year after year since HOQ were suspended in Japan. However, it is also apparent that there still are many countries were HOQ is not withdrawn.

DISCUSSION AND CONCLUSION

The results of our surveys clearly indicate that the number of cases of HOQ intoxication have increased annually outside Japan although the number is not as great as it had been in Japan. However, in Japan a special research commission was established in 1969 and the nationwide survey was carried out four times to discover 11,007 SMON cases (3). Therefore, it is possible that if other countries would establish such special research commissions to carry out more detailed surveys, more cases of HOQ intoxication might be revealed. Moreover, it is quite possible that the number of the sufferers will continue to increase if HOQ is used without rigid regulation.

Another question is whether HOQ should be entirely banned or whether their use should be severely restricted. According to the surveys, opinions are divided outside Japan. To elucidate this problem, the following facts should be considered:

In Mexico in 1958, Kean and Waters studied the preventive effect of clioquinol, neomycin and lactose (placebo) on travellers' diarrhea using American students in a double-blind study. Diarrhea occurred in 38.6% of those taking clioquinol, 20.1% of those on neomycin and 33.6% of those on placebo. The difference between neomycin and placebo was significant and clioquinol was apparently no more effective than the placebo (4).

In the U.S.A. in 1960, the F.D.A. cast serious doubt on the efficacy and safety of Entero-Vioform in common diarrhea and advised limiting the use of the drug to amebic dysentery. Ciba Ltd. accepted the advice in 1961 (5). After the sale of HOQ was suspended in Japan in 1970, Ciba-Geigy Ltd. withdrew Entero-Vioform from the U.S. market in 1972.

In Sweden in 1968, serious doubts were cast on the preventive and therapeutic effects of HOQ in travellers' diarrhea. An epidemiological study revealed that Swedish tourists visiting Mediterranean countries who regularly took HOQ prophylactically had a significantly higher incidence of Salmonella infections than those who did not take the drug. The same thing was demonstrated experimentally in mice (6). The National Laboratory of Drugs, having received this report, recommended in 1969 not to use HOQ as a prophylactic for diarrhea. Ciba-Geigy Ltd. withdrew the register of Entero-Vioform in 1975 because, according to Dr. Anna-Karin Furhoff, zinc preparations were found to be effective on acrodermatitis enteropathica, for which only HOQ were considered useful previously (7).

In Norway in 1973, the Board of Drugs withdrew all oral preparations containing HOQ from the market after January 1974, the reasons being their possible adverse reactions and 'the lack of evidence of therapeutic effect'.

In Denmark, the regulation against the use of HOQ has gradually strengthened since 1972, and HOQ were withdrawn from the market in May 1978 because 'better drugs are available also against amebic dysentery, notably metronidazole, --------- and acrodermatitis enteropathica, which can now be treated with zinc preparations' (8).

Although these findings and decisions had already been expressed, Dr. Pinto and Dr. Burley of Ciba-Geigy did not positively admit the relationship between HOQ and SMON, claiming that the evidence for the efficacy of Entero-Vioform had been clearly shown in travellers' diarrhea, in amebiasis, as well as in other infestations and infections (9). However, Dr. Wright of Charing Cross Hospital Medical School pointed out that there were 'inherent shortcomings' and defects in the studies cited by them (10). They have not yet responded to this.

In conclusion, our opinion is that prohibition of at least internal use of HOQ should be seriously considered in those countries were HOQ are still in use.

SUMMARY

Between January 1970 and September 1978 114 cases were reported as SMON or intoxication with halogenated oxyquinoline derivatives (including suspected cases) in 55 articles published outside Japan. Detailed studies and discussions of 74 cases in 42 articles were given after excluding 'uncertain' cases. Further, inquiries on the use of halogenated oxyquinoline derivatives revealed an increase in the number of countries where these preparations were regulated or prohibited after 1970.

ACKNOWLEDGEMENTS

We thank the health authorities concerned of the 41 countries which kindly answered our questions. We also thank Dr. Itsuzo Shigematsu, chairman of the SMON Research Commission, for his kind advice and support of our research.

REFERENCES

1. Tsubaki, T., Honma, Y. and Hoshi, M. (1971): *Lancet, 1*, 696.
2. Nakae, K., Yamamoto, S., Shigematsu, I. and Kono, R. (1973): *Lancet, 1*, 171.
3. Nakae, K., Yamamoto, S., Shigematsu, I., Yanagawa, H., Kawaguchi, T. and Ohtani, M. (1976): *Report of S.M.O.N. Research Committee in Fiscal 1975*, p. 238.
4. Kean, B.H. and Waters, S.R. (1959): *New Engl. J. Med., 261*, 71.
5. Personal communication from C.H. Sullivan of Ciba Co. to M.L. Yakowitz of F.D.A. (1961): Documentary evidence of S.M.O.N. Lawsuit Tokyo District Court. Koh-201-2.
6. Ringerts, O. and Mentzing, L.O. (1968): *Acta path. microbiol. scand., 74*, 367.
7. Summary of interview with Dr. Anna-Karin Furhoff/Swedish Adverse Drug Reaction Committee), enclosed in personal communication dated September 6, 1976.
8. Pedersen, A. (1978): *Ugeskr. Laeg., 140*, 1181.
9. Pinto, O. De S. and Burley, D. (1977): *Lancet, 1*, 1256.
10. Wright, D.J.M. (1977): *Lancet, 2*, 197.

REFERENCES Tables 2a,b,c

1. McEwen, L.M. (1971): *Brit. med. J., 4*, 169.
2. Spillane, J.D. (1971): *Lancet, 2*, 1371.
3. Cambier, J., Masson, N., Berkman, N. and Dairou, R. (1972): *Nouv. Presse méd., 1*, 1991.
4. Grenier, B., Rolland, J.-C., Kiffer, A. and Maupas, Ph. (1973): *Nouv. Presse méd., 2*, 1073.
5. Castaigne, P., Rondot, P., Lenoel, Y., Raibadeau Dumas, J.-L. and Autret, A. (1973): *Thérapie, 28*, 393.
6. Latterre, E.C., Stevens, A., Goffin, L. and Velghe, L. (1973): *Nouv. Presse méd., 2*, 2550.
7. Gendre, J.-P., Barbanel, Cl., Degos J.-D. and Le Quintrec, Y. (1974): *Nouv. Presse méd., 3*, 2395.
8. Vitale, C., Feldmann, J.L., Hubault, A., Weisbecker, J., Bechetoille, A. and De Sèze, S. (1974): *Ann. Méd intern., 125*, 941.
9. Froissart, M., Morcamp, D. and Mizon, J.-P. (1976): *Nouv. Presse méd., 5*, 863.
10. Kaeser, H.E. and Wüthrich, R. (1970): *Dtsch. med. Wschr., 95*, 1685.
11. Boergen, K.P. (1973): *Klin. Mbl. Augenheilk., 163*, 217.
12. Heilig, P. and Thaler, A. (1974): *Klin. Mbl. Augenheilk., 164*, 386.
13. Mamoli, B., Thaler, A., Heilig, P. and Siakos, G. (1975): *J. Neurol., 209*, 139.
14. Osterman, P.O. (1971): *Lancet, 2*, 544.
15. Hansson, O. (1978): *Läkartidningen, 75*, 3064.
16. Jensen, J.P.A. and Bryndum, B. (1972): *Ugeskr. Laeg., 134*, 1523.
17. Kjaersgaard, K. and Christiansen, N. (1972): *Ugeskr. Laeg., 134*, 1526.
18. Dahl, K.B. (1974): *Ugeskr. Laeg., 136*, 263.
19. Van Beeck, J.A. and Scholten, J.B. (1972): *Ned. T. Geneesk., 116*, 1621.
20. Bron, H.L.N.M., Korten, J.J., Pinckers, A.J.L.G. and Majoor, C.L.H. (1972): *Ned. T. Geneesk., 116*, 1615.
21. Yamamoto, K. and Okamoto, S. (1972): *Clin. Neurol., 12*, 632.
22. Danis, P. (1972): *Bull. Soc. belge Ophtalmol., 159*, 671.
23. Otte, G. (1976): *Acta neurol. belg., 76*, 331.
24. Fabiani, F. and Sinibaldi, L. (1977): *Lancet, 2*, 555.
25. Derakhshan, I. and Forough, M. (1978): *Lancet, 1*, 715.
26. Wadia, N.H. (1973): *Neurol. India, 21*, 95.

27. Wadia, N.H. (1977): *J. Neurol. Neurosurg. Psychiat., 40*, 268.
28. Selby, G. (1972): *Lancet, 1*, 123.
29. Reich, J.A. and Billson, F.A. (1973): *Med. J. Aust., 2*, 593.
30. Pittman, F.E. and Westphal, M. (1973): *Lancet, 2*, 566.
31. Behrens, M.M. (1974): *J. Amer. med. Ass., 228*, 693.
32. Fleisher, D.I., Hepler, R.S. and Landau, J.W. (1974): *Pediatrics, 54*, 106.
33. Carr, W.G.L., Bowen, R.A. and Horner, F.A. (1977): *Can. med. Ass. J., 116*, 251.
34. Reich, H. (1973): *Klin. Wschr., 51*, 1024.
35. van Balen, A.Th.M. (1971): *Ophthalmologica, 163*, 8.
36. Drukker, J. and Lindenburg, P.A.W. (1972): *Ned. T. Geneesk., 116*, 1618.
37. Papuzinski, M. and Wilmowska-Pietruszynska, A. (1974): *Pediat. Pol., 49,* 1393.
38. Idriss, Z.H. and Der Kaloustian, V.M. (1973): *Clin. Pediat., 12*, 393.
39. Garcia-Perez, A., Castro, C., Franco, A. and Escribano, R. (1974): *Brit. J. Dermatol., 90*, 453.
40. Kaeser, H.E. and Scollo-Lavizzari, G. (1970): *Dtsch. med. Wschr., 95*, 394.
41. Kjaersgaard, K. (1971): *Lancet, 2*, 1086.
42. Ferrier, T.M. and Eadie, M.J. (1973): *Med. J. Aust., 2*, 1008.

NOTE ADDED IN PROOF

1. Ciba-Geigy directed to delete ‘prophylaxis’ and ‘non-specific diarrhea’ from the indications for the products containing halogenated hydroxyquinolines for oral use in April, 1978.
2. Since completing this paper, a study by G. Baumgartner et al. *(J. Neurol. Neurosurg. Psychiat.,* 1979, *42,* 1073) has come to our attention. This report is an analysis of 220 cases of possible neurotoxic reactions to halogenated hydroxyguinolines reported from outside Japan between 1935 and 1978.

Discussion

Chairman: Now, we have a combined discussion on the papers by Dr. Hansson, Dr. Berggren, Dr. Dukes and Dr. Katahira, and first I am asking if any speakers have questions or comments to Dr. Hansson's paper.

Tsubaki: Dr. Hansson and Dr. Berggren, the signs and symptoms of patients with clioquinol intoxication reported by you seem to differ from those of Japanese patients. The latter have more severe sensory complaints. But your cases show only an optic atrophy and I would like to ask you why is this?

Hansson: In Sweden we have the whole spectrum of neurological symptoms and signs of clioquinol damage. Some of the cases are exactly comparable with the severe SMON cases. Most of them have sensory disturbances of varying degrees. In some cases optic atrophy is the only manifestation of oxychinoline intoxication. I doubt that a real difference exists between the Japanese and the Swedish cases. But obviously severe cases predominate in Japan.

Tsubaki: You mean that your cases had paresthesia in the lower limbs, while I thought that most of your cases had only optic atrophy.

Berggren: I think that you have misunderstood. The case with acrodermatitis enteropathica had optic atrophy. The other cases which Dr. Hansson presented were SMON cases.

Tsubaki: In Japanese cases, the most characteristic signs are very severe sensory changes with paresthesia, by which SMON patients can be diagnosed correctly. If the sensory changes are not so severe, it is difficult to differentiate it from Devic's disease or some other neuropathy due to nutritional deficiency. I think that the sensory changes of Japanese cases with SMON are very severe and characteristic.

Dukes: Both Dr. Hansson and Dr. Katahira referred to the fact that clioquinol is still being sold and used on a large scale in many parts of the world. Now, this use obviously reflects a widespread belief that the product is effective for diarrhea, and has great relevance in many countries for many people. Are there any recent, reliable publications demonstrating its inefficacy in the treatment of diarrhea?

Chairman: Can anybody answer that question? This matter appears to be of no interest to the people who promote the drug. Are there any more questions to the papers by Dr. Hansson and Dr. Berggren or by Dr. Dukes?

Hansson: I do not know of any recent investigation that tests the efficacy or inefficacy of clioquinol to treat diarrhea. Given present knowledge of the potential risks of irreversible neurological injuries, it is clearly impossible to do such an investigation on ethical grounds.

Böttiger: I think with regard to Dr. Dukes's question that a Swedish study should be mentioned that was published in the late '60s (by Ringertz et al.) showing that clioquinol ('Enterovioform') was ineffective against travellers' diarrhea, and also that there were indications that the risks for travellers' infections increased after the use of the drug because the normal bacteria in the gut were killed. There are very few drugs which are not only ineffective but also harmful.

Oakley: 1. Perhaps the reason why the isolated optic atrophy seems more common outside Japan is because most of the cases reported were children. Perhaps the children were too young to report the paresthesia. What is the incidence in pediatric patients of non-optic nerve neuropathy? 2. Many human teratogens affect the nervous system. Were there pregnant SMON patients who took clioquinol? What was the outcome of those pregnancies? Were there birth defects?

Hansson: Concerning your first question, one of our two children with optic atrophy in the acute stage had signs of polyneuropathy or myelopathy, but that was reversible because happily the drugs were stopped.

Takano: I would like to raise a question with Dr. Dukes. You reported that in the Netherlands there are various assessing committees and these are considered to be the doctors' responsibility. But what do you consider to be the responsibility of pharmaceutical companies for providing the information? My personal view is that as soon as this sort of information comes to the pharmaceutical companies then that information should be disseminated throughout the country, throughout the world, as soon as possible. Then, the center can be the WHO or an equivalent organization.

Dukes: I agree that drug companies should pass on the information they have, but one should not oblige them to pass on every suspicion of an adverse reaction to every physician – this would be confusing. A company should report all possible adverse reactions and further notification of serious suspicion should be passed on (e.g. in amended data sheets, approved by the authorities) to physicians.

Hanakago: I have been involved in rehabilitation of many SMON patients and recently I have encountered two cases with acrodermatitis enteropathica. I have an impression that children with acrodermatitis enteropathica and SMON show somewhat different signs and symptoms compared with adult SMON cases: their paresthesia seemed to be rather milder and the motor and optic disturbances more severe. I propose collecting cases of this sort from both Japan and Western countries in a joint study for comparison. We have carried out such a study in Japan and a synopsis has already been distributed.

Kurahashi: Dr. Hansson, you refer to 16 patients in Sweden. Did you say that the administration period was less than 10 days in some cases?

Hansson: There is one patient with 10 days only. And there is one with an acute intoxication with retrograde amnesia, who took oxyquinoline for just one day. All others had taken oxyquinoline for more than 10 days.

Kurahashi: In Okayama, 75% of SMON patients received chinoform as a drug prescribed by doctors. Does this also apply in Western countries? I would ask Dr. Hansson therefore: In Sweden, Chinoform was probably sold in various ways. What was the most common way of selling chinoform, as over-the-counter drug or prescribed drug or otherwise?

Hansson: Firstly it is now banned in Sweden. When it was used in Sweden, in most cases I think it was an over-the-counter drug, and very seldom was it prescribed by doctors. Occasionally doctors recommended it to patients if they were going abroad but it was not prescribed. They just recommended that the patient buy it. It was not commonly used I think in hospitals, for example.

Chairman: Thank you everybody for the very interesting discussion.

Clinical study of clioquinol intoxication in dogs and cats

P. HANGARTNER

5 Marc-Dufour, Lausanne, Switzerland

It is a great honour and pleasure to have the opportunity to report here the facts concerning the toxicity of Entero-Vioform, and indeed of all drugs containing clioquinol, in dogs and cats.

From 1958, I observed cases of severe convulsions, epileptiform attacks and psychic disorders. Starting from this point and seeking the case history, it was revealed that in all these animals Entero-Vioform had been used to control gastrointestinal diseases such as enteritis, gastroenteritis or common diarrhoea.

In veterinary medicine, dog and cat owners frequently give their animals drugs which are effectively used in man. One such drug is Entero-Vioform. At present, Entero-Vioform as well as several other drugs containing clioquinol is sold on the Swiss market without prescription.

Later cases in which Entero-Vioform was the sole drug were selected. According to the owners, the animals had been in previously perfect health. These data were published in 1965. At the same time, it became evident that Mexaform, Intestopan and Colenter were also toxic in dogs, as judged in my practice in 1958.

HISTORY

Various reports on clinoquinol toxicity were published at Ciba Geigy, from 1970 on, e.g. Brückner (1), Hess (2–4,6), Thomann (5), Krinke (7), Worden (8) and co-workers.

Initially no toxicity of clioquinol was apparent, but as research progressed the toxicity, especially its epileptogenic properties in acute intoxication, became apparent. The authors revealed neuropathy of the central, but not peripheral, nervous system after prolonged administration. Others independently observed toxicity of clioquinol in the central nervous systems of dogs and cats with epileptiform crises.

Schantz and Wikström (9) described oxychinoline intoxication in dogs and Müller (10) epilepsy and haematuria after Mexaform. Püschner and Frankhauser (11) found nervous symptoms and necrosis of neurons in the Ammon's horn in mice. Lannek (12) and Kammermann-Lüscher (13) reported intoxication induced by halogenated oxychinolines, Entero-Vioform and Mexaform in dogs.

MATERIAL

Animals: 10 dogs (7 female; 3 male) of various breeds including poodle, Scotch terrier, cairn terrier, pomeranian, hound, pincher, Bernese sheepdog and 1 cat. Ages ranged from 1 to 14 years.

CASE HISTORIES

All dogs were given Entero-Vioform per os for simple diarrhoea or more severe gastroenteritis (in one case a bloody stool was present).

At the time, distemper with nervous complications frequently occurred. Distemper, or other infectious diseases with nervous troubles, present characteristics which cannot clinically be confused with simple diarrhoea or gastroenteritis without underlying disease.

The dogs received between 2 and 5 tablets of Entero-Vioform. The cat (3.5 kg) licked approximately 0.7 g Vioform powder out of its fur.

SYMPTOMATOLOGY

It should be mentioned that in my practice I was mostly called in for 'emergency' for epileptiform attacks. It is evident that more *acute cases* are seen and it is rare to be able to follow a case over a long period – even as far as death – and observe chronic disorders.

In general, three kinds of epileptiform crisis were observed: (1) crises of neural infectious disease; (2) crises of unknown aetiology occurring irregularly in healthy dogs; (3) crises due to toxins with specific or non-specific neural actions such as metaldehyde or Entero-Vioform (clioquinol).

The crisis starts abruptly, without preliminary tonic-phase signs: the stare becomes fixed, with a spastic lid-reflex, pupils dilate in mydriasis, the head rises and the animal sits down and falls on its side, remaining in lateral decubitus with opisthotonus. Sometimes, it cries briefly.

The clonic phase follows: muscles tighten and legs stretch. Salivation and jaw movements are accompanied by uncontrolled rapid swimming and running movements of the legs and generalized shivering. Respiration is almost imperceptible and shallow. The tongue becomes cyanotic blue. Excretory functions are disturbed. Pulse is flying and hard. The crisis lasts from a few seconds to several minutes with relapses after hours or days, or there may be complete recovery.

The shock of such events sometimes induces owners to request euthanasia for the dog.

The end of the crisis is marked by progressive disappearance of the leg spasms and cyanosis, the breathing recommences and becomes deeper, and consciousness returns; the dog is not yet able to stand up, appearing tired and exhausted. Finally when it does stand, its walk is hesitating, swinging and atactic-like. After some time (1–2 hours) recovery is complete.

Besides these classical encephalopathy symptoms, there may be, during the attack, abnormal body torsion, torpor, glassy stare, gnashing of the jaws, unsteady walking and restless running. With repeated crises the psychic faculties are greatly reduced, ending even in prostration, stupor, complete apathy and anorexia. Fever is not recorded, except during the crisis as a result of tetany or tremor.

Entobex, a Mexaform component, leads to haematuria.

DIAGNOSIS

None of the symptoms is pathognomonic. The epileptiform crisis is indicative of encephalopathy and is non-specific, resulting from oedema of the brain and/or injury to the hippocampus. Therefore, the diagnosis is only possible after obtaining a complete case history. Laboratory tests are unknown.

I never encountered the chronic condition characterized by anorexia, weight loss, muscle weakness and emaciation, with neural disorders as described for human SMON by Tateishi and Otsuki (15) and Worden (8); the latter author did not find peripheral neural disorders.

DIFFERENTIAL DIAGNOSIS

Fankhauser (14) defines epileptiform crises as:

1. *Primary epilepsy:* without detectable structural deteriorations in brain, or
2. *Secondary epilepsy:* with structural and/or biochemical alterations in brain.

Secondary epilepsy may result from:

a. *Primary brain disease*
   Encephalitis (distemper, toxoplasmosis, virus, hepatitis, by septicaemia; mycosis)
   Tumours of the brain
   Metabolic disorders of the brain (leukodystrophy, lipidosis)
   Hydrocephalus and other deformities
b. *Direct injury of the brain*
   Trauma (brain injuries and wounds; brain swelling; brain haemorrhage)
   Lack of oxygen
   Intoxication
c. *Indirect injury of the brain*
   Disordered blood circulation
   Blood diseases
   Liver diseases
   Hypoglycaemia

PATHOGENESIS

In the cases observed, the primary condition for therapy with clioquinol was gastrointestinal disorder, free of underlying infectious disease. This type of gastroenteritis is well known to veterinarians and creates neither emergency nor danger for the central or peripheral nervous systems.

Absorption by the gut is a problem. In all clinical cases, acute intoxication was present revealing absorption of significant quantities of toxic material by the disturbed gut mucosa, not quantitatively related to the dose taken orally.

There are great differences in sensitivity to clioquinol and these vary with breed and individual. The epileptogenic properties of clioquinol (halogenated oxychinoline) are evident. In acute stages, the symptoms indicate general brain but especially hippocampal (Ammon's horn) problems.

Experiments on mice (11) showed oedema and necrosis of the hippocampal pyramidal cells with oedema and necrosis of ganglionic and glial cells. These changes are akin to the cell degeneration provoked by ischaemia (lack of oxygen for neurons as a result of reduced blood flow or by hypoxia).

Intestinal lesions thus seem to be one of the main conditions for clioquinol intoxication; the injured gut mucosa allows passage of high quantities of toxin. Diarrhoea is the main symptom of defence by the gut, but, on the other hand, the disturbed gut mucosa may become unphysiologically permeable to many other drugs and to toxins.

CONCLUSION

Entero-Vioform and drugs containing clioquinol have been used in veterinary medicine without trouble, but it is clear that clioquinol is toxic and is especially neurotoxic and epileptogenic in dogs and cats.

So long as clioquinol is used in veterinary medicine, accidents will occur. The only way to avoid further accidents, is to *STOP* the use of clioquinol and all quinolines.

REFERENCES

1. Brückner, R., Hess, R., Pericin, C. and Tripod, J. (1970): Tierexperimentelle Untersuchungen bei langdauernder Verabreichung von hohen Dosen von Jod-chlor-8-hydroxychinolin mit besonderer Berücksichtigung möglicher toxischer Augenveränderungen. *Arzneimittel-Forsch., 20,* 575.
2. Hess, R., Keberle, H., Koella, W.P., Schmid, K. and Gelzer, J. (1972): Clioquinol: absence of neurotoxicity in laboratory animals. *Lancet, 2*, 424.
3. Hess, R., Koella, W.P., Krinke, G., Pericin, C., Petermann, H., Sachsse, K. and Thomann, P. (1974): Detection and evaluation of neurotoxicity. In: *Proceedings, European Society for the Study of Drug Toxicity, Vol. XV, Zürich, 1973*. Excerpta Medica, Amsterdam.
4. Hess, R., Koella, W.P., Krinke, G., Petermann, H., Thomann, P. and Zak, F. (1973): Absence of neurotoxicity following prolonged administration of iodochloro-8-hydroxyquinoline to Beagle dogs. *Arzneimittel-Forsch., 23,* 1566.
5. Thomann, P., Koella, W.P., Krinke, G., Petermann, H., Zak, F. and Hess, R. (1974): The assessment of peripheral neurotoxicity in dogs: Comparative studies with acrylamide and clioquinol. *Agents and Actions, 4/1.*
6. Hess, R., Thomann, P. and Krinke, G. (1977): The assessment of neurotoxicity in laboratory animals. Paper presented at: I International Congress on Toxicology, Toronto, 1977.
7. Krinke, G., Pericin, C., Thomann, P. and Hess, R. (1978): Toxic encephalopathy with hippocampal lesions. *Zbl. Vet.-Med. A., 25,* 277.
8. Worden, A. N., Heywood, R., Prentice, D.E., Chesterman, H., Skerrett, K. and Thomann, P.E. (1978): Clioquinol toxicity in the dog. *Toxicology, 9*, 227.
9. Schantz, B. and Wikström, B. (1965): Suspected poisoning with oxychinoline preparation in dogs. *Svensk. vet. Tidn., 17*, 106.
10. Müller, L.F. (1967): Die Mexaformvergiftung des Hundes (klinische Demonstration). *Kleintierpraxis, 12*, 51.

11. Püschner, H. and Fankhauser, R. (1969): Neuropathologische Befunde bei experimenteller Vioform-Vergiftung der weissen Maus. *Schweiz. Arch. Tierheilk.*, *111*, 371.
12. Lannek, B. (1974): Toxicity of halogenated oxychinolines in dogs. A clinical study. *Acta vet. scand.*, *15*, 219.
13. Kammermann-Lüscher, B. (1974): Entero-Vioform- und Mexaformvergiftung beim Hund. *Tierärztl. Prax.*, *2*, 59.
14. Fankhauser, R.: Ueber die Epilepsie des Hundes. In: *100 Jahre Kynologische Forschung in der Schweiz*, pp. 161–172.
15. Tateishi, J. and Otsuki, S. (1975): Experimental reproduction of SMON in animals by prolonged administration of clioquinol: Clinico-pathological findings. *Jap. J. med. Sci. Biol.*, *28*, 165.

Reproduction of experimental SMON in animals by oral administration of clioquinol

JUN TATEISHI

Department of Neuropathology, Neurological Institute, Kyushu University, Medical School, Fukuoka, Japan

To investigate the neurotoxicity of clioquinol, long-term oral administration of the drug to mongrel dogs, beagle dogs, cats, monkeys, rats and mice was repeated in our laboratory on several occasions. The results of these animal experiments are summarized below and compared with SMON in Japanese patients.

ACUTE INTOXICATION

As reported by Hangartner (1), Schantz and Wikström (2) and Müller (3), some mongrel dogs and cats died of general weakness and/or convulsions soon after administration of clioquinol (4). Autopsy of these animals revealed only non-specific changes such as small hemorrhages and congestion of the brain and necrobiotic changes in the nerve cells. Many mice given increasingly larger doses of clioquinol (daily doses of 380 mg/kg for 55 days, 1900 mg/kg for 20 days and 3800 mg/kg for 115 days) showed selective disappearance of nerve cells in the hippocampus (Fig. 1). This pathological change, probably due to convulsive seizure, was reported by Püschner and Fankhauser (5) but was seen more clearly in our experiment.

Convulsions and delirious state were reported in some human cases of acute clioquinol intoxication (6).

CHRONIC INTOXICATION

To avoid acute death in animals, the daily dosage of clioquinol was increased gradually in our early experiments (4). This had the great advantage of elevating the blood level of unconjugated clioquinol and causing chronic intoxication. The fixed-dose method, however, also produced the same syndrome in beagle dogs (7). The number of animals that receive clioquinol, the daily dose required to cause neurological symptoms, and the results of pathological examinations are summarized in Table 1.

The daily dose given to mongrel dogs ranged from 60 to 144 mg/kg, which was 1.5 to 7 times higher than the average dose of clioquinol (20 to 40 mg/kg) administered to many SMON patients in Japan. Combined procedures causing prolonged constipation, and hepatic and renal dysfunction seemed to lower the

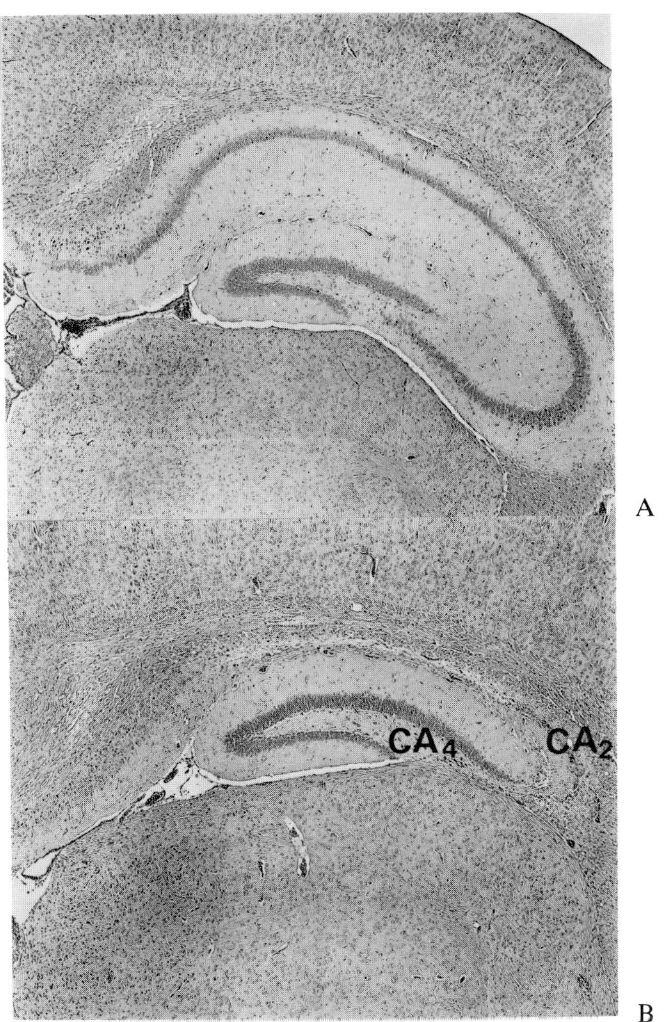

Fig. 1. (A) Hippocampus of a control mouse. H-E stain. (B) The same area of a mouse intoxicated with clioquinol. Note total loss of nerve cells in CA_1 and CA_3, while a few nerve cells are preserved in CA_2 and CA_4. H-E stain.

threshold of clioquinol intoxication. This fact may explain the individual susceptibility to the neurotoxicity of the drug. In rats and mice, daily doses were gradually increased to a maximum of 900 mg/kg and 3800 mg/kg, respectively, during 190 days. Chronic intoxication symptoms, however, were not observed in rats and mice. These facts strongly suggest the existence of differences in strains as well as in species of animals with regard to neurotoxicity. These differences depend on the concentration ratio of unconjugated clioquinol, a neurotoxic form, in the blood of animals.

Chronic intoxication in many dogs and cats consisted of distinct neurological signs that began with side-swaying of the hips and ataxic gait followed by muscle

TABLE 1. *Clioquinol administration*

Animals	No. of animals	Daily dose (mg/kg)	Lesions(No.of animals)	
			Spinal cord	Optic tract
Beagle dogs	17	250–400	15	14
Mongrel dogs	21	60–144	15	11
Cats	27	90–250	22(5)*	9
Japanese monkey	1	324	1	0
Rats	4	900**	0	0
Mice	5	3800**	0	0

* Mild change.
**Maximum doses administered.

weakness in the hindlegs. The longer the period of administration, the more severe the symptoms became. Forelegs that had remained healthy for a long period, however, later developed slight weakness. Visual acuity was also impaired in long-surviving animals. Cessation of administration produced a decrease in the neurological signs except for ataxic weakness of the hindlegs.

As already reported (8), the most pathognomonic changes of chronic intoxication were found in the spinal cord and optic tracts of dogs and cats. In the spinal cord, degenerative changes were most advanced in the posterior fasciculus, especially in Goll's tract in the upper cervical cord (Fig. 2), and were less severe in the corticospinal tract of the lumbar cord. These changes were mostly distal, diffuse, continuous and symmetrical, damaging axons first, then myelin sheaths. Axonal changes varied from swelling, vacuolization and fragmentation to total disappearance. Degeneration and complete loss of myelin sheaths accompanied by neutral fat droplets occurred later. Plump and often binucleated astrocytes were seen, although proliferation of glial fibers was not marked. Burdach's tract in the upper cervical cord and the proximal portion of Goll's tract at the lumbar level later showed similar but milder changes.

The same advanced changes as in Goll's tract in the cervical cord occurred bilaterally in the optic tracts of long-surviving dogs and cats. Similar but milder changes were seen in the chiasm and optic nerves. Neither inflammatory nor vascular lesions were found in these areas.

The nature and distribution of these changes were specific, simulating system degeneration, composing a definite pathological entity, and corresponding well with those of SMON in humans (9). The results of our animal experiments were confirmed by many researchers in Japan and abroad (10) including Ciba-Geigy, AG, laboratories (11).

Histological changes seen in other nervous regions, such as peripheral nerves, autonomic nerves, the spinal root ganglia, ganglion cell layer of the retina, spinal roots, anterior spinal horn, brainstem, and some gray matter in the cerebrum, were occasional, mild, and non-pathognomonic.

The pathology of visceral organs in our animals was non-specific, but intestinal abnormalities, such as invagination, volvulus and megacolon, were noteworthy concerning the untoward abdominal effects of this substance (see below).

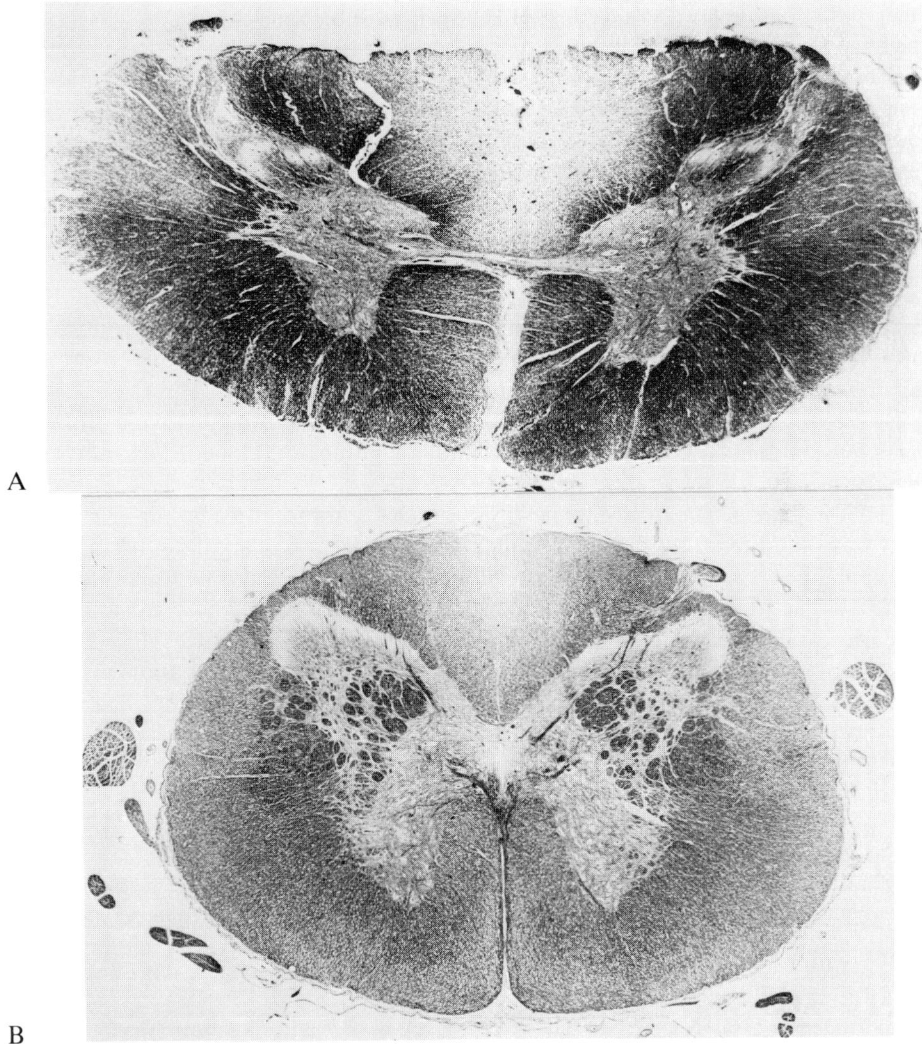

Fig. 2. (A) Thoracic cord of a 57-year-old man who died from SMON, showing degeneration of the long tracts in the posterior and lateral fasciculi. Woelcke stain. (B) Cervical cord of a mongrel dog intoxicated with clioquinol. Woelcke stain.

ABDOMINAL SYMPTOMS

After administration of clioquinol, many SMON patients suffered from abdominal symptoms, such as abdominal pain, diarrhea and/or constipation, and vomiting, simulating ileus (12). To disclose the cause of this distress we conducted physiological experiments on 8 mongrel dogs (8). It was observed that abnormal, periodic constriction occurred in the small intestine 30 to 90 min after intraduodenal instillation of clioquinol. This constriction did not disappear even when all the splanchnic nerves were severed, but disappeared only when the vagal nerve trunks were cut bilaterally in the cervical region or when the animals were decerebrated at the mesencephalon. Therefore, the effect of clioquinol on the intestinal tract appeared to be associated with excitation of the parasympathetic center in the diencephalon. The abdominal symptoms seen in many SMON patients might be explained by this effect of clioquinol.

SUMMARY

1. Long-term oral administrations of clioquinol in dogs and cats reproduced the SMON syndrome with a high incidence.
2. The daily dose of clioquinol given to mongrel dogs was 1.5 – 7 times higher than the average dose administered to many SMON patients. Animals with prolonged constipation or dysfunction of the liver and/or kidney developed the syndrome at lower dosage.
3. The major pathological change produced by chronic intoxication in dogs and cats was predominantly distal axonopathy in the posterior and lateral fasciculi of the spinal cord and in the optic tracts which corresponded well with that in SMON patients. The results of our animal experiments were confirmed by many researchers in Japan and abroad including the Ciba-Geigy, AG, laboratories.
4. After instillation of clioquinol in the small intestine of dogs, a marked increase in intestinal movements was observed which might explain the abdominal symptoms in SMON patients following clioquinol intake.

REFERENCES

1. Hangartner, P. (1965): Troubles nerveux observés chez le chien après absorption d'Entéro-Vioforme Ciba. *Schweiz. Arch. Tierheilk. 107*, 43.
2. Schantz, B. and Wikström, B. (1965): Suspected poisoning with oxyquinoline preparation in dogs. *Svensk. vet. T., 17,* 106.
3. Müller, L.F. (1967): Die Mexaformvergiftung des Hundes (klinische Demonstration). *Kleintierpraxis, 12*, 51.
4. Tateishi, J., Kuroda, S., Saito, A. and Otsuki, S. (1972): Experimental myelo-optic neuropathy induced by clioquinol. *Acta neuropath., 24*, 304.
5. Püschner, H. and Fankhauser, R. (1969): Neuropathologische Befunde bei experimenteller Vioform-Vergiftung der weissen Mäuse. *Schweiz. Arch. Tierheilk., 3,* 371.
6. Kaeser, H.E. and Wüthrich, R. (1970): Zur Frage der Neurotoxizität der Oxychinoline. *Dtsch. med. Wschr., 33*, 1685.
7. Tateishi, J., Kuroda, S., Ikeda, H. and Otsuki, S. (1975): Neurotoxicity of iodoxy-quinoline: a further study on beagle dogs. *Jap. J. med. Sci. Biol., 28, Suppl.,* 187.
8. Tateishi, J., Kuroda, S., Ikeda, H. and Otsuki, S. (1977): In: *Neurotoxicology*, pp. 345–351. Editors: L. Roizin, H. Shiraki and N. Grečević. Raven Press, New York.
9. Shiraki, H. (1971): Neuropathology of subacute myelo-opticoneuropathy, 'SMON'. *Jap. J. med. Sci. Biol., 24*, 217.
10. Heywood, R., Chesterman, H. and Worden, A.N. (1976): The oral toxicity of clioquinol (5-chloro-7-iodo-8-hydroxyquinoline) in beagle dogs. *Toxicology, 6*, 41.

11. Schaumburg, H.H., Spencer, P.S., Krinke, G., Thomann, P. and Hess, R. (1978): The CNS distal axonopathy in dogs intoxicated with clioquinol. *J. Neuropath. exp. Neurol., 37*, 686.
12. Sobue, I. and Ando, K. (1972): Abdominal symptoms in SMON: Analysis of correlations of clioquinol medication to the onset of the neurological symptoms. *Igakuno Ayumi, 82*, 354.

Discussion

Chairman: Now, I would like to open the floor for questions and answers on the presentations by Dr. Hangartner and Dr. Tateishi.

Mashford: I would like to congratulate Dr. Tateishi on the delightful presentation and ask him two questions.

Firstly, do you have any evidence that the species variability in toxicity which you described is due to variations in absorption or cellular susceptibility?

Secondly, do the periodic increases in tone of the innervated ileal loops represent an increase in tone or do they represent propagated peristaltic waves? If the former applies, could the actions of clioquinol on diarrhea therefore reflect a toxic effect on the nervous system expressing itself in the gut rather than by acting (if it does) in an antibacterial fashion as usually stated?

Tateishi: As to the first question, as Prof. Tamura mentioned, the difference in absorption of clioquinol seems to explain the species difference in susceptibility.

Regarding your second question, the pathologic ileal movement was observed only in the innervated gut and blocked by vagal section or decerebration. Therefore, our experiments show that abdominal symptoms of SMON patients are caused by toxic actions of clioquinol on the CNS, the effect of which was mediated by the vagus nerve. On the other hand, the efficacy of clioquinol, if it exists, may be explained as follows: Prof. Otsuka demonstrated that clioquinol has a local anesthetic action on the intestinal mucosa. Therefore I believe it is possible that such a local anesthetic action may alleviate the intestinal tone and be effective in some cases with diarrhea but not due to antibacterial effect.

Matsunami: I have a question for Prof. Tateishi.

In the pre-war period 2-phenyl-quinolin-carbonic-acid was used and it was found to induce gastric and intestinal ulcers in some patients. SMON patients often display gastro-intestinal ulceration. In view of this, I suspected that clioquinol induced such ulceration. Now, from that point of view, concerning the mechanism of the gastro-intestinal system ulceration, the most probable explanation would be the constriction or convulsion of the gastro-intestinal system after the administration of clioquinol. And if these two theories and investigative results are combined, then interesting conclusions may be reached.

Tateishi: As for the Atophan case, I have no idea what it means. Our own experiment revealed no hyperactivity in the stomach but increases in the movement of the intestinal loop were seen. I do not know what the cause of the gastric ulceration is.

Lannek: I would like to ask Dr. Hangartner some questions.

1. How many cases of oxyquinoline poisoning have you had since your publication in 1965, and was the clinical picture always the same? What about heart and liver disorders and post-mortem findings?

2. Have you taken liver biopsies and started the historical picture in those cases who

recovered and what were your findings?
3. Have you investigated the cerebrospinal fluid?
4. Have you made any later investigations of those patients who recovered from the acute poisoning – do you know if there were later neurological symptoms? In my clinical and experimental material about 30% have existing neurological disorders several years later.

I would like to ask Dr. Tateishi about his experiments on dogs. You have worked with acute and specially chronic poisoning in healthy experimental dogs. I have worked mostly with spontaneous cases of oxyquinoline poisoning in dogs and experiments where I have tried to imitate the relations in the clinical cases. In my material the heart and liver injuries were dominant compared with the neurological disorders and changes in the patients' temper and mood.

Hangartner: After investigations at the Universities of Bern and Zurich, I must point out that there seems to be NO statistics available on the clioquinol cases in Switzerland. Dr. Kammermann of Zurich reported on 41 cases of intoxication with Entero-Vioform and Mexaform (40 dogs and 1 cat) between 1966 and 1973; nearly all recovered and none of them came back for control.

The Toxicology Center of Zurich reported about 5 dogs and 1 cat intoxicated with Mexaform since 1969. In my own practice, I recall having had 3–4 cases (clioquinol); the last one in 1978 (Reasec-Plus). One case was recorded by a colleague in Lausanne (Entero-Vioform).

I could never see a correlation of toxicity between the liver and the myocardial disorders. Liver disorders occur frequently in diarrhea.

Neither in Bern, nor in Zurich, were liver biopsies taken. This also applies to my practice (cases which recovered).

Lannek: Have you investigated the cerebrospinal fluid?

Hangartner: I did not analyse the cerebrospinal fluid. This also applies to Bern and Zurich. One of my cases had a final, lethal epilepsy after 4 months (mentioned in my report 1965).

Chairman: May I invite Dr. Tateishi to respond to the questions.

Tateishi: In chronically intoxicated dogs degeneration or degenerative changes in the liver and kidney are sometimes seen. However, no such findings were found in the heart. No differences or changes were seen in cerebro-spinal fluid.

There is a question that I would like to ask Dr. Hangartner. Do you think that acute intoxication in dogs and cats is caused by the primary neurotoxic effects? Because the early reports of Ciba-Geigy explained that it was not due to a direct neurotoxic effect, but rather to a secondary neurotoxic action resulting from the pulmonary edema.

Secondly, concerning the gastrointestinal system of dogs, it is said that clioquinol is absorbed through damaged mucosa of the gastrointestinal tract of dogs with diarrhea. But I think that even healthy dogs can absorb clioquinol. And when cats lick up these agents, no gastrointestinal disturbances take place. So, in this regard, I would like to invite your comments.

Hangartner: In the cases I have examined since 1958, I have only seen acute cases. It is impossible for me to ascertain today whether acute intoxication was the effect of the primary neurotoxicity or not. The autopsies done at that time showed just edema of the brain in one case. But in Zurich, Dr. Kammermann reported edema of the brain as an effect of intoxication with Entero-Vioform and Mexaform, and it looks as if the toxicity is a primary edematising and secondary necrosing effect on the neurons. The successful therapy was to infuse 30% urea and very few patients died. This might be an indication for secondary neurotoxicity.

I once found edema of the lungs, but this was considered to be an effect of the excessive dyspnea during the crises. In the clinic, the pulmonary edema is probably due to cardiac insufficiency with nephritis; I never found a relationship with epilepsy.

It is evident that clioquinol is absorbed from the normal gastrointestinal tract. But I believe that diarrhea is a primary condition which produces the intoxication: in other words, diarrhea greatly enhances absorption of the drug through the gut and, therefore, epilepsy is then likely to occur.

In the cat, there was inflammation of the gut at autopsy. The cat had no clinical symptoms besides an eczema crustosum all over the body. It licked up a lot of pure Vioform powder on the fur, and, hence, the intoxication occurred in absence of gastro-intestinal disorders, but just in skin disease. It is possible that clioquinol is absorbed through the skin, but this is an open question.

Clinical chemistry of clioquinol*

ZENZO TAMURA

Hospital Pharmacy, Faculty of Medicine, University of Tokyo, Tokyo, Japan

The etiology of SMON had not been clarified, while the number of new patients had been increasing annually up to 1970, when Professor Toyokura noticed that the feces and the fur on the tongue of SMON patients were often colored green. At last 2 patients were found to excrete green urine in May of 1970.

The green urine was offered to us for identification of the green pigment. The urine was turbid and contained a dark-green sediment. Under a microscope, the sediments displayed green amorphous substances, together with many pale-yellowish long crystals. The urine was sterilized and separated as shown in Figure 1. The crystals were extracted into non-polar organic solvents such as n-hexane and benzene, and recrystallized by evaporation (A and B). In total, more than 100 mg of the crystals were obtained from 500 ml of the urine. On the other hand, the green pigment was difficult to extract and only 1 mg of it was obtained. Therefore the crystals were first investigated by many kinds of analytical methods and identified as 5-chloro-7-iodo-8-quinolinol. The compound is called clioquinol or chinoform.

According to the nature of clioquinol, the coexisting green pigment was supposed to be its ferric complex. So the complex was synthesized and compared with the

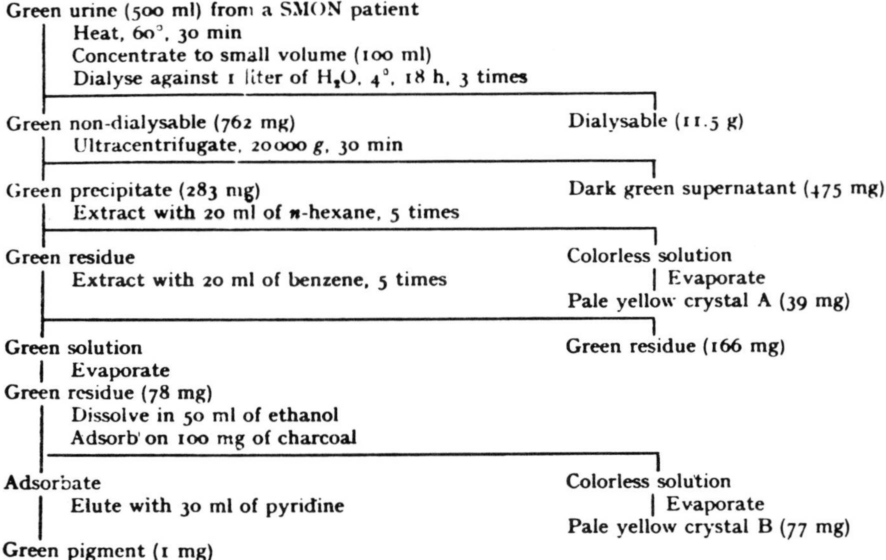

Fig. 1. Isolation of clioquinol in green urine of a SMON patient.

*Reprinted from *Proceedings of 6th Asian Congress of Pharmaceutical Sciences, Jakarta, 1976,* by courtesy of the Federation of Asian Pharmaceutical Associations.

TABLE 1. *Incidence of SMON in groups of patients with or without clioquinol administration*

Authors	Clioquinol administration	SMON (%)	Non-SMON	Remarks
Yoshitake et al. (1970)	Yes	34 (43.6)	44	Post-surgery
	No	0 (0.0)	77	
Kuratsune et al. (1971)	Yes	5 (4.3)	110	Enteric disorders
	No	0 (0.0)	217	P<0.005
Aoki et al. (1971)	Yes	17 (3.2)	515	Enteric disorders
	No	4 (0.1)	3,782	P<0.001
Tsubaki et al. (1971)	Yes	29 (11.0)	234	Enteric disorders
	No	0 (0.0)	706	P<0.001

pigment. The complex and the pigment were identical in the visible absorption spectra of their solutions, and in the chromatograms on a thin-layer plate (1).

These findings led to epidemiological surveys by Professor Tsubaki and others. The results (Table 1) indicated that SMON had mainly occurred in persons who were administered clioquinol. Especially post-surgery, more than 40% of patients became susceptible to SMON when treated with clioquinol while no SMON occurred in untreated patients.

The Ministry of Health and Welfare decided to prohibit the sale of clioquinol on September 8th, 1970. As a result, the occurrence of SMON rapidly decreased, and since 1974 almost no case has been reported (Fig. 2). The results strongly indicated clioquinol as the main etiological agent.

Further support for the etiology was presented by Professor Tateishi and others from animal experiments, using dogs, cats and monkeys. The animals showed paralysis and pathological changes in the spinal cord similar to SMON within a

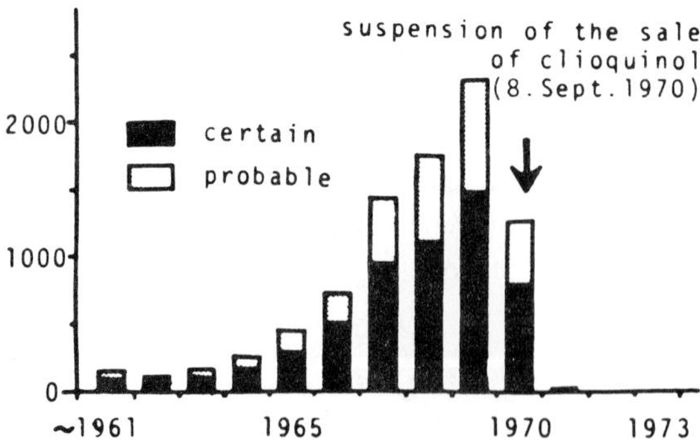

Fig. 2. Annual occurrence of SMON patients.

month of continuous administration of clioquinol. However, the doses were much higher than those in SMON patients.

A gas-chromatographic method for determination of clioquinol and its main metabolites, the glucuronide and sulfate, in biological materials was developed by us (2). In this method, clioquinol itself was extracted with a mixture of pyridine and benzene, purified on a Florisil column, acetylated and analyzed by gas chromatography with the aid of an electron-capture detector. The glucuronide of clioquinol remained in the aqueous phase. It was hydrolyzed with β-glucuronidase to produce clioquinol which was analyzed as mentioned above. Then the sulfate was hydrolyzed with hydrochloric acid and treated similarly.

By the method, about 10 μg of clioquinol was detected in 1 ml of the serum of a SMON patient (No. 4 in Table 2) after 1-month suspension of clioquinol. Moreover, from another SMON patient (No. 6) who had not been treated with clioquinol in the record, a similar amount of clioquinol was detected (1).

In Patient 1 in Table 3, about 0.1 μg of clioquinol was found in 1 g of a fresh sample of the sciatic nerve, and a greater quantity was detected in the liver and fat tissue after 9 months suspension of the drug, although more rapid disappearance was observed in the other cases (1). Similar retention of clioquinol in the nervous system was also observed in an intoxicated dog (No. 615, Table 4) after 1 month suspension of the drug (3). Quite different doses were required for man, dogs and monkeys to obtain similar levels of clioquinol in serum as shown in Table 5, which will explain the species difference of intoxication doses shown in the table (4).

Professor Yonezawa cultivated fetal posterior ganglia of rats or mice in a medium of 25% calf serum since clioquinol is fairly soluble in serum. With a medium containing 6 ~ 10 μg of clioquinol per ml, mitochondria in the axon degenerated, swelled and filled with vacuoles after several days, and the axon and myelin sheath were destroyed. These changes were similar to the histological changes in nerves seen in SMON patients (5).

Fig. 3 summarizes the main pathway of clioquinol in man. Since clioquinol is

TABLE 2. *Clioquinol content in 1 ml of serum*

Patient No.	Diagnosis	Clioquinol administration	I/Cl	Clioquinol
4	SMON	yes	4.5×10^{-3}	ca. 10 μg
6	SMON	no	2.8×10^{-3}	ca. 10 μg
15	Normal	no	1.0×10^{-5}	not detected

TABLE 3. *Retention of clioquinol in organs of SMON patients (μg/g)*

Patient	Period after treatment	Liver	Kidney	Fat	Nerve
1	9 months	0.5	ND	0.3	0.1
2	3 months	0.05	ND	0.05	ND
3	1 month	0.05	ND	0.05	ND

ND = not detected.

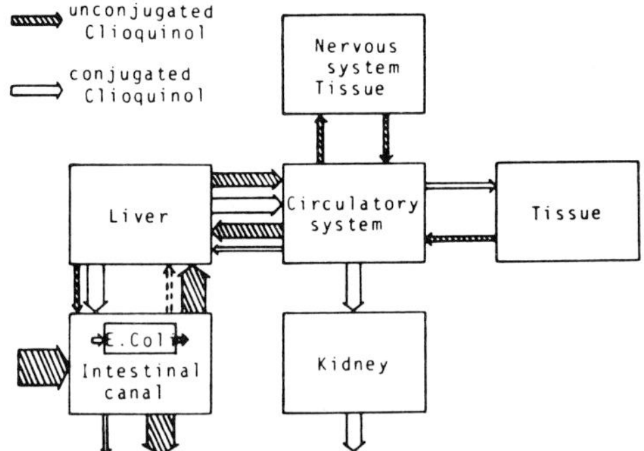

Fig. 3. Main pathway of clioquinol.

toxic to cells, and detoxication by conjugation in the body is incomplete, as shown in the figure, continuous high dose administration of the drug, e.g. more than 1 g/day, is thought to be an essential factor in causing SMON.

TABLE 4. *Clioquinol levels in the nervous system*

Dog No.		611	623	615
Frontal lobe of cerebrum			5.0	3.8
Cerebellum			7.7	2.4
Hypophysis		34.6	18.6	*
Cervical spinal cord		5.0	13.7	*
Thoracic spinal cord			6.4	*
Lumbar spinal cord		3.7	7.0	*
Spinal ganglia			13.9	*
Sciatic nerve		14.8	15.8	3.2
Optic nerve		13.4	10.3	*
Sural nerve			10.1	*
Subcutaneous fat		14.1		
Perirenal fat			78.5	
Liver		19.7		
Kidney		7.0		
	Clioquinol	10.0	4.3	0
Serum	Glucuronide metabolite	4.2	0.9	0
	Sulfate metabolite	8.3	2.2	0.3
	Clioquinol		5.4	0.3
Urine	Glucuronide metabolite		large	1.8
	Sulfate metabolite		large	> 10

* trace

611 At appearance of symptoms

623 1 month after appearance of symptoms

615 After 1 month suspension of clioquinol

n mole/g or n mole/ml

TABLE 5. *Maximum serum levels of clioquinol*

	Man	Dog	Monkey
Dose (mg/kg)	7 – 9	200	500
Serum clioquinol (μg/ml)	3 – 6*	3 – 10	6 – 6.5
Comparison with conjugates	C>G>S	C>S>G	G>S>C
Intoxication dose (mg/kg/day)	10 – 40	60 – 300	200 – 1000

* About 10 μg of clioquinol was detected in 1 ml of serum of a SMON patient after 1 month suspension.

REFERENCES

1. Tamura, Z., Yoshioka, M., Imanari, T., Fukaya, J., Kusaka, J. and Samejima, K. (1973): Identification of green pigment and analysis of clioquinol in specimens from patients with subacute myelo-optico-neuropathy. *Clin. chim. Acta, 47*, 13.
2. Chen, C.T., Samejima, K. and Tamura, Z. (1976): A gas chromatographic determination method of 5-chloro-7-iodo-8-quinolinol and its conjugates in biological fluids. *Chem. pharm. Bull., 24*, 97.
3. Hayakawa, K., Imanari, T., Tamura, Z., Kuroda, S., Ikeda, H. and Tateishi, J. (1977): Relationship between neurological symptoms and concentration of clioquinol in serum and nervous systems of beagle dogs. *Chem. pharm. Bull., 25*, 2013.
4. Chen, C.T., Kodama, H., Egashira, Y., Samejima, K., Imanari, T. and Tamura, Z. (1976): Serum levels of 5-chloro-7-iodo-8-quinolinol and its toxicity in various animals. *Chem. pharm. Bull., 24*, 2007.
5. Yonezawa, T., Saida, T., Nakano, A. and Hasegawa, M. (1977): Neurotoxic effects of chinoform, studied on nervous tissue maintained in vitro. In: *Neurotoxicology*, pp. 361 – 369. Editors: S. Roizin and Grečević. Raven Press, New York
6. Yoshitake, Y. and Igata, A. (1970): On the SMON cases following abdominal surgery-relationship of chinoform administration. *Igaku-no-Ayumi (Progr. Med.), 74,* 598 (in Japanese).
7. Kuratsune, M., Yoshimura, T., Tokudome, S., Kouchi, S., Matsuzaka, J., Nishizumi, M. and Mori, S. (1973): An epidemiological study on the association between SMON and Chinoform. *Nippon Eiseigaku Zasshi (Jap. J. Hyg.), 28,* 450 (in Japanese, with English summary).
8. Aoki, K., Ohtane, M., Sobue, I. and Ando, K. (1972): Clinico-epidemiological study on the occurrence of subacute myelo-optico-neuropathy (SMON) in relation to clioquinol. *Nippon Koshu Eisei Zasshi (Jap. J. publ. Hlth.), 19,* 305 (in Japanese, with English summary).
9. Tsubaki, T., Honma, Y. and Hoshi, M. (1971): Neurological syndrome associated with clioquinol. *Lancet, 1,* 696.

DISCUSSION

Chairman: Before moving on to the General Discussion, we would like to have questions and comments on Professor Tamura's paper.

Yokota: Up to now, I get an impression that there are differences between Caucasians or Europeans and the Japanese in susceptibility to toxicity of clioquinol. At the same time, while listening to Professor Tateishi's presentation I got an impression that there are also species differences in animals. You also mentioned age and sex differences. You explained the move or transition of clioquinol within the serum. I would like to hear your comments about these differences in man, animal species, age and sex factors etc. Also, since SMON was caused by the intake of clioquinol, was the appearance of the SMON syndrome due to species and racial differences or simply to differences in dosage or administration of the drug?

Tamura: A species difference in absorption of clioquinol does exist. However, there have been many investigators who tested the blood level of clioquinol administered orally. I compared our data with those of Swiss workers, but found no differences between the Japanese and the Swiss.

One of the reasons for age and sex preferences in SMON can be explained by a greater retentive capacity of the fat tissue for clioquinol than muscle tissue. I consider that the nervous tissue succumbs to degeneration if the clioquinol level rises above a certain threshold for a certain period of time.

Ishizaki: I should like to put a couple of questions to Dr. Tamura. First of all, the pharmacokinetics of clioquinol would be the determining factor in producing high plasma levels, and thereby accumulation in the nervous tissue. Do you have any information about the bioavailability, in other words, the first-pass effect, in the liver? Secondly, if this is so, the higher frequency of SMON in elderly people could be explained by impaired renal function. Both these factors possibly heighten the plasma level of the drug, and thereby accumulation in the nervous tissue. Do you have any information about the pharmacokinetic parameters of this drug?

Tamura: There is a great variation in absorption of clioquinol. Thus, in terms of pharmacokinetics, there will be no clear-cut data to substantiate it. Roughly speaking, in humans, 20% of what is ordinarily administered is excreted in the urine as glucuronide. The sulfate conjugated form circulates within the body, and probably some is excreted in the bile along with the free form. But this is an analogy from animal experiments. Part of it would go via the enterohepatic circulation.

Also, there is a wide fluctuation in absorption seen in animal experiments. In dogs administered one dose of clioquinol, the plasma level of the drug often showed two peaks. Probably dogs took meals in between and the bile acid would be excreted, thus accelerating absorption.

SMON: General discussion

Chairman: First, I would like to invite Professor Lenz to express some general views on SMON.

Lenz: I am not in a position to speak on SMON as an expert, but having been interested in drug problems for quite a few years, I would like to make some general remarks. I want first to congratulate everybody who has contributed to this magnificent work, which I feel is a great service to humanity and which has demonstrated beyond reasonable doubt that claims of non-toxicity sometimes advanced may prove to be entirely false.

Today is the second day after the Easter holiday. In Germany we have a famous drama, *Faust*, written in 1831 by Johann Wolfgang von Goethe. In the most famous part of this work, the Easter Walk, Faust tells of the experience of his father who was a 'doctor', an Alchemist. In the original words of Goethe:

'Hier war die Arzenei, die Patienten starben
Und niemand fragte: wer genas?
So haben wir mit höllischen Latwergen
In diesen Thälern, diesen Bergen,
Weit schlimmer als die Pest getobt.
Ich habe selbst den Gift an Tausende gegeben.
Sie welkten hin, ich muss erleben
Dass man die frechen Mörder lobt.'

('Here was the medicine, the patients died
And no one asked: Who thrived?
So have we with hellish electuaries
In these valleys, these mountains,
Raged worse than any plague.
I have myself given the poison to thousands.
They withered, I must live to see
The impudent murderers praised.')

This of course is an old story, but Goethe knew something of iatrogenic diseases which had been recognized for centuries. I have tried to point out 3 types of errors in which doctors may become involved: (1) weakness of pre-marketing research on drugs, (2) insufficient attention to side-effects, and (3) insufficient preventive measures even when side-effects have become known.

What are the conclusions? (1) Doctors should never lose a keen critical attitude towards claims about the merits and non-toxicity of drugs. (2) Doctors should always bear in mind the possibility that what they see in a patient may be the result of the drug treatment or that the drug they prescribe may harm the patient. (3) Doctors should never keep silent about any observed bad effect of a drug. They should not only immediately notify those responsible for production, distribution and supervision of the drug but also insist on an honest and complete response.

If these principles had been adhered to in the past by all doctors, I believe that neither the thalidomide nor the SMON catastrophes would have happened. If these principles are adhered to in the future, the power of decision will be taken away from the drug companies, where it should not remain, and be entrusted to those to whom it rightfully belongs, namely responsible doctors.

There is another German saying which is based on rather ancient wisdom: 'Happiness is not the highest human good, but guilt is the worst of evils.' Let us be aware of guilt.

Chairman: Thank you very much, Professor Lenz. Would anybody like to make further comments or ask questions?

Böttiger: It seems almost a shame to make any comments after Dr. Lenz's nice remarks! Much has been said about SMON in Japan and Sweden, and there was also a question from the floor about the possible differences between Japanese and Caucasians with regard to clioquinol absorption. I think further comments are required about the differences in the numbers of cases and in the apparent severity of the clinical picture. In Europe, clioquinol, or Entero-Vioform, has usually been taken by healthy persons for a short period, generally 1 week, for prophylaxis during holiday visits to the Mediterranean area, whereas in Japan clioquinol has been given mainly for therapeutic purposes, chiefly for gastrointestinal disorders or in the postoperative period. Gastrointestinal disease may, of course, lead to increased absorption of the drug. So, I think these factors are more likely to explain the differences than differences in genetic constitution between Caucasian and Japanese patients.

Takano: I would like to put a question to Dr. Yakowitz. One of the measures taken by the U.S. FDA in the late 1950's and early 1960's, was their insistence that Ciba-Geigy Co. should limit the indications for the use of clioquinol to amebic dysentery. What was the main reason for making this kind of request to the drug manufacturing company? This is the first question. The FDA, I believe, is not obliged to make such information available to other countries. But if it were known to the Japanese Ministry of Health and Welfare, it should have taken measures to control the use of clioquinol in Japan. Because of the lack of such measures, we have come to face the disastrous incidence of SMON. I would like Dr. Yakowitz to comment.

Yakowitz: The FDA recommended in 1960 that Ciba-Geigy restrict Vioform to the prescription drug class. This recommendation was based on the views of the FDA medical officers at that time. In 1960 there was no FDA program for notifying other countries of its medical views, such as the decision about Vioform. Perhaps countries should now be informed of the views of the FDA in all important cases.

Shin: To add to the many excellent scientific and technical presentations, I would like to make some general comments on the SMON tragedy and other potential similar drug hazards.

Several points seem to me to be important: (1) Drug companies should not manufacture and sell such drugs. (2) Physicians should not prescribe such drugs. (3) Patients should not take such drugs even though they are prescribed by their physicians. (4) (Perhaps most important) Such drugs should not have been approved by the government controlling agency in the first place.

But how can these ends be achieved? Who is actually responsible for such cases as SMON – the drug company, the physicians, the patients, the government controlling agency, or society as a whole which generally accepts the sale of such drugs? This is not an easy problem, but I believe that if we become more honest rather than seeking to make money as a first priority, even by harming others, we will probably be better off and may become more immune from such hazards in the future.

Hung: It seems to me that there are two types of subjective sensory symptoms suffered by the Japanese SMON patients: (1) a rather steady numbness, or pins and needles, and (2) a rather abrupt and severe burning or excruciating pain which is often brought about by external stimuli or by changing posture. The second type is like 'causalgia'. Do you have any experience that chemical or surgical block of the lumbar sympathetic ganglia could alleviate this type of pain?

Tsubaki: It is the general opinion of Japanese neurologists that there is only one type of sensory change in SMON. However, as Professor Hung pointed out, it sometimes resembles causalgia, and some neurologists have tried a spinal ganglion block. The effect was slight and only temporary.

Melmon: Despite the idealist hopes we all share that there will never be another SMON or thalidomide tragedy, we would do well to remember the limitations of available methodology. No system can prevent the possibility of another disaster rearing its head. We should be dedicated to systematic post-marketing surveillance that will minimize its extent.

It takes very few experiments to prove or disprove the efficacy of a new drug. Society then wants to use it. We have no right to withhold the drug if the efficacy is substantial. We have no way, however, of guaranteeing its safety or that unintended effects will not emerge during use. Rare events that are biologically important cannot be detected in the same time that it takes to establish a drug's effectiveness.

To point an accusing finger at industry, physicians or government create an illusion that these are the devils and we are the saints. Saints do not promise what cannot be done. We may wish to resolve to do our utmost to prevent any widespread tragedy, but at the same time we should educate ourselves and others that we cannot provide efficacious drugs in a timely manner without requiring society to face substantial risks.

Chairman: Thank you very much, Dr. Melmon. We would like to close this General Discussion. Thank you very much for your cooperation and attention.

PLENARY SESSION

Plenary session

CO-CHAIRMEN: W.H.W. INMAN and T. SODA

Chairman (Inman): With your very kind cooperation we have come to the last part of our program and I would like to introduce the first part of this last plenary session. This consists of the summary reports by the three session organizers and by the Chairmen of the Panel Discussion. So, may I first of all invite Dr. Sakuma for Session I?

Sakuma: In Session I we had 19 reports, from the standpoint of medical and pharmaceutical sciences, about what has been done, what is being done and what remains to be done to prevent drug hazards.

For the sake of foreign participants, there was an introductory report on drug-induced sufferings in Japan and the countermeasures taken by the Japanese government in the past 20 years.

Following this, the problem of predicting the behavior of drugs in the human body from the results of animal experiments was discussed. Three reports dealt with pharmacodynamic and pharmacokinetic studies. Although not complete, qualitative predictions are now possible, but predictions of what may be expected by the use of drugs under special conditions or those of a quantitative nature are still far from satisfactory.

At present we can learn retrospectively about the cause-effect relation and its mechanism only after some type of clinical problem has developed with a drug. We would like to know the problem in advance. Rapid progress in predictive studies has been noted, but we experience a lack of specialists as well as of financial support, which must be promptly resolved for future progress.

In relation to methodological considerations about extrapolation and prediction, we also discussed the extent to which preclinical investigations should be elaborated. Our society is always seeking both for more effective drugs and for safer drugs. The solution of this paradox is the fundamental problem.

One suggested solution was that carcinogenicity tests may become replaced, at least in part, by mutagenicity tests. Another suggestion was to replace classic compartment models by non-classic physioanatomical models in order to improve pharmacokinetic predictability. A report was given on whole body microautoradiography, a method for determining the possible sites of toxicity in the body. A thorough statistical study of biochemical individuality was recommended to aid precise clinical judgements on the safer use of drugs.

In relation to clioquinol, we had presentations on the epidemiological method to clarify the cause-effect relation in drug mishaps, and on the analysis of dose-response curves utilizing the life table analysis. In general, administrative action has only been taken after noticing adverse effects of a drug and finding a causative relationship. Delay causes unnecessary hazards, catastrophes and victims. This point was illustrated by a report on the thalidomide tragedy.

The intentional publication of misleading data in medical journals or the deliberate suppression of data can lead to a big mishap. In principle all the raw data should be available to those who need them without any changes.

Although not directly connected with drug hazards, the collection and analysis of data on clinical trials in Japan was discussed. A lack of medical biostatisticians and related specialists was noted.

Traditionally, drugs have been administered with such instructions as 'three times a day' or 'two tablets after each meal'. Recent pharmacokinetic studies have pointed to more rational individual dose regimens. For some drugs, these have been successful at maximizing the beneficial effects while suppressing the unwanted ones. Along the same line, another report stressed the necessity of avoiding hazards from useless drugs. Here again, the lack of specialists and funds to promote this aspect of therapeutics was noted.

A drug is often compared to a double-edged sword. It has good effects as well as bad effects; risks are always inherent in its use. To obtain a drug which is completely and absolutely safe is impossible. Thus the risk-benefit balance is central to approval for marketing and use. We have to think critically about for whom a drug will be beneficial and for whom it is going to be hazardous.

Recently, WHO specialists have prepared a list of essential drugs. A report was given about how the risk-benefit principle was applied to this work. There were discussions about the number of drugs available and the amounts used, which in many ways appeared to be too numerous and too voluminous, respectively.

A drug is a chemical substance, but one in which various functions and information are concealed. There is a tendency to regard a drug as a single entity. Yet from the standpoint of safety not only investigations but also manufacturing, supply and consumption processes are potential sources of danger. A presentation stressed that defective products as well as those giving deficient or distorted information are liable to cause mishaps.

All drugs pass through a line of manufacturers, government experts, pharmacists, physicians and patients. We had three reports about the transmission of drug information. They referred to the role of doctors, the role of patients, and the quality and quantity of information. There were lively discussions among participants on the self-awareness of doctors and on the information to be conveyed to patients. The principle seemed generally to be accepted that all information about drugs ought to be passed to patients, even though there might be exceptions.

Yesterday, we distributed questionnaires about what should be explained to the patient upon medication. Of 60 answers, 57 were in agreement that all information should be passed and 3 agreed but added conditions.

Lastly we learned about the post-marketing monitoring of drugs as was discussed in Session II. It was emphasized that some adverse effects are easily detected and at the same time some are easily overlooked depending on their frequency, severity and nature.

Throughout the session many problems had been pointed out and emphasized in order to prevent drug hazards. Among them were: (1) Newer methods should be developed and adopted as quickly as possible in preclinical studies in order to improve extrapolation and prediction. (2) All data, particularly those on drug toxicity, should be made available, with alteration, for those who need them.

(3) Physicians must always weigh the risk-benefit balance, fully utilizing the available information and must take professional responsibility for prescribing the treatment which is most beneficial to each particular patient. (4) As for the exchange and dissemination of information, we have various unsolved problems of international cooperation, communication to doctors and instruction to patients.

Chairman: I would like to ask Dr. Sunahara to make the report on Session II.

Sunahara: The presentations made in this Session can be classified into those related to pharmaceutical administration and those related to post-marketing surveillance.

In Japan, the amendment to the Drug Affairs Law and the Law for the Relief of the Victims of Drug-Induced Sufferings are being proposed in the Japanese Diet. Therefore, on the first day, officials and those related to the Ministry of Health and Welfare presented an overview and the major amendments of these laws. Lawyers involved in the litigation over drug-induced sufferings and researchers in health sociology voiced their criticisms of these proposed amendments. It was agreed that although some improvement has been achieved by the amendments, in essence they were still less than satisfactory.

It was stated that in order to satisfy the ethical and scientific requirements of clinical trials, clearer stipulations must be made, and also that the requirements to publicize all the materials had not been fully stipulated. As for the Relief Law of the Victims of the Drug-Induced Sufferings, removal of the stipulation for health and welfare undertakings, and the lack of any stipulations on non-fault responsibility, were pointed out as shortcomings.

From the United States, United Kingdom, Federal Republic of Germany and the European Community, various amendments to the Drug Affairs Laws were described. The Japanese amendments were compared with these amendments proposed in other countries.

At the same time, some people pointed out that although legal requirements and stipulations are quite important, these stipulations may hinder the development and marketing of necessary new drugs. In relation to such national policies, the problems entailed in clinical trials were raised. None of the presentations dealt with the ethical and scientific difficulties entailed in the establishment of pre-marketing safety or with practical measures to overcome these difficulties. I believe these aspects were dealt with in Session I. However, post-marketing surveillance is closely related to pre-marketing trials. To be ideal, even if the pre-clinical or pre-marketing trial is repeated, the confirmation of safety should not be postponed until after the marketing of the drug. Otherwise a slight error may lead to a large catastrophe. Nevertheless, in this Conference, post-marketing surveillance attracted much attention. I believe this reflects the difficulties of pre-clinical trials and the various efforts made to ensure safety of drugs at the pre-clinical stage. Even so, clinical trials should not be slighted. If we review the drug-induced sufferings, it is clear that more thorough pre-clinical and clinical trials might have been able to detect the hazards earlier, and the stipulations of ethical requirements which are indispensable for clinical trials have not been sufficiently observed in many of the countries of the world.

At any rate, because of the difficulties entailed in clinical trials, we are now looking to post-marketing surveillance. We are, however, faced with even greater difficulties. From Sweden, The Netherlands, the United States, Australia and Great Britain, Federal Republic of Germany and Japan, the present status and problems of monitoring have been reported. Spontaneous monitoring is quite widely used in many countries. But the responsibility for reporting is not clearly defined. It is necessary to have as many doctors as possible making honest and sincere reports.

In Sweden, although no punitive actions have been taken, doctors are required to make reports. However, compulsory reports do not always function well. It is necessary to educate doctors and also to give them the clinical and pharmacological information. At the same time the format of the reports must be simplified to facilitate cooperation by the physicians. In spontaneous monitoring the problems lie in the quality of the report submitted.

At present, the establishment of a causal relationship cannot be left to individual doctors. We must assure them that to report a suspected case will not involve them in medical litigation. It is thus necessary to have public organizations for establishing the causal relationship based upon adequate clinical and pharmacological knowledge. We need some kind of organization that can make early decisions without any undue delay.

Some countries already have such a public organization. Companies which neglect or delay reporting of unfavorable drug reactions should be condemned. A difficulty is that many of the adverse reactions cannot easily be differentiated from the symptoms of the underlying disease.

Premature disclosure of uncertain or unproven information to the mass media may cause some confusion to the society and should be avoided. In order to fill the shortcomings of spontaneous monitoring, various proposals have been made. If the patient is aware that he is being monitored, that may affect the outcome of the investigation. In that sense, prospective post-marketing trials are very difficult. Therefore, some people insisted that more should be done in the field of retrospective post-marketing trials.

In the United States, the Commission on Prescribed Drug Use is now planning to conduct a systematic survey on 100 of the most commonly used drugs. In this survey, they do not intend to use any single formalistic method. Experimental or non-experimental methods will depend upon the investigated drugs. This was quite useful information for us.

We try to obtain information about adverse reactions in routine clinical settings. In such circumstances, if the reality is far removed from the ideal, the effort is meaningless. Research in clinical medicine is not like freely painting a picture on a blank sheet of paper. We have to find out how we can search for the truth, or in some cases relative truth, under very complicated conditions.

Listening to the papers on post-marketing monitoring, my awareness of the difficulties in establishing the safety of drugs was re-awakened. But no matter how difficult it may be, we cannot get away from it. We have to ask all doctors to become actively involved. The state and society should become aware that legislation alone does not create safe drugs. More realistic and pragmatic approaches should be continued.

The discussion conducted in Session II may be summarized in the following two items. First, it was pointed out that the Drug Affairs Law must take a more active attitude vis-à-vis the procedures for approval and post-marketing surveillance. Secondly, various suggestions were put forward to overcome the difficulties encountered in post-marketing surveillance. I hope these proposals and suggestions will be brought to fruition in the near future.

Last, but not least, I would like to express my heartfelt gratitude to those people who made presentations in Session II, to the Chairmen, and also to the discussants. With this I conclude my brief summary.

Chairman: Now, we would like to move to the report from Mr. Izumi for Session III.

Izumi: The report, presentations and discussions of Session III can roughly be divided into two categories. The first issue is what should be done to prevent drug-induced sufferings. The second is how to relieve the victims promptly.

One of the most effective methods in the prevention of drug-induced sufferings is to transmit information as widely and as quickly as possible.

The discussion of the report by Dr. Silverman was extremely pertinent on this issue. He reported that the number of adverse drug reactions in the United States had been estimated to be at least 30,000 and perhaps as many as 130,000 annually, of which 80% was predictable and, in the main, preventable.

In Japan I believe the situation is similar, or may even be more serious.

To the view that the same advice may not always be appropriate in all countries was added the important suggestion that accurate information concerning the safety, adverse effects and efficacy of drugs must be distributed to all people of all nations. Many doctors pointed out that a lack of sensitivity towards adverse effects was a reason for the mass outbreak of SMON in Japan. It was commented that the highest incidence of SMON was observed among large general hospitals. This involved a very serious issue. It was also emphasized that physicians needed to select and utilize the important and correct information from the flood or material to prevent adverse effects of drugs.

The importance of the exchange of information was recognized by all the participants. For example, the papers and reports by Dr. Berggren and Dr. Hansson on the optic atrophy caused by clioquinol were extremely effective weapons for the relief of all SMON patients in Japan. Similarly, the results of the SMON litigation in Japan will contribute to the relief of SMON patients in Sweden.

Mr. Tuveson reported on the assistance he received from Professor Shapiro in Connecticut in this litigation concerning the injection of Kontrast-U. Victory in this litigation, which will come in the very near future, will greatly contribute to the relief of large numbers of potential victims in Japan. The information concerning other drugs such as chloramphenicol was similarly useful.

As the result of this Conference, we hope to establish a system for mutual exchange of information.

The second part of Session III dealt with actual occurrences of drug-induced sufferings. Under such circumstances, early relief of the victims is most important. On this point, we must revise our thinking about the classical theory of negligence. Product liability, which is not acknowledged under the Japanese law, is one possible legislative solution. Some members suggested that, if legal revision is delayed, we should proceed on a presumption of negligence.

Concerning drug-induced sufferings, the trial is often prolonged by the argument over scientific problems and early relief is extremely difficult to obtain. Therefore, recognition of non-fault liability and formal, practical and essential revision of laws are indispensable.

In order to relieve plaintiffs of mass litigation, it is necessary to recognize the foreseeability as easily as possible. One report emphasized that the system of provisional disposition is extremely useful for those patients who are suffering over a prolonged period.

In the thalidomide and SMON cases, the litigations of the same kind were filed in many district courts in Japan and this entailed further difficulties. If there is a consensus among the parties, it is possible to introduce a *de facto* model suit in one particular court.

Another means devised by attorneys in the SMON case was to establish clear standards to judge the degrees of severity and the sum of damages for application to all patients throughout the country.

One controversial issue was the liability of the state. One problem was raised by the fact that compensation by the state is paid by the taxpayer. If joint responsibility is placed on the state and the pharmaceutical company, there may be cases where no payment is made by the pharmaceutical company and the total sum is paid by the state.

There are some countries where no liability is placed on the state. Some views were expressed that it would be more advantageous for the victims if the state was not the accused, but was in a position to persuade the defendant companies to relieve the victims.

At the same time, there were sharp comments indicating a liaison between administrative authorities and companies. Under such circumstances, doubts were expressed whether the state could protect and guarantee the welfare of the victims.

As pointed out in the key-note speech, there must be sufficient philosophical discussion to bring about a national consensus on the Act for a Fund to Relieve the Victims of Drug-Induced Sufferings.

Next, I would like to deal with the roles of the press or mass media. Some believed this to be very important. There was a general consensus that the press can be utilized to relieve the patients and victims, on humane grounds.

Finally, there were detailed reports by researchers of the situation of the victims, and about their restoration to the original state. A report on the permanent policies, that is the policies for the SMON patients concerning rehabilitation, research into medical treatment and expenses after the realization of the settlement, was useful.

I would like to express our appreciation to the overseas and domestic participants for their efforts towards the solution of this problem. The determination to provide cooperation beyond national boundaries and across the ocean for the relief of victims who themselves have not much power or financial ability, has led to the success of this Conference.

Chairman: This concludes the summary reports by three session organizers. And in this Conference, along with the three Sessions, we organized a special Panel Discussion on SMON, which was the cause of especially disastrous sufferings in Japan.

Kono: The Panel Discussion on SMON was held under the co-chairmanship of Dr. Lenz and myself and I am sure it is still new in your memory, but I would like to summarize the discussions.

First, Professor Tsubaki who originated the clioquinol causation theory reported about the epidemics in Kushiro City in Hokkaido, in which he himself was involved. He also elucidated the clinical picture of SMON and the autopsy findings which motivated him to designate the disease as subacute myelo-opticoneuropathy.

Further, he described how, in the search for the etiology of SMON, in earlier studies, the finding of a greenish fur on the tongue and the chemical analysis of green urine made clioquinol a suspicious agent. By an epidemiological survey in hospitals, he said he then became convinced that clioquinol was the cause.

The second presentation was made by Dr. O. Hansson from Sweden. He stated that in 1934 Ciba-Geigy started to market oral clioquinol as Enterovioform, and that already in 1935 cases of neurological disturbances had been reported in Argentina. In 1962, its acute toxicity in dogs was observed. Therefore, the myth that clioquinol was insoluble and thus not absorbed by the gut and not greatly toxic, was disproved.

Dr. Hansson himself, together with Professor Berggren, reported the first cases of optic nerve atrophy in 1966 and called them to the attention of Ciba-Geigy, but the caution was ignored and led to the disaster of SMON.

Even after 1970, when the Japanese SMON cases came to be known outside Japan, cases continued to occur in 25 countries and Dr. Hansson dealt with 22 cases in Sweden. Accordingly, in countries where clioquinol is not regulated, it is evident that SMON cases continue to be produced.

Moreover, clioquinol hardly has any benefit as a pharmaceutical drug. He therefore concluded that it is unforgivable that many pharmaceutical companies, including Ciba-Geigy, continue to sell clioquinol. The questionnaire survey reported by Dr. Katahira supplemented reports by Dr. Hansson and others. By means of a mail survey, the world-wide regulations of clioquinol have been studied and it appears that there are only 6 countries in which clioquinol is completely regulated. Reviewing the medical literature and by mail surveys, he could list 207 patients with SMON from 28 countries.

Dr. Dukes referred to the 5 cases in The Netherlands which had occurred after the toxicity of clioquinol had become known, and questioned the ethics of the doctors involved.

The report by Dr. Berggren dealt with acrodermatitis enteropathica patients. Besides the follow-up studies on the first case of optic nerve atrophy after long-term administration of clioquinol, Dr. Berggren already in 1968 noticed that a fair amount of clioquinol was absorbed through the gut. The knowledge of this fact in Japan would have facilitated the settlement of SMON matters, which indicates the importance of exchange of information.

Dr. Hangartner's report on the discovery of the toxicity of clioquinol to dogs and cats, antecedent to the human report, emphasized the importance of exchange of information between human and veterinary medicine in preventing drug-induced sufferings.

Professor Tateishi succeeded in inducing chronic intoxication by giving clioquinol to dogs which was regarded as a complete reproduction of the SMON syndrome clinically as well as pathologically. He pointed out the difference in the requisite dosage between mongrel and beagle dogs. Apart from the nervous system, he often observed intestinal volvulus and invagination. In other experiments in dogs, he found that clioquinol stimulated intestinal movements indirectly through the central nervous system via the vagus nerve, and he thus confirmed that the abdominal symptoms preceding the onset of neurological symptoms of SMON was also an adverse effect of clioquinol.

Lastly, Professor Tamura analysed the greenish urine of SMON patients in which he detected the iron chelate of clioquinol. He established the method for quantitative analysis of clioquinol conjugated with glucuronic acid and sulfuric acid, and he found, even 1 month after the suspension of clioquinol administration, 10 μg of clioquinol in 1 g of the liver tissue of a SMON patient.

It was demonstrated that there are 3 forms of clioquinol within the body, and their pharmacokinetic states were also explained by Professor Tamura. These experimental studies concerning the toxicity of clioquinol strongly support the clioquinol theory for SMON.

In the general discussion, the Chairman, Professor Lenz, cited lines from the Easter Walk from Goethe's *Faust*. He commented that: 'physicists must not lose their critical minds and whenever they see a patient, must always wonder whether a symptom might be the result of a drug and, if an adverse reaction happens to be discovered, should never keep their mouths closed about it'.

Chairman: Before we start the Final Session of General Discussion, there are two announcements to be made and I would like to call first on Dr. Herxheimer.

Herxheimer: I would like to tell everyone here that the foreign participants in this Conference wish to make a public statement about clioquinol and the damage that it can cause (see opposite page).

Chairman: The second statement will be by Mr. Kaneda.

Kaneda: Representing the 1900 plaintiffs who fought in the Tokyo District Court, I would like to make the following recommendations: At this International Conference, we have the participation of many people from Japan and abroad, and for this fact I would like to express my heartfelt gratitude to those who organized and prepared this Conference, to congratulate you on its success, and also to express my hope for the future success and continuation of this kind of work.

The pharmaceutical Affairs Law to be amended in Japan, where the thalidomide catastrophy was followed by the SMON disaster which affected even more victims, should include more strict stipulations than those found in other countries to ensure the safety and efficacy of pharmaceutical products. At the conclusion of this memorable Conference, attended by the experts and authorities from all over the world, we, the victims of SMON, urgently wish that a recommendation be made to incorporate the following items in the proposed amendment of the Pharmaceutical Affairs Law of Japan:

1. The criteria for approving new drugs shall satisfy the following conditions: (a) The efficacy of the drug shall be substantially proved by strictly controlled clinical

STATEMENT

The evidence is overwhelming that medicines containing certain hydroxyquinoline compounds, such as clioquinol, cause serious and irreversible injury to the nervous system. We urge those manufacturers who are still selling these products, either to provide clear evidence that there are benefits which justify the risks, or to withdraw them. In our opinion, the reassessment of these drugs is an urgent task for national drug regulatory authorities and international organizations.

April 18, 1979

Lennart BERGGREN *(Sweden)*
Lars. E. BÖTTIGER *(Sweden)*
Teoh Pek CHUAN *(Singapore)*
Iwan DARMANSJAH *(Indonesia)*
M.N.G. DUKES *(Netherlands)*
Paul HANGARTNER *(Switzerland)*
Olle HANSSON *(Sweden)*
Freya HERMANN *(U.S.A.)*
Andrew HERXHEIMER *(United Kingdom)*
Tsu-Pei HUNG *(Taiwan)*
K.H. KIMBEL *(F.R. of Germany)*
Birgitta LANNEK *(Sweden)*
Widukind LENZ *(F.R. of Germany)*
Åke LILJESTRAND *(Sweden)*
N.D.W. LIONEL *(Sri Lanka)*
P.K.M. LUNDE *(Norway)*
Mia LYDECKER *(U.S.A)*
M.L. MASHFORD *(Australia)*
Mohd Zaini bin Abdul RAHMAN *(Malaysia)*
Hyun Duk SHIN *(R. of Korea)*
Milton SILVERMAN *(U.S.A.)*
Gianni TOGNONI *(Italy)*
Michael TUVESON *(Sweden)*
Alexander WALKER *(U.S.A)*
Barbro WESTERHOLM *(Sweden)*

---

trials. (b) The approval of a new drug shall be rejected if the safety of the drug is not supported with substantial evidence. (c) Upon application for approval, all possible evidence, both favorable and unfavorable, shall be submitted by the manufacturer.
2. All the material examined and submitted when applying for new drugs shall be made public after the approval is granted.
3. After the approval is granted, the Government will collect, record and analyse the information on the efficacy and safety of the drugs, with the cooperation of physicians and manufacturers and take appropriate measures.

Last but not least, I hope that you will adopt this recommendation unanimously.

Chairman: We now have a period of one hour for free discussion. May I make one or two suggestions before we start? This Conference has been heavily slanted towards the tragedy of SMON. We must not forget that we must look to the future and that the majority of drugs are mercifully safe. I suggest that at least some of our thoughts should be concerned with the balance between risk and benefit. I am sure that we will admit that, as Sir Henry Dale once said, 'Bias is a normal function of the human mind.' We all have our biases, scientists, lawyers, journalists and patients. We are all fallible, and I hope that none of us will fear the possibility of loss of face if we make mistakes in the future, as we have in the past.

So, I would like to throw the floor open to anybody who cares to raise his hand.

Dukes: I am very glad that you referred to the balance between safety and efficacy, because this has already been raised during this meeting. It is quite clear that the continuing large-scale use of clioquinol in some areas of the world continues to reflect the belief of a lot of people, physicians, patients and, presumably, manufacturers, that clioquinol is effective and necessary for some conditions. I have myself tried during this meeting, by talking to people, to assess the evidence that clioquinol is of any value. As far as I can see, there has been no serious controlled work, since that which was already available at the time of the clioquinol ban in Japan 9 years ago, as regards the value of clioquinol in diarrhea. This is surprising, since any company which continues to believe that clioquinol is effective might have been expected to have undertaken this work if their belief were an honest and substantial one. This would appear to put paid to the view that the product is effective in diarrhea. In addition, however, we have heard impressive evidence that clioquinol also causes diarrhea in man, for a reason which is evident from pharmacological and veterinary studies. I think, therefore, we can forget clioquinol as a treatment for diarrhea. The same arguments seem to apply to amebic dysentery. A drug that causes diarrhea is not suitable for use in that condition. And for amebic dysentery I think we now also have better and safer drugs.

Finally, the remaining indication, acrodermatitis enteropathica, which would provide a marginal reason for the drug to remain on the market, appears now to have been discredited. It appears that the drug was simply acting as a zinc carrier in a condition where zinc should be given. So the evidence raised during these 3 days takes away the therapeutic bases for the continued use of this drug. If this conclusion is accepted and propagated, this must surely affect the use of this drug throughout the world.

Chairman: I find the continued presence of clioquinol on the international markets extremely strange and I have wondered whether there might be some obscure medico-legal reason for it. It occurred to me that if I were a lawyer advising the manufacturers, I might suggest they should not make any change in marketing policy until the litigation has been decided. Can any of the legal people present here tell me whether this is a myth or has some substance?

Ohasi: I have no direct evidence, but in the case of the lawyers for Ciba in Japan I am sure that they were not sincere in proceeding with the litigation. I am not sure whether they actually gave the advice or not, but it is always a possibility for lawyers to discuss such matters with the executives of the company.

Yamashita: This issue must be very carefully studied. This is a basic question not for lawyers but for companies. It is only in Japan that these drug-induced sufferings occurred; there was no problem in foreign countries. This was what they asserted by their evidence in court. The basic attitude of the pharmaceutical companies is probably also reflected by the lawyers.

Ballin: A minor question to Dr. Dukes. Clioquinol has not been available for systemic use in the United States for more than a decade. But I understand that it is still available in topical form for an alleged antibacterial and anti-infective action. I am not aware of the evidence in support of such a function, but I wonder if your blank condemnation of this drug included its topical use.

Dukes: I was thinking only of the oral use.

Hansson: It may be of interest for you to know that clioquinol is absorbed through the skin and can be detected in the blood. So, there may be some risk in using it topically.

Kono: Yesterday in the Panel Discussion on SMON, no reference was made to some of the experimental results and I would like to add some remarks.

Dr. Tateishi pointed out that clioquinol increases intestinal movement. It exerts its influence locally on the intestine and this sometimes reduces the intestinal movement. So it may have some symptomatic effect in some diarrhea cases. However, an antibacterial action is, in our view, unlikely. One experiment was conducted in Sweden in which clioquinol was administered for traveller's diarrhea. Larger amounts of Salmonella were found in the feces than in untreated subjects.

Herxheimer: I wonder if I could mention one point that came out in one session I was listening to, namely that of the whole problem of judging scientific issues in a court of law. I think everybody agreed that this was a totally inappropriate way of settling scientific questions related to drug-induced illness. You have special reasons for the many litigations concerned with this problem in Japan. But that emphasizes the importance of making a special effort to get the problems sorted out outside the legal framework. I wonder whether an additional measure would be to organize some seminars in clinical pharmacology for lawyers and for judges, because judges are notorious for getting scientific questions back to front.

Chairman: It sounds like an excellent suggestion. Could I suggest that, as questions are coming rather slowly, we might address ourselves to the future and perhaps widen the scope to cover drugs other than clioquinol, and express some views how we might try to prevent this type of accident or at least speed up the identification of new problems. How, for example, can we overcome the apparent reluctance of doctors to part with useful data?

Westerholm: I think you bring up an immense problem which starts with the education of medical students. We have to teach them to look at the events, to follow what happens to each patient and ask 'Is this the result I expected?' Or 'What went wrong? Was it my treatment which made it go wrong?' At least in my country, this approach is not very well taught. Perhaps it is best taught by giving examples of things that happended in the past. I think that other medical personnel and even patients also need this kind of training. 'Why didn't I get well?' But we are short of people who can teach.

Chairman: I agree. I think there are many young people who could make very good drug monitors but because many of the monitoring centers are located in the government this involves becoming a civil servant. Many suitable people do not like the idea of accepting the constraints of the civil service, such as restriction of scientific freedom, and so on.

Mashford: I see the roles of gathering data about adverse drug reactions and education as being closely interconnected. I think we are missing a very great opportunity if we do not combine them. If a hospital has, say, an intensive monitoring unit, this will influence the procedures in the hospital and the training of doctors, nurses, pharmacists and medical students. I think we need also to view the spontaneous monitoring programs in this light. They must not be judged solely in terms of the information which they obtain, but also by the effect they have on the system which they are setting out to observe. It is our experience that having monitors in the ward asking questions makes people think and modifies prescribing. I cannot definitely say that it reduces adverse effects but it certainly reduces the number of drugs which are given.

Yamashita: I was involved in the SMON litigation and I would like to learn from all of you. My question is related to drugs. I believe that drugs exist to promote health of man. What I learned through this litigation was that drugs, in one sense, are toxic by their nature. Now is this true? If it is so, we must communicate this to every human being on earth. What are your views?

Chairman: Well, I think that one has to accept that practically everything we do is dangerous. There is an old saying in England that 'Everything I do is either illegal, immoral or fattening.'

Takano: I was very fortunate to have heard these very significant reports. I have been studying drug sufferings in Japan largely because they developed alongside high economic growth; examples include Minamata and Itai-itai disease, which are well known environmental diseases that occurred concurrently. Both scientific and medical methods were applied, but not altogether successfully.

In Japan, however, drug induced sufferings took a litigational course and it became very clear that pharmaceutical companies had much information about dangers and risks which was not revealed to physicians. As pointed out by Dr. Hansson, such facts were accumulated and known by multinational companies but they were not passed on to other countries so that very serious drug induced suffering occurred.

In Japan, this took place during a very unique and conspicuous stage of development with high economic growth. Italy and other countries have experienced similar events.

Natural science research is of course necessary but at the same time, information of pharmaceutical companies must not be concealed; false advertisement or claims must not be made and misleading promotion by pharmaceutical companies must be monitored and controlled internationally. Otherwise, drug induced sufferings may not be eliminated even if scientists make the utmost efforts.

I believe that this has been learned from the cases in Japan, and I hope such experiences can be utilized, and I hope that my comments contribute to the solution of your problems.

Chairman: Of course, in many European countries there is no great problem as far as drug marketing is concerned but it is, nevertheless, essential that all adverse drug reactions or suspected adverse reactions are reported to the National Center. In our own center, since the introduction of legal obligations, information from industry about drugs has increased from about 3% of the total input to about 20%, although this has not materially altered the reports of serious adverse reactions; most seem to come directly from the doctors who witnessed them.

Tognoni: I would like to make some general comments about the point concerned with learning about risks in the future. I agree that doctors are pivotal to the process, but I suspect that in many countries the education of doctors will take a long time. In addition, I think that doctors are not given the education, rather they comply with instructions, but if they are aware of the requirements of public opinion (from scandals and general education) promoted by the mass media then benefits will ensue. In Italy for example the mass media more or less decided issues in a number of such accidents.

The point I now wish to make is that we, in the medical profession, and as international or national bodies keeping surveillance and communicating on side effects, must search for ways to communication with the mass media.

A pertinent example occurred in Sweden where in general links with the mass media are not good.

As the public becomes increasingly anxious they believe both in excessive safety and in excessive damage, and further biases in the doctor's practice are imposed. In ways similar to those Dr. Herxheimer proposed for judges, I think that there is now a case for some kind of ethical standard being required for the mass media internationally. Also the medical profession must establish international links to facilitate transference of information to mass media regarding drugs and the environment.

These aspects were central to previous discussions. My own view following Dr. Dukes' comments is that in developing countries where clioquinol containing products are widely used, and in which diarrhea remains common, such conclusions cannot readily be incorporated into an educational program on diarrheal diseases. There is a clioquinol risk, but in general, how does one deal with a major health problem, such as diarrheal disease, while discouraging the use of an effective drug? In some countries, I encountered great surprise from doctors when the risk associated with clioquinol containing products was mentioned.

Westerholm: Regarding the mass media, there is a two way passage of information between doctors and the mass media people. Journalists comprise balanced scientific individuals and those of a more sensational bent, and it is necessary for us to encourage both types of coverage.

Chairman: Following on Dr. Tognoni's comments, I found that in New Delhi clioquinol is freely available, and that it is proposed over the next few years to give villagers (1/1000 of the population or 600,000 villagers overall) a simple, basic medical training. This seems to me to be the beginnings of progress for the people of the third world.

Dukes: We might add perhaps that the moment is now ripe for these approaches to be applied in many parts of the world. There is a tendancy as a result of nuclear accidents and environmental pollution etc. to be somewhat suspicious of all man-made solutions to problems and even man-made remedies. We in Europe have particularly noticed these aspects. The public response has been tremendous with respect to drug usage and abuse. Even the benzodiazepines, which in many countries are becoming almost a daily habit for very many people, and which are generally safe drugs, have their risks if only in the sense of emotional function.

I recall that when we produced television spots to discourage the use of sleeping tablets and recruit mass media assistance, there was a tremendous response, apparently despite the fact that these drugs were given on doctor's prescription and were being asked for at the doctor's surgery by patients; there were many people seriously worried about being virtually addicted and who were prepared to listen and take general advice about their use of these products.

Kimbel: It is clear that proper documentation is essential for the evaluation of drug risks. Hospital computers and data banks of course store information on patients, but information and evidence on drug risks are rarely documented in this way. The same largely applies to the notes kept by general practitioners. Most drug monitoring just duplicates the reports which should already be in a good patient history. The litigation in the clioquinol cases revealed that many patients were unaware that they had ever taken clioquinol. Professor Lenz tells the story that when he went to mothers of thalidomide babies, they often denied having taken thalidomide, but the drug was found in her medicine chest. I thus feel that all data pertinent to drug risks should be recorded in a standardized and routine form, to produce a complete history for hospital in-patients, and by standardizing general practitioners' notes perhaps the evaluation for drug risks would be facilitated.

There is one obstacle I anticipate. Many countries have laws that protect data. In Germany for example one cancer registry was officially and legally sealed for two years although a newly created law has permitted access to those data. The benefits of revealing versus protecting patients' data must be weighed carefully but in most cases, the consent of the patient may be gained easily provided he is clearly informed.

Chairman: In our country over the years something like 1 million standard forms for reporting adverse reactions have been distributed but over 15 years only 60,000 reports have appeared.

Nagai: As a pharmacologist, I wish to emphasize aspects of the patient-oriented pharmacy. All actions should be directed towards the patients, unlike previously when drugs were corrective agents and not something potentially harmful. Medical care in Japan often involves discussion which in a way disregards patients. For instance, in medical institutions doctors encounter territorial conflicts leading to many unpleasant situations. Such disputes ignore the patients. Another example is the Japan Medical Association, which is a very powerful organization that can be a very strong pressure group to which even government ministers bow. This has both merits and disadvantages, for if particular organizations become too powerful, they can pursue self-interest rather than the interests of patients.

Doctors and paramedicals have often been at the center of medical care but in the future teamwork is essential, avoiding one boss, so that the patients are central. Historically man has executed various splendid programs, such as the Apollo Project in the United States, as a result of teamwork, and it should now be our aim to apply such endeavors to medical care.

Darmansjah: There have been some papers concerning exaggerated claims of drug companies in their drug information pamphlets. One factor that has been ignored in this respect is the efforts of marketing departments in pharmaceutical companies.

Frequently medical directors work in the marketing divisions and, in some companies, not necessarily in developing countries, those in medical departments cannot always prevent marketing departments from over-promoting. I wonder if anything can be done about this such as not allowing medical directors to be under marketing control. Is this possible?

Chairman: I spent 6 years working for a very reputable company in which the Medical Director had as much say, if not more, than anybody else. I am rather interested to hear what Dr. Dukes, who has had similar experience, might have as comment.

Dukes: Well, the circumstances of medical people in the drug industry vary enormously. There are some indeed, who enjoy great independence while others unfortunately do not. The drug industry has always been organized idiosyncratically; this will continue irrespective of what we say. I suppose we should be very glad that so many excellent medical people work in the drug industry and we should encourage the maintenance of the highest possible medical standards.

The general organization within a company will not change very much. The main thing is, whether the medical man there is prepared to maintain the highest ethical standards of his profession in this situation.

Herxheimer: It strikes me that one very simple solution might be to publish the names of the companies in which the medical people are under the marketing department so that mere publication would improve the reputation of these companies.

Shin: I would like to raise some general questions about future trends and programs. To be frank, before I came here, I really didn't know what drug induced suffering meant.

About thirty countries are represented here, courtesy of Japanese sponsors, but in the future I suggest that, since the Japanese sponsored this Conference, some kind of clearing house for the information be established to reduce the problems such as SMON and by creating a corresponding headquarters or equivalent perhaps will repeat such meetings.

Are there any particular programs we should consider?

Soda: In Japan there are opinions concerning such services. It would however involve responsibilities beyond individual ones and encompass the Government and would require cooperation from various sides. It is not possible now but with the cooperation of medical with pharmaceutical and administrative circles, such a service for Asia or Southeast Asia could be established.

Silverman: I wish to say a few words in defense of the drug companies. Some of the people in these companies are my friends, I think there are four or five. They are all in the Research Division. Some of the products are very good. I lived to reach this advanced age because some of them saved my life.

This terminates the nice things I have to say about the drug industry. There is another aspect which I had hoped to hear discussed before the end of this meeting; it concerns the claims of most of the multi-nationals, that society in general, and governments in particular, are making too many demands on them. We are insisting on more data, more careful trials, more expensive trials, lower prices, and the companies say that if we continue to make these demands, that at the very most, we may drive these companies out of business, at the very least we will force them to cut down on their extensive research programs.

Most of this is nonsense. In the United States we have heard the companies make these claims since 1906. Every time the Federal Government proposes any kind of change in drug relations, we hear the same chorus. 'You will cause us, you will force us to cut down on our research'. And oddly enough although we have changed and toughened our drug laws in the United States since 1906, the companies have not gone out of business, they have not cut down on their research, in fact they have increased it, and they have not had lower profits, as a matter of fact they have had higher profits. But over 90% of this attitude of the industry is (I hope there is a suitable Japanese word) 'garbage'; it is not 100% garbage however. We may reach the point at which we will force the industry to cut down, not merely their unimportant research, but their important research. Their attempts to find drugs for the future that are more effective, more safe, more economical, that I hope will control diseases, which cannot now be controlled will be restricted. If we force companies to retrench to that point, we will have committed a tragic disservice to future generations.

Chairman: Having as it were lived on both sides of the fence for a number of years, I can understand the industry worrying about expenditure of vast sums of money on animal experiments which turn out not to be very reliable predictors of human toxicity and I personally would like to feel that the industry could be persuaded to provide more funds for post-marketing surveillance and perhaps save some on these animal experiments, which are undoubtedly enormously expensive.

Yamashita: In Algeria, there was an International Lawyers Conference attended by lawyers from the developing nations. Doctor Hansson talked about 'drug imperialism' in Latin America and in South East Asian nations. The results of this Conference, through WHO should be conveyed accurately to the people of Latin America, Asia and other parts of the world.

Chairman: I am sure, Dr. Soda, that through your Organizing Committee you will be able to convey these requests to the appropriate people.

Mashford: With reference to that last point, I wonder if the Committee or anybody else has collated the package inserts for clioquinol throughout the world and drawn attention to the various disparities. I myself have no information about this, but I think it would be a useful maneuver to point out the various attitudes adopted by companies in different areas.

Chairman: A very useful suggestion.

Herxheimer: Such a survey was undertaken by the International Organization of Consumer Unions in which I was involved. We obtained package inserts from between 30 and 40 countries, compared and tabulated them, and demonstrated the chaos that existed at that time. The survey was published as a special report in 1976 and it also appeared as an article in the *Journal of Antimicrobial Therapy*. It would be useful to see whether any changes have occurred since then. However, it would be a fair amount of work and since we already have some data, perhaps this should not have high priority.

Sonoda: Mr. Izumi very well summarized the discussions of the Third Session, in which I made a presentation. The two major issues were to prevent drug-induced sufferings and how to relieve the victims when such suffering occurred.

In listening to the Plenary Session, I believe that the second issue, i.e. the relief of victims, has not been discussed. Therefore, I would like to ask you to do the following:

In Japan, and probably in other countries, victims of drug-induced sufferings must usually resort to litigation to obtain settlement or compensation. But how can the victims who are not actually the parties to litigation be relieved? At present, 4700 SMON patients are engaged in litigation and this is less than half of the 11,000 recognized by the Ministry of Health and Welfare. Does this mean that the victims who are not party to litigations have no problems regarding their lives, physical impairments etc.?

We find no differences between the victims engaged in litigation and the others. The reasons why some do not participate in the litigation are often because they cannot bear the cost or they cannot get medical documents from the doctors. At the same time they may be very reluctant to file a suit against the State or the doctors, and if they take part in litigation, they believe that other people will treat them as sick.

Some say that they were not asked to participate in the litigation and they do not know how to do so. Many gave such reasons. To solve these issues, more positive measures for relief of the patients must be taken on the part of the State. Potential victims who are not yet recognized by the SMON group or the Ministry of Health and Welfare must be notified by the doctors so that they can be checked by the group of experts.

Chairman (Inman): I would like to pick you up on one phrase you used. You talked about 'prevention of drug-induced suffering'. We will never completely prevent drug-induced suffering because all drugs with any worthwhile therapeutic effects have side-effects which are manifested in some people.

I am sure the best we can ever hope to achieve is to identify new problems rapidly and to alleviate them. But you will never completely eliminate drug-induced suffering.

It now falls upon me to try and summarize this Conference. More than 60 papers have been read, I clearly have an impossible task. Fortunately, the various Session Chairmen have done this very effectively for us. So I will just express my gratitude for the opportunity to make a few personal comments. I shall start and finish on the theme of communication, which is what the Conference was all about.

I believe the public has a right to know about the benefits and dangers of drugs. And I believe that it also has a right to expect that the information which is passed to it is meaningful and accurate. Unfortunately bad news is more likely to be printed than good news. The media are sometimes very skilful in converting mere suspicions, even fiction, into fact. I agree with those who said that we must have better liaison between scientists, doctors, lawyers, patients and the media in order to make sure that the information which is produced does more good than harm. With better communication it may be possible to avoid the need for action groups that have been used on occasion to secure recognition of the needs of disabled people.

Most of my remarks will apply to drugs in general but with regard to SMON, I am still impressed by the differences between the Japanese experience and that of the rest of the world. Whenever publicity has been given to problems with widely-used drugs such as oral contraceptives, phenformin or beta-blockers, this has nearly always led to the discovery of large numbers of previously unrecognized cases. This did not happen with SMON. Clioquinol undoubtedly causes neurotoxicity, especially when used in doses in excess of those recommended and, indeed, small numbers of cases have been reported outside of Japan in a number of countries. In my own country, the United Kingdom, the drug has been used for about 30 years by millions of people and neither the publicity nor the hope of compensation has produced numbers of cases on a scale that remotely approaches that in Japan. Possibly, as Dr. Böttiger told us yesterday, Europeans rarely use the drug for more than a short period, perhaps one or two weeks, while they are on holiday. I was the one who suggested in the Conference that, as far as the English were concerned, they couldn't afford a holiday of more than one or two weeks!

Why, then, is it variously estimated that between 10,000 and 30,000 cases have occurred in Japan? Has more clioquinol been used more frequently or in greater doses in Japan than in other parts of the world? Have non-Japanese got a higher threshold for toxicity? Is there a genetic factor? Are there some as yet unidentified co-factors? I think it is important to consider whether SMON has been overdiagnosed. Obviously these are strong possibilities. We saw yesterday that other diagnoses may masquerade as SMON if clioquinol has been taken. I do not believe all these questions have been answered; perhaps some of them never will be. But the general deduction is quite clear. Clioquinol is a cause of neurological damage. I personally believe that prolonged and high dosage may be the simplest explanation of what has happened.

Now, Japanese law does not distinguish the following statements: (1) clioquinol is *a* cause of SMON and (2) clioquinol is *the* cause of SMON. Scientifically, the distinction is important and I was delighted to hear from Professor Kono, and most heartily agree with him, when he said that scientists rather than lawyers should make this kind of decision.

But rather than argue endlessly about the cause of SMON it seems to me to be far more important to ask ourselves what we are going to do about other people with similar disability, whether drug-induced or not. Some of the Japanese SMON cases did not have clioquinol, so it seems likely that the drug is not the cause of all the problems. But these people need just as much help.

We must never forget SMON or thalidomide or practolol. But I do feel we must look to a future in which accidents of this kind, and we will certainly never prevent them completely, will be dealt with rapidly and preferably by some form of no-fault insurance rather than by expensive law suits which may prevent the patients getting the help they need for 5 or 10 years.

Next, with regard to the role of industry, we must not forget the good things that they have done, such as the virtual elimination in some countries of tuberculosis, malaria, poliomyelitis, and control of many chronic diseases. Industry frequently has acted in a responsible manner. It is motivated by profit and it cannot afford disasters or bad publicity. From time to time it has undoubtedly been guilty of sharp commercial practice, especially in developing countries. I am a doctor and not a lawyer, so I try not to take sides. I personally would not refer to the industry or to any corporation as the enemy. I should prefer to reform it rather than to execute it.

Now, natural justice would demand that compensation should be paid only to those damaged by these drugs and, in the normal course of events, it would be reasonable to suggest that each patient should be examined by a panel of independent neurological experts, who could decide if they have been damaged by the drug. Professor Tsubaki listed 11 items in the differential diagnosis of SMON. But with so many cases this is clearly impracticable. I believe, therefore, that the governments and not the patients should be the plaintiff. This should remove the appaling anxiety that is added to the burden of disability of the sufferers. I am sure there have been many errors of judgement in the marketing of drugs, and probably also in the interpretation of the tests which have been conducted on them. It is always very enjoyable to be proved right. It is very honorable to be proved wrong and to it admit freely.

Before I finish, I would like to turn to the SMON sufferers themselves. Some of them have joined us at KICADIS. Quite by chance, I have spent about 60% of my life in a wheelchair. I try not to identify myself with disability except when it suits. I do know that most disabled people come to accept their misfortune with dignity and almost always with humor. Looking at the faces of the sufferers that surrounded us I think this is very true of them. Quite frankly, however, I saw little that was dignified and nothing that amused me in the film which we were shown on Saturday and I regret that it was thought necessary to produce a film like this to achieve the objective that was desired. I have seen many films about disabled people and about their strange way of extracting the greatest possible enjoyment from lives which, to the ignorant ablebodied, appear to be a total disaster. I am very pleased to see that our disabled colleagues who are present today have retained both their dignity and their humor.

Without forgetting the past, we must obviously look forward. We must introduce, I hope through insurance rather than litigation some means of dealing with the tragedies which will inevitably occur in the future. Above all, I think we must continue to communicate with each other as colleagues and human beings and we must avoid confrontations of the kind which we witnessed on Saturday. SMON and other tragedies occurred on a large scale because we do not yet have effective methods for post-marketing surveillance. This, I think, is the fundamental defect that we must correct. We will never eliminate the risk, but we must do everything we can to minimize it.

To conclude, although certain moments in the Conference did nothing to lower my blood pressure, I have enjoyed it very much. I know I can speak for the invited participants in extending a very warm vote of thanks to our Japanese hosts. I congratulate them on the choice of meeting place, on the extremely high quality of their organization and on the meticulous attention to detail, not only in organizing the Conference itself but for our comforts and our enjoyment of the meeting and, above all, I thank them for the chance to make new friendships and to achieve new understandings. I would like to record very special thanks to our interpreters who have delighted our senses in at least two ways – first, our sense of hearing and, secondly, for those like myself who have spent some time looking at their little windows, they have delighted our eyes.

May the cherry trees continue to bloom in Japan and may the message of this meeting spread to other parts of the world.

Closing remarks

TAKEMUNE SODA

Institute of Public Health, Tokyo, Japan

This Kyoto International Conference Against Drug-Induced Sufferings which we organized has now come to a successful close. We were delighted to have 37 participants from 9 European countries and the United States and 10 participants from 7 South-East Asian countries. Together with the Japanese participants, nearly 500 of our colleagues and the people who shared the common aspirations – 492, to be exact – congregated here. From the 14th of April to the 18th, today, we have had very active discussions. We discussed various experiences of drug-induced sufferings caused by various drugs such as thalidomide, clioquinol and others, and the preventive measures were elucidated further. The detailed aspects have already been reported by the representatives in each session and by the Chairman of the SMON Panel, as well as by Dr. Inman who has just given us a comprehensive general summary. So, I shall not repeat what has already been said. But in any country, not only knowledgeable people and unfortunate victims, but also everyone who abhors drug-induced sufferings and who wishes their eradication should join hands. We can then make the utmost efforts to implement the most effective and appropriate measures in relation to time and place. Even though one case may be successfully dealt with in one country, the experience cannot be automatically applied to other countries. Experience in various countries should, however, be conveyed immediately to other countries, so that each can learn from the lessons. In that way, measures can be taken which are befitting to the situation prevailing in each country. At the same time, we should not suppress the future development of further effective new drugs out of excessive fear of drug hazards.

It was pointed out that measures of control, caution and surveillance would be needed to prevent further disastrous drug hazards. We have not yet discovered any measure which can be universally applied. However, we hope that with unceasing caution and effort we can prevent and eliminate the major and disastrous hazards. To that end, we should continuously try to pursue scientific truth and also to develop a technology through which the outcome of research can be utilized for the sake of the health and welfare of mankind. The right information needs to be conveyed to everyone and to be understood by everyone.

Medical administrators, pharmaceutical manufacturers, doctors, pharmacists, consumers, educators, mass media and journalists should fulfil their duties and be fully aware of each one's responsibility.

All this has been discussed. During this Conference, to me as President of the Organizing Committee, and also to the Secretariat, various comments were sent testifying to the impact of holding KICADIS. We must appreciate the efforts made by journalists in disseminating KICADIS through radio, newspapers, TV and so forth. A typical comment was as follows: 'I am glad that this sort of conference is being held. I lost my wife recently. I don't know the exact cause, but it seemed like the adverse effect of the drug she took'. Numerous such letters were received. They show that so far there has been no forum to which these people could appeal. In the past, there were conspicuous major cases of SMON and thalidomide but there were other similar untold cases. We should not forget the many who are suffering from unknown kinds of drug injuries. Through doctors and clinics we have established a system of reporting drug-induced hazards. We are asking doctors to provide us with the information, but this is still far from being sufficient. Each person affected wants to find somebody who can warn others of the possible hazards. But they feel hesitant about telling the doctors, because they feel obliged to them for their care. We must provide a place where these people can go.

During the past 5 days we have discussed many matters, but we should not just leave them at lip service. We must ensure that our discussions will be reflected in our daily practice. That is a problem we should follow up from now on.

The present Conference will soon be over and everybody will be dispersing to their homes. But in each place, an effort must be made to put the results of our Conference into practice. I hope that our efforts will bear fruit and that at some time in the future we can again meet somewhere in the world to report the outcome.

Lastly, I would like to express our heartfelt gratitude to all the speakers, discussants, and participants, for the cooperation and patience which have brought us to this successful ending. I would also like to express my appreciation to the people in the Secretariat who worked so hard behind the scenes at the logistics. At the same time, along with Dr. Inman, I would like to thank the simultaneous interpreters who facilitated the communication, which can be a very difficult task, between the Japanese and European language speakers. The Japanese language is said to be the linguistic orphan of the world having a unique grammatical structure and different terminology.

With this, I would like to conclude this KICADIS meeting. Thank you all very much. We hope to see you again in the near future.

Subject Index

Prepared by H. Kettner, M.D., Middelburg

Author Index